Manual of

Valvular Heart Disease

Manual of

Valvular Heart Disease

Craig R. Asher, MD, FACC, FASE
The Robert and Suzanne Tomisch Department of Cardiology
Heart and Vascular Institute
Cleveland Clinic
Weston, Florida

Brian P. Griffin, MD, FACC
Section Head
Cardiovascular Imaging
Vice Chairman
The Robert and Suzanne Tomisch Department of Cardiovascular Medicine
Heart and Vascular Institute
Cleveland Clinic
Cleveland, Ohio

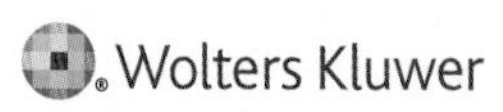

Philadelphia • Baltimore • New York • London
Buenos Aires • Hong Kong • Sydney • Tokyo

Senior Acquisitions Editor: Sharon Zinner
Development Editor: Ashley Fischer
Editorial Coordinator: Lauren Pecarich
Marketing Manager: Rachel Mante Leung
Production Project Manager: Linda Van Pelt
Design Coordinator: Holly McLaughlin
Manufacturing Coordinator: Beth Welsh
Prepress Vendor: S4Carlisle Publishing Services

9 8 7 6 5 4 3 2 1

Printed in China

Library of Congress Cataloging-in-Publication Data

Names: Asher, Craig R., editor. | Griffin, Brian P., 1956– editor.
Title: Manual of valvular heart disease / [edited by] Craig R. Asher, Brian P. Griffin.
Description: Philadelphia: Wolters Kluwer Health, [2018] | Includes bibliographical references.
Identifiers: LCCN 2017022873 | ISBN 9781496310125 (paperback)
Subjects: | MESH: Heart Valve Diseases | Heart Valves—surgery
Classification: LCC RC685.V2 | NLM WG 260 | DDC 616.1/25—dc23 LC record available at https://lccn.loc.gov/2017022873.

LWW.com

RRS1708

CONTRIBUTORS

Craig R. Asher, MD
Staff Cardiologist
Department of Cardiology
Cleveland Clinic Florida
Weston, Florida

Roger Byrne, MD
Advanced Imaging Fellow
Department of Cardiovascular Medicine
Cleveland Clinic
Cleveland, Ohio

Joseph Campbell, MD
Interventional Cardiology Fellow
Department of Cardiology
Massachusetts General Hospital
Boston, Massachusetts

Patrick Collier, MD, PhD
Staff Cardiologist
Section of Imaging
Department of Cardiovascular Medicine
Cleveland Clinic
Cleveland, Ohio

Paul C. Cremer, MD
Staff Cardiologist
Section of Imaging
Department of Cardiovascular Medicine
Cleveland Clinic
Cleveland, Ohio

Milind Y. Desai, MD
Staff Cardiologist
Section of Imaging
Department of Cardiovascular Medicine
Cleveland Clinic
Cleveland, Ohio

Eoin Donellan, MD
Fellow in Cardiovascular Medicine
Cleveland Clinic
Cleveland, Ohio

A. Marc Gillinov, MD
Chairman
Department of Thoracic and Cardiovascular Surgery
Cleveland Clinic
Cleveland, Ohio

Andrew L. Goodman, MD
Staff Cardiologist
Centennial Hospital
Nashville, Tennessee

Brian P. Griffin, MD
Section Head
Imaging
Department of Cardiovascular Medicine
Cleveland Clinic
Cleveland, Ohio

Richard A. Grimm, DO
Director
Echocardiography Laboratory
Section of Imaging
Department of Cardiovascular Medicine
Cleveland Clinic
Cleveland, Ohio

Divya Gumber, MD
Resident in Internal Medicine
Cleveland Clinic
Cleveland, Ohio

Serge C. Harb, MD
Advanced Imaging Fellow
Department of Cardiovascular Medicine
Cleveland Clinic
Cleveland, Ohio

Terence Hill, MD
Fellow in Cardiovascular Medicine
Cleveland Clinic
Cleveland, Ohio

Syed T. Hussain, MD
Staff Surgeon
Department of Thoracic and Cardiovascular Surgery
Cleveland Clinic
Cleveland, Ohio

Christine L. Jellis, MD, PhD
Staff Cardiologist
Section of Imaging
Department of Cardiovascular Medicine
Cleveland Clinic
Cleveland, Ohio

Douglas R. Johnston, MD
Surgical Director
Aortic Valve Center
Department of Thoracic and Cardiovascular Surgery
Cleveland Clinic
Cleveland, Ohio

Brandon M. Jones, MD
Interventional Cardiology Fellow
Department of Cardiovascular Medicine
Cleveland Clinic
Cleveland, Ohio

Samir R. Kapadia, MD
Director
Sones Cardiac Catheterization Laboratory
Section Head
Interventional Cardiology
Department of Cardiovascular Medicine
Cleveland Clinic
Cleveland, Ohio

Srikanth Koneru, MD
Fellow in Cardiovascular Medicine
Cleveland Clinic
Cleveland, Ohio

Amar Krishnaswamy, MD
Associate Program Director
Interventional Cardiology
Department of Cardiovascular Medicine
Cleveland Clinic
Cleveland, Ohio

Deborah H. Kwon, MD
Staff Cardiologist
Section of Imaging
Department of Cardiovascular Medicine
Cleveland Clinic
Cleveland, Ohio

Stephanie L. Mick, MD
Staff Surgeon
Department of Thoracic and Cardiovascular Surgery
Cleveland Clinic
Cleveland, Ohio

Gian M. Novaro, MD
Director
Echocardiography Laboratory
Department of Cardiology
Cleveland Clinic Florida
Weston, Florida

Jayendrakumar S. Patel, MD
Fellow in Cardiovascular Medicine
Cleveland Clinic
Cleveland, Ohio

Gösta B. Pettersson, MD, PhD
Vice Chairman
Department of Thoracic and Cardiovascular Surgery
Cleveland Clinic
Cleveland, Ohio

Dermot Phelan, MD, PhD
Director
Sports Cardiology
Department of Cardiovascular Medicine
Cleveland Clinic
Cleveland, Ohio

Lourdes R. Prieto, MD
Director
Pediatric Catheterization Laboratory
Department of Pediatric Cardiology
Cleveland Clinic
Cleveland, Ohio

Grant W. Reed, MD
Interventional Cardiology Fellow
Department of Cardiovascular Medicine
Cleveland Clinic
Cleveland, Ohio

L. Leonardo Rodriguez, MD
Associate Director
Echocardiography Laboratory
Section of Imaging
Department of Cardiovascular Medicine
Cleveland Clinic
Cleveland, Ohio

Ellen Mayer Sabik, MD
Staff Cardiologist
Section of Imaging
Department of Cardiovascular Medicine
Cleveland Clinic
Cleveland, Ohio

William J. Stewart, MD
Staff Cardiologist
Section of Imaging
Department of Cardiovascular Medicine
Cleveland Clinic
Cleveland, Ohio

Balaji Tamarappoo, MD, PhD
Staff Cardiologist
Cedar Sinai Medical Center
Los Angeles, California

Maran Thamilarasan, MD
Staff Cardiologist
Section of Imaging
Department of Cardiovascular Medicine
Cleveland Clinic
Cleveland, Ohio

E. Murat Tuzcu, MD
Chairman
Department of Cardiovascular Medicine
Cleveland Clinic Abu Dhabi
Abu Dhabi, United Arab Emirates

Patrick R. Vargo, MD
Fellow in Thoracic and
Cardiovascular Surgery
Cleveland Clinic
Cleveland, Ohio

PREFACE

From the time the most elementary stethoscopes became available, physicians have been fascinated with valvular heart disease. Early on in training, medical students throughout the ages have been challenged to learn the signature sounds and signs of heart valve lesions. During the 20th century, the anatomy, pathophysiology, and natural history of most valvular heart diseases were well elucidated. Heart valve surgery became commonplace, though medical therapy, randomized trials, and nonsurgical therapies lagged far behind other cardiac conditions, like coronary artery disease.

But times have changed. In the 21st century, valvular heart disease has rapidly emerged as an exciting and successful area of growth in the field of medicine. This resurgence is largely credited to the growth in multimodality cardiac imaging and earlier, lower risk interventions through percutaneous procedures and less invasive surgical options. The importance of valve disease is further illustrated by the development of valve clinics in medical centers throughout the country, a growing number of high-impact peer-reviewed manuscripts, courses and websites on the topic, guideline statements from major societies, and expanded coverage on many certifying examinations (general cardiology, interventional and echocardiography boards). Therefore, clinicians (cardiologists, cardiothoracic surgeons, cardiac anesthesiologists, and trainees) and ancillary personnel (technicians, sonographers, nurses, and physician assistants) caring for these patients require focused and up-to-date knowledge of the subject.

The Cleveland Clinic is a leading center in the United States for the evaluation and treatment of valve disease. With this expertise, we have compiled an easily readable and referenced manual written by faculty at the institution. The *Manual* comprises 23 chapters including native and prosthetic valves; percutaneous pediatric and adult interventions and surgical procedures; cardiac imaging with three-dimensional echocardiography, computed tomography, and cardiac magnetic resonance imaging; echocardiography and cardiac catheterization laboratory hemodynamics, formulae, and cases; and a catheterization laboratory atlas, all specifically pertaining to valve disease. There are plentiful figures and tables, key points, guideline statements, and even a question bank to review each chapter.

We hope that this first edition of the *Manual of Valvular Heart Disease* will serve as an educational resource for caretakers providing the latest and best care for their patients. As two former program directors, we must always acknowledge the unyielding motivation, patience, and inspiration of our own families and our extended Cleveland Clinic family, most notably a superb cast of fellows and staff who contributed in countless ways to the production of this work and our careers.

Craig R. Asher, MD, FACC, FASE
Brian P. Griffin, MD, FACC

CONTENTS

SECTION II

Special Conditions 169

SECTION III

Percutaneous and Surgical Valve Procedures 189

SECTION IV

Multimodality Imaging and Cardiac Catheterization Laboratory Assessment 287

SECTION I

Native and Prosthetic Valve Diseases

CHAPTER 1

Divya Gumber
Eoin Donellan
Patrick Collier

Aortic Stenosis

I. INTRODUCTION

Aortic stenosis (AS) is a common treatable cardiovascular problem whose prevalence is on the increase because of our aging population. From aortic sclerosis (focal areas of thickening and/or calcification) through worsening degrees of obstructive AS (characterized by more advanced valve thickening and calcification), the disease leads to ventricular dysfunction, symptoms, and death if untreated. The prevalence of aortic sclerosis is age dependent, ranging from 9% in a study in which the mean age was 54 years to 42% in a study in which the mean age was 81 years. Similarly, the prevalence of AS is age dependent, estimated at 1% of those aged over 65 years, 2.5% of those aged 75 years, and 8% of those aged 85 years.

II. ETIOLOGY

Age-related degenerative calcific disease (>50% of cases) is the most common etiology underlying AS, followed by congenital bicuspid aortic valve disease (30%–40% of cases) and postinflammatory rheumatic disease (<10% of cases). Bicuspid aortic valve disease is the most common underlying etiology in patients needing surgery who are younger than 70 years, because of the high frequency of this congenital disease in the general population (estimated prevalence of 0.9%–2%) and the younger age of presentation of those with such anatomy (Fig. 1.1).

Tracking historical temporal changes in etiologic factors for patients with AS referred for aortic valve replacement has shown that the relative frequency of degenerative calcific aortic valve disease has increased considerably, mainly in place of postinflammatory rheumatic aortic valve disease. Multiple factors have likely driven this changing trend, including better primary and secondary prevention of rheumatic fever, improvements in life expectancy in the general population, alterations in patient referral practices, and an increased willingness of surgeons to operate on older patients with newer safer techniques for higher risk patients.

Radiation heart disease, although a rare overall cause of AS, deserves special mention because recognition of this as an underlying etiology has significant implications for prognosis and therefore management. Thickening of the aortomitral curtain should raise suspicions of radiation heart disease, which can cause pancarditis via latent changes in interstitial cells to a more profibrotic and procalcific phenotype (Fig. 1.2). Prior radiation exposure significantly increases perioperative morbidity and mortality above and beyond standard risk stratification scores (particularly with redo surgery), the implication being that surgical intervention should be delayed for as long as possible and any such intervention should aim to minimize the likelihood of reoperation.

Subvalvular AS is a congenital condition that may become manifest later in life, whereby fixed obstruction of the left ventricular outflow tract results from a discrete membrane or a tunnel-like orifice most likely as a maladaptive adaptation to abnormal localized flow dynamics. Shone syndrome refers to the association of subvalvular AS with sequential left-sided obstructive lesions. Transesophageal echocardiography is the most useful technique to distinguish this pathology from dynamic obstruction, namely hypertrophic

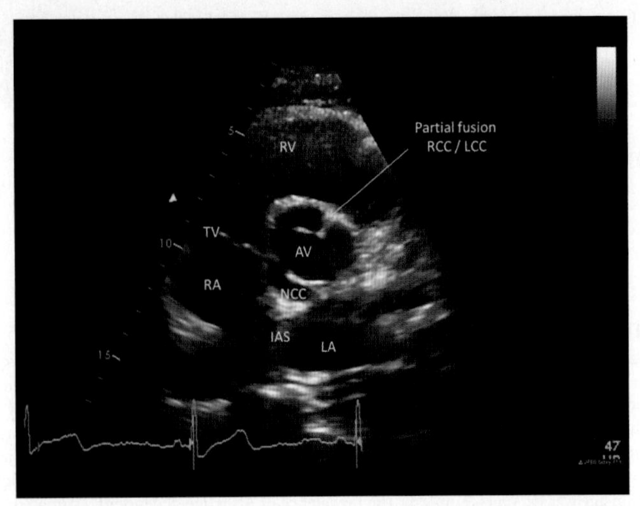

FIGURE 1.1 Bicuspid aortic valve morphology as imaged by transthoracic echocardiography. Fusion of the right and left coronary cusps represents the most common bicuspid morphologic variant. The right cusp is typically the most anterior cusp (closest to the chest wall), whereas the noncoronary cusp is most posterior and lies adjacent to the interatrial septum. AV, aortic valve; IAS, interatrial septum; LA, left atrium; NCC, noncoronary cusp; RA, right atrium; RCC/LCC, right/left coronary cusps; RV, right ventricle; TV, tricuspid valve.

cardiomyopathy. Recurrence postresection has been described, whereas subvalvular AS may also result in a high-velocity, forward-flow jet lesion that may cause secondary aortic regurgitation. Even the presence of a mild leak should prompt consideration of the need for surgical intervention because it may be possible to concomitantly preserve/repair the aortic valve after resecting the membrane.

Supravalvular AS is a characteristic feature of Williams syndrome, which was first identified in 1961 by New Zealander J. C. P. Williams. It is much rarer than subvalvular AS and occurs in approximately 1 in 20,000 births. In general, supravalvular AS is caused by deletions or incompletely penetrant autosomal dominant mutations in the *ELN* gene that cause downregulation of the protein tropoelastin, an elastin precursor, fibers of which make up approximately 50% of the aorta. A compensatory increase in aortic smooth muscle cells ultimately leads to aortic narrowing.

Unicuspid aortic valve is a rare cause of congenital AS (estimated prevalence of 0.02% in the adult population) most commonly presenting with congestive heart failure in infancy. Most often, this is a retrospective rather than a preoperative diagnosis, more often made at pathologic examination of the surgically excised valve or at autopsy. Other associated anomalies are common and include aortic coarctation (~37%), ventricular septal defect (~12%), patent ductus arteriosus (~5%), and aortic aneurysm (~5%). It shares many of the features of bicuspid aortic valve, including valvular dysfunction, aortic dilation, aortic dissection, and dystrophic calcification, and indeed has been classified as a subset of bicuspid valve. Surgery for unicuspid aortic valve in adults is most commonly performed for mixed stenosis and regurgitation with combined aortic repair in a majority of cases. In contrast, the rarer quadricuspid valve phenotype (estimated prevalence of 0.01% in the adult population) is more commonly associated with aortic regurgitation rather than stenosis.

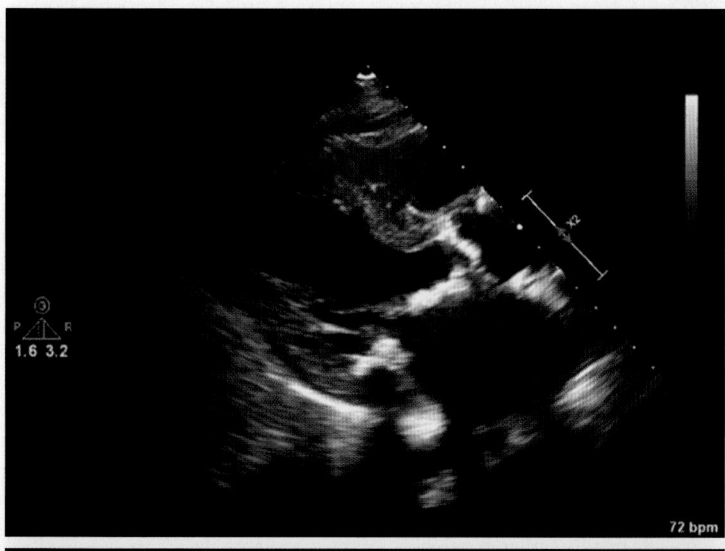

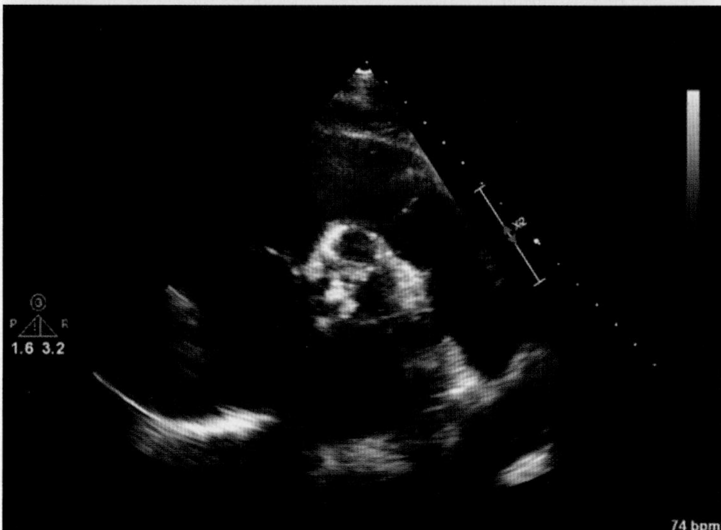

FIGURE 1.2 Aortic stenosis caused by radiation heart disease. Echo findings of marked thickening of the aortomitral curtain as well as the presence of concomitant severe calcific mitral stenosis point to this rare but important underlying etiology.

III. GENETICS

Aortic valve calcification is a common feature of advancing aortic valve pathology with both genetic and nongenetic causes. (The latter include standard cardiovascular risk factors, namely, age, diabetes, hypertension, obesity, dyslipidemia, smoking, and male gender.) The strongest genetic evidence predisposing to aortic valve calcification to date has come from a study that looked at more than 2.5 million gene variants, called single-nucleotide polymorphisms, in more than 6,900 people of white European background and found that a variant in the lipoprotein(a) [Lp(a)] gene locus (rs10455872) was strongly associated with having aortic valve calcification on cardiac tomography (CT) scanning. Findings were confirmed among thousands of patients from a range of ethnic backgrounds. This variant, found in 7% of the general population, also increased the risk of developing AS by more than 50%. Mediated by Lp(a) levels, this gene discovery supports a causal role for Lp(a), although it remains unanswered whether potential targeting of Lp(a) levels might reduce the incidence or progression of aortic valve disease.

Potential genetic markers of accelerated valvular calcification have also been investigated in family members with calcific bicuspid aortic valve disease. Here, linkage studies identified a nonsense mutation in *NOTCH1* on chromosome 9q34-35 as a susceptibility locus. This finding was supported by the discovery of a *NOTCH1* frameshift mutation in an unrelated family with similar aortic valve disease, suggesting that haploinsufficiency of *NOTCH1* is a genetic cause of aortic valve malformations and calcification. Decreased *NOTCH* signaling has been linked to a molecular pathway for aortic valve calcification, via increased expression of bone morphogenic protein 2 as well as RUNX2 (a central transcriptional regulator of osteoblast-specific genes), with the net result of increased aortic valve calcification.

Supravalvular AS, as discussed earlier, is a characteristic feature of Williams syndrome and is caused by a hemizygous deletion of about 26 genes (including the elastin gene) from the long arm of chromosome 7, resulting in a distinctive "elfin" phenotype, an unusually cheerful demeanor and ease with strangers, developmental delay coupled with strong language skills, and transient hypercalcemia.

IV. PATHOLOGY

Pathologic mechanisms underlying degenerative aortic valve disease are complex and likely involve multiple genetic and environmental factors. Nonetheless, most current theories addressing degenerative aortic valve disease pathology invoke abnormal pathologic responses to increased mechanical stresses including activation of transforming growth factor beta, cytokine elaboration, mononuclear cell infiltration, and myofibroblast-induced matrix remodeling. These pathologic processes have many similarities with the inflammatory intimal remodeling seen in atherosclerotic vascular disease such as deposition of low-density lipoprotein cholesterol, Lp(a), and ultimately calcium. Distinguishing inciting factors from contributors to progression has not yet been fully elucidated. Ultimately, valve thickening and calcification lead to increased aortic valve leaflet compliance and loss of elasticity as a result of ongoing chronic inflammation.

V. NATURAL HISTORY

It seems likely but is not definitively proven that patients who develop AS progress through aortic sclerosis initially. According to the 2014 American Heart Association/American College of Cardiology (AHA/ACC) guidelines, the transition from sclerotic to stenotic change is defined by the presence of mild obstruction to blood flow, characterized by increased transaortic valve velocities with a cutoff point defined as a peak aortic jet velocity of 2 m/s or greater (Fig. 1.3). It is estimated that aortic sclerosis progresses to clinical AS at a rate of <2% per year. Despite this low rate of progression to stenosis, aortic sclerosis is associated with a significantly increased risk of cardiovascular morbidity and mortality: 68% increased risk of coronary events (hazard ratio [HR]: 1.68; 95% confidence interval [CI]: 1.31–2.15); a 27% increased risk of stroke (HR: 1.27; 95% CI: 1.01–1.60), a 69%

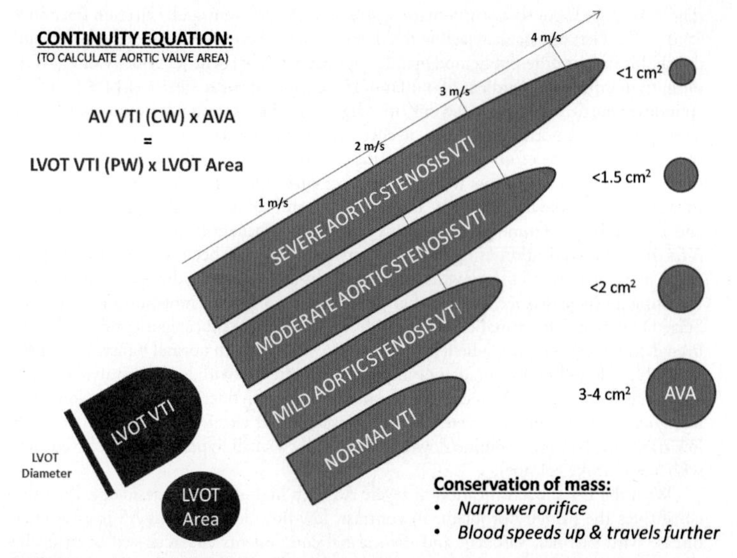

FIGURE 1.3 Visual representation of the conservation of mass that underlies estimation of aortic valve area in the continuity equation. AVA, aortic valve area; AV VTI, aortic valve velocity time integral; CW, continuous wave Doppler; LVOT VTI, left ventricular outflow tract velocity time integral; PW, pulse wave Doppler.

increased risk of cardiovascular mortality (HR: 1.69; 95% CI: 1.32–2.15), and a 36% increased risk of all-cause mortality (HR: 1.36; 95% CI: 1.17–1.59).

Once AS is present, it appears to progress inexorably over time. With moderate AS, the average annual rate of progression is estimated as a decrease in valve area of 0.1 cm^2, which roughly corresponds to an increase in velocity of 0.3 m/s, and an increase in mean pressure gradient of 7 mm Hg. However, while progression may be more rapid in older patients and in those with more severe leaflet calcification, there can be marked individual variability in progression rates, mandating regular clinical and echocardiographic follow-up in all patients with asymptomatic mild-to-moderate AS. When severe AS is detected in patients without symptoms, the likelihood of overt symptom development is high, with 50% to 70% of patients experiencing an adverse cardiovascular event within the next 2 years. Therefore, patients with asymptomatic severe AS require particularly frequent monitoring for progressive disease not least because symptom onset may be insidious and may indeed go unrecognized by the patient. With bicuspid aortic valve disease, severe AS remains the most common reason for intervention.

VI. PATHOPHYSIOLOGY

Recent ACC/AHA valve guidelines have, for the first time, applied a more detailed staging system for disease progression, similar to that used in heart failure. Stage A refers to "at risk" asymptomatic patients with risk factors for development of AS (aortic sclerosis or bicuspid aortic valve). Stage B covers "progressive" asymptomatic AS (namely, mild-to-moderate severity AS with peak aortic jet velocity of 2 to 2.9 m/s and 3 to 3.9 m/s, respectively)

(Fig. 1.3). Stage C covers asymptomatic severe AS (C1 if left ventricular ejection fraction is ≥50%; C2 if left ventricular ejection fraction is <50%). Severe AS is defined at or beyond thresholds in four different hemodynamic parameters: peak aortic jet velocity of ≥4 m/s, mean transaortic valve gradient of ≥40 mm Hg, estimated aortic valve area of ≤1 cm^2, or an indexed aortic valve area ≤0.6 cm^2/m^2 (Fig. 1.3). These thresholds do not completely overlap; in fact, at normal flow rates, an aortic valve area of 0.8 cm^2 correlates with a mean aortic valve gradient of 40 mm Hg, but the rationale for using this higher threshold is that the prognosis of patients with AS is poorer when the aortic valve area is <1.0 cm^2 (hence, some people use the term "moderately severe" for aortic valve area between 0.8 and 1.0 cm^2 because some patients in this category may benefit from valve intervention). A further subclassification using the term "very severe" AS has been advocated when peak aortic jet velocity is ≥5 m/s or when the mean transaortic valve gradient is ≥60 mm Hg, reflecting an increased recognition that prognosis is worse with more advanced disease. Stage D refers to symptomatic patients with severe AS, three subcategories of which have been defined: D1—high-gradient symptomatic severe AS (with normal transvalvular flow rates); D2—low-flow, low-gradient symptomatic severe AS (with low transvalvular aortic volume flow rates caused by reduced left ventricular ejection fraction); and D3—low-flow, low-gradient symptomatic severe AS and left ventricular ejection fraction ≥50% (with low transvalvular aortic volume flow rates caused by a small hypertrophied left ventricle with a low stroke volume).

With the D1 subclassification of severe AS with high-gradient physiology, the valve constitutes the primary problem. In contrast, low-flow, low-gradient AS is a systemic disease with valvular, vascular, and myocardial components characterized by typically slower progression of transvalvular gradients, yet worse clinical outcomes as a result of concomitant impaired systolic function (D2) or diastolic dysfunction (D3). Of suspected cases of low-flow, low-gradient AS (either D2 or D3), 30% turn out on subsequent testing to be pseudostenosis (discussed later), in which the severity of the valvular component is actually mild or indeed moderate.

In more detail, the D2 subclassification refers to the scenario when true symptomatic severe AS is determined to be present on the basis of an estimated aortic valve area ≤1 cm^2 or an indexed aortic valve area ≤0.6 cm^2/m^2, yet corresponding gradients are lower than anticipated (mean transaortic valve gradient is <40 mm Hg) because of low flow (stroke volume index <35 mL/m^2) resulting from reduced left ventricular ejection fraction (<50%). Dobutamine stress echocardiography is particularly useful to help distinguish D2 from "pseudosevere AS" whereby a combination of primary myocardial function and afterload mismatch in the presence of mild-to-moderate AS results in incomplete opening of stiffened aortic leaflets, which can be overcome by augmenting flow rates, a scenario that may not benefit from surgical intervention over intensive medical therapy and close follow-up. D2 is diagnosed if a peak aortic jet velocity of ≥4 m/s can be recorded along with an estimated aortic valve area ≤1 cm^2 at any pharmacologically augmented flow rate. Transesophageal echocardiography and/or noncontrast CT scan can also play a differentiating role by simply getting a better look at valve anatomy—D2 is more likely if the valve is severely calcified (defined by CT as an aortic valve calcification score >1,000 Agatston units) (Fig. 1.4). Another consideration that may account for discrepant severe-range aortic valve area, yet moderate range gradients, is underestimation of the left ventricular outflow tract diameter (not uncommon in bicuspid aortic valve); such an error may result in an exponential underestimation of aortic valve area—better visualization of the left ventricular outflow tract by transesophageal echocardiography or noncontrast CT scan can aid measurement of this parameter.

The D3 subclassification refers to the so-called paradoxic low-flow, low-gradient symptomatic severe AS, wherein low flow (stroke volume index <35 mL/m^2) occurs despite left ventricular ejection fraction ≥50% and is presumed to be because of a combination of small left ventricular chamber size and increased afterload. The prevalence of this

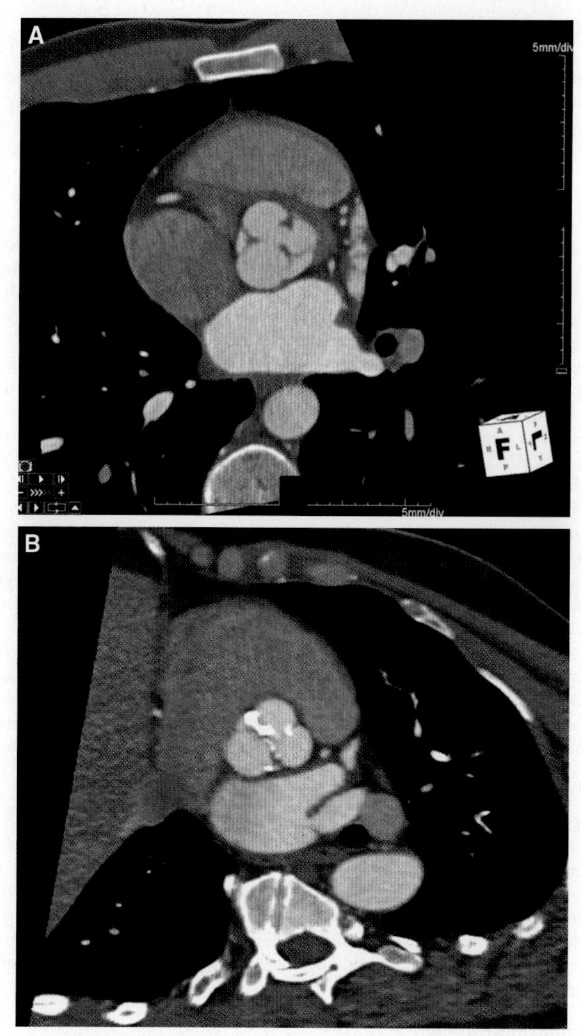

FIGURE 1.4 Examples of the utility of CT scanning in the preoperative assessment of aortic stenosis. Aortic valve repair remains an option for some patients with bicuspid aortic valve regurgitation, particularly in the absence of aortic valve calcification **(A)**. Leaflet calcification is an important determinant of aortic stenosis progression, which is more rapid in patients as leaflet calcification becomes more severe **(B)**.

subclassification varies widely between studies and is estimated at between 5% and 25% of cases of severe AS. Use of dobutamine stress echo for D3 has been assessed only in a small cohort of patients and currently is not guideline recommended, pending validation in larger series of patients.

VII. CLINICAL MANIFESTATIONS

Overt symptom development is typically a late phenomenon (reflecting stage D disease, as discussed). Nonetheless, all patients with AS that are being followed routinely are advised to report any new symptoms. Such symptoms may involve fatigue, lack of energy, reduced exercise capacity, shortness of breath, angina, syncope, and/or fluid overload/congestion. From the perspective of prognosis, heart failure carries the most concern (50% 2-year mortality without aortic valve replacement), followed by syncope (50% 3-year mortality without aortic valve replacement) and angina (50% 5-year mortality without aortic valve replacement).

Syncope in AS typically occurs with exertion and may relate to an inability to compensate for decreased peripheral arterial resistance caused by a relatively fixed cardiac output state. Other potential mechanisms include a secondary vasodepressor response of the left ventricle in response to significantly increased intraventricular pressures and arrhythmias. Angina can occur in AS independently of coronary artery disease because of supply–demand mismatch, particularly in the setting of significant left ventricular hypertrophy. Some patients with AS experience gastrointestinal bleeding because of angiodysplasia of the colon, which is called Heyde syndrome. The underlying mechanism of this bleeding has been discovered to relate to an acquired shear stress–dependent depletion of von Willebrand factor by the protease ADAMTS13 resulting from increased turbulence around the stenotic valve that typically resolves postaortic valve replacement.

An important point to consider is that most patients when first diagnosed with AS are asymptomatic because the diagnosis is often picked up as an incidental finding. Once patients with or at risk of AS are identified, an annual history and physical examination are recommended. At the time of initial detection (or during serial follow-up thereafter), patients with AS may neither fully appreciate nor report the extent of their limitations, reflecting the gradual progression of the disease and the insidious nature of the more common early symptoms of AS (such as fatigue, lack of energy, and reduced exercise capacity). Given that the presence or absence of symptoms is paramount for staging and decisions about treatment, a careful history is of great importance in the evaluation of such patients. In addition, because greater than 20% of the AS patients who claim to be asymptomatic have been shown to exhibit exercise-limiting symptoms during exercise testing and to have worse outcomes: exercise testing has been proposed to confirm symptom status. Serial measurement of exercise tolerance (metabolic equivalents [METS] achieved) during exercise testing, particularly for patients with asymptomatic severe AS (stage C disease), provides an objective measure to aid determination of clinical stability versus often subtle deterioration.

For patients in whom surgical intervention is being planned, careful assessment to determine symptoms and signs of comorbidities and frailty is paramount. Signs of frailty include inability to perform activities of daily living (dependence in feeding, bathing, dressing, transferring, toileting, urinary continence, etc.) and reduced gait speed, grip strength, and muscle mass.

VIII. PHYSICAL DIAGNOSIS

Auscultation of a heart murmur during routine clinical examination (often at the time of a noncardiac presentation) is a common scenario in which AS may first be detected. A detailed physical examination should be performed to diagnose and assess the severity of valve lesions based on a compilation of findings on palpation and with auscultation.

The pulse in AS has characteristic features including a small volume (parvus), a notched upstroke (anacrotic), and a reduced pulse pressure (plateau) that with more advanced disease may become late peaking (tardus). The apex beat may be hyperdynamic and slightly displaced, and there may be a palpable systolic thrill over the base of the heart (aortic area—second right intercostal space). In the presence of AS, it takes more time to achieve higher peak left ventricular systolic pressure (aortic valve gradient plus the systolic blood pressure), resulting in delayed aortic valve closure causing a single second heart sound or even reversed splitting (ordinarily, S2 is split because of a relative delay of the A2 component). This sign may also relate to left bundle branch block but is typically absent in advanced fibrocalcific disease where A2 is typically soft or inaudible. The murmur of AS is classically described as ejection systolic (crescendo–decrescendo), is typically loud and harsh sounding, particularly in full expiration with the patient sitting forward, and radiates to both carotid arteries. It can be distinguished from the dynamic murmur of hypertrophic cardiomyopathy and the pansystolic murmur of mitral regurgitation in a number of different ways including with maneuvers—characteristically diminishing in response to hand grip (increased afterload) and the Valsalva strain phase (decreased preload) and becoming louder with squatting or leg raise (increased preload).

Physical examination findings specific (but not very sensitive) for the presence of severe AS are a delayed and diminished carotid pulse, an absent second heart sound, and a late-peaking murmur. Presence of an S4 (only if in sinus rhythm, because of a late-diastolic, high-pitched, high-pressure atrial wave reflecting from a noncompliant left ventricle) or signs of heart failure reflect advanced disease. In contrast, a soft ejection systolic murmur audible in the aortic area but not over the carotids, with a normal second heart sound and pulse, would be typical of aortic sclerosis.

Clues with regard to the etiology of the AS may be identified by physical examination. With suspected infective endocarditis, examination of the hands may reveal signs such as tender Osler nodes, painless Janeway lesions, splinter hemorrhages, and/or clubbing. In cases of rheumatic AS, concomitant mitral stenosis is common, and auscultation may reveal a soft first heart sound, early opening snap, a long diastolic murmur, atrial fibrillation, and/or signs of pulmonary hypertension. An ejection systolic click after the first heart sound at the beginning of the ejection murmur can be heard in congenital valvular AS produced with opening of stenosed but pliable aortic valve leaflets. Subvalvular AS can result in a concomitant jet lesion of aortic regurgitation resulting in an early diastolic decrescendo murmur (absence of silence after S2). As discussed earlier, the distinctive phenotypic features of Williams syndrome (the so-called elfin facial appearance including a broad forehead, widely set eyes, and a pointed chin) are associated with supravalvular AS.

IX. DIAGNOSTIC TESTING

For preoperative patients with AS, laboratory testing plays an important role in the detection of a wide range of potential blood dyscrasias and comorbid diseases including liver or kidney functional abnormalities. Although routine measurement of biomarkers is not currently recommended by latest valve disease management guidelines, a number of such biomarkers have undergone investigations with regard to their potential role in risk stratification and prognosis in patients with AS, of which B-type natriuretic peptide (BNP) has received the most attention. In asymptomatic patients with AS and preserved left ventricular ejection fraction, higher serial change in BNP levels portends a higher likelihood of the development of a class I indication for aortic valve replacement. Thereafter, following transcatheter or surgical aortic valve implantation, plasma BNP is a strong independent predictor of all-cause mortality and cardiovascular mortality. Because atherosclerotic risk factors are associated with aortic valve disease, patients identified with such degenerative changes should undergo testing to assess lipid profile and glucose levels.

An electrocardiogram is useful to confirm heart rhythm, assess for left ventricular hypertrophy, and detect underlying conduction system disease (a common comorbid finding in patients with AS). Occasionally, a chest X-ray (CXR) may first indicate the presence of AS either directly in the presence of gross aortic valve calcification or indirectly via detection of cardiomegaly or pulmonary congestion. A CXR may also detect comorbid lung pathology.

CT imaging plays an increasingly important role in preoperative testing for aortic valve calcification scoring or for patients undergoing redo surgery (to assess proximity of structures to the sternum for portal of entry planning and to assess the degree/location of ascending aorta calcification for cross-clamp placement) (Fig. 1.4). Dedicated CT and cardiac magnetic resonance imaging have also been developed for patients being considered for transcatheter valve replacement, in particular to assess anatomic considerations for valve sizing and vascular access. Because of its high negative predictive value, CT angiography may be appropriate as an alternative test to preoperative screening coronary angiography in order to exclude high-grade coronary artery disease, particularly in those with low or intermediate pretest likelihood of disease (men <40 years of age and premenopausal women with no atherosclerotic risk factors). It could also be considered for patients undergoing preoperative evaluation that have acute aortic dissection, large aortic valve vegetations, or occlusive prosthetic thrombosis, although the presence of tachycardia (especially atrial fibrillation) and/or dense coronary calcifications poses particular diagnostic challenges.

X. ECHOCARDIOGRAPHY

An echocardiogram is indicated for first-degree relatives of patients with bicuspid aortic valve and/or in patients with symptoms or signs suggestive of AS in order to confirm the diagnosis, establish etiology, determine severity, assess hemodynamic consequences, determine prognosis, and evaluate for timing of intervention. For those in whom AS is identified, it is recommended that echocardiography is performed at least every 3 to 5 years in patients with mild AS, at least every 1 to 2 years in patients with moderate AS, and every 6 to 12 months in patients with (asymptomatic) severe AS. Repeat echocardiography should be considered in patients with AS undergoing serial follow-up that experience a change in symptoms and/or those that are identified as having new signs on physical examination to determine whether the etiology of the symptoms is a progression in the valve lesion, deterioration of the ventricular response to the pressure overload, or something else.

In addition to grading aortic valve stenosis and informing about aortic valve morphology, transthoracic echocardiography can assess for other concomitant valvular disease (particularly of the mitral and/or tricuspid valves), left ventricular hypertrophy, left ventricular dysfunction (typically diastolic but occasionally also systolic), and other associated abnormalities such as aortic dilation, left atrial dilation, pulmonary hypertension, and abnormalities of the right ventricle.

Measurements of peak velocity, as well as calculation of the dimensionless index, valve gradients, and valve area (often indexed to body surface area), may help characterize the severity of the AS. Multiple windows should be obtained and the peak velocity recorded, because such Doppler/velocity measurements are so angle dependent (indeed, peak gradients are often recorded at the right sternal border or the suprasternal notch view rather than in standard apical views). Use of the nonimaging Pedoff probe may also aid in peak velocity measurement, but correlation should always be made to jet profile and timing as well as aortic valve morphology to avoid the possibility of mistakenly detecting spurious Doppler profiles (such as mitral or tricuspid regurgitation, or rarely waveforms because of a restrictive ventricular septal defect or an arterial stenosis). The dimensionless index refers to the decimal ratio of the blood profile (maximum or mean velocity, or velocity time integral) in the left ventricular outflow tract (using pulsed wave Doppler) versus at the aortic valve (using continuous wave Doppler), with a value below 0.25 considered severe. Estimation of the aortic valve area is done using the continuity equation, a concept based on preservation of flow in a closed system, by multiplying the left ventricular outflow tract area by the ratio of the left ventricular outflow/aortic valve velocity time integrals (Fig. 1.3).

Hemodynamic measurements can be performed at rest and during provocation. As discussed, it is particularly useful in low-flow states to be able to pharmacologically augment per-beat flow via inotropic and vasodilator effects of low-dose dobutamine in order to distinguish true versus pseudosevere (moderate) AS. The absence of contractile reserve (whereby stroke volume does not augment by >20% in response to dobutamine) is not a contraindication to aortic valve replacement, but rather indicates a poor prognosis with surgical therapy and an especially poor prognosis with medical therapy.

An investigative role of newer echocardiographic parameters such as left ventricular global longitudinal strain has been shown to independently predict mortality and to provide incremental prognostic utility in patients with severe AS with preserved left ventricular ejection fraction, in addition to standard clinical and echocardiographic parameters.

XI. CARDIAC CATHETERIZATION

These days, the most common reason to perform cardiac catheterization in patients with severe AS is to assess for high-grade coronary artery disease that would provide an indication to perform coronary artery bypass surgery at the time of aortic valve replacement. Rarely, despite thorough noninvasive imaging, there remains uncertainty regarding the severity of AS. If there are inconclusive, noninvasive data, particularly in symptomatic patients, or if there is a discrepancy between the noninvasive tests and clinical findings, a hemodynamic cardiac catheterization should be considered (although crossing a stenotic calcified valve risks cerebral emboli). Transaortic valve gradients via a pullback technique are typically less than simultaneous gradients measured by echocardiography. Aortic valve area may be calculated with the Gorlin formula, using a Fick or thermodilution cardiac output measurement. For patients that have low cardiac output, repeat measurement of gradients and cardiac output can be obtained with concomitant administration of dobutamine. For symptomatic patients in whom there is a concern that the AS severity is underestimated, although rarely done clinically, it remains possible to perform exercise hemodynamics at the time of catheterization.

XII. MEDICAL TREATMENT

In short, there is no medical therapy currently proven to alter the natural history of AS. Nonetheless, guideline-directed medical therapy is advised for common comorbidities such as hyperlipidemia, diabetes mellitus, and hypertension. Antihypertensive medications should be initiated at low dose and gradually titrated, particularly in patients with severe AS. Patients with severe AS and severe decompensated heart failure may benefit from medical stabilization using careful afterload reduction prior to urgent aortic valve replacement. Despite experimental models and retrospective clinical studies suggesting that statin therapy might prevent disease progression, three subsequent well-designed large randomized controlled trials failed to show a benefit, either in terms of changes in hemodynamic severity or in clinical outcomes of patients with mild-to-moderate valve obstruction. Rheumatic fever prophylaxis and infective endocarditis prophylaxis should be given to appropriate groups as per guidelines.

XIII. SURGICAL/PERCUTANEOUS INTERVENTION

Table 1.1 summarizes the current 2014 ACC/AHA indications and level of evidence for surgical/percutaneous aortic valve replacement. At this time, surgical aortic valve replacement is indicated for low- or intermediate-risk patients who meet an indication for aortic valve replacement. Transcatheter aortic valve replacement is indicated for patients with prohibitive surgical risk with a life expectancy >12 months or as an alternative procedure for patients deemed at intermediate or high surgical risk as assessed by a Heart Valve Team. Percutaneous aortic balloon valvuloplasty may be considered as a bridge to surgical or transcatheter aortic valve replacement in stage D patients (symptomatic severe AS).

TABLE 1.1 Current 2014 American College of Cardiology/American Heart Association Indications and Level of Evidence for Surgical/Percutaneous Aortic Valve Replacement

Aortic valve replacement is *recommended/indicated* (class I/evidence level B) in:

- Stage D1 (symptomatic severe high-gradient aortic stenosis)
- Stage C2 (asymptomatic, severe aortic stenosis and left ventricular ejection fraction [LVEF] <50%)
- Stage C or D (severe aortic stenosis) when undergoing other cardiac surgeries

Aortic valve replacement is *reasonable* (class IIa/evidence level B or C) in:

- Stage C1 (asymptomatic, severe aortic stenosis) if aortic stenosis is very severe and low surgical risk
- Stage C1 (asymptomatic, severe aortic stenosis) if abnormal exercise test
- Stage D2 (symptomatic low-flow, low-gradient severe aortic stenosis) after dobutamine stress
- Stage D3 (symptomatic low-flow, low-gradient severe aortic stenosis, preserved LVEF)
- Stage B (moderate aortic stenosis) when undergoing other cardiac surgeries

Aortic valve replacement *may be considered* (class IIb/evidence level C) in:

- Stage C1 (asymptomatic, severe aortic stenosis) if rapid progression and low surgical risk

KEY PEARLS

- Despite high clinical prevalence, assessment of AS remains complex as there is no single parameter that reliably indicates aortic valve stenosis severity.
- Multiple factors need to be considered, including anatomic and physiologic valve parameters (e.g., aortic valve area, calcification, valve compliance, gradients, transaortic valve flow) as well as other patient factors (left ventricular function/remodeling, afterload, body size, comorbidities, etc.).
- Treatments for AS are highly effective but remain invasive for the foreseeable future (surgical/transcatheter).
- The ongoing and successful progress of transcatheter aortic valve replacement technologies has provided a strong impetus for further research, which continues to spawn a rapidly increasing amount of clinical knowledge of the wider field including complementary yet diverse areas such as multimodality imaging and heart management teams.
- Better methods of risk stratification are required for patients with severe AS to help guide who would be best served by surgery, transcatheter therapies, or a conservative approach.

SUGGESTED READINGS

Aronow WS, Ahn C, Kronzon I, et al. Prognosis of congestive heart failure in patients aged > or = 62 years with unoperated severe valvular aortic stenosis. *Am J Cardiol.* 1993;72:846–848.

Baliga RR. From clinical observation to mechanism—Heyde's syndrome. *N Engl J Med.* 2013;368:579.

Clavel MA, Ennezat PV, Maréchaux S, et al. Stress echocardiography to assess stenosis severity and predict outcome in patients with paradoxical low-flow, low-gradient aortic stenosis and preserved LVEF. *JACC Cardiovasc Imaging.* 2013;6:175–183.

Coffey S, Cox B, Williams MJ. The prevalence, incidence, progression, and risks of aortic valve sclerosis: a systematic review and meta-analysis. *J Am Coll Cardiol.* 2014;63:2852–2861.

Dorn GW II. Shared genetic risk for sclerosis of valves and vessels. *N Engl J Med.* 2013;368:569–570.

Ennezat PV, Maréchaux S, Iung B, et al. Exercise testing and exercise stress echocardiography in asymptomatic aortic valve stenosis. *Heart.* 2009;95:877–884.

Garg V, Muth AN, Ransom JF, et al. Mutations in NOTCH1 cause aortic valve disease. *Nature.* 2005;437:270–274.

Herrmann S, Fries B, Liu D, et al. Differences in natural history of low- and high-gradient aortic stenosis from nonsevere to severe stage of the disease. *J Am Soc Echocardiogr.* 2015;28(11):1270.e4–1282.e4.

Kusunose K, Goodman A, Parikh R, et al. Incremental prognostic value of left ventricular global longitudinal strain in patients with aortic stenosis and preserved ejection fraction. *Circ Cardiovasc Imaging.* 2014;7:938–945.

Lindman BR, Breyley JG, Schilling JD, et al. Prognostic utility of novel biomarkers of cardiovascular stress in patients with aortic stenosis undergoing valve replacement. *Heart.* 2015;101:1382–1388.

Lindroos M, Kupari M, Heikkila J, et al. Prevalence of aortic valve abnormalities in the elderly: an echocardiographic study of a random population sample. *J Am Coll Cardiol.* 1993;21:1220–1225.

Nishimura RA, Otto CM, Bonow RO, et al. 2014 AHA/ACC guideline for the management of patients with valvular heart disease: a report of the American College of Cardiology/American Heart Association Task Force on Practice Guidelines. *J Am Coll Cardiol.* 2014;63:e57–e185.

Otto CM, Pearlman AS, Gardner CL. Hemodynamic progression of aortic stenosis in adults assessed by Doppler echocardiography. *J Am Coll Cardiol.* 1989;13:545–550.

Pellikka PA, Sarano ME, Nishimura RA, et al. Outcome of 622 adults with asymptomatic, hemodynamically significant aortic stenosis during prolonged follow-up. *Circulation.* 2005;111:3290–3295.

Thanassoulis G, Campbell CY, Owens DS, et al. Genetic associations with valvular calcification and aortic stenosis. *N Engl J Med.* 2013;368:503–512.

CHAPTER 2

Roger Byrne
Dermot Phelan

Aortic Regurgitation

I. INTRODUCTION.

I. INTRODUCTION. Aortic regurgitation (AR), despite being one of the more common forms of valvular heart disease, remains clinically challenging with regard to accurate assessment of severity and management. When closed, the normal three leaflets of the aortic valve (AV) overlap their neighbors by 2 to 3 mm, forming a tight seal against backflow of blood despite substantial diastolic pressure in the aorta. However, disruption of either the valve leaflets or the surrounding aortic root may cause leaflet malcoaptation, leading to AR.

The etiology and clinical presentation of acute AR differ significantly from those of chronic AR. Acute AR is challenging to diagnose by both physical examination and echocardiography and so requires a high index of suspicion and understanding of the specific clinical and imaging characteristics.

Chronic severe AR leads to both volume and pressure overload of the left ventricle (LV), leading to compensatory ventricular dilation and eccentric hypertrophy before finally resulting in systolic dysfunction that may not be reversible.

Surgical AV replacement (AVR) remains the only effective treatment option for the majority of patients with severe AR. Medical therapy has limited effect, and AV repair is suitable only for a small number of patients. Timing of surgery in chronic AR requires weighing the risks/benefits of surgery versus watchful waiting, while trying to avoid irreversible systolic dysfunction.

Advanced echocardiographic imaging utilizing three-dimensional (3D) imaging and two-dimensional (2D) strain imaging may improve diagnostic accuracy and identify patients who may benefit from early intervention. Multimodality imaging, including cardiac magnetic resonance (CMR) imaging and cardiac computed tomography (CCT), is increasingly being utilized in the assessment of AR.

II. ETIOLOGY

The etiologies of AR may be divided into two main categories: primary (valvular leaflet abnormalities) and secondary (aortic root abnormalities) (Fig. 2.1). Common primary causes include congenital abnormalities of the valve leaflets, such as a bicuspid aortic valve (BAV), and acquired valvular lesions, such as degenerative/calcific changes, endocarditis, or rheumatic disease. Common secondary causes leading to dilation of the aortic root include degenerative changes usually related to age, atherosclerosis, or long-standing hypertension, and genetic aortopathies such as Marfan syndrome or Loeys–Dietz syndrome. Additionally, there are mixed primary and secondary etiologies that result in AR by multiple mechanisms; these include aortic dissection and blunt chest trauma.

Clinically, the causes of AR may also be divided into pathologies that result in either chronic or acute AR (Table 2.1).

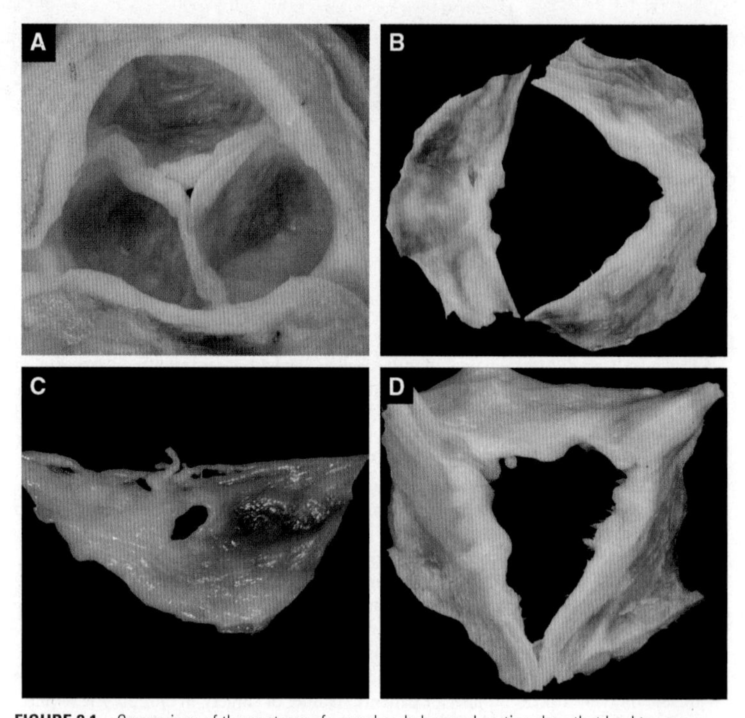

FIGURE 2.1 Comparison of the anatomy of normal and abnormal aortic valves that lead to severe aortic regurgitation. **A:** Normal aortic valve. A cephalad view of a normal aortic valve from a young adult is shown. The size of the cusps and the distance between each of the commissures are roughly equal. **B:** Regurgitation secondary to dilated aortic root and bicuspid aortic valve. The excised valve shows a bicuspid aortic valve with the larger conjoint cusp shown on the right side. There is mild thickening of the free edge without calcification. **C:** Regurgitation secondary to healed endocarditis. A semilunar valve cusp shows a large central perforation as a sequela of infective endocarditis. **D:** Trileaflet aortic valve with regurgitation. A trileaflet aortic valve shows marked thickening and retraction of cusps. The cusp retraction by fibrous tissue results in failure of coaptation at the center of the valve. The fusion in two of the three commissures also results in valve stenosis. Abundant Lambl excrescences are present at the free edge of the cusp on the right. (Courtesy of Drs. E. Rene Rodriguez and Carmela D. Tan at www.e-heart.org.)

III. PATHOPHYSIOLOGY

A. Chronic aortic regurgitation

The primary hemodynamic effect of AR is an increase in LV end-diastolic volume (preload) due to leaking of blood from the aorta back into the LV during diastole. Increased LV end-diastolic volume (LVEDV) results in increased wall tension. In AR, the sum of the regurgitant volume and the normal forward stroke volume (SV) is ejected forward into the high-pressure aorta during systole. The increase in the ejected forward SV causes systolic hypertension (increased afterload), and together with the decrease in diastolic pressure (owing to the drop in the aortic diastolic pressure) results in the classic finding of a wide pulse pressure. Conversely, in mitral regurgitation (MR),

TABLE 2.1 Etiologies of Aortic Regurgitation

General	Specific	Condition	Acute	Chronic
Primary (valvular abnormality)	Congenital	Bicuspid, quadricuspid, unicuspid aortic valve		X
	Degenerative	Age-related thickening/calcification		X
		Myxomatous degeneration		X
		Membranous subaortic stenosis (turbulent jet causes leaflet damage)		X
		Acute prosthetic valve dysfunction	X	
	Infectious/inflammatory	Bacterial endocarditis	X	X
		Nonbacterial endocarditis	X	X
		Rheumatic valvular heart disease		X
	Traumatic	Iatrogenic (post–percutaneous aortic balloon dilation or cardiac catheterization)	X	
		Traumatic rupture	X	
	Neoplastic	Papillary fibroelastoma		X
	Toxic	Anorexigen exposure		X
		Drugs: fenfluramine, phentermine, ergots		X
		Radiation heart disease		X
Secondary (aortic root abnormality)	Genetic	Marfan syndrome		X
		Loeys–Dietz syndrome		X
		Ehlers–Danlos syndrome		X
		Turner syndrome		X
		Familial thoracic aortic aneurysm syndrome		X
	Degenerative	Age		X
		Hypertension		X
		Atherosclerosis		X
	Infectious	Syphilis		X
		Salmonella		X
		Staphylococci		X
		Mycobacteria		X

(continued)

TABLE 2.1 Etiologies of Aortic Regurgitation *(continued)*

General	Specific	Condition	Acute	Chronic
	Inflammatory	Giant cell arteritis		X
		Takayasu arteritis		X
		Rheumatoid arthritis		X
		Spondyloarthropathies		X
		Reactive arthritis		X
	Traumatic	Aortic dissection (type A)	X	
		Leaflet tear or disruption of leaflet support at the aortic root	X	
	Other	Supracristal ventricular septal defect: may cause leaflet prolapse		X

the regurgitant SV flows retrogradely into the low-pressure left atrial (LA) chamber; therefore, MR is characterized by volume overload *only*, whereas AR is characterized by *both volume and pressure overload*. The Law of Laplace states that wall tension is proportionate to pressure times radius and inversely proportionate to wall thickness, and so, to maintain normal wall tension, compensatory eccentric hypertrophy occurs. The ratio of ventricular wall thickness to cavity radius is maintained in order to keep wall stress near normal despite the larger LVEDV.

In the majority of patients with AR, the disease course is chronic, characterized by slowly progressive LV adaptation via chamber dilation and eccentric hypertrophy. Eventually, the myocytes reach maximum sarcomeric elongation so that further volume increases result in reduced contractility (Frank–Starling mechanism). A concurrent, progressive reduction in LV compliance, as a result of interstitial fibrosis, leads to a chronic decompensated state.

Oxygen supply/demand mismatch resulting in the symptom of angina may occur because of (1) decreased aortic diastolic pressure and elevated left ventricular end-diastolic pressure (LVEDP), resulting in decreased coronary perfusion pressure, (2) shorter diastolic time as a result of reflex tachycardia, and (3) reduced coronary blood flow reserve in the hypertrophied myocardium.

LV distention may induce mitral annular dilation with resultant functional MR, further increasing the LA pressure and pulmonary capillary wedge pressure (PCWP), which may eventually increase pulmonary artery pressures and ultimately compromise right ventricular function.

The end result of chronic volume overload is eccentric hypertrophy, chamber enlargement (increase in end-systolic and diastolic volumes), increased LVEDP, and a progressive decrease in left ventricular ejection fraction (LVEF) and cardiac output (CO).

B. Acute aortic regurgitation

The sudden volume overload into a noncompliant, nondilated LV seen in acute AR causes an acute rise in LVEDP, subsequently increasing the LA and PCWP, causing pulmonary edema.

The acute afterload increase, resulting from the combination of elevated blood pressure and increased wall stress, leads to an acute decrease in SV and LVEF, causing hypotension and cardiogenic shock. A compensatory reflex tachycardia helps maintain CO.

Diastolic pressure between the LV and aorta equilibrates rapidly because of the acute rise in LVEDP and drop in aortic diastolic pressure. The drop in the diastolic gradient between the aorta and LVEDP (i.e., the myocardial perfusion pressure) may cause subendocardial hypoperfusion and myocardial ischemia. This rapid equilibration also results in (1) a short early diastolic murmur of AR that rapidly becomes quiet on auscultation, and (2) early diastolic preclosure of the mitral valve, and later diastolic MR (owing to severely elevated LVEDP). Acute AR may therefore be difficult to appreciate both by auscultation and by color and spectral Doppler echocardiography. Because the LV does not have time to dilate (which would increase the SV), classic physical findings of chronic AR such as a wide pulse pressure and a displaced point of maximum impulse are not present. In addition, rapid LV distention may dilate the mitral annulus, causing functional MR, further increasing the LA pressure and PCWP. Acute AR is usually a hemodynamic emergency, and urgent diagnosis and rapid intervention can be lifesaving. A known history of aortic aneurysm, Marfan disease, or BAV may point toward the diagnosis.

IV. GENETICS

The most common congenital cardiac anomaly is a BAV, which is seen in 0.5% to 2% of the population. Even individuals with a normal tricuspid AV in families with BAV disease that have associated genes such as *NOTCH1* may be at risk for AV calcification or thoracic aorta aneurysm. This may lead to mixed AV disease through sclerosis and aortic root dilation.

Genetic aortopathies should be suspected in young patients with AR as a result of aortic root dilation. The most common of these is Marfan syndrome (autosomal dominant), a connective tissue disorder with a characteristic phenotypic expression defined by the revised Ghent criteria. Cardiovascular features include dilation of the aortic root at the level of the sinuses of Valsalva, aortic regurgitation and MR, and mitral valve prolapse. *FNB1* mutations are identified in over two thirds of cases. *TGFBR2* mutations have also been identified in patients with Marfan-like phenotypes. Patients with *FBN1* mutations were found to have more extensive skeletal involvement, whereas patients with *TGFBR2* mutations had more severe aortic phenotypes. Marfan syndrome patients also may exhibit findings such as ectopia lentis (lens dislocation) and dolichostenomelia (long limbs) that are not seen in Loeys–Dietz syndrome.

Loeys–Dietz syndrome (autosomal dominant) has a continuum of presentations that generally include both vascular and skeletal. It is caused by mutations in the *TGFBR1, TGFBR2, SMAD3, TGFB2,* or *TGFB3* genes. Patients have widely spaced eyes and a bifid uvula not seen in vascular (or cardiac valvular) type Ehlers–Danlos syndrome.

Ehlers–Danlos syndrome vascular type (autosomal dominant) is attributable to a mutation in *COL3A1*. Midsize arteries are usually involved, with arterial rupture being the most common cause of sudden death. Valvular complications emerge during adulthood. Ehlers–Danlos cardiac valvular type is a very rare variant and relatively mild on the spectrum of clinical phenotypes resulting from *COLIA2* mutations.

Finally, 91 patients with lone AR were studied by human leukocyte antigen (HLA) typing for HLA-B27 (an immunogenic marker present in 8% of the world's white population associated with seronegative spondyloarthropathies). HLA-B27 was found to be present in 88% of the male patients with AR and severe conduction system disease.

V. NATURAL HISTORY

A. Chronic aortic regurgitation

Chronic AR has a variable progression, but in the majority of patients, the disease course is chronic and slowly progressive.

Bonow et al. studied 104 asymptomatic patients with severe AR and normal LVEF. The rate of attrition (defined as death, symptoms, or asymptomatic LV dysfunction) was <5% per year over a 11-year follow-up. The rate of sudden death was only 0.4%

per year. At 11 years, 58% of patients remained asymptomatic with normal LV systolic function. Borer et al. (*Circulation* 1998;97:525) found similar results in 104 different patients monitored for a mean of 7.3 years. The rate of attrition was 6.2% per year and was predicted by the change in LVEF, or LVEF adjusted for wall stress from rest to exercise. At 5 years, 75% of patients remained free of death, symptoms, or LV dysfunction.

Dujardin et al. (*Circulation* 1999;99:1851) investigated the fate of 246 patients with moderately severe or severe AR with a mean follow-up time of 7 years. Unlike the two prior studies, these patients were not all asymptomatic with normal LV systolic function. The 10-year mortality rate was 34%, with independent predictors of survival being age, functional class, comorbidity index, atrial fibrillation, LV end-systolic diameter, and LVEF. Patients with greater New York Heart Association (NYHA) functional class or LV end-diastolic diameter (LVEDD) >25 mm/m^2 had an adverse prognosis. Taken together, these studies indicate that asymptomatic patients with normal LV function generally have a favorable prognosis and that decline in LVEF on serial follow-up may identify patients who will require surgical intervention.

In asymptomatic patients with normal LV function and compensated severe AR, the progression rate to symptoms is <6% per year, and the progression to LV dysfunction is 3.5% per year. Risk of sudden death is very low in asymptomatic patients (<0.2% per year). Once LV dysfunction develops, symptoms will likely occur within 3 years (>25% per year); once symptoms develop, the rate of mortality increases to >10% per year.

B. Acute aortic regurgitation

Acute severe AR is generally a surgical emergency, with outcomes dependent on the underlying substrate, etiology, and early management.

VI. CLINICAL MANIFESTATIONS

A. Chronic aortic regurgitation

Chronic AR is usually well tolerated, and patients are frequently diagnosed on routine clinical examination prior to the development of any symptoms. The development of symptoms is generally due to pulmonary congestion and decreased CO. Initial symptoms include dyspnea on exertion and a decrease in exercise tolerance. Later, symptoms of orthopnea and paroxysmal nocturnal dyspnea usually occur as LV systolic function begins to decline. Angina (also nocturnal angina) may uncommonly occur regardless of obstructive coronary artery disease owing to decreased myocardial perfusion pressure causing subendocardial ischemia, as described earlier.

B. Acute aortic regurgitation

Acute AR presents with symptoms and signs of sudden hemodynamic instability (dyspnea, syncope, altered mental status) or frank cardiogenic shock. Concomitant chest pain should raise the suspicion of aortic dissection as part of the differential diagnosis for cardiogenic shock.

VII. PHYSICAL DIAGNOSIS

A. Chronic aortic regurgitation

1. Peripheral pulse examination

AR is characterized by a hyperdynamic pulse and wide pulse pressure as a result of a brisk systolic upstroke (caused by increase in LV SV) followed by a rapid diastolic collapse (caused by reversal of flow in the aorta). It is best appreciated by raising the arm abruptly and feeling the radial pulse. This hyperdynamic pulse was thought to result in the many classic eponymous signs of AR (Table 2.2); however, a 2003 review by Babu et al. of the peer-reviewed literature found only four signs with sufficient original literature for review, and overall, there was little published evidence to support their usefulness in AR. It is important to note that the signs of a hyperdynamic circulation are not specific to AR and can be seen in other conditions associated with a hyperdynamic circulation (anemia, thyrotoxicosis,

TABLE 2.2 Eponymous Physical Signs Historically Associated with a Hyperdynamic Pulse in Chronic Aortic Regurgitation

Sign	Description
Austin Flint murmur	Low-pitched, mid-to-late diastolic rumble at apex, often with presystolic accentuation. Best heard at the apex, with the bell of the stethoscope, with the patient in the left lateral position, on expiration. Sensitivity 52–100%, specificity not available (6 studies, 90 patients).
Corrigan sign	"Water hammer" pulse—i.e., rapid rise/fall or distention/collapse of the carotid pulse (or other pulses). Palpation of the radial artery while elevating the wrist. Positive if the pulse increases in amplitude. Sensitivity 100%, specificity 16% (1 study, 1 patient).
Duroziez sign	Intermittent to-and-fro femoral artery systolic and diastolic murmur generated by light compression with the bell of a stethoscope. Sensitivity 0%, specificity 35–100% (1 study, 5 patients).
Hill sign	Popliteal systolic blood pressure – brachial systolic blood pressure ≥20 mm Hg: this sign is an artifact of lower limb indirect (sphygmomanometric) blood pressure measurement. Sensitivity 75–100%, specificity 71–100% (2 studies, 14 patients).
Traube sound	"Pistol shot" double sound heard over the femoral artery when it is compressed distally.
de Musset sign	Head-nodding with each heart beat (low sensitivity).
Müller sign	Pulsations of the uvula.
Becker sign	Arterial pulsations visible in the retinal arteries.
Rosenbach sign	Pulsatile liver.
Gerhardt sign	Enlarged spleen.
Mayne sign	Diastolic blood pressure drop of >15 mm Hg with arm raised.
Lincoln sign	Pulsatile popliteal.
Sherman sign	Dorsalis pedis pulse unexpectedly prominent in age >75 y.
Landolfi sign	Alternating constriction and dilation of the pupil.
Lighthouse sign	Blanching and flushing of the forehead.
Quincke pulses	Subungual capillary bed pulsations (low sensitivity).

beriberi, large arteriovenous fistula, and patent ductus arteriosus). A bisferiens (twice-beating) carotid arterial pulse may also occur in severe AR. Paradoxically in decompensated AR, the pulse pressure narrows because of a decreasing LV systolic function and forward SV.

2. **Palpation**

   In severe AR, the apical impulse may be diffuse, laterally and caudally displaced (owing to eccentric hypertrophy of the LV), sustained, and hyperdynamic. A diastolic thrill may be felt in the second left intercostal space, and if there is a large increase in SV, a systolic thrill may be present because of the increased aortic flow.

3. **Auscultation**
    a. **Heart sounds**
    - S_1: may be soft, early, and less forceful owing to preclosure of the mitral valve as a result of elevated LVEDP. Generally, a soft S_1 is associated with an elevated LVEDP.
    - S_2: is soft (A_2 may be reduced owing to poor coaptation, P_2 may be normal but obscured by the diastolic murmur), narrowly split, or paradoxically split because of protracted ejection time.
    - S_3: may be present owing to increased early diastolic filling into a noncompliant LV. If present, suggests LV volume overload/decreased LV systolic function.
    - S_4: may be present owing to atrial contraction into a noncompliant, hypertrophied LV.
    - Ejection click: may be present related to abrupt opening of a bicuspid AV.

    b. **Murmurs**

    The classic murmur of chronic AR is a "blowing," high-frequency/pitched, decrescendo, early diastolic murmur starting immediately after A_2, best heard at the left sternal border (third and fourth intercostal space), and radiating toward the apex. If soft, the murmur is augmented by (1) using the diaphragm of the stethoscope, (2) sitting the patient forward (brings the base of the heart close to the chest wall), (3) expiration (increased flow through the left heart), (4) bilateral isometric handgrip for 20 to 30 seconds (increased peripheral resistance), (5) squatting (increased peripheral resistance *and* venous return), (6) inflating bilateral arm blood pressure cuffs above systolic pressure (increased peripheral resistance), and (7) administering a vasopressor (increased peripheral resistance).

    The severity of AR is generally proportional to the duration of the murmur except in mild chronic AR and late very severe AR (where other signs of very severe AR should be present). Classically, a diastolic murmur radiating to the right sternal border indicates aortic dilation with secondary AR, and at the left sternal border indicates a primary valvular AR. Increased forward flow across the valve results in a short ejection systolic murmur at the base of the heart radiating to the neck.

    Rarely, a low-pitched, mitral stenosis–like murmur (Austin Flint murmur), which is a mid-to-late diastolic rumble at the apex, often with presystolic accentuation, may occur. In this scenario, the diastolic jet of AR strikes the anterior mitral valve, impeding opening, and results in functional mitral stenosis. There may also be a coexisting murmur of aortic stenosis if mixed AV disease exists.

B. **Acute aortic regurgitation**

The physical examination of acute severe AR differs significantly from that of chronic severe AR (Table 2.3). The primary clinical feature is usually cardiogenic shock. Other notable features include:

1. **Peripheral pulse examination**

    The typical chronic AR signs of a hyperdynamic circulation may be absent in acute AR. If aortic dissection is suspected, the blood pressure should be measured in all four extremities.

2. **Palpation**

    The apical impulse is typically nondisplaced because the LV has not had time to dilate.

3. **Auscultation**
    a. **Heart sounds**
    - S_1: is soft or absent owing to early preclosure of mitral valve.
    - A_2: is often soft.
    - P_2: is increased secondary to postcapillary pulmonary hypertension.
    - S_3: is common and reflects cardiac decompensation.

TABLE 2.3 Comparison of Selected Clinical and Hemodynamic Findings in Severe Chronic versus Acute Aortic Regurgitation (AR)

	Chronic AR	Acute AR
Clinical presentation	Often asymptomatic	Pulmonary edema, heart failure
Systolic aortic pressure	Increased	Normal or slightly decreased
Diastolic aortic pressure	Decreased	Normal or slightly decreased
Pulse pressure	Increased	Normal or slightly increased
Heart rate	Normal or slightly increased	Increased
Cardiac output	Normal	Decreased
Point of maximal impulse	Displaced laterally	Normal position
Murmur	Diastolic decrescendo	Short and quiet, may not be audible
Left ventricular (LV) size	Significantly dilated	Normal to near normal
Left ventricular end-diastolic pressure (LVEDP)	Normal to near normal	Significantly elevated
Aortic pressure	Rapid upstroke: augmented LV contractility (Frank–Starling law) Increased systolic pressure secondary to increased forward stroke volume Rapid decrease in diastolic aortic pressure caused by regurgitation Wide pulse pressure Near-equalization of aortic and LV pressures at end-diastole caused by continuous regurgitation	Reduced aortic systolic pressure caused by decreased forward stroke volume Pulse pressure narrowed more than normal
LV pressure	Left ventricular end-diastolic volume (LVEDV) increased with normal or near-normal LVEDP because of increased LV compliance LV systolic pressure may be normal or elevated because of increased diastolic volume and augmented LV contractility	Steep rise in LV diastolic pressures with a markedly increased LVEDP caused by an increased LVEDV without increased LV compliance
Left atrial pressure	LA pressures and waveform usually normal. May have prominent "a" wave if associated with LVH (similar to that in aortic stenosis)	LA pressure elevated Small "a" and "v" wave, and the nadir of the "x" and "y" descents is less than normal

b. Murmurs

There is a low-pitched, quiet, and short early diastolic murmur owing to rapid equilibration of the LV and aortic diastolic pressures limiting the volume and duration of AR. There may not be any audible murmur in very severe acute AR.

VIII. DIAGNOSTIC TESTING

A. Laboratory testing

Beyond assessment of LV volumes and LVEF, there is a need for early identification of systolic dysfunction so that patients can either be followed more closely or be potentially referred for early intervention, before the onset of permanent LV systolic dysfunction. B-type natriuretic peptide (BNP) levels are higher in symptomatic than in asymptomatic patients. In patients with severe asymptomatic AR and normal LV function, BNP is an independent marker for a combined endpoint of subsequent symptoms/LV dysfunction/death. A cutoff BNP value ≥130 pg/mL categorizes a higher-risk subgroup.

B. Electrocardiography

The ECG changes seen in chronic AR reflect the adaptive morphologic changes that occur in the LV as a result of volume and pressure overload, typically with findings of LV hypertrophy (LVH).

1. Characteristic findings include LVH in the lateral precordial leads (V5, V6). Because blood is an excellent conductor of electricity, a dilated LV with increased blood volume magnifies the transmural activation front and results in high-voltage QRS complexes (the so-called Brody effect). The dilated LV cavity lies closer to the chest wall, which also contributes to the increased amplitude.
2. Generally, there is an absence of ST- or T-wave changes; however, these may occur if there is associated LV dysfunction.
3. Left axis deviation and LA enlargement are commonly associated with chronic AR. Rarely, negative U waves have been reported in LV volume overload and other cardiac conditions.
4. Conduction abnormalities are not common and generally only occur late in the course of chronic AR, when LV dysfunction occurs. Premature atrial and ventricular complexes are common.

C. Chest X-ray

Radiographic findings are generally nonspecific; these include:

1. Increased cardiac–thoracic ratio. There are no specific signs for LV enlargement on chest X-ray; however, the LV enlarges inferiorly and in a leftward direction. Therefore, the vertical diameter increases more than the lateral diameter.
2. LA enlargement in AR does not occur unless there is significant LV dysfunction. If present in mild AR, it suggests coexisting mitral valve disease.
3. Ascending aorta dilation suggests secondary nonvalvular AR.
4. Calcification of the AV suggests mixed AV disease.
5. Linear calcifications in the aortic wall are classically described in cases of syphilitic aortitis.

IX. ECHOCARDIOGRAPHY

Transthoracic echocardiography (TTE) is the test of choice in the initial evaluation of a patient suspected to have AR. 2D and Doppler echocardiography will confirm the presence and assess the mechanism and severity of AR (Table 2.4). Echocardiography also provides vital information on the hemodynamic effect of the AR through quantification of LV size, systolic function, LVEDP (short deceleration time of the mitral inflow E wave, premature closure of the mitral valve, and/or diastolic MR are features suggestive of an elevated LVEDP), LA size, and pulmonary pressures. These data provide important prognostic information. In symptomatic patients undergoing aortic valve replacement

TABLE 2.4 Assessment of Valvular Regurgitation by Echocardiography

	Mild	Moderate	Severe
Qualitative			
Valve morphology	Normal/abnormal	Normal/abnormal	Abnormal/flail/large coaptation defect
Color Doppler regurgitant jet	Small in central jets	Intermediate	Large in central jets, variable in eccentric jets
CW signal of regurgitant jet	Incomplete/faint	Dense	Dense
Diastolic flow reversal in descending aorta			Holodiastolic flow reversal (end-diastolic velocity >20 cm/s)
Diastolic mitral regurgitation			May be present
Semiquantitative			
VC width (cm)	<0.3		>0.6
Pressure half time (ms)	>500		<200
Quantitative			
ERO (cm^2)	<0.1	0.1–0.29	≥0.3
R Vol (mL)	<30	30–59	≥60
RF (%)	<30	30–49	≥50
Jet width/LVOT width (%)	<25	25–64	≥65
+ LV (and LA) size			Enlarged

CW, continuous wave; VC, vena contracta; ERO, effective regurgitant orifice area; R Vol, regurgitant volume; RF, regurgitant fraction; LV, left ventricle; LA, left atrium; LVOT, left ventricular outflow tract.

(AVR), preoperative LV systolic function and end-systolic dimension (ESD) or volume are significant determinants of survival and functional results after surgery. Symptomatic patients with normal LVEF have significantly better long-term postoperative survival than those with depressed systolic function. Associated pathologies, such as aortic dilation or dissection, coarctation associated with a bicuspid valve, and other associated valvular lesions, can be evaluated by echocardiography, as might be the case with infective endocarditis or rheumatic valvular disease.

A. Qualitative assessment of AR by 2D echocardiography

1. Aortic valve morphology

a. May define a primary (valvular) etiology (e.g., bicuspid valve, prolapse, perforation, vegetations, or rheumatic changes).

b. Flail segments or valves with large coaptation defects suggest severe AR (Fig. 2.2).

2. Aortic root morphology

a. May define a secondary etiology: for example, aortic dilation or dissection.

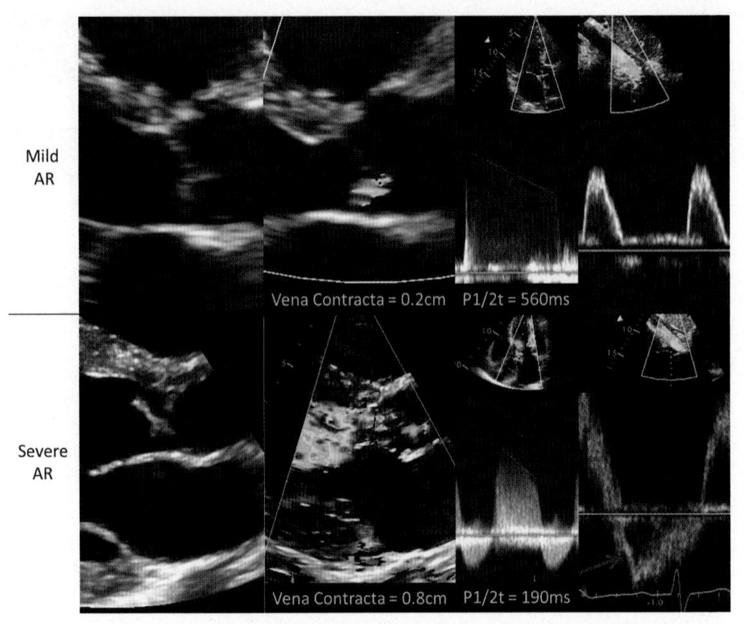

FIGURE 2.2 Comparison of mild versus severe aortic regurgitation (AR) using qualitative and semiquantitative parameters. Compared to mild AR, which shows a mildly sclerotic valve, small vena contracta (VC), a shallow pressure half time (P1/2t), and a small amount of early diastolic flow reversal in the abdominal aorta, severe AR demonstrates complete lack of central coaptation on two-dimensional imaging because of disruption from endocarditis, a large proximal flow convergence and VC, a dense jet of AR on continuous wave Doppler with a steep P1/2t, and holodiastolic flow reversal in the abdominal aorta *(red arrow)*.

   b. May indicate a secondary indication for valvular surgery in nonsevere AR: for example, aneurysmal aortic dilation or endocarditis.

3. **Color Doppler:** Presence of a proximal isovelocity surface area (PISA) at a standard color Doppler aliasing velocity of 50 to 60 cm/s suggests at least moderate AR.
4. **Continuous wave (CW) Doppler signal:** The density and pressure half time (PHT) of the AR envelope help quantify AR. If the density of the envelope is equal to or greater than the forward flow spectral envelope, this suggests severe AR.
5. **Diastolic flow reversal in the descending thoracic aorta or proximal abdominal aorta:** Assessing duration of reversed flow during diastole in the aortic arch and abdominal aorta provides a quick semiquantitative estimate of severity. Significant holodiastolic flow reversal, a diastolic velocity time integral (VTI) similar to systolic VTI, and a high end-diastolic velocity >20 cm/s suggest severe AR.
6. **Left ventricular size and systolic function (LVEF)**
   a. Chronic severe AR is almost invariably associated with LV dilation. LV size and LVEF will inform decision making for valve surgery. The 2014 American College of Cardiology (ACC)/American Heart Association (AHA) valvular guidelines define severe dilation as LVESD >50 mm or indexed LVESD >25

mm/m^2 by linear measurement. LV linear dimensions should be acquired in the parasternal long-axis view, perpendicular to the LV long axis, and measured at the level of the mitral valve leaflet tips by 2D echocardiography.

b. LV volume measurements using 3D acquisition or, if not available/reliable, the 2D biplane method of disks should be used to confirm dilation and as a means of following the progress of LV dilation over time. The 2015 American Society of Echocardiography/European Association of Cardiovascular Imaging chamber quantification guidelines define LV dilation as:

- 2D linear dimensions: LVEDD ≥59 mm or LVESD ≥40 mm (male), and LVEDD ≥53 mm or LVESD ≥35 mm (female).
- 2D volumes: LVEDV ≥75 mL/m^2 (male), and ≥62 mL/m^2 (female). Generally, measurement of LV volumes by the biplane method of disks is the recommended technique to assess LV size rather than relying on linear dimensions (which are representative of size *only* in normally shaped ventricles).
- 3D volumes: LVEDV ≥80 mL/m^2 (male), and ≥72 mL/m^2 (female).

7. Left atrial size

a. By 2D echocardiography, the LA is dilated if LA end-systolic volume index is >34 mL/m^2 for both genders by 2D biplane disk summation.

B. Semiquantitative assessment of AR severity

1. Vena contracta width (VCW): Defined as the narrowest regurgitant jet width *(parasternal long-axis view or TEE [transesophageal echocardiography] 135 degrees three-chamber view only)*; >0.6 cm suggests severe AR (Fig. 2.2).

2. Pressure half time

a. PHT is measured from the CW Doppler signal of the regurgitant jet, usually obtained from the apical five-chamber or apical three-chamber views. This is a measure of how quickly the pressure gradient across the AV in diastole is reduced by half. Rapid reduction in the pressure gradient (PHT <200 ms) indicates rapid equilibration of LVEDP and the aortic diastolic pressure and suggests severe AR. Slow reduction in the pressure gradient (PHT >500 ms) suggests mild AR. Unfortunately, PHT is dependent on multiple changeable variables (systemic vascular resistance, aortic compliance, LV compliance, systolic blood pressure, chronicity of regurgitation), which limits this measurement's utility. For example, AR PHT is shortened with (1) increasingly severe LV diastolic dysfunction, (2) vasodilator therapy, and (3) dilated compliant aorta.

C. Quantitative assessment of AR by 2D echocardiography

Several important *quantitative* measurements are used to grade AR severity. These include the regurgitant volume, the regurgitant fraction, and the effective regurgitant orifice area (EROA). There are multiple methods of calculating these. We will briefly discuss two main methods used by echocardiography: the continuity method and the PISA method (Fig. 2.3). EROA ≥0.3 cm^2, regurgitant volume ≥60 mL/beat, and regurgitant fraction ≥50% all suggest severe AR.

D. Continuity method

The continuity method is based on the principle of conservation of mass: total flow across the regurgitant valve is equal to the sum of the forward flow and the regurgitant flow. Calculation of the regurgitant volume is based on the calculation of the SV through the AV and the SV throughout a second and competent valve, usually the mitral valve, assuming there is *no or minimal* MR. The volume of AR can then be calculated by subtracting the flow through the mitral valve from the total flow through the AV. A small error in measurement can strongly affect the calculations, and so this method is rarely used clinically.

1. Hydraulic orifice formula

- Flow *rate* = Cross-sectional area (CSA) × Velocity
- Flow *volume* = CSA × VTI

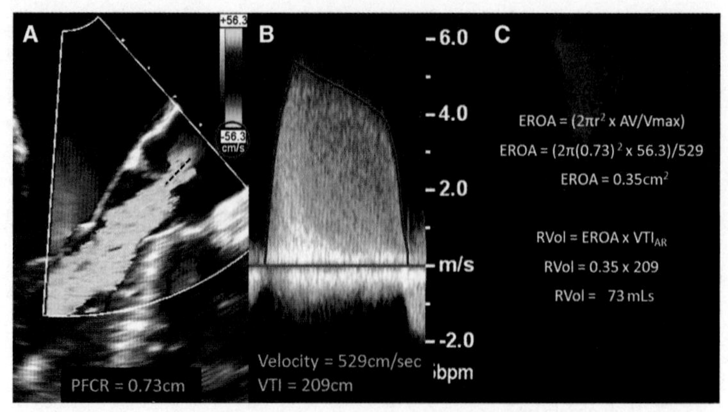

FIGURE 2.3 Quantitative assessment of aortic regurgitation. **A:** The proximal isovelocity surface area radius or proximal flow convergence region is measured from the first aliasing velocity to the leaflet. **B:** Continuous wave Doppler is used to calculate the VTI. **C:** Calculation of effective regurgitant orifice area (EROA) and regurgitant volume (Rvol). AV, aliasing velocity; PFCR, proximal flow convergence region; VTI, velocity time integral.

$$\text{Regurgitant volume (mL/beat)} = \text{Q total (total SV)} - \text{Q systemic (forward SV)}$$

$$= \text{Total } \textit{incompetent} \text{ valve flow} - \text{Total } \textit{competent} \text{ valve flow}$$

$$\text{Therefore,} = \text{LVOT flow} - \text{Mitral inflow}$$

$$= (\text{LVOT CSA} \times \text{VTI}) - (\text{MV CSA} \times \text{VTI})^*$$

$$\text{Regurgitant fraction (\%)} = (\text{Regurgitant aortic volume/Total aortic flow}) \times 100\%$$

$$\text{RF} = (\text{Regurgitant volume/LVOT SV}) \times 100\%$$

E. Proximal isovelocity surface area method

The PISA method of quantifying AR is another application of the principle of the conservation of mass based on the fact that flow acceleration proximal to a narrowed orifice occurs in isovelocity shells (Fig. 2.3). If the AR is sufficiently severe, color Doppler will reveal an area of proximal flow convergence (PFC). The aliasing velocity defines the velocity of the hemisphere where there is a color change from red to blue. Unlike the continuity method, the *presence of* MR *will not affect* the quantitation of AR. In patients with a dilated ascending aorta, the flow convergence zone may occupy >220 degrees around the AV leaflets, leading to *underestimation* of EROA and regurgitant volume by this method.

1. By the **conservation of mass principle**:
   - Flow at hemisphere surface = $2\pi \times r^2 \times V_r$, where r = PISA radius, and V_r = aliasing velocity

---

*Note: Because the MV annulus is saddle shaped, a more accurate mitral annular cross-sectional area can be measured using its minor axis radius (long-axis "three-chamber" MV radius) and the major axis radius ("bicommissural" two-chamber MV radius) using the area of an ellipse formula: MV CSA = 3.14 × (minor radius) × (major radius). The pulmonic valve SV (RVOT CSA × VTI) may also be used as the competent valve in this calculation, *assuming no or minimal pulmonary regurgitation*. Its usefulness is limited by the difficulty in accurate right ventricular outflow tract CSA calculation.

2. By the **hydraulic orifice formula**, as in 1:

Flow through regurgitant orifice = ERO × Peak regurgitant velocity

Therefore, ERO = Flow rate/Peak AR velocity

3. Combining both formulas:

$$\text{Regurgitant orifice area (cm}^2\text{) or ERO} = \frac{2\pi \times (r\ (\text{cm}))^2 \times (\text{Aliasing velocity [cm/s]})}{(\text{Peak AR}_{CW}\ \text{velocity [cm/s]})}$$

$$\text{ERO} = \text{Regurgitant volume (mL/beat)/AR}_{CW}\text{VTI (cm), as above}$$

Therefore,

$$\text{Regurgitant volume (mL/beat)} = \text{ERO} \times \text{AR}_{CW}\text{VTI}$$

And again,

$$\text{Regurgitant fraction (\%)} = (\text{Regurgitant volume/LVOT SV}) \times 100\%$$

F. **Advanced cardiac mechanics**

Advanced imaging methods to assess regional and global systolic function, such as global peak longitudinal strain, may prove to be more sensitive than LVEF in identifying patients who are at higher risk for developing subsequent symptoms and/or LV dysfunction. In one study by Olsen et al. of 64 patients with chronic severe AR, reduced myocardial systolic strain, systolic strain rate, and early diastolic strain rate by speckle-tracking echocardiography predicted persistent symptoms or LV dysfunction after surgery, and also predicted the development of symptoms or worsening LV function during conservative management. Clinical utility may be limited by the finding that with increasing LV size (LVEDVI >97 mL/m^2), the LVEF and all deformation parameters were found to decrease.

G. **3D Echocardiography**

3D echocardiography represents a major innovation in cardiovascular ultrasound, and should be used as standard in all examinations. 3D echocardiography has superior and more reproducible quantification of LV size, mass, and systolic function than standard 2D echocardiography. Direct measurement of the anatomic regurgitant orifice area (AROA) and of the vena contracta area may be performed for AR quantification. 3D is superior to 2D for planimetry of the AV area and the elliptical LVOT. 3D should also be used for aortic root measurements in cases of secondary AR, or mixed AV disease. By current convention, the AV volume 3D image should be displayed with the right coronary cusp located inferiorly at the 6 o'clock position.

1. **Quantitative assessment of AR by 3D echocardiography**

   a. Anatomic regurgitant orifice area

   This is a direct quantification of the size of the anatomic regurgitant orifice, without the use of color Doppler. It is measured by multiplanar reformatting of an acquired 3D volume to obtain an *en face* view of the AROA, and then measuring the area by direct planimetry (Fig. 2.4). This technique is limited because measurements can be affected by gain settings. Note: the AROA is theoretically larger than the EROA.

   b. Vena contracta area (VCA)

   3D echocardiography (TTE and TEE) enables direct measurement of the VCA using a 3D color full-volume acquisition of the AR jet, with offline multiplanar reformatting to obtain an *en face* view of the vena contracta. The VCA may then be measured by planimetry. Because the VCA is measured without any flow or geometric assumptions, it is especially useful for eccentric jets or noncircular regurgitant orifices. The use of multibeat

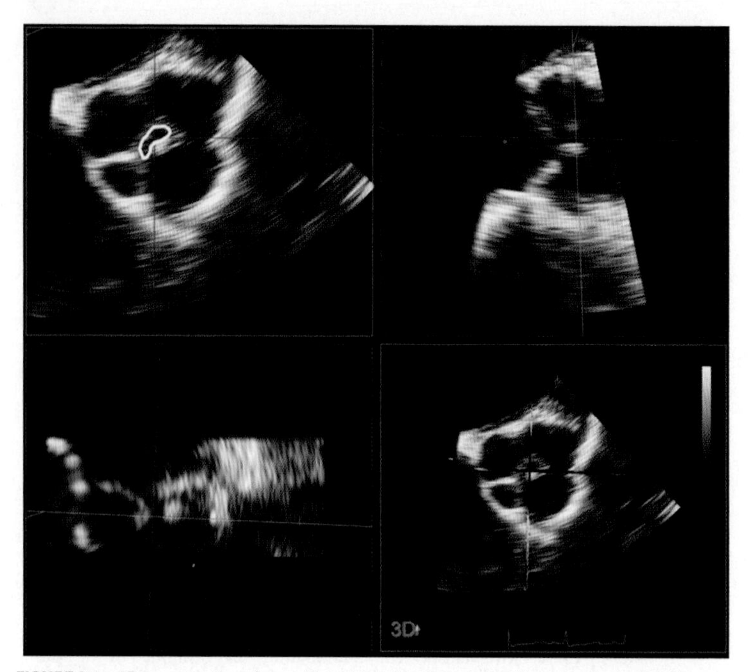

FIGURE 2.4 3D reconstruction of a quadricuspid aortic valve using multiplanar reformatting. The anatomic orifice area is identified at the leaflets tips and indicates severe aortic regurgitation.

3D volumes to improve spatial resolution predisposes to stitching artifact. Non-multibeat 3D acquisitions may partially overcome this at the cost of worsening an already relatively low spatial and temporal resolution compared to a 2D acquisition.

c. Proximal isovelocity surface area

3D PISA-based EROA provides the ability to measure the 3D surface area of the PFC without geometric shape assumptions; this is especially important for nonhemispherical PISA. Indeed, recent technological advancements permit calculation of the PISA at every single diastolic frame, which are then summed and divided by the number of diastolic frames to provide a more accurate assessment of AR, particularly in nonholodiastolic jets.

d. Regurgitant volume and regurgitant fraction

The measured 3D AROA or 3D VCA or 3D PISA-based EROA *all* can be used with the AR VTI (obtained from 2D CW Doppler) to calculate regurgitant volume, exactly as in the 2D techniques described earlier.

$$\text{Regurgitant volume (mL/beat)} = \text{ROA} \times \text{AR}_{\text{CW}}\text{VTI}$$

The use of 3D measurements may increase the accuracy of the PISA EROA calculation compared to the standard 2D technique. 3D echocardiography also has provided a better appreciation of the variability in the shape of the PFC.

Additionally, a 3D full-volume acquisition can be used to measure the 3D LV SV (and LVEF) and thus to calculate the RF:

Regurgitant fraction (%) = (Regurgitant volume/LV SV) × 100%

e. Direct measurement
Finally, a novel method is to use 3D color Doppler to measure mitral inflow and LV outflow SV and to use the difference to obtain the regurgitant volume. This method integrates flow velocities across the entire aortic and mitral orifice to calculate SV without LVOT or mitral annular geometry assumptions. A significant time commitment is required to quantify SV across each valve. Further studies are needed before this technique can be used clinically for AR or MR quantification.

H. Focused transthoracic echocardiographic analysis of chronic AR
The parasternal long-axis, apical five-chamber, and apical three-chamber images are first viewed, with and without color Doppler, to identify the presence of AR and its mechanism. Next, any *specific signs* of severe AR should be noted. If no *specific signs* are noted, the study is reviewed systematically to decide on overall severity using multiple parameters (including M-mode and 3D), and relying on quantitative measurements where possible. Note that by definition the absence of *specific signs* does not imply that the AR is not severe. Finally, the study is directly compared with the immediate prior study, and also the most remote study available. If image quality is suboptimal, then consider TEE.

1. Specific signs of severity in chronic AR

a. Fluttering of the anterior mitral valve leaflet (M-mode or 2D) can be seen with both acute and chronic moderate-to-severe AR. In severe AR, premature closure of the mitral valve may also be seen. Later, diastolic MR (attributable to significantly elevated LVEDP) may be seen on color M-mode or 2D color Doppler.

b. Effective regurgitant orifice area ≥0.3 cm^2, regurgitant volume ≥60 mL/beat, and regurgitant fraction ≥50% (usually PISA method) are indicative of severe AR.

c. Holodiastolic flow reversal in the descending thoracic aorta or proximal abdominal aorta and an end-diastolic velocity of >20 cm/s suggest severe AR.

d. LVOT jet width of ≥65% of the LVOT width suggests severe AR.

e. VCW >0.6 cm suggests severe AR.

I. Focused transthoracic echocardiographic analysis of acute AR
In acute AR, the LVEDP and the aortic diastolic pressure equilibrate rapidly in diastole. Acute AR may therefore be difficult to appreciate by color and spectral Doppler echocardiography. A high suspicion of acute AR in cardiogenic shock with normal LV size and systolic function should prompt a search for specific echocardiographic signs of acute AR.

1. Specific signs of severity in acute AR

a. Fluttering of the anterior mitral valve leaflet (M-mode or 2D) with both acute and chronic moderate-to-severe AR.

b. Premature closure of the mitral valve and, later, diastolic MR (when seen with AR) caused by significantly elevated LVEDP.

c. Diastolic flow reversal in the descending thoracic aorta or proximal abdominal aorta.

J. Indication for echocardiography in the assessment of AR
Echocardiography is indicated for the initial diagnosis of AR to quantify AR severity and LV systolic function at baseline, for changing signs and symptoms, and in routine follow-up both pre- and post-AV surgery (Table 2.5). The prognosis of chronic AR is closely associated with the degree and pace of LV remodeling, even in the absence of symptoms. Independent predictors of death or development of symptos

TABLE 2.5 Indication for Echocardiography in the Assessment of Aortic Regurgitation (AR)

Clinical Status	Indication
	Initial Diagnosis
Signs or symptoms of aortic regurgitation	Transthoracic echocardiography (TTE) is indicated in patients with signs or symptoms of AR (stages A to D) for accurate diagnosis of the cause of regurgitation, regurgitant severity, and left ventricular size and systolic function, and for determining clinical outcome and timing of valve intervention
Dilated aortic sinuses or ascending aorta or with a bicuspid aortic valve	TTE is indicated in patients with dilated aortic sinuses or ascending aorta or with a bicuspid aortic valve (stages A and B) to evaluate the presence and severity of AR
	Changing Signs or Symptoms
Previously documented mild or moderate AR	New-onset dyspnea or angina may indicate that AR has progressed in severity and repeat TTE is indicated If AR remains mild (*symptom–severity discordance*), further investigation for other etiologies is indicated.
Previously documented severe AR	Onset of symptoms is an indication for surgery (class I). Repeat TTE is indicated to determine the status of the aortic valve, aorta, and left ventricle preoperatively.
	Routine Follow-up
Mild-to-moderate AR	Yearly clinical assessment 2-y echocardiogram
Severe AR	6-mo clinical and echocardiogram assessment
Post–bioprosthetic AVR	Baseline post-op TTE Yearly clinical assessment Yearly TTE after 10 y
Post–mechanical AVR	Baseline post-op TTE Yearly clinical assessment Repeat TTE if change in clinical status

in a multivariate analysis of asymptomatic patients with AR and normal LV systolic function on serial echocardiography were (1) age, (2) initial end-systolic dimension (LVESD) and rate of change in ESD, and (3) rest LVEF and rate of decrease of LVEF. Because asymptomatic patients with significant chronic AR can experience poor outcomes, including sudden death, serial echocardiography is indicated to assess for LV dilation and dysfunction so as to identify patients progressing toward the threshold for surgery.

X. STRESS ECHOCARDIOGRAPHY

The role of stress (exercise) echocardiography is less well established in patients with chronic severe AR than in those with MR. It is most frequently employed in patients with equivocal symptoms or discrepancies between the severity of symptoms described and the severity of AR noted on resting echocardiography (*symptom–severity discordance*).

A. Reasonable indications for stress echocardiography in assessment of AR

1. Asymptomatic severe AR to assess objective functional capacity.
2. Asymptomatic severe AR in which LV size and function do not meet surgical criteria to unmask poor prognostic signs.
   a. Lack of contractile reserve as defined by a failure to increase LVEF during exercise or a fall in LVEF on exercise is less predictive of occult contractile dysfunction in severe AR than in MR. In AR, afterload often increases significantly with exercise, resulting in a fall in EF. An increase in LVEF in patients with LV dysfunction suggests a better likelihood of improvement in LV function postsurgery.
   b. Inducible LV dilation.
   c. Increase in AR.
   d. Increase in estimated RVSP to >60 mm Hg.

B. Inappropriate indications for stress echocardiography in assessment of AR

These patients should be referred for surgery without stress testing:

1. Symptomatic patients with severe AR.
2. Patients with depressed LVEF.
3. Patients with severe LV dilation.

XI. TRANSESOPHAGEAL ECHOCARDIOGRAPHY

There are few data on the comparative value of TEE and TTE in measuring the severity of AR. A combination of transthoracic and transesophageal imaging is often warranted for accurate assessment of LV size and systolic function and optimal visualization of the AV, especially in cases where transthoracic image quality is suboptimal or for complex pathology such as endocarditis, aortic dissection, or prosthetic valve dysfunction.

TEE is highly sensitive to even trivial degrees of AR, and the vena contracta can be easily measured. TTE is generally superior to TEE for measuring the AR jet VTI by CW Doppler owing to the technical difficulties in accurately aligning the ultrasound beam with the jet direction in TEE. Descending aortic flow reversal by PW Doppler can be identified by both TTE and TEE.

Evaluation of AR in patients with an AVR is particularly challenging. In general, if less than 10% of the sewing ring is noted to be involved in the short-axis view, this suggests mild regurgitation, whereas 10% to 20% suggests moderate regurgitation, and greater than 20% involvement suggests severe regurgitation, especially when the regurgitation is associated with rocking of the prosthesis. This is obviously a crude assessment because a wide orifice that involves 10% of the sewing ring may result in far more AR than a thin linear orifice that involves >20% of the ring.

3D TEE with and without color Doppler provides incremental data. *En face* imaging of the AV with live or with offline manipulation allows improved anatomic localization of pathologies such as perforations, and paravalvular regurgitation. VCA by planimetry may improve quantitation of AR compared to 2D VC or conventional Doppler methods. Real-time 3D peak and integrated PISA measurements may also improve quantitation. 3D enables direct measurement of the LVOT and aortic annulus areas, by planimetry, required for transcatheter aortic valve replacement (TAVR) planning. 3D TEE planimetered method underestimates these cross-sectional areas by 10% compared to cardiac CT, while a 2D TEE calculated circular method underestimates areas by 13% to 26%.

The reported sensitivity and specificity of TTE for diagnosis of aortic dissection are only 60% to 80% and 60% to 90%, respectively, whereas TEE has a sensitivity of 95% to 99% and a specificity of 92% to 97%, respectively.

XII. CARDIAC MAGNETIC RESONANCE IMAGING

CMR has a class 1 indication in patients with moderate or severe AR (stages B, C, and D) for the assessment of systolic and diastolic LV volumes, and measurement of AR severity in patients with suboptimal echocardiographic images. In addition to its value in patients with suboptimal echocardiographic images, CMR is useful for evaluating patients in whom there is discordance between clinical assessment and severity of AR by echocardiography. Phase contrast imaging measures both forward systolic flow and backward diastolic flow. The regurgitant fraction is the ratio of backward to forward flow (Fig. 2.5). The presence of diastolic flow reversal in the proximal descending aorta can also be assessed. CMR measurement of regurgitant severity is less variable and more precise than echocardiographic measurement, although not necessarily more accurate. In addition, CMR is the gold standard for assessment of LV volumes (and dimensions) and LVEF. Because of its superior signal-to-noise and contrast-to-noise ratio, CMR also allows for accurate assessment of AV morphology, and accurate serial quantification of aortic root and ascending aortic dimensions without the use of ionizing radiation. Despite published superior inter- and intraobserver variability in the assessment of LV size and function compared to echocardiography, the benefit of following patients with

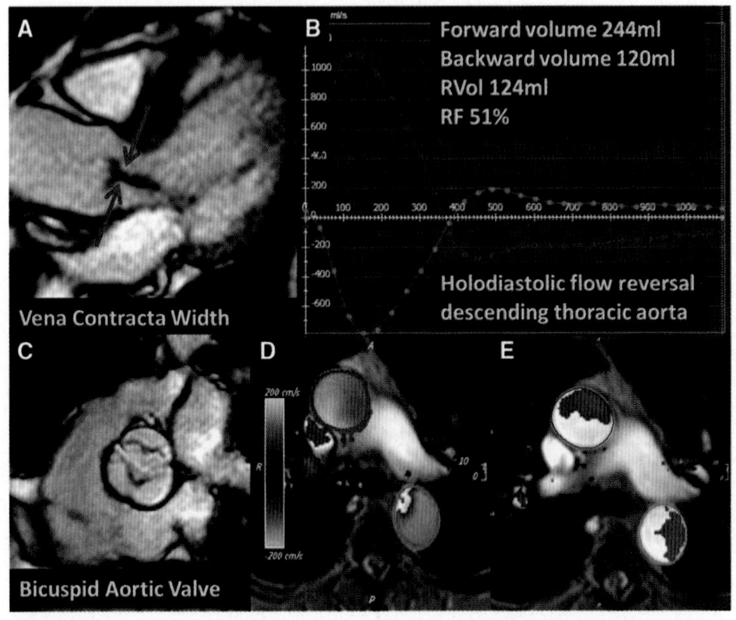

FIGURE 2.5 Assessment of aortic regurgitation using cardiac magnetic resonance imaging. **A:** Flow void caused by dephasing protons creates a vena contracta seen on this left ventricular outflow tract view using steady-state free precession (SSFP) cine imaging during a diastolic phase. **B:** Flow quantification at the midascending *(red)* and descending thoracic aorta *(green)* with holodiastolic flow reversal in both consistent with severe AR. **C:** SSFP image at the level of the aortic valve demonstrating clear anatomic definition of a bicuspid aortic valve in systole. **D:** Systolic phase with forward flow in the ascending aorta *(red)* and descending aorta *(blue)* at the level of the pulmonary bifurcation. **E:** Diastolic phase with flow reversal seen in both the ascending *(blue)* and descending *(red)* segments.

severe AR with serial CMRs to assess for increasing regurgitant fraction, progressive LV dilation, or deteriorating EF has not been fully assessed.

A. Quantitative assessment of AR by CMR

1. Anatomic regurgitant orifice area

The AROA may be planimetered directly using short-axis steady-state free precession (SSFP) or fast gradient-recalled echo (GRE) cine imaging. This technique is limited by issues with spatial resolution, partial volume effects, and/or calcium artifact unless the orifice is very large.

2. Vena contracta width and area

The dephasing of protons as they pass through the regurgitant orifice into the LV produces a flow void visible as a diastolic jet of regurgitation, best seen on MRI cine imaging. This flow void is better visualized using fast GRE cine imaging than the now more commonly used SSFP cine imaging (lower sensitivity to flow caused by short repetition and echo times). This allows a qualitative assessment of jet origin, direction, and jet severity. The flow void width can be measured, similar to a vena contracta width, with long-axis GRE cines. The flow void area can also be measured, similar to a vena contract area, using short-axis GRE cines just below the AV or with through-plane phase contrast imaging.

3. Regurgitant volume and regurgitant fraction

These may be obtained using direct and indirect methods. A significant clinical limitation of quantifying AR using CMR is that it remains unclear whether the regurgitant volume and regurgitant fraction cutoffs to classify AR severity using the standard echocardiographic guidelines can be applied to CMR measurements.

4. Direct method

a. Phase contrast imaging: through-plane phase-encoding velocity (and flow) imaging with the imaging slice placed just above the AV can directly measure (1) forward volume, (2) regurgitant volume, (3) SV, and (4) the regurgitant fraction. The phase sequence most commonly used is a one-dimension, one-directional technique, which has good reproducibility.

b. Significant underestimation of the stroke and regurgitation volumes may occur (1) if the flow is not orthogonal to the slice position and (2) if movement of the valve toward the LV apex during systole allows blood to flow into the gap between the imaging plane and the valve. This blood may return to the ventricle during diastole and not flow through the imaging plane, thus being lost to measurement. This tendency is exacerbated by several factors: aortic distention during systole, a dilated aortic root (resulting in greater volume between the imaging plane and the valve), and vigorous longitudinal contraction of the LV (common in significant AR). Future CMR abilities may include valve tracking to move the imaging plane accordingly.

5. Indirect methods

The regurgitant volume is calculated on the basis of the difference between:

a. The LV SV and right ventricular SV, obtained by planimetry of a stack of breath-held short- or long-axis cine images through the RV and LV.

b. Aortic outflow volume and mitral inflow volume using phase contrast imaging.

The indirect methods are not accurate if other coexisting valvular lesions or intracardiac shunting is present. The RF can be calculated as:

$$\text{Regurgitant fraction (\%)} = (\text{Regurgitant volume/ LV SV}) \times 100\%$$

XIII. CARDIAC COMPUTED TOMOGRAPHY

Using ECG prospectively triggered or retrospectively gated protocols at about 75% of the RR interval (diastole) allows for offline 3D reconstruction of the AV. The valve morphology and the ascending aorta are easily assessed, because of the excellent spatial resolution of CT. If there is significant central coaptation failure, the AROA can be directly measured by planimetry. In addition, CT provides the most rapid and accurate approach to diagnose aortic dissection. Dynamic imaging of the moving valve leaflets is feasible with the current newer generation of scanners because of their improved temporal resolution. A retrospective, ECG-gated, 4D acquisition of the AV is performed, at the cost of increased radiation. Valvular motion and morphology can be assessed. The AV and LVOT areas can be measured in associated aortic stenosis (useful in TAVR planning). 4D dynamic CT can be used to assess mechanical valve leaflet motion in suspected leaflet dysfunction.

Theoretically, regurgitant volume and regurgitant fraction can be measured by indirect methods, similar to CMR, by calculating the difference between left and right ventricular SVs. In practice, this requires modification of the intravenous contrast administration to ensure simultaneous opacification of both ventricles and results in higher radiation exposure, because this must be a retrospective gated acquisition. In view of the technical difficulties, limitations in temporal resolution, and use of ionizing radiation, this is rarely used clinically in a patient who has no contraindications to a CMR examination. Valvular flow assessment is not possible with current CT technology.

XIV. CARDIAC CATHETERIZATION

Generally, coronary catheterization is indicated to assess coronary anatomy pre-AVR in all patients >50 years of age. Emergency valve surgery *should not* be delayed for coronary angiography for acute severe AR with hemodynamic instability. Invasive aortography may be useful to assess the degree of AR when echocardiography and clinical findings are discordant and alternative noninvasive imaging, such as CMR, is contraindicated. Aortography is performed in the LAO position with the pigtail catheter approximately 2 cm above the aortic leaflets. The flow injector settings are usually set with about 60 mL of contrast at 20 to 25 mL/s. Aortography enables assessment of AV movement and the number of leaflets, coexisting aortic pathology (aneurysm or dissection), and regurgitation severity. Assessment of AR severity is based on the amount of opacification of the ventricle compared to that of the aortic root two complete cardiac cycles after injection. The semiquantitative angiographic AR grading system is similar to that of MR. Aortography may underestimate the severity of AR in the setting of acute severe AR owing to rapid equalization of diastolic aortic and LV pressure. Intracardiac pressure measurements may also be useful. Selected hemodynamic findings in chronic and acute AR are listed (Table 2.3).

A. Semiquantitative assessment

1+ (mild)—Minimal LV opacification, clears with each beat
2+ (moderate)—Mild chamber opacification < aortic root, >1 beat to clear
3+ (mod–severe)—LV contrast density equal to aortic root, intermediate clearing
4+ (severe)—Dense LV opacification on first beat, density > aortic root density, slow clearing

B. Quantitative assessment of AR severity by angiography and right heart study

Requires estimating (1) an angiographic LV SV and (2) a forward SV.

1. Angiographic LV SV can be estimated by performing left ventriculography using a single plane (30 degrees RAO usually) or a biplane (30 degrees RAO and 60 degrees LAO). End-diastolic and end-systolic volumes can be then calculated. Angiographic SV = EDV − ESV.
2. The CO is measured invasively by the Fick technique (gold standard) or the thermodilution technique (if no tricuspid regurgitation present). Forward SV is CO divided by the heart rate.

Regurgitant volume (mL/beat) = SV angiographic minus SV forward (assuming no MR, other coexisting regurgitant valvular lesions, or intracardiac shunt).

Regurgitant fraction (%) = (SV angiographic minus SV forward)/SV angiographic.

1+ (mild)	<20%
2+ (moderate)	20%–40%
3+ (moderate–severe)	40%–60%
4+ (severe)	>60%

XV. TREATMENT

A. Acute aortic regurgitation

In acute severe AR, surgery should not be delayed, especially if there is evidence of cardiogenic shock or pulmonary edema. Numerous studies have demonstrated improved in-hospital and long-term survival in such patients if they are treated with prompt AVR. The goal of medical therapy is hemodynamic stabilization; to maximize forward CO and minimize any aortic dissection progression before proceeding with urgent surgical correction. Leading causes of severe acute native valve AR include type A aortic dissection, infective endocarditis, blunt chest trauma, and iatrogenic complications of cardiac catheterization/balloon valvotomy. Causes of acute prosthetic AR include valve thrombosis or endocarditis.

1. **Surgical management**

   Immediate surgical evaluation should be performed for acute AR resulting from aortic dissection or chest trauma. The surgical approach depends on the cause of AR. For example, in type A aortic dissection, preservation of the native AV may be attempted with valve resuspension (+/− valve repair) together with ascending aorta graft replacement.

2. **Medical management**

   a. Vasodilators, such as IV nitroprusside, are the mainstay of medical therapy to reduce LV afterload via reduction in systemic vascular resistance. This will decrease the volume of regurgitation.

   b. **β-blockers** may be cautiously used in treating AR resulting from type A aortic dissection. They reduce arterial d*P*/d*t*. It is important to note that *β-blockers should not be used in treating other, nondissection causes of acute AR* because preventing the compensatory tachycardia may lead to a marked decrease in CO. In addition, increasing diastolic time will exacerbate acute AR. Administration of cardiac glycosides (e.g., digoxin) for rate control may in rare cases be necessary.

   c. Inotropic support (+/− chronotropic support) may be temporarily necessary for hemodynamic support of the failing heart.

   d. If acute AR is associated with endocarditis, antibiotic therapy should be started as soon as all culture specimens are obtained.

3. **Percutaneous therapy**

   a. Intra-aortic balloon pump counterpulsation is *absolutely contraindicated* with acute severe AR. Augmentation of the aortic diastolic pressure will increase the aortic regurgitant volume, thereby elevating the LV filling pressures and decreasing forward output.

   b. Unlike in severe aortic stenosis, transcatheter AV implantation is not approved for the treatment of severe AR.

B. Chronic aortic regurgitation

Chronic AR may be classified into four stages based on clinical and echocardiographic findings (Table 2.6).

1. **Medical management**

   The primary goal is to alleviate symptoms and to treat associated conditions such as systemic hypertension and heart failure.

   a. Vasodilators (dihydropyridine calcium channel blockers, angiotensin-converting enzyme (inhibitors/angiotensin receptor blockers, or hydralazine) are used

TABLE 2.6 2014 AHA/ACC Guideline for the Management of Patients with Valvular Heart Disease

Stage	Definition	Valve Anatomy	Valve Hemodynamics	Hemodynamic Consequences	Symptoms
A	At risk of AR	Bicuspid aortic valve (or other congenital valve anomaly) Aortic valve sclerosis History of rheumatic fever or known rheumatic heart disease IE	AR severity: none or trace	None	None
B	Progressive AR	Mild-to-moderate calcification of a trileaflet valve, bicuspid valve (or other congenital anomaly) Dilated aortic sinuses Rheumatic valve changes Previous IE	**Mild AR:** Jet width <25% of LVOT Vena contracta <0.3 cm RVol <30 mL/beat RF <30% ERO <0.10 cm^2 Angiography grade 1+ **Moderate AR:** Jet width 25%–64% of LVOT Vena contracta 0.3–0.6 cm RVol 30–59 mL RF 30–49% ERO 0.10–0.29 cm^2 Angiography grade 2+	Normal LV systolic function Normal LV volume or mild LV dilation	None
C	Asymptomatic severe AR		**Severe AR:** Jet width ≥65% of LVOT Vena contracta >0.6 cm	C1: Normal LVEF (≥50%) and mild-to-moderate LV dilation (LVESD ≤ 50 mm)	None; exercise testing is reasonable to confirm symptom status

			Holodiastolic flow reversal in the proximal abdominal aorta RVol ≥60 mL/beat RF ≥50% ERO ≥0.3 cm^2 Angiography grade 3+ to 4+ In addition, diagnosis of chronic severe AR requires evidence of LV dilation	C2: Abnormal LV systolic function with depressed LVEF (<50%) or severe LV dilation (LVESD >50 mm or indexed LVESD >25 mm/m^2)	
D	Symptomatic severe AR	Calcific valve disease Bicuspid valve (or other congenital abnormality) Dilated aortic sinuses or ascending aorta Rheumatic valve changes Previous IE with abnormal leaflet closure or perforation	**Severe AR:** Jet width ≥65% of LVOT Vena contracta >0.6 cm Holodiastolic flow reversal in the proximal abdominal aorta RVol ≥60 mL/beat RF ≥50% ERO ≥0.3 cm^2 Angiography grade 3+ to 4+ In addition, diagnosis of chronic severe AR requires evidence of LV dilation	Symptomatic severe AR may occur with normal systolic (LVEF >50%), mild-to-moderate LV dysfunction (LVEF 40–50%), or severe LV dysfunction (LV <40%) Moderate-to-severe LV dilation is present	Exertional dyspnea or angina or more severe HF symptoms

AR, aortic regurgitation; IE, infective endocarditis; LVOT, left ventricular outflow tract; RVol, regurgitant volume; RF, regurgitant fraction; ERO, effective regurgitant orifice; LV, left ventricular; LVEF, left ventricular ejection fraction; LVESD, left ventricular end systolic dimension; HF, heart failure.

Adapted from Nishimura RA, Otto CM, Bonow RO, et al. 2014 AHA/ACC Guideline for the Management of Patients With Valvular Heart Disease: Executive Summary. A Report of the American College of Cardiology/American Heart Association Task Force on Practice Guidelines. *J Am Coll Cardiol.* 2014;63(22):2438–2488, with permission from Elsevier.

for LV afterload reduction. They are indicated in severe chronic AR with (1) symptoms, (2) LV dysfunction, or (3) hypertension. They are generally used if the patient is not an operative candidate or while the patient is waiting for surgical AVR.

b. In mild-to-moderate secondary AR attributable to aortic root dilation (>4.5 cm), β-blockers may be used carefully to decrease wall stress; however, a relative bradycardia may worsen the AR. In low LVEF, β-blockers may be considered.

c. If chronic AR is associated with endocarditis, antibiotic therapy should be started as soon as all culture specimens are obtained.

2. Percutaneous therapy

a. Intra-aortic balloon pump counterpulsation is *absolutely contraindicated* as per management of acute AR.

b. Unlike in severe aortic stenosis, transcatheter AV implantation is not approved for the treatment of severe AR.

3. Surgical therapy

In appropriate patients, AV surgery remains the only definite treatment for AR. Despite advances in primary AV repair, especially in young patients with BAV, the experience at a few specialized centers has not yet been replicated at the general community level; therefore, performance of AV repair should be concentrated in those centers with proven expertise. In these specialized centers, freedom from reoperation for AV surgery is 78% at 10 years post–AV repair. Valve-sparing replacement of the aortic sinuses and ascending aorta (modified David procedure) is a possible strategy in patients with AR caused by aortic root dilation in which a trileaflet or bicuspid valve is not severely thickened, deformed, or calcified. The vast majority of patients who require surgery for chronic severe AR will require AVR. In broad terms, there are two categories of valves that include mechanical and bioprosthetic valves; the choice of which valve to use should be individualized (Table 2.7).

TABLE 2.7 2014 American College of Cardiology (ACC)/American Heart Association (AHA) Summary of Recommendations for Aortic Valve Replacement and Prosthetic Valve Choice in Severe Aortic Regurgitation (AR)

Recommendations	Class of Recommendation	Level of Evidence
AVR is indicated for symptomatic patients with severe AR regardless of LV systolic function (stage D)	I	B
AVR is indicated for asymptomatic patients with chronic severe AR and LV systolic dysfunction (LVEF <50%) (stage C2)	I	B
AVR is indicated for patients with severe AR (stage C or D) while undergoing cardiac surgery for other indications	I	C
AVR is reasonable for asymptomatic patients with severe AR with normal LV systolic function (LVEF ≥50%) but with severe LV dilation (LVESD >50 mm) (stage C2)	IIa	B

TABLE 2.7 2014 American College of Cardiology (ACC)/American Heart Association (AHA) Summary of Recommendations for Aortic Valve Replacement and Prosthetic Valve Choice in Severe Aortic Regurgitation *(continued)*

Recommendations	Class of Recommendation	Level of Evidence
AVR is reasonable in patients with moderate AR (stage B) who are undergoing other cardiac surgery	IIa	C
AVR may be considered for asymptomatic patients with severe AR and normal LV systolic function (LVEF ≥50%, stage C1) but with progressive severe LV dilation (LVEDD >65 mm) if surgical risk is low	IIb	C
Choice of valve intervention and prosthetic valve type should be a shared decision process	I	C
A bioprosthesis is recommended in patients of any age for whom anticoagulant therapy is contraindicated, cannot be managed appropriately, or is not desired	I	C
A mechanical prosthesis is reasonable for AVR or MVR in patients <60 y of age who do not have a contraindication to anticoagulation	IIa	B
A bioprosthesis is reasonable in patients >70 y of age	IIa	B
Either a bioprosthetic or mechanical valve is reasonable in patients between 60 y and 70 y of age	IIa	B
Replacement of the aortic valve by a pulmonary autograft (the Ross procedure), when performed by an experienced surgeon, may be considered in young patients when VKA anticoagulation is contraindicated or undesirable	IIb	C

NOTE: In patients with aortic root dilation with significant AR, progression of the aortic diameter to ≥50 mm is generally accepted as an indication for aortic root and aortic valve surgery (lower threshold ≥45 mm should be considered for patients with Marfan disease or bicuspid aortic valve, especially if the rate of dilation is accelerated).

AVR, aortic valve regurgitation; LV, left ventricle; LVEF, left ventricular ejection fraction; LVEDD, left ventricular end-diastolic diameter; MVR, mitral valve regurgitation; VKA, vitamin K antagonist.

Adapted from Nishimura RA, Otto CM, Bonow RO, et al. 2014 AHA/ACC Guideline for the Management of Patients With Valvular Heart Disease: Executive Summary: A Report of the American College of Cardiology/American Heart Association Task Force on Practice Guidelines. *J Am Coll Cardiol.* 2014;63(22):2438–2488, with permission from Elsevier.

AVR, aortic valve replacement; LV, left ventricle; LVEDD, left ventricular end-diastolic diameter; LVEF, left ventricular ejection fraction; LVESD, left ventricular end-systolic dimension; MVR, mitral valve replacement; VKA, vitamin K antagonist

C. Timing decisions for AR surgery depend on the following factors:

1. Severity of AR

a. Surgery performed for severe AR.

b. Moderate AR is surgically treated only when the patient is undergoing cardiac or aortic surgery for another primary indication.

2. **Symptoms**
   a. Symptomatic severe chronic AR is an indication for surgery irrespective of LV size or systolic function.
   b. Symptoms include angina, exertional dyspnea, and other presentations of heart failure.
3. **Left ventricular size and systolic function**
   a. Asymptomatic patients with severe chronic AR—indication for surgery if:
      i. LVEF <50%.
      ii. LVEF is normal (>50%) but there is LV dilation: LVESD >50 mm, or LVEDD >65 mm. Evidence for the ESD cutoff is stronger than the EDD value. Note that there are no suggested LV *volume* cutoffs for defining need for surgery in the 2014 ACC/AHA valvular guidelines.
4. **Need for other primary cardiac surgery**
   a. If patient is undergoing cardiac surgery for other indications, AV surgery should be considered in all patients with moderate or severe AR irrespective of symptoms, LV size, or systolic function.

D. Postoperative prognosis

The LV end-diastolic diameter and end-diastolic volume usually decrease in the immediate postoperative period. The EF tends to increase postoperatively in patients with preexisting LV systolic dysfunction. It may also decrease following surgery because of decreased preload. Patients with preoperative LV systolic dysfunction may have continued improvement in the EF in the months to years following AV surgery. The degree of increase in EF correlates with the decrease in end-diastolic diameter. Patients with severe preoperative symptoms or reduced exercise tolerance and those with severe or long-standing LV dysfunction tend to have higher operative mortality and worse recovery of LV systolic function.

KEY PEARLS

- Abnormalities of either the aortic valve leaflets (primary aortic regurgitation [AR]) or the surrounding aortic root (secondary AR) may cause leaflet malcoaptation leading to regurgitation.
- The etiology and clinical presentation of acute AR differ significantly from chronic AR. Acute AR may be very difficult to appreciate both by auscultation and by color and spectral Doppler echocardiography owing to rapid equilibration of the left ventricular end-diastolic pressure and the aortic diastolic pressures. A high degree of clinical suspicion is required.
- Chronic severe AR leads to both volume and pressure overload of the left ventricle, leading to compensatory ventricular dilation and eccentric hypertrophy before finally resulting in systolic dysfunction that may not be reversible.
- Chronic severe AR is usually well tolerated with a low mortality until the development of symptoms, when mortality significantly increases to >10% per year.
- Two-dimensional echocardiographic quantification of chronic AR is challenging. Assessment should be approached in a qualitative, semiquantitative, and quantitative manner. Chronic severe AR is almost invariably associated with left ventricular dilation.
- Three-dimensional echocardiography with and without color Doppler should be performed in all patients with AR (transthoracic echocardiography and transesophageal echocardiography) if possible.
- Specific echocardiographic signs of *acute* AR include fluttering of the anterior mitral valve leaflet, premature mitral valve closure and later diastolic mitral regurgitation (in the presence of AR), and diastolic flow reversal in the proximal abdominal aorta or the descending thoracic aorta.

- Multimodality imaging using mainly cardiac magnetic resonance and, more rarely, invasive angiography or cardiac CT is useful for further assessment of AR in patients with symptom–severity discordance by echocardiography or in cases of suboptimal echocardiographic acoustic windows. The lack of a gold standard for *quantifying* AR limits the absolute superiority of any one modality over the other.
- The decision regarding timing of aortic valve replacement is based on severity of AR, presence of symptoms, hemodynamic effect on the left ventricle, and whether the patient is undergoing other cardiac or aortic surgery.
- Histopathologic and genetic analysis of explanted aortic tissue from patients with secondary AR should be performed for diagnosis and future familial screening for genetic conditions such as Marfan and Loeys–Dietz syndromes.

SUGGESTED READINGS

Babu AN, Kymes SM, Carpenter Fryer SM. Eponyms and the diagnosis of aortic regurgitation: what says the evidence? *Ann Intern Med.* 2003;138(9):736–742.

Bergfeldt L. HLA-B27-associated cardiac disease. *Ann Intern Med.* 1997;127(8, part 1):621–629.

Bergfeldt L, Insulander P, Lindblom D, et al. HLA-B27: an important genetic risk factor for lone aortic regurgitation and severe conduction system abnormalities. *Am J Med.* 1988;85(1):12–18.

Bonow RO, Carabello BA, Chatterjee K, et al. 2008 Focused update incorporated into the ACC/AHA 2006 guidelines for the management of patients with valvular heart disease: a report of the American College of Cardiology/American Heart Association Task Force on Practice Guidelines (writing committee to revise the 1998 Guidelines for the Management of Patients With Valvular Heart Disease): endorsed by the Society of Cardiovascular Anesthesiologists, Society for Cardiovascular Angiography and Interventions, and Society of Thoracic Surgeons. *Circulation.* 2008;118(15):e523–e661.

Leon MB, Piazza N, Nikolsky E, et al. Standardized endpoint definitions for transcatheter aortic valve implantation clinical trials: a consensus report from the Valve Academic Research Consortium. *Eur Heart J.* 2011;32(2):205–217.

Meredith EL, Masani ND. Echocardiography in the emergency assessment of acute aortic syndromes. *Eur J Echocardiogr.* 2009;10(1):i31–i9.

Murphy-Ryan M, Psychogios A, Lindor NM. Hereditary disorders of connective tissue: a guide to the emerging differential diagnosis. *Genet Med.* 2010;12(6):344–354.

Myerson SG. Heart valve disease: investigation by cardiovascular magnetic resonance. *J Cardiovasc Magn Reson.* 2012;14:7.

Ng AC, Delgado V, van der Kley F, et al. Comparison of aortic root dimensions and geometries before and after transcatheter aortic valve implantation by 2- and 3-dimensional transesophageal echocardiography and multislice computed tomography. *Circ Cardiovasc Imaging.* 2010;3(1):94–102.

Nishimura RA, Otto CM, Bonow RO, et al. 2014 AHA/ACC guideline for the management of patients with valvular heart disease: executive summary: a report of the American College of Cardiology/American Heart Association Task Force on Practice Guidelines. *J Am Coll Cardiol.* 2014;63(22):2438–2488.

Olsen NT, Sogaard P, Larsson HB, et al. Speckle-tracking echocardiography for predicting outcome in chronic aortic regurgitation during conservative management and after surgery. *JACC Cardiovasc Imaging.* 2011;4(3):223–230.

Pizarro R, Bazzino OO, Oberti PF, et al. Prospective validation of the prognostic usefulness of B-type natriuretic peptide in asymptomatic patients with chronic severe aortic regurgitation. *J Am Coll Cardiol.* 2011;58(16):1705–1714.

Shiga T, Wajima Z, Apfel CC, et al. Diagnostic accuracy of transesophageal echocardiography, helical computed tomography, and magnetic resonance imaging for suspected thoracic aortic dissection: systematic review and meta-analysis. *Arch Intern Med.* 2006;166(13):1350–1356.

CHAPTER 3

Gian M. Novaro
Craig R. Asher

Bicuspid Aortic Valve Disease

I. INTRODUCTION

Bicuspid aortic valve (BAV) disease is the most commonly encountered defect among adult congenital heart diseases. Complications are common and can be related to valve disease, including aortic stenosis, aortic regurgitation, and infective endocarditis, or can be the result of BAV-related aortopathy, which can result in ascending aortic dilatation, aneurysm formation, and aortic dissection. With heterogeneous presentations and variable phenotypes, the surveillance and decision making in BAV disease remain challenging in view of the parallel considerations given to the valve and the aorta. Recent investigations have provided a better appreciation of clinical outcomes, improved the timing of surgical interventions, and enhanced our understanding of the biology and genetics behind BAV disease.

II. PREVALENCE

The most common congenital heart malformation, BAV has a prevalence between 0.5% and 2% in the general population. There is a clear male predominance of at least 3:1. Recently, racial variations have been reported with a very low rate of BAV among African-Americans, noted in echocardiographic and surgical cohort studies.

III. ASSOCIATED CONDITIONS

The majority of BAVs occur in isolation, but in certain groups, they may be associated with other cardiac and congenital anomalies (Table 3.1). The most common cardiac abnormality is dilatation of the ascending aorta (the aortic root, ascending portion, and/or arch), which is present in 50% to 60% of cases.

Among the most common associated congenital conditions is coarctation of the aorta. About 50% to 75% of patients with coarctation of the aorta have a BAV. Numerous congenital defects can also coexist with BAV, including ventricular septal defects, patent ductus arteriosus, atrial septal defects, sinus of Valsalva aneurysms, and coronary artery anomalies. Genetic syndromes that include a BAV may occur; among them are Shone syndrome, Turner syndrome (~30% have BAV), Loeys–Dietz syndrome (~20% have BAV), and Williams syndrome.

IV. ETIOLOGY AND GENETICS

The exact etiology of BAV remains unknown, but evidence predominantly favors an underlying genetic abnormality leading to a developmental defect early in valvulogenesis. This model, the genetic theory, is more widely accepted as opposed to the hemodynamic molding theory of altered or diminished blood flow through the valve during valvulogenesis. The aortic valve and ascending aorta develop from the remodeled endocardial cushions, with involvement of migrating cardiac neural crest cells. Valve and outflow tract formation in this early stage relies on molecular signaling pathways to regulate development, and perturbations during this time likely result in the altered formation or septation of the leaflet primordia.

TABLE 3.1 Bicuspid Aortic Valve and Associated Conditions

Coexisting cardiovascular abnormalities	
	Dilatation of the ascending aorta and arch
	Aneurysm of the ascending aorta
	Dissection of the ascending aorta
	Left coronary artery dominance
	Short left main trunk
	Dilatation of the pulmonary root
	Cervicocephalic artery dissection or aneurysms
	Intracranial aneurysms
Coexisting congenital defects	
	Coarctation of the aorta
	Ventricular septal defect
	Patent ductus arteriosus
	Sinus of Valsalva aneurysm
	Atrial septal defect
	Interrupted aortic arch
Genetic syndromes with bicuspid aortic valve	
	Shone complex
	Turner syndrome
	Williams syndrome
	Hypoplastic left heart syndrome
	Loeys–Dietz syndrome
	Andersen–Tawil syndrome

In support of a predominant genetic component, pedigree-based reports have demonstrated the heritability of BAV. Familial clustering of BAV disease occurs with an estimated prevalence of 9% among first-degree relatives, and 24% to 37% of families have at least one other affected relative; these studies suggest an inheritance pattern that is autosomal dominant with reduced penetrance and variable expressivity.

In addition to BAV, family members of BAV probands have high heritability for other cardiac and congenital heart defects including ascending aortic abnormalities. Despite these findings, most BAVs occur as sporadic cases. Even though most accept a genetic basis for BAV, the identification of a specific gene abnormality has not been consistent. From both human studies and animal models, there have been a number of identified gene mutations linked to BAV. The recognized genes include *NOTCH1, NOS3, KCNJ2, GATA5, HOXA1, NKX2.5, ACTA2, TGFB1, TGFB2, FGF8, AXIN1,* and *UFD1L*. In addition, family-based linkage studies have found associations between BAV and chromosomes 18q, 5q, and 13q.

Given its apparent genetic heterogeneity, it seems that BAV disease is the result of a polygenic disease complicated with variable patterns of penetrance and expressivity, influenced by epigenetic and environmental factors.

V. VALVE ANATOMY (CLASSIFICATIONS)

The normal aortic valve is a trileaflet (tricuspid) valve, made up of three leaflets (cusps) named by their association with the coronary arteries (left, right, and noncoronary cusps). A BAV results from defective cusp development, leading to a valve possessing two asymmetric leaflets (due to fusion of two cusps) and two commissural attachments. The larger conjoined leaflet typically has a central raphe or a false commissure, a fibrous ridge of tissue where the cusps failed to divide or remained fused. The anatomic variations of BAV have been well described and depend on which commissures remain fused (Fig. 3.1).

The most common BAV morphology is fusion of the right and left coronary cusps (type 1, RL pattern; 70% to 85% of cases), which results in a horizontal commissure and leaflets oriented in an anterior–posterior location. The RL pattern is the most common BAV associated with coarctation of the aorta. The second most common morphology is fusion of the right and noncoronary cusps (type 2, RN pattern; 15% to 25% of cases), which results in a vertical commissure and leaflets oriented in a right–left position. The RN-pattern BAV usually leads to significant valvular dysfunction. Finally, the LN pattern, fusion of the left and noncoronary cusps, is rare (type 3, less than 5% of cases). In over 90% of BAVs, the two cusps are unequal in size, with the fused cusp always being the larger cusp. Finding a BAV with symmetric cusps and no raphe, the so-called "pure" BAV, is rare.

A leaflet classification scheme has been proposed by Sievers and Schmidtke, which includes three major types, first categorized by raphe(s), followed by leaflet orientation and type of valve dysfunction. For example, Sievers type 1, L/R, S refers to a BAV with 1 raphe, LR cusp fusion and aortic stenosis, whereas type 0, L/R, N is a BAV with no raphe, LR fusion, and normal valve function.

VI. BICUSPID AORTIC VALVE–RELATED AORTOPATHY

It is now well recognized that BAV is associated with dilatation of the ascending aorta. Once thought to be the result of "poststenotic" dilatation, BAV-related aortic enlargement is predominantly attributed to a genetic basis. In support of a genetic underpinning, aortic dilatation can be seen early in life with BAV, without stenosis, and, in children, aortic dimensions increase at a greater rate than in matched controls with a trileaflet aortic valve.

In adults with BAV, aortic dilatation is present in approximately 50% to 60% of cases. The adult ascending aorta at all levels (annulus, sinuses, midascending) is larger in BAV subjects compared with their trileaflet valve counterparts. BAV aortic dilatation can be present in those without valvular dysfunction and can progress despite having undergone valve replacement surgery. Finally, dilated aortas are prevalent in first-degree relatives of probands with a BAV.

Although not considered the primary reason, there is evidence that altered hemodynamics contribute, perhaps in combination, to the primary BAV aortopathy. Even a normally functioning BAV wrinkles, domes, and folds during the cardiac cycle, leading to turbulent flow currents that can impose increased shear stress on the ascending aortic wall. In aortic regions enduring the most increased wall stress, greater degrees of medial matrix disruption are found. These eccentric flow patterns across a BAV will vary depending on leaflet orientation. Visualized using four-dimensional flow magnetic resonance imaging (MRI), the RL-pattern BAV directs a turbulent jet in the direction of the right anterior greater curvature (right-handed flow), whereas the RN-pattern BAV promotes flow toward the posterior aortic wall and proximal arch (left-handed flow). In small populations, these two BAV subtypes were associated with distinct patterns of aortic dilatation, midtubular dilatation, and distal ascending and arch dilatation, respectively.

Because not all BAVs will develop a dilated aorta, the hemodynamic alterations alone are insufficient to fully explain the developing aortopathy. Histologically, BAV-related aortopathy is associated with distinct intrinsic alterations of the aortic wall that reduce its structural integrity. Abnormalities in the aortic media of BAV patients are commonly identified and consist of vascular smooth muscle cell apoptosis, elastic fiber fragmentation, increased matrix metalloproteinase activity, and matrix disruption. These changes notably

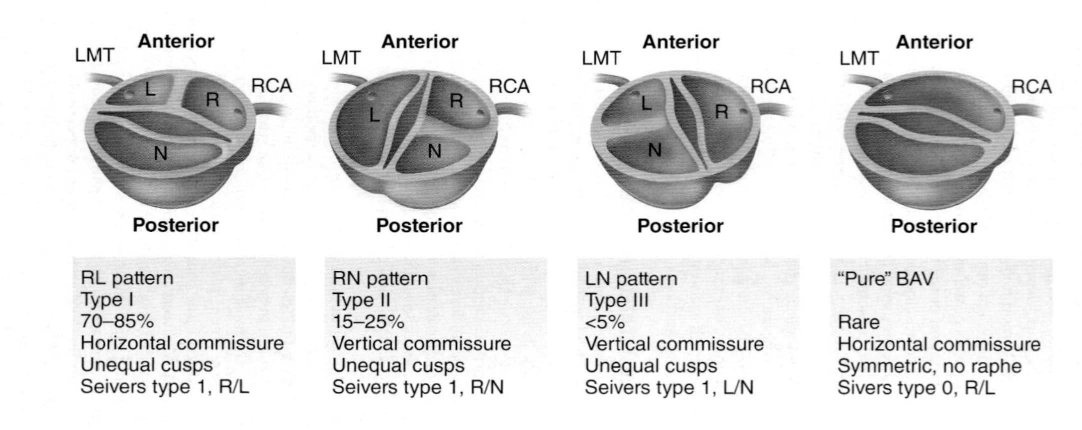

FIGURE 3.1 Anatomic variations in bicuspid aortic valves as viewed from a surgical perspective.

differ in pattern from those seen in diseased dilated aortas of patients with trileaflet aortic valves. The degenerative medial process in the aortic wall is thought to result from an imbalance between tissue concentrations of matrix metalloproteinases and their endogenous tissue inhibitors, specifically an increase in matrix metalloproteinase 2 relative to tissue inhibitor of metalloproteinase 1. Moreover, fibrillin-1, the glycoprotein that functions abnormally in Marfan syndrome, has been found in lower amounts in BAV aortas. It has thus been speculated that abnormal signaling of transforming growth factor β may also play a role in BAV aortopathy.

As BAVs differ in morphotype, so do their dilated aortas (Fig. 3.2A–C). Although there is no widely accepted classification scheme, there are three principal patterns of aortic dilatation:

- The most common pattern, **type 1** (tubular or ascending phenotype with the ST junction > brachiocephalic artery origin), involves predominant dilatation of the midtubular ascending aorta along the convexity of the aorta, with mild degrees of aortic root involvement. This pattern is most often associated with R–L fusion, aortic stenosis, and older age.
- **Type 2** (diffuse or arch phenotype with the diameter at the ST junction < brachiocephalic artery origin) encompasses dilatation of the midtubular ascending aorta with variable degrees of aortic arch involvement. This pattern is most often associated with R–N fusion.
- **Type 3** (root phenotype) is the least common aorta pattern and involves isolated dilatation of the aortic root at the sinuses of Valsalva. This pattern is most often associated with younger men.

An alternative classification scheme, one based on hierarchical cluster analyses, has been proposed, which describes four distinct patterns of aortic dilatation. Cluster I involved dilatation limited to the aortic root, cluster II involved the tubular ascending aorta, cluster III involved the tubular ascending aorta extending to the aortic arch, and cluster IV involved the aortic root and tubular ascending aorta with tapering across the aortic arch. Three-fourths of BAV patients were categorized into clusters III and IV. Together, these aortic patterns highlight the variability in phenotype of BAV aortopathy and underscore the need to adapt the surgical strategies in aortic repair.

VII. ECHOCARDIOGRAPHY

With modern-day echocardiography, the diagnosis of a BAV can be made routinely and reliably, with an accuracy greater than 90% by transthoracic studies. Distinguishing between a trileaflet valve and a BAV can be made difficult by the presence of a raphe, which can mimic a commissure if seen during diastole. To confirm the diagnosis, the valve must be seen on the short axis during systole and the persistently fused commissure appreciated. Also in systole, the orifice should have an elliptical shape, giving it its "fish-mouthed" description. When a BAV is seen in the long axis, there is an eccentric line of coaptation in diastole and leaflet doming in systole.

By transthoracic echocardiography, the aortic root and proximal-midascending aorta must be visualized and inspected for signs of dilatation. Often, movement of the transducer 1 to 2 interspaces up may improve visualization of the more distal segments of the aorta. Also, right parasternal and suprasternal notch imaging may be useful. When transthoracic imaging is inadequate, transesophageal echocardiography may be needed to better define aortic valve cusp anatomy and to visualize the entire ascending aorta. For more definitive visualization of the midascending aorta and arch, computed tomography (CT) or MRI is often utilized.

VIII. NATURAL HISTORY AND CLINICAL MANIFESTATIONS

The clinical presentation of BAV has heterogeneous manifestations and ultimately will depend on the status of aortic valve function and the occurrence of complications related to the aorta and valve. The timing of presentation also varies, from severe valve disease during infancy or adolescence to the incidental detection in older adulthood. Nonetheless, most patients with a BAV will develop a complication during their lifetime.

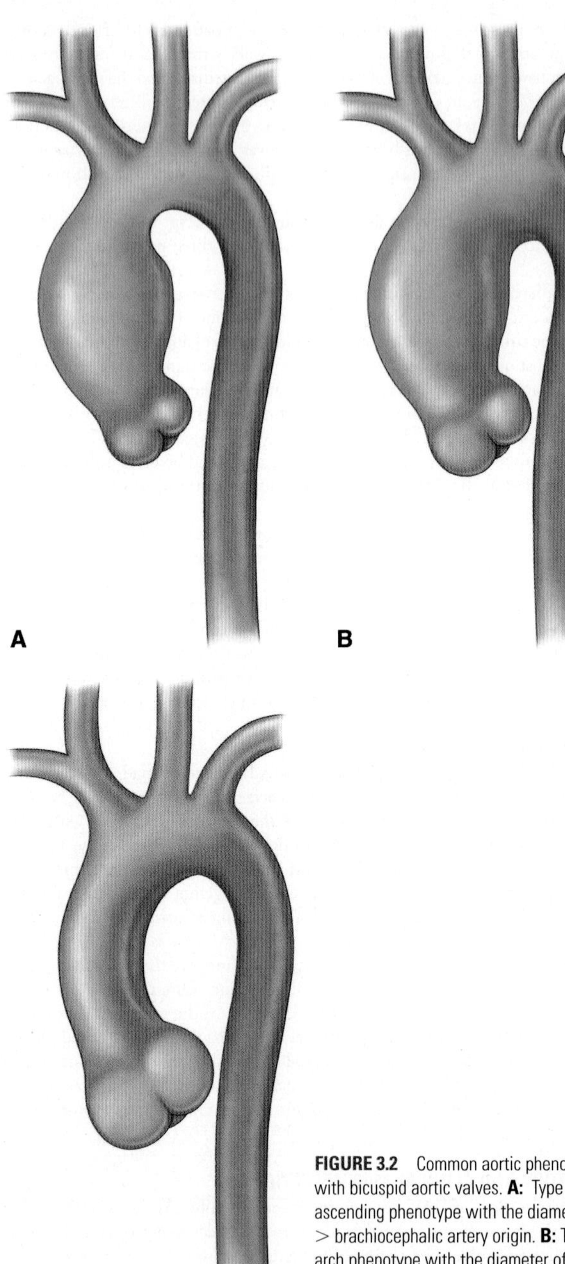

FIGURE 3.2 Common aortic phenotypes associated with bicuspid aortic valves. **A:** Type 1, tubular or ascending phenotype with the diameter at the ST junction > brachiocephalic artery origin. **B:** Type 2, diffuse or arch phenotype with the diameter of the ST junction < brachiocephalic artery origin. **C:** Type 3, root phenotype.

A. Aortic stenosis

By far, the most frequent complication of BAV is aortic stenosis. Although uncommon, stenotic aortic valve disease can develop during infancy and can be found in up to 2% of adolescent BAVs. In adults <65 years of age with aortic stenosis, a BAV is present in a large majority. In the United States, BAV accounts for half of all aortic stenosis cases and 60% of aortic valve replacements in those under 70 years of age.

The pathogenesis of aortic stenosis is the result of an active calcification process influenced by clinical, genetic, and anatomic factors. Similar to what is observed in trileaflet aortic valves, the development of BAV leaflet calcification involves a highly regulated process of cellular-mediated inflammation, lipoprotein infiltration, and a pro-osteogenic environment. The calcification process is certainly premature in BAV likely because of the increased mechanical stress incurred from abnormal leaflet folding and resultant turbulent flow. Accordingly, BAV cuspal calcification is common by middle age. Clinical factors are associated with the development of aortic stenosis in BAV and include hypercholesterolemia, elevated lipoprotein (a) levels, tobacco use, hypertension, and female gender. Anatomic features may also play a role in propensity for aortic stenosis among those with a BAV. Several series have noted that the type 2 BAV, RN cusp pattern, is associated more with stenosis in children and adults and with more rapid progression of aortic stenosis.

B. Aortic regurgitation

Aortic regurgitation occurs less commonly than stenosis in BAV. Although varying degrees of aortic regurgitation occur at a significant prevalence, isolated severe aortic regurgitation only develops in upward of 15% of cases. BAV regurgitation can develop as a result of primary leaflet abnormalities or be secondary to aortic root dilatation. BAV leaflets can prolapse from redundancy (typically, the conjoined cusp with a distal raphe cleft), become retracted from fibrosis, or become damaged as a result of endocarditis. The aortic root, usually with increasing age, can dilate at the sinotubular junction and lead to aortic leaflet malcoaptation, causing secondary aortic regurgitation. In addition, an incompetent BAV can develop as a result of balloon valvuloplasty performed during infancy or childhood.

C. Infective endocarditis

Endocarditis is a highly morbid complication of BAV and can be the initial manifestation of the valvular lesion. Endocarditis can cause valve destruction via leaflet tears or perforations, or can lead to abscess formation in the aortic root. When valve damage occurs, the resultant lesion is invariably aortic regurgitation, and the need for surgical intervention is high. In case series of native valve endocarditis, a BAV is found to comprise approximately 15% of the total cases, and is considered an important underlying risk factor. Because of reporting bias in older studies, the rates of endocarditis have been historically considered high, but contemporary estimates are low, placing the risk at approximately 2%. As a result of this low risk, the more recent American Heart Association/American College of Cardiology (AHA/ACC) Valvular Heart Disease Guidelines no longer recommend endocarditis prophylaxis for patients with a BAV.

D. Aortopathy

The most feared complications of BAV are ascending aortic aneurysm formation and its potential by-product, acute aortic dissection. BAV is a certain independent risk factor for dilatation of the ascending aorta and aortic dissection; for example, a BAV is present in approximately 5% to 10% of all aortic dissection cases in clinical series and upward of approximately 20% of dissections in the young (<40 years of age).

Ascending aortic dilatation and aneurysm formation are harbingers of risk and the best predictor of acute dissection. When dissection occurs in BAV, it almost always originates in the ascending aorta. The average BAV aorta dilates unpredictably but at an average rate that is greater than for those with trileaflet aortic valves; growth estimates range from 0.2 to 1.2 mm/y, with rates up to 1.9 mm/y in aneurysmal disease. Dilatation rates of the BAV tubular ascending aorta are comparable to dilatation rates of the aortic root in patients with Marfan syndrome. In contrast to Marfan patients, however, approximately 40% of BAV aortas fail to progressively dilate.

The best available predictors of more rapid aortic dilatation are increasing age, aortic valve dysfunction, elevated blood pressure, and larger aortic diameter at baseline. The best predictors of aortic dissection include larger aortic size, family history of aortic dissection, aortic regurgitation, and aortic stiffness.

Although the historical risk of BAV-related aortic dissection was considered high (up to ninefold in early studies), modern era estimates are considerably lower but remain higher than in the general population. In two contemporary series of BAV, the incidence of aortic dissection was 0.1% per patient-year of follow-up in one study and 3.1 cases per 10,000 patient-years in the other, resulting in an age-adjusted relative risk of 8.4 compared with the general population. In these series, the occurrence of dissection was strongly related to baseline aortic size. During follow-up, there were no dissections in those with a baseline aortic diameter <4.5 cm. In two BAV aortic registries, the average ascending aortic diameter at the time of dissection was 5.4 and 5.2 cm, respectively.

Although the modern-day clinical practice of aortic imaging and prophylactic surgery has likely lowered dissection rates, it has in turn highlighted the morbidity associated with BAV-related aortopathy. In a population-based study of BAV patients, the 25-year risk of developing an aortic aneurysm was 23%, and the risk of undergoing an aortic surgery was 26% (Fig. 3.3).

The ascending aorta of BAV patients remains at risk of further dilatation and dissection even after aortic valve replacement, a circumstance that is absent in those with trileaflet aortic valves. In a group of BAV patients undergoing aortic valve replacement, the 15-year risk of aortic complications was strongly related to aortic size at the time of surgery. Those with aortic diameters <4.0 cm at aortic valve replacement enjoyed

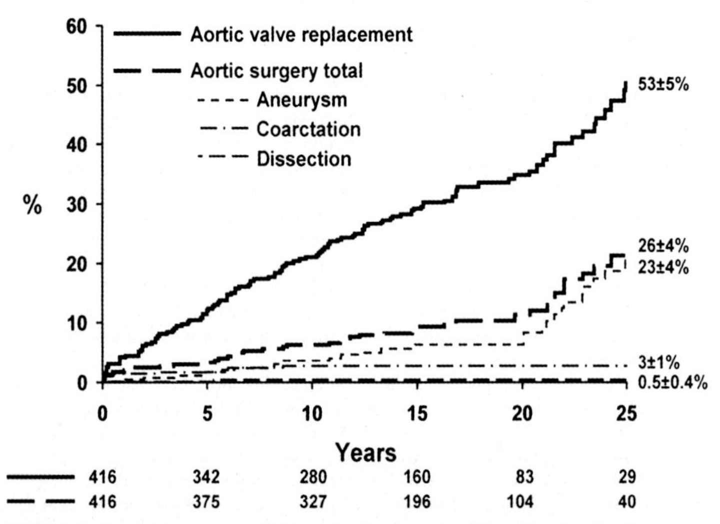

FIGURE 3.3 Twenty-five-year natural history after the diagnosis of bicuspid aortic valve. Percentage of patients requiring aortic valve replacement or aortic procedures based on etiology.
From Michelena HI, Prakash SK, Della Corte A, et al. Bicuspid aortic valve. *Circulation* 2014;129:2691–704.

a 15-year freedom rate from aortic complications of 86%, as compared with only 43% in those with an aortic diameter of 4.5 to 4.9 cm. An additional study suggested that freedom from aortic complications after aortic valve replacement was considerably lower in those with a root phenotype and predominant aortic regurgitation, a notable finding given the younger age of this patient subgroup.

IX. MEDICAL MANAGEMENT AND SURVEILLANCE

There are no specific medical agents recommended for long-term therapy of BAV disease. The use of statin drugs to slow the progression of calcific aortic stenosis in those with BAV has been studied and was found to have no effect on the rate of progression. Accordingly, the 2014 AHA/ACC Valvular Heart Disease Guidelines do not support the use of statins for the treatment of aortic stenosis.

Although there is a biologic rationale for the use of renin–angiotensin–aldosterone system inhibition to prevent the progression of AS, a small randomized study of eplerenone did not show benefit. For BAV with aortic regurgitation, vasodilator therapy is recommended only in the setting of treating hypertension. As previously mentioned, endocarditis prophylaxis for patients with a BAV is no longer recommended.

Medical therapy may have its greatest role in BAV-related aortopathy. When aortopathy is present, hypertension should be well managed with preferred agents, specifically β-blockers, angiotensin receptor blockers, and angiotensin-converting enzyme inhibitors. Extrapolated from the benefits seen in Marfan syndrome, β-blockers are used to reduce aortic stress and slow the rate of aortic progression. Also extrapolated from small studies in Marfan patients, angiotensin receptor blockers have been shown to attenuate aortic root dilatation. Thus, when hypertension is present, it seems reasonable to choose one of the agents that has theoretical advantages. A clinical trial evaluating the benefit of a β-blocker and an angiotensin receptor blocker in BAV-related aortopathy is ongoing.

In regard to the routine imaging and surveillance of BAV disease, serial imaging of the valve should be determined by the extent of valve dysfunction (i.e., stenosis, regurgitation) and change in symptoms, for instance, annually when valve dysfunction is at least moderate.

BAV patients should be advised in regard to participation in physical activity, weighing the combined risk of valve disease and aortopathy. Because the most concerning threat is aortic dissection, high-intensity sport, contact sport, and intense isometric exertion should be restricted when an aortic diameter is >4.0 cm. Strenuous weight lifting should probably be avoided altogether in any patient with a BAV. If the aorta is <4.0 cm and there is no significant valve dysfunction, then participation in competitive or high-intensity sport is permitted. BAV patients should also be advised to pursue screening of their first-degree family members. An echocardiogram is the test of choice for screening for the presence of a BAV and ascending aortic disease, even in the absence of BAV.

For surveillance of the ascending aorta, annual imaging is recommended when the aortic diameter is >4.0 cm at any level. At baseline when aortopathy is present, CT or MRI scanning should be performed to survey the entire ascending aorta and arch. When an aortic diameter reaches 4.5 to 5.0 cm, cardiac imaging should be performed every 6 to 12 months. Particular attention should be paid not just to the absolute aortic diameter but also to the rate of change (≥0.5 cm/y is considered high risk) and the ratio of aortic cross-sectional area to body height (>10 cm^2/m is considered high risk). In a normal-sized BAV aorta with a diameter <4.0 cm, serial imaging can be performed every 2 to 3 years.

The 2014 AHA/ACC Valvular Heart Disease Guidelines state that it is "clearly appropriate" to screen family members of BAV patients if they have aortopathy. They state that there is uncertainty with regard to cost-effectiveness of screening all first-degree relatives of patients with BAV.

Pregnancy is safe and well tolerated in most women with BAV. However, those with significant aortic stenosis or aortopathy with ascending aortic diameter >4.5 cm should be advised against pregnancy because of the risk of complications according to the AHA/ACC 2008 Guidelines for the Management of Adults with Congenital Heart Disease.

In addition, referral to a pediatric cardiologist experienced in fetal echocardiography is recommended by the same guidelines to assess for cardiac defects in the fetus.

X. SURGICAL TREATMENT—VALVULAR AND AORTIC CONSIDERATIONS

In general, BAV patients with severe aortic stenosis or severe aortic regurgitation who are symptomatic or have depressed left ventricular function or abnormal ventricular dimensions should be considered for aortic valve replacement surgery. Specific indications for aortic valve surgery in BAV patients are similar to those in patients with trileaflet aortic valves as outlined in the 2014 AHA/ACC Valvular Heart Disease Guidelines. On average, aortic valve surgery occurs a couple of decades earlier than in patients with trileaflet aortic valves. In a BAV population–based study, the 25-year risk of requiring aortic valve replacement was 53% (Fig. 3.3).

BAV patients with isolated severe aortic regurgitation with a redundant conjoined cusp and noncalcified leaflets may be candidates for aortic valve repair. Although the long-term results of valve repair are variable, the technique remains an option for select BAV patients, particularly those undergoing concomitant valve-sparing aortic root replacement surgery. Specific to the pediatric population with BAV and aortic stenosis, balloon valvuloplasty remains an attractive option when performed by experienced operators. Given the coupled considerations of the valve and the aorta, the timing of surgery can be challenging; it is estimated that 20% to 30% of BAV patients require aortic surgery at the time of aortic valve replacement.

Consideration for aortic surgery in patients with BAVs (root repair or ascending replacement) has been recently updated with the ACC/AHA Task Force on Clinical Guidelines—Statement of Clarification. This statement aimed to clarify discrepancies between the 2010 Thoracic Aortic Disease Guidelines and 2014 Valvular Heart Disease Guidelines (Table 3.2).

TABLE 3.2 ACC/AHA Task Force on Clinical Guidelines—Statement of Clarification on Surgery for Aortic Dilatation in Patients with Bicuspid Aortic Valves

Class 1—asymptomatic ≥5.5 cm
Class 2a—asymptomatic ≥5 cm + 1 risk factor (change in size ≥0.5 cm/y or family history of aortic dissection or sudden death) or experienced team or short stature (using indexed cutoffs based on body surface area or aortic cross-sectional area/patient height ratio >10 cm^2/m)
Class 2a—aortic valve replacement and >4.5 cm

KEY PEARLS

- Bicuspid aortic valve (BAV) has a prevalence of 0.5% to 2% in the general population, with a male predominance of at least 3:1 and a lesser occurrence in African-Americans compared with whites.
- BAV is associated with ascending aortic dilatation in 50% to 60% of cases and with various congenital and genetic syndromes. The most common congenital disorders associated with BAV include coarctation of the aorta, patent ductus arteriosus, and ventricular and atrial septal defects.
- The exact etiology of BAV remains unknown, but evidence predominantly favors an underlying genetic abnormality leading to a developmental defect early in valvulogenesis. In support of a predominant genetic component, pedigree-based reports have demonstrated the

heritability of BAV. Familial clustering of BAV disease occurs with an estimated prevalence of 9% among first-degree relatives.

- The most common BAV morphology is fusion of the right and left coronary cusps (70% to 85% of cases), which results in a horizontal commissure and leaflets oriented in an anterior–posterior location. The second most common morphology is fusion of the right and noncoronary cusps (15% to 25% of cases), which results in a vertical commissure and leaflets oriented in a right–left position. The LN pattern, fusion of the left and noncoronary cusps, is rare (less than 5% of cases).
- Dilatation of the aorta in patients with BAV is thought to be primarily due to genetic underpinnings, although altered hemodynamics likely also contribute.
- Although there is no widely accepted classification scheme, there are three principal patterns of aortic dilatation in patients with BAV.
  - *Type 1* involves predominant dilatation of the midtubular ascending aorta along the convexity of the aorta, with mild degrees of aortic root involvement (tubular or ascending phenotype with the ST junction > brachiocephalic artery origin).
  - *Type 2* encompasses dilatation of the midtubular ascending aorta with variable degrees of aortic arch involvement (diffuse or arch phenotype with the diameter at the ST junction < brachiocephalic artery origin).
  - *Type 3* is the least common aorta pattern and involves isolated dilatation of the aortic root at the sinuses of Valsalva (root phenotype).
- The clinical presentation of BAV has heterogeneous manifestations related to the aortic valve function and aorta. Aortic stenosis is by far the most common complication and accounts for half of all aortic stenosis cases and 60% of aortic valve replacements in those under 70 years of age. The most feared complications of BAV are ascending aortic aneurysm formation and its potential by-product, acute aortic dissection.
- There are no specific medical agents recommended for long-term therapy of BAV disease. The use of statin drugs to slow the progression of calcific aortic stenosis in those with BAV has been studied and found to have no effect on the rate of progression. When aortopathy is present, hypertension should be well managed with preferred agents, specifically β-blockers, angiotensin receptor blockers, and angiotensin-converting enzyme inhibitors.
- Imaging of the ascending aorta should be done in all patients with BAV. If echocardiography is suboptimal or aortic dimension is >4.0 to 4.5 cm, the entire ascending aorta, aortic arch, and descending aorta should be visualized by computed tomography or magnetic resonance imaging.
- In general, BAV patients with severe aortic stenosis or severe aortic regurgitation who are symptomatic or have depressed left ventricular function or abnormal ventricular dimensions should be considered for aortic valve replacement surgery.
- Consideration for aortic surgery in patients with BAVs (root repair or ascending replacement) has been recently updated with the ACC/AHA Task Force on Clinical Guidelines—Statement of Clarification (summarized in Table 3.2).

SUGGESTED READINGS

Biner S, Rafique AM, Ray I, et al. Aortopathy is prevalent in relatives of bicuspid aortic valve patients. *J Am Coll Cardiol.* 2009;53:2288–2295.

Cripe L, Andelfinger G, Martin LJ, et al. Bicuspid aortic valve is heritable. *J Am Coll Cardiol.* 2004;44:138–143.

Michelena HI, Desjardins VA, Avierinos JF, et al. Natural history of asymptomatic patients with normally functioning or minimally dysfunctional bicuspid aortic valve in the community. *Circulation.* 2008;117:2776–2784.

Michelena HI, Prakash SK, Della Corte A, et al. Bicuspid aortic valve: identifying knowledge gaps and rising to the challenge. From the International Bicuspid Valve Consortium (BAVCon). *Circulation.* 2014;129:2691.

Sievers HH, Schmidtke C. A classification system for the bicuspid aortic valve from 304 surgical specimens. *J Thorac Cardiovasc Surg*. 2007;133:1226–1233.
Siu SC, Silversides CK. Bicuspid aortic valve disease. *J Am Coll Cardiol*. 2010;55:2789–2800.
Svensson LG, Kim KH, Lytle BW, et al. Relationship of aortic cross-sectional area to height ratio and the risk of aortic dissection in patients with bicuspid aortic valves. *J Thorac Cardiovasc Surg*. 2003;126:892–893.
Tzemos N, Therrien J, Yip J, et al. Outcomes in adults with bicuspid aortic valves. *JAMA*. 2008;300:1317–1325.
Verma S, Siu SC. Aortic dilatation in patients with bicuspid aortic valve. *N Engl J Med*. 2014;370:1920–1929.
Wojnarski CM, Svensson LG, Roselli EE, et al. Aortic dissection in patients with bicuspid aortic valve-associated aneurysms. *Ann Thorac Surg*. 2015;100:1666.

CHAPTER 4

L. Leonardo Rodriguez

Mitral Stenosis

I. INTRODUCTION.

I. INTRODUCTION. Rheumatic disease remains the predominant cause of mitral stenosis (MS). However, this etiology is declining in the United States, and other causes of MS should also be considered (Table 4.1).

In general, MS progresses slowly, and once symptoms begin to develop, there follows a period of about 7 years before they become severe. Once debilitating symptoms develop, the 10-year survival rate without intervention is <15%.

II. CLINICAL PRESENTATION

A. Signs and symptoms

1. There is a long asymptomatic course in patients with MS. Most patients tend to develop symptoms in the fourth or fifth decade of life.
2. Predominant symptoms are exertional dyspnea, followed by paroxysmal nocturnal dyspnea and orthopnea. In general, patients with chronic MS are able to tolerate higher left atrial (LA) pressures. Patients with very high pulmonary vascular resistance may never experience paroxysmal dyspnea.
3. Precipitating factors, such as exercise, pregnancy, infection, emotional stress, or atrial fibrillation with a rapid ventricular response, worsen symptoms by increasing transvalvular gradients and LA pressure. Atrial fibrillation with rapid ventricular response is a typical exacerbating factor and can lead to pulmonary edema, even in those with moderate MS.
4. Hemoptysis can occur and likely represents rupture of small bronchial veins from elevated LA pressure. Hemoptysis is now relatively uncommon, but it can present as sudden unexpected profuse hemorrhage, blood-stained sputum associated with acute pulmonary venous congestion, pink frothy sputum accompanying acute pulmonary edema, and frank hemoptysis due to pulmonary infarction (rare). Acute bronchitis in the winter months is also a common finding.
5. LA dilation and stasis, particularly in the context of atrial fibrillation (persistent or paroxysmal), predispose to thrombus formation and embolic events. Sometimes, embolic events are the presenting symptoms in patients with MS. Embolic events can involve cerebral (most common), coronary, or peripheral circulation. The thickened and deformed valve is predisposed to the development of endocarditis. Ortner syndrome refers to hoarseness caused by the dilated LA impinging on the recurrent laryngeal nerve.
6. With long-standing MS with pulmonary hypertension, symptoms of right ventricular (RV) failure may develop. Anginal chest pain can be present in patients with tight MS and may reflect low cardiac output. Fatigue is a common expression of reduced cardiac output. In patients with pulmonary hypertension, it may be secondary to increased RV oxygen demand.

B. Physical findings

1. **Inspection and palpation:** Patients may have a malar facial flush, which is nowadays uncommon. The jugular venous pulse can demonstrate a prominent a-wave if there is elevated pulmonary vascular resistance and the patient is still in sinus

TABLE 4.1 Etiologies of Mitral Stenosis

Rheumatic	Most common
Calcific	Most often in elderly, renal failure, radiation
Postsurgical	Small annuloplasty ring
Congenital	Parachute mitral valve, supravalvular ring, etc.
Postinflammatory	Lupus, rheumatoid arthritis
Postendocarditis	Residual leaflet thickening, restriction, densities
Infiltrative	Mucopolysaccharidosis

rhythm. Jugular venous pressure is elevated in RV failure. In advanced cases with low cardiac output, peripheral cyanosis occurs. The carotid upstrokes are of low amplitude when there is low cardiac output. The apex beat is not displaced, and the impulse and first heart sound can be palpable. An apical diastolic thrill may be felt in the lateral decubitus position in a third of patients. If there is pulmonary hypertension, a parasternal RV lift with a palpable P_2 is present. A RV lift is seen in about 60% of the patients.

2. **Auscultation:** The main auscultatory findings are shown in Figure 4.1.
   - **a.** S_1 is usually loud except in patients with associated significant mitral regurgitation (MR). The diastolic opening snap (OS) is the most characteristic auscultatory hallmark of MS. However, as the mitral valve becomes more calcified and immobile, the OS may no longer be present. It may also be absent in patients with associated moderate to severe MR. An OS should be differentiated from an S_3 gallop (Table 4.2).
   - **b.** The murmur of MS is typically a low-pitched rumbling mid-diastolic murmur, heard best with the bell of the stethoscope with the patient in the left lateral decubitus position. Presystolic accentuation is more often present in sinus rhythm (although it can be occasionally heard in patients with atrial fibrillation) and is not related to the severity of MS. Auscultation after a brief period of exercise may accentuate the murmur of MS as the increased output and heart rate increase the transvalvular gradient. The length of the murmur correlates better with the severity of MS than its loudness. The longer the murmur and the shorter the time interval from S_2 to the OS, the more severe the MS.
   - **c.** Diminished flow across the mitral valve in cases of congestive heart failure, pulmonary hypertension, and aortic stenosis may reduce the diastolic murmur. The presence of a loud S_1 may be the only clue to the presence of MS in these cases.
   - **d.** Other conditions that may simulate the clinical presentation of MS include LA myxoma and cor triatriatum. The tumor plop of a myxoma may be mistaken for an OS, and tumor obstruction of the valve leads to a diastolic murmur. In this condition, the physical findings will vary with changes in position.

     Other conditions in which a diastolic rumble may be present include large atrial septal defect or ventricular septal defect, the Austin-Flint murmur of aortic regurgitation, which is typically preceded by an S_3, and tricuspid stenosis. (The murmur is heard at the left sternal border and typically increases with inspiration.) Patients with severe MR may have a short diastolic rumble also preceded by S_3, but the loud holosystolic murmur is the predominant finding.

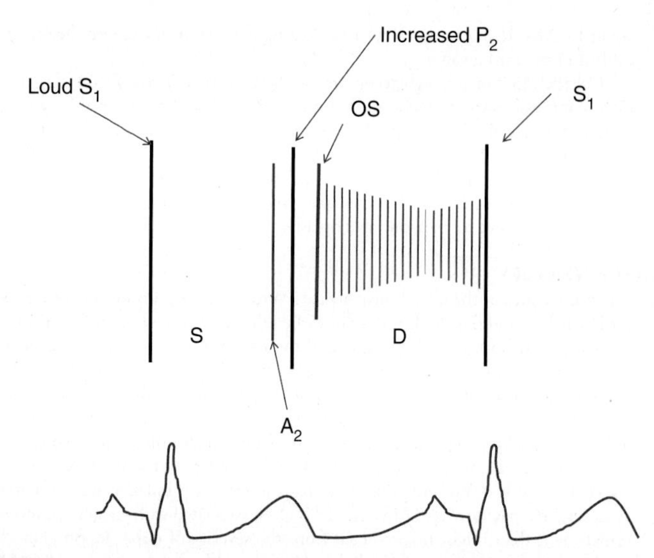

FIGURE 4.1 Finding on auscultation in mitral stenosis. Increased first sound. Louder pulmonary component of the second sound in patients with pulmonary hypertension. OS followed by diastolic rumble with presystolic accentuation. In patients with mild MS, the rumble may be present only at the beginning of diastole and after atrial contraction (points of maximal diastolic gradients). D, diastole; OS, opening snap; S, systole.

TABLE 4.2 Differences between Opening Snap and Third Heart Sound on Auscultation

	Opening Snap	S_3
Relation to second sound	Very close to A_2	Early diastole
Characteristics	Shorter, higher pitch	Longer, lower pitch
Location	Left sternal border	Apex

III. ETIOLOGY (TABLE 4.1)

A. It is important to remember that up to 50% of patients with rheumatic MS are not aware of a history of rheumatic fever. Although the incidence of rheumatic fever is roughly equal between men and women, rheumatic MS develops two to three times more frequently in women.

1. Thickening and fibrosis of leaflets with commissural fusion is the pathognomonic finding. Commissural and chordal fusion and chordal shortening contribute to the development of stenosis. Calcium deposition occurs on the leaflets, chordae, and annulus, decreasing valvular excursion. As a result of these changes, the mitral valve becomes funnel-shaped with a decreased orifice size.

B. Causes of nonrheumatic MS include extensive annular calcification in the elderly, congenital malformation, radiation heart disease, lupus, and restrictive mitral valve repair for MR. In addition, valvular thickening may result in MS after healed endocarditis of the mitral valve.

Calcific MS is increasingly recognized in the aging population. Frequently, but not always, it is associated with chronic kidney disease, but is also seen in elderly patients with aortic stenosis. The morphology of the mitral valve in calcific MS differs from rheumatic disease. The commissures are spared and the obstruction is caused by severe calcification of the mitral annulus, reducing the mobility of the leaflets and reducing the annular area. Management of these patients is different from those with rheumatic MS. There is no role for balloon valvuloplasty, and surgery is technically more difficult.

IV. PATHOPHYSIOLOGY

A. The normal area of the mitral valve orifice is 4 to 6 cm^2. A pressure gradient between the left atrium and the LV (LA) develops when the valve area is <2 cm^2. As the orifice area decreases, both the LA pressure and the transmitral pressure gradient increase (Fig. 4.2). Although the transmitral pressure is a useful indicator of MS severity, it is critically affected by the cardiac output and duration of diastolic filling period (gradient increases as the square of flow). The cross-sectional area of the mitral valve orifice is basically independent of flow considerations and thus can be considered a more robust measure of the severity of MS. The severity of the stenosis needs to be assessed in terms of not only the valve area and gradients but also symptomatology and exercise capacity. Mixed MS and MR is often associated with greater symptomatic impairment than might be predicted from the severity of either lesion alone. The current American College of Cardiology/American Heart Association (ACC/AHA) guidelines in Valvular Heart Disease define four stages of MS (Table 4.3).

B. Increased LA pressure is transmitted to the pulmonary vasculature, resulting in symptoms of pulmonary congestion. The passive increase in pulmonary venous pressure may elevate pulmonary vascular resistance (reactive pulmonary hypertension). Patients with increased pulmonary vascular resistance are less prone to pulmonary edema. Pulmonary hypertension is usually reversible if the stenosis is relieved. However, in long-standing, severe MS, irreversible obliterative changes in pulmonary vasculature may occur. Severe pulmonary hypertension can cause RV dysfunction and right-sided heart failure.

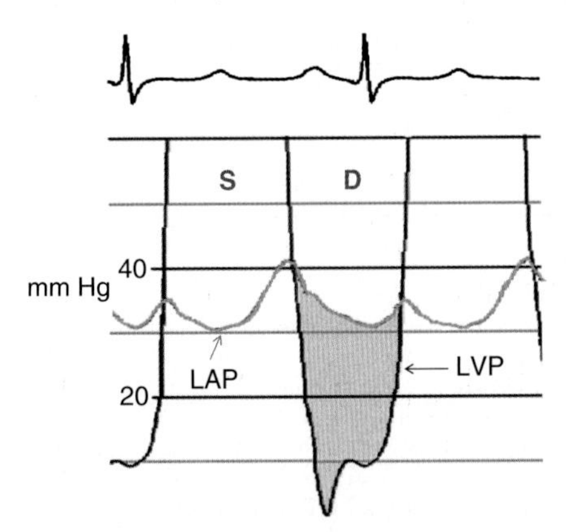

FIGURE 4.2 Simultaneous left atrial and left ventricular pressure showing elevated diastolic pressure gradient. This is the hemodynamic hallmark of mitral stenosis. D, diastole; LAP, left atrial pressure; LVP, left ventricular pressure; S, systole.

TABLE 4.3 Stages of Mitral Stenosis as Proposed in the 2014 American College of Cardiology/American Heart Association Guidelines

	Valve Anatomy	Valve Hemodynamics	Hemodynamic Consequences
Stage A	Patients at risk of developing mitral stenosis (MS)	Mild diastolic doming of the mitral valve	Normal left atrial (LA) size
Stage B	Progressive MS	Increase transmitral velocities and valve area >1.5 cm^2	Mildly enlarged LA; normal resting pulmonary pressures
Stage C	Severe asymptomatic MS	Severe MS defined as valve area ≤ 1.5 cm^2 and very severe MS as valve area ≤ 1.0 cm^2	Severe LA enlargement and elevated pulmonary systolic pressures
Stage D	Severe symptomatic MS	Mitral valve area ≤ 1.5 cm^2 and very severe MS as valve area ≤ 1.0 cm^2	Same as stage C + decreased exercise tolerance and exertional dyspnea

C. Decreased LV ejection fraction can be seen in up to a third of patients as a result of **either** decreased preload or a rheumatic myocarditis. In patients with severe pulmonary hypertension with enlarged RV, ventricular interdependence may also contribute to LV dysfunction.

D. In severe MS, low cardiac output may contribute to peripheral hypoperfusion. Chronically depressed cardiac output causes a reflex increase in systemic vascular resistance and increased afterload with further impairment in LV performance.

V. DIAGNOSTIC TESTING

A. Electrocardiogram. LA enlargement (P mitrale) is usually present in patients in sinus rhythm. Signs of RV hypertrophy are seen with pulmonary hypertension. Atrial fibrillation is common, and the fibrillatory waves are usually coarse.

B. Chest radiography. LA enlargement is apparent with a double density along the right heart border. A convexity can be apparent below the pulmonary artery, representing the LA appendage. Radiographic elevation of the left main bronchus and posterior displacement of the esophagus at barium swallow examination also reflect LA enlargement. Kerley B lines may be present from increased pulmonary venous pressure. RV enlargement (decreased retrosternal air space on the lateral radiograph) may be seen. Evidence of mitral valve calcification, or rarely LA calcification (McCallum patch), has been described.

C. Echocardiography has a critical role in the evaluation of MS for initial diagnosis, determination of severity, LV and RV function, presence of pulmonary hypertension, and identification of concomitant valve lesions. It is also of paramount importance in the evaluation and selection of patients considered for percutaneous balloon mitral valvuloplasty.

1. M-mode is now less often relied upon for diagnosis, and findings include dense echoes and decreased excursion of the mitral valve. Anterior motion of the posterior leaflet and decreased E–F slope on the anterior leaflet are M-mode hallmarks of MS. However, decreased E–F slope can be seen in other conditions too and is not directly related to the severity of MS.

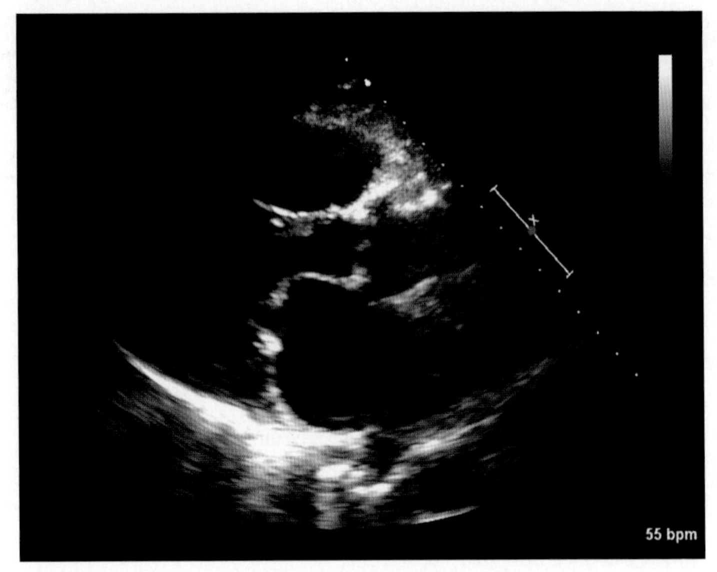

FIGURE 4.3 Mitral valve diastolic doming. Parasternal long-axis view.

2. **Two-dimensional (2D) echocardiography**. The morphologic diagnosis of MS can be made with 2D imaging. Typical findings include restricted motion and diastolic doming of leaflets (hockey stick sign) in the parasternal long-axis view (Fig. 4.3). The posterior mitral leaflet mobility is more impaired than the anterior leaflet and is often fixed. In the short-axis view, the mitral valve reveals commissural fusion with a fish-mouth appearance. The leaflets are thickened and are often calcified in older patients. Chordae are also thickened and shortened.
3. **Doppler echocardiography** is an integral part of the noninvasive evaluation of stenosis severity. The mean transvalvular gradient using continuous-wave (CW) Doppler of the mitral inflow provides an estimate of the severity of stenosis. A mean gradient <5 mm Hg is typically present in mild stenosis. Moderate stenosis is associated with a mean gradient between 5 and 10 mm Hg. A gradient >10 mm Hg suggests severe MS. However, it should always be kept in mind that these gradients are flow dependent.
4. **Estimating mitral valve area (MVA)**
   a. Planimetry. Direct planimetry of the orifice can be performed in the parasternal short-axis view. Optimal positioning is initially done from the parasternal long-axis view, placing the mitral valve orifice in the center of the scan plane. The transducer is then rotated 90 degrees to obtain the short-axis view. Measurements are obtained at the tips of the mitral leaflets during maximal diastolic opening. Finding the tips of the mitral valve requires careful scanning from base to apex.
   b. Poor-quality 2D images and a thick, calcified subvalvular apparatus can make it difficult to obtain accurate measurements. Improper orientation of the scanning plane can produce oblique cuts across the valve and lead to overestimation of valve area. In vertical hearts, a proper short-axis view of the mitral valve may be impossible to obtain. Dense fibrosis or calcification at the margins of

the valve orifice can lead to underestimation of the valve area. Optimal gain settings are important to avoid over- or underestimation. Planimetry is less reliable in patients with a history of commissurotomy. Although planimetry remains the preferred method to assess the MVA by means of echocardiography, it requires technical expertise to achieve accuracy.

c. Pressure half-time method. The smaller the mitral valve orifice, the longer it takes for the decline in transvalvular pressure gradient. This prolongs pressure half-time (time it takes for pressure to fall to one-half the starting value, which equates with the time for the velocity to decrease to 70% of peak velocity [peak velocity/$\sqrt{2}$]). The slope of the mitral inflow E wave is used in the calculation. Because it is in general easier to obtain the pressure half-time, it is probably the most common method for estimation of MVA.

An empiric pressure half-time has been shown to correlate with valve area, such that MVA (in cm^2) = 220/pressure half-time.

If a software package to perform the calculations is not available, pressure half-time can be calculated by multiplying the deceleration time by 0.29. If atrial fibrillation is present, 5 to 10 consecutive beats are obtained and averaged.

Limitations of pressure half-time method need to be kept in mind.

- The pressure half-time method is inaccurate if there are rapid changes in LA hemodynamics and atrioventricular compliance, such as immediately after balloon valvuloplasty.
- The pressure half-time method may be difficult to apply if sinus tachycardia is present (E–A fusion) and in cases of nonlinear slope of the E wave velocity decay. Severe aortic insufficiency also fills the LV in diastole, decreases pressure half-time, and may lead to overestimation of the MVA.

i. Continuity equation or the proximal convergence area method.

The continuity equation is calculated as:

$$\text{MVA} = \text{LVOT area} \times \text{VTI}_{\text{LVOT}}/\text{VTI}_{\text{MV}}$$

where *LVOT* is left ventricular outlet obstruction and *VTI* is velocity time interval.

However, if more than mild mitral or aortic regurgitation is present, the continuity equation will not be accurate and should not be used.

ii. The proximal convergence method for MS is calculated as:

$$\text{MVA} = 2\pi r^2 \times \frac{V_{\text{nyqst}}}{V_{\text{Max}}} \times \frac{\alpha^\circ}{180^\circ}$$

where r is the radius of the diastolic flow convergence on the atrial side, V_{Max} is the peak diastolic mitral valve CW velocity, and α is the angle subtended by the leaflets. If the angle measurement is not available, an empiric angle of 115 to 120 degrees can be used.

5. **Three-dimensional echocardiography (3DE)** provides a 3D data set to determine the MVA and should be used if available. This method allows correct alignment of the cut-plane at the level of the mitral valve tips. Using real-time 3D transesophageal technology, visualization of the mitral valve *en face* from the left atrium or LV is possible at the time of percutaneous balloon mitral valvuloplasty with visualization of the commissures before and after each balloon inflation. The degree of commissural splitting (unilateral or bilateral) appears to have prognostic value.
6. **Stress echocardiography** is a useful diagnostic tool in the evaluation of patients with symptoms when the resting study is discrepant with symptoms or clinical findings (ACC/AHA class I). Gradients can be assessed during (supine bicycle) or immediately after (treadmill) exercise. Measurement of tricuspid regurgitation velocity is used to estimate pulmonary pressures before and with stress. A rise in pulmonary pressures during exercise is closely related to net atrioventricular compliance.

7. **Transesophageal echocardiography (TEE)** is indicated to exclude LA thrombus and assess severity of MR before valvuloplasty. If LA thrombus is present, anticoagulation for at least 1 month is undertaken with repeat TEE to confirm resolution. TEE is also used if the transthoracic echocardiography (TTE) data are suboptimal (ACC/AHA class I), but is not indicated routinely if TTE data appear adequate. In some catheterization laboratories, TEE is routinely used to guide the balloon valvuloplasty procedure.
8. Echocardiographic follow-up in *asymptomatic patients.* Follow-up echocardiography is recommended every 3 to 5 years in patients with MVA >1.5 cm^2, every 1 to 2 years with MVA 1.0 to 1.5 cm^2, and every year in patients with MVA <1.0 cm^2.

D. Cardiac catheterization

The indication for cardiac catheterization is when echo-Doppler and clinical findings are discrepant or when echocardiographic findings are inconsistent or suboptimal. In cases where symptoms are mainly exertional and out of proportion to resting hemodynamic severity, data could be obtained during exercise. Hemodynamic measurements obtained in the cardiac catheterization laboratory are used to assess the severity of stenosis and direct measurement of pulmonary pressures. Simultaneous measurement of LV end-diastolic pressure, LA pressure (either directly or more commonly with pulmonary capillary wedge pressure [PCWP] as a surrogate), cardiac output (Fick method or thermodilution), heart rate, and diastolic filling period (seconds per beat) is required. LV pressure and PCWP (or LA pressure) tracings are made simultaneously and mean transmitral gradient is then measured. The PCWP/LV pressure gradient frequently overestimates the true severity of MS owing in part to a phase shift in PCWP. Therefore, tracing ideally should be realigned by 50 to 70 m to the left to account for the time delay in transmission of LA pressure to the pulmonary venous beds. Calculation of MVA is done using the Gorlin formula.

1. **The Gorlin formula**

   MVA = Cardiac output/Diastolic filling period × Heart rate/37.7 × √Mean transmitral pressure gradient

   Gorlin derived the empiric constant of 37.7, which is the Gorlin constant (44.3) multiplied by 0.85 (the correction factor for the mitral valve) to account for the coefficients of velocity loss and orifice contraction.
2. A simplified version of the Gorlin formula proposed by Hakki et al. has been validated and provides a reasonable approximation of the valve area. Hakki equation:

   $$\text{MVA} = \text{Cardiac output}/\sqrt{\text{Mean mitral gradient}}$$

3. Cardiac catheterization laboratory pitfalls are important to consider. PCWP should not be used if the patient has pulmonary venous occlusive disease. Oximetric confirmation that the catheter is properly wedged should be performed. The gold standard for cardiac output determination is the Fick principle, in which cardiac output is O_2 consumption divided by the difference between arterial and venous O_2. Thermodilution is less accurate particularly in patients with severe tricuspid regurgitation. Immediately after valvuloplasty, the presence of significant MR or atrial septal defect may lead to inaccurate estimations of mitral flow.

VI. MEDICAL THERAPY. The management of patients with MS should integrate symptom status, degree of stenosis, and suitability of the valve for percutaneous balloon mitral valvuloplasty. Other aspects to be considered in management are the presence of atrial fibrillation and pulmonary hypertension.

A. Patients without symptoms who have mild MS (valve area >1.5 cm^2 and mean gradient <5 mm Hg) need no specific treatment and, in accordance with current AHA guidelines, do not require endocarditis prophylaxis. In patients with rheumatic valve disease, guidelines for the prevention of rheumatic fever should be applied. Secondary prophylaxis for rheumatic fever should be used for at least 10 years after the last episode or until the patient is 40 years old (whichever is longer).

B. Patients with only mild symptoms of exertional dyspnea can be treated with diuretics and salt restriction to lower LA pressure. Published studies in general do not support the general use of heart rate control in patients with MS and normal sinus rhythm. However, heart rate control with β-blockers in patients with sinus rhythm may be considered when symptoms markedly worsen with exercise (class IIb). In pregnant women, metoprolol is the β-blocker of choice.

C. Atrial fibrillation can clearly exacerbate symptoms, and cardioversion or rate control measures are important to maintain diastolic filling time. Embolism is a much feared complication of MS and occurs in up to 20% of patients. Advancing age and atrial fibrillation are major risk factors.

1. Digitalis and β-blockers are the preferred agents to achieve rate control.
2. Anticoagulation with warfarin is mandatory for patients with atrial fibrillation (paroxysmal, persistent, or permanent) because they are at high risk for thromboembolism. It is also indicated in those with a history of prior embolism or known LA thrombus (ACC/AHA class I). It remains controversial whether anticoagulation should be used in patients with sinus rhythm but should be considered with dense spontaneous echo contrast on TEE or a severely enlarged atrium. The targeted international normalized ratio (INR) is typically between 2.0 and 3.0. At the present time, use of novel oral anticoagulants in patients with MS has not been investigated and should not be used. A case has been reported of a large LA thrombus in a patient with MS and atrial fibrillation taking dabigatran.
3. Pulmonary vein ablation has been performed in conjunction with balloon valvuloplasty for the treatment of atrial fibrillation.

D. Percutaneous balloon valvuloplasty. This technique has had a considerable impact on the management of patients with severe MS and is the procedure of choice in patients with favorable anatomy and no contraindications to the procedure. Favorable anatomy is defined as a pliable and relatively thin valve with a small amount of calcification and less than severe involvement of the subvalvular apparatus.

1. An echocardiographic score has been developed to help select patients who may be candidates for percutaneous valvuloplasty. The score has four components: mobility, leaflet thickening, subvalvular thickening, and calcification, each one ranging from 0 to 4. A score of 4 represents mild rheumatic involvement, and a score of 16 represents an immobile valve with fibrosis involving the entire leaflet and subvalvular apparatus and severe superimposed calcification. In general, extensive subvalvular disease results in a poorer outcome with valvuloplasty. Patients with extensive or asymmetric mitral valve calcification appear to have worse outcomes after percutaneous therapy. A total echocardiographic score of >11 is associated with an unfavorable outcome and a suboptimal increase in valve area, a higher incidence of heart failure and restenosis, and higher mortality. For patients with high scores, surgery is a better alternative if they are not at high risk of surgical complications.
2. Optimal results of balloon valvuloplasty are usually achieved when the echocardiographic score is 8 or less.
3. A modified score has been proposed with increased predictive value for acute success after balloon valvuloplasty. This score includes initial valve area, diastolic mitral leaflet displacement, commissural area ratio, and subvalvular thickening (Table 4.4).
4. The technique of percutaneous balloon valvuloplasty involves placement of a balloon-tipped catheter across the mitral valve through a transseptal puncture. The balloon is inflated in order to split the commissures. One or multiple balloon inflations are performed until there is significant improvement in mitral gradients or there is worsening MR.
   a. Typically, there is an increment in valve area of 1 cm^2, mainly as a result of splitting of the fused commissures. The mean valve area usually doubles with a 50% to 60% reduction in transmitral gradient. Favorable initial results, defined as valve area $\geq$1.5 cm^2 with MR $<$ moderate, are achieved in more than 80% of cases.

TABLE 4.4 New Score Proposed to Include Commissural Morphology

Variable	Assessment	Points
Mitral valve area $<1.0\ cm^2$	By planimetry	2
Maximal apical leaflet displacement ≤1.2 cm (doming height)	In the four-chamber view from the annulus to the tip of the mitral valve in diastole	3
Commissural area ratio >1.25	Measured in short axis. Planimetry of the medial half and lateral half of the valve. Ratio of larger/smaller half area	3
Subvalvular thickening	Absent or mild versus extensive thickening	3

NOTE: Low score is 0 to 3, intermediate score is 5, and high score is 6 to 11.
From Nunes MCP et al. *Circulation.* 2014;129:886.

b. This procedure is generally contraindicated in patients with > moderate MR or in whom there is an LA thrombus. Presence of concomitant severe aortic or tricuspid valve disease or coronary artery disease is a relative contraindication to the procedure. Major complications of percutaneous mitral valvuloplasty include procedural mortality (0.5% to 4%), hemopericardium (0.5% to 10%), embolism (0.5% to 5%), and severe regurgitation (2% to 10%).

5. Percutaneous balloon valvuloplasty or surgical therapy is indicated in patients with moderate or severe symptoms (New York Heart Association [NYHA] class II or greater) (Table 4.5). Balloon valvuloplasty is preferred to surgery if anatomy is favorable. Asymptomatic patients, with very severe MS and evidence of pulmonary hypertension at rest or with exercise, should also be considered for percutaneous therapy if the valve is suitable. Surgery should be reserved for more severe symptoms (functional class III to IV). Although significant pulmonary hypertension (pulmonary arterial systolic pressure >60 mm Hg) is not part of the current guidelines, it should be taken into account when considering the indication for mechanical treatment, along with presence of symptoms or significant decrease in functional capacity.

Rarely, for patients with asymptomatic MS, percutaneous intervention or surgery may be warranted. Indications include the following:

a. Patients with very severe MS (MVA $<1.0\ cm^2$) with favorable anatomy for balloon valvuloplasty

b. New-onset atrial fibrillation and favorable valve morphology (IIb)

c. Patients undergoing other cardiac surgery

d. Patients with repeated embolism despite anticoagulation, who may be considered for surgical intervention with LA appendage ligation performed simultaneously (class IIb indication)

e. In women with severe MS contemplating to become pregnant, valvuloplasty is an option. Percutaneous mitral balloon commissurotomy is also recommended (class I) before pregnancy for asymptomatic patients with severe MS (MVA $\leq 1.5\ cm^2$, stage C) who have valve morphology favorable for percutaneous mitral balloon commissurotomy.

6. TEE can be used during valvuloplasty to rule out LA and appendage thrombus as well as significant MR and for procedural guidance. If thrombosis is present, anticoagulation for at least 1 month is undertaken with repeat TEE to confirm

TABLE 4.5 Indications for Intervention in Patients with Mitral Stenosis (MS) According to the 2014 ACC/AHA Guidelines

Class I

Percutaneous mitral balloon valvuloplasty (PMBV) is indicated in ***symptomatic*** patients with severe MS and favorable anatomy and no contraindications.

Mitral valve surgery is indicated in ***severely symptomatic*** patients (New York Heart Association class III/IV) with severe MS who are not high risk for surgery and who are not candidates for or failed previous PMBV.

Concomitant mitral valve surgery is indicated for patients with severe MS undergoing other cardiac surgery.

Class IIa

PMBV is *reasonable* in ***symptomatic patients*** with severe MS and favorable anatomy and no contraindications.

Mitral valve surgery is *reasonable* in ***symptomatic patients*** with severe MS who could otherwise undergo PMBV but have other operative indications (tricuspid regurgitation, coronary artery disease).

Class IIb

PMBV could be considered for ***asymptomatic patients*** with severe MS and favorable valve morphology who have new onset of atrial fibrillation in the absence of contraindications.

PMBV may be considered for ***severely symptomatic*** patients with severe MS who have suboptimal valve anatomy and are not candidates for surgery or at high risk for surgery.

Concomitant mitral valve surgery may be considered for patients with moderate MS (mitral valve area 1.6–2.0 cm^2) undergoing other cardiac surgery.

Mitral valve surgery and excision of the left atrial appendage may be considered for patients with severe MS (symptomatic or not) who have had recurrent embolic events while receiving adequate anticoagulation.

resolution before valvuloplasty. TEE can also help guide balloon positioning and assess the gradient and degree of MR after each balloon inflation. Postprocedure MR is not well predicted by echocardiographic scores. The use of real-time 3DE has allowed evaluation of the commissural splitting. Bilateral commissural splitting is a surrogate for a successful procedure and has been related to better outcomes. The pressure half-time method is typically unreliable until 24 to 48 hours after the procedure. Postprocedure echocardiography should also assess for pericardial effusion and tamponade.

7. The frequency of restenosis of the valve is variable, depending on the age of the patient and the immediate procedural increment in valve area. Data from the National Heart, Lung, and Blood Institute registry of all functional classes of patients show an 84% survival rate 4 years after treatment. Advanced age, higher echo score, higher NYHA functional class, presence of atrial fibrillation, smaller initial MVA, higher pulmonary arterial pressure, and substantial tricuspid regurgitation are associated with poorer long-term results. These variables identify a population with more serious illness that frequently necessitates intervention and should not preclude valvuloplasty. More postprocedural MR and lower postprocedural MVA or lack of commissural splitting is associated with poorer long-term results.

VII. SURGICAL TREATMENT

Closed **commissurotomy** was the earliest surgical approach used to treat MS. It was performed through a thoracotomy (without cardiopulmonary bypass), and an atriotomy was performed by using a valve dilator or finger insertion to split the commissures. This procedure is rarely used in the United States and has been replaced by open mitral valvotomy, which involves direct visualization of the mitral valve on cardiopulmonary bypass, debridement of calcium, and splitting of fused commissures and chordae. In older patients, commissurotomy is rarely performed, and patients usually undergo mitral valve replacement. Randomized studies of balloon valvuloplasty versus open commissurotomy in ideal patients suggest equal improvement in valve area and symptoms immediately postprocedure and in medium-term follow-up.

Mitral valve repair is more difficult but can be performed in selected cases with commissurotomy when there is mixed MS/MR. In these cases, MS is in general not severe. Several factors favor the need for mitral valve replacement, including coexistent disease in other valves (e.g., aortic stenosis or aortic regurgitation) and extensive fibrosis and calcification, or concomitant MR.

For patients with long-standing atrial fibrillation, a combined Maze procedure (either surgical or using an intraoperative ablation catheter) can be performed in conjunction with the valve operation. LA appendage exclusion should also be added to reduce future cardioembolic risk. Left atrial appendage excision should be preferred to ligation given the high incidence of residual communication with LA cavity.

Patients who have undergone balloon valvuloplasty or operations for MS should undergo baseline echocardiography, preferably >72 hours after the procedure. Clinical follow-up examination should be performed at least once a year and more often if symptoms develop. It has become common practice at many centers for patients to undergo follow-up echocardiography on a yearly basis, although it may be less often in asymptomatic patients.

KEY PEARLS

- Mitral stenosis (MS) is predominantly due to rheumatic heart disease in the United States, though the prevalence is declining and other etiologies such as calcific disease of the annulus/leaflets are increasingly seen in the elderly population.
- There is a long asymptomatic course in patients with rheumatic MS, with most patients developing symptoms in the fourth or fifth decade of life. The most common symptoms are exertional dyspnea and decreasing exercise capacity.
- The auscultatory hallmark of rheumatic MS is the opening snap (OS) associated with a murmur, which is a low-pitched mid-diastolic rumble. Severe MS is associated with a longer duration murmur and a shorter duration A_2 (aortic second heart sound) to OS interval.
- The classic appearance of rheumatic MS by two-dimensional echocardiography is doming of the leaflets, reduced leaflet mobility, thickening and calcification of the leaflets and subvalvular apparatus, commissural fusion, and a fish-mouth appearance of leaflet opening.
- Determination of mitral valve area (MVA) can be obtained with (1) planimetry, (2) pressure half-time, (3) continuity equation, or (4) proximal convergence methods. Each method has limitations. Three-dimensional echocardiography–guided planimetry should be used if available.
- Assessment of severity of MS in the cardiac catheterization laboratory should be performed when there is discordance between clinical and echocardiographic information or suboptimal echocardiographic data. MVA is determined using the Gorlin or Hakki equations. Use of pulmonary capillary wedge pressure as a surrogate of LA pressure has limitations and often overestimates gradients and therefore overestimates severity of stenosis.

- Medical management of symptomatic MS is primarily with diuretics, β-blockers, and anti-coagulation for atrial fibrillation or select patients in sinus rhythm. Antibiotic prophylaxis for dental procedures is not recommended by current guidelines, though secondary prophylaxis for rheumatic fever should be used for 10 years or after the last episode or until the patient is 40 years old (whichever is longer).
- The 2014 American College of Cardiology/American Heart Association Valvular Heart Disease Guidelines define severe MS as an MVA of $\leq$1.5 cm^2 and very severe MS as a valve area of $\leq$1.0 cm^2.
- Percutaneous mitral balloon valvuloplasty (PMBV) is indicated in *symptomatic* patients with severe MS and favorable anatomy and no contraindications (class 1 recommendation).
- Mitral valve surgery is indicated in *severely symptomatic* patients (New York Heart Association class III/IV) with severe MS who are not high risk for surgery and who are not candidates for failed previous PMBV (class 1 recommendation).

SUGGESTED READINGS

Chandrashekhar Y, Westaby S, Narula J. Mitral stenosis. *Lancet.* 2009;374:1271.

Cheriex EC, Pieters FA, Janssen JH, et al. Value of exercise Doppler-echocardiography in patients with mitral stenosis. *Int J Cardiol.* 1994;45:219–226.

Gorlin WB, Gorlin RJ. A generalized formulation of the Gorlin formula for calculating the area of the stenotic mitral valve and other stenotic cardiac valves. *Am Coll Cardiol.* 1990;15:246–247.

Leavitt JI, Coats MH, Falk RH. Effects of exercise on transmitral gradient and pulmonary artery pressure in patients with mitral stenosis or a prosthetic mitral valve: a Doppler echocardiographic study. *J Am Coll Cardiol.* 1991;17:1520–1526.

Muñoz S, Gallardo J, DiazGorrin J, et al. Influence of surgery on the natural history of rheumatic mitral and aortic valve disease. *Am J Cardiol.* 1975;35:234–242.

Reyes VP, Raju BS, Wynne J, et al. Percutaneous balloon valvuloplasty compared with open surgical commissurotomy for mitral stenosis. *N Engl J Med.* 1994;331:961–967.

Sagie A, Freitas N, Padial LR, et al. Doppler echocardiographic assessment of long-term progression of mitral stenosis in 103 patients: valve area and right heart disease. *J Am Coll Cardiol.* 1996;28:472.

Schlosshan D, Aggarwal G, Mathur G, et al. Real-time 3D transesophageal echocardiography for the evaluation of rheumatic mitral stenosis. *JACC Cardiovasc Imaging.* 2011;4:580.

Thomas JD, Wilkins GT, Choong CY, et al. Inaccuracy of mitral pressure half-time immediately after percutaneous mitral valvotomy: dependence on transmitral gradient and left atrial and ventricular compliance. *Circulation.* 1988;78:980–993.

Wilkins G, Weyman A, Abascal M, et al. Percutaneous balloon dilatation of the mitral valve: an analysis of echocardiographic variables related to outcome and the mechanism of dilatation. *Br Heart J.* 1988;60:299–308.

CHAPTER 5

Serge C. Harb
Brian P. Griffin

Mitral Regurgitation

I. INTRODUCTION

A. **Mitral valve anatomy** (**Fig. 5.1**). The mitral valve (MV) consists of two leaflets—the anterior and posterior leaflets.

1. The **anterior leaflet** is triangular in shape and larger and thicker than the posterior leaflet, accounting for most of the closing surface area of the mitral orifice. Its broad surface is divided into anterior and posterior areas. The anterior leaflet attaches at its base to the mitral annulus in continuity with the aortic valve through the fibrous aortic–mitral curtain.
2. The posterior leaflet is crescent shaped and has a longer attachment to the mitral annulus, compared to the anterior leaflet. It is segmented into three scallops that are separated by clefts: segment 1 is anterolateral, segment 2 is in the middle, and segment 3 is posteromedial.
3. The anterior and posterior leaflets meet at two commissures: the posteromedial and anterolateral commissures. The mitral annulus is a C-shaped fibromuscular ring at the base of the left ventricle (LV) to which the MV leaflets attach. It has a three-dimensional (3D) saddle shape with its "lowest points" at the level of both commissures.

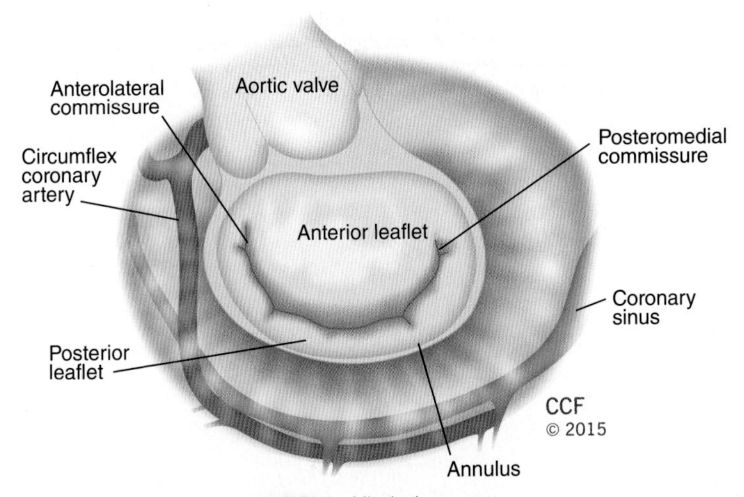

FIGURE 5.1 Mitral valve anatomy.

4. The chordae tendineae are thin fibrous structures that attach the leaflets to the two papillary muscles in the LV. Normal chordae vary widely in number and appearance, and are designated according to their insertion site on the leaflet.
   a. Primary chordae (marginal chordae) insert on the free margins of the leaflets. They play a major role in leaflet coaptation and prevent prolapse.
   b. Secondary chordae (basal or strut chordae) insert on the leaflets' ventricular surface, providing structural support and preventing leaflet billowing.
   c. Tertiary chordae insert on the mitral annulus and posterior leaflet base and also contribute to leaflet structural support.
   d. Of note, there are also commissural chordae (distinct from the leaflet chordae), which insert into the free margins of the two commissures.
5. The papillary muscles (anterolateral and posteromedial) originate from the LV free wall between the apex and middle third of the ventricular cavity. The anterolateral papillary muscle has usually two heads, anterior and posterior, whereas the posteromedial papillary muscle usually has three heads, anterior, intermediate, and posterior.

   Anatomic variations in papillary muscle anatomy, including their origin, shape, and number of heads, have important pathologic consequences. For instance, anterior displacement of the papillary muscles may cause leaflet slack and increased residual leaflet length, which may have an impact on the production of systolic anterior motion.

   The posteromedial papillary muscle has a single blood supply usually from the posterior descending artery, whereas the anterolateral papillary muscle is supplied by both the left anterior descending artery and left circumflex artery. Because of differences in blood supply, the posteromedial papillary muscle is more vulnerable to rupture than the anterolateral papillary muscle in the setting of myocardial infarction.

B. **Surgical classification.** A segmental anatomy of the mitral leaflets proposed by Carpentier helps with the description of the localization of specific MV lesions. Because the posterior leaflet is naturally segmented by clefts at the free edge into three scallops, the Carpentier classification divides the posterior leaflet into three corresponding segments (P1, P2, and P3) from lateral to medial (P1 is the most lateral and P3 is the most medial). The anterior leaflet (devoid of clefts) is then also divided into three segments (A1, A2, and A3) that are opposing each of the corresponding posterior scallops (the segment opposing P1 is A1, the segment opposing P2 is A2, and the segment opposing P3 is A3)—see Figure 5.2.

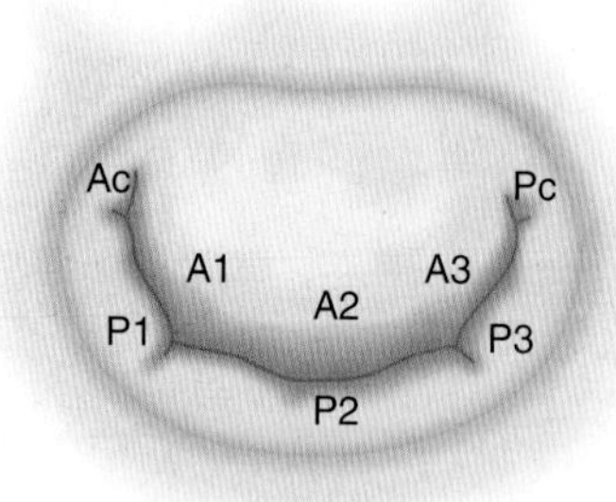

FIGURE 5.2 Segmental anatomy of the mitral leaflets. Ac, anterior commissure; Pc, posterior commissure.

In most cases, transthoracic echocardiography (TTE) is sufficient to visualize all three segments and the commissures; however, in some instances, advanced echocardiographic techniques (3D echocardiography [3D echo] and transesophageal echocardiography [TEE]) are required for a better understanding of the MV anatomy, especially when surgery is contemplated.

II. PATHOPHYSIOLOGY

A. Pathoanatomy (Fig. 5.3). The pathologic causes of mitral regurgitation (MR) can be classified anatomically as follows:

1. **Leaflet abnormalities,** which in turn may be subclassified into:
   - Excessive leaflet motion due to MV prolapse (MVP) or as seen in leaflet, chordal, or papillary muscle disruption. In these cases, the jet of MR is directed away from the affected leaflet.
   - Normal leaflet motion, as seen in cases of leaflet perforation due to endocarditis, or in congenital MV disorders (cleft MV, double orifice MV [DOMV]). In these situations, the MR jet may be central or eccentric.
   - Restricted leaflet motion from distortion/scarring as seen in rheumatic valvular disease, connective tissue disorders, ischemic MR (IMR), and in the healing phase of endocarditis. In such instances, the jet of MR is directed toward the affected leaflet.
2. **Mitral annular abnormalities**
   - **a.** Annular dilation from left atrium (LA) or LV enlargement with resultant loss of adequate leaflet coaptation.
   - **b.** Mitral annular calcifications causing restricted motion of the annulus and loss of its sphincter activity.
3. **Chordal abnormalities**
   - **a.** Chordal elongation and in severe forms chordal rupture (flail) due to myxomatous degeneration as seen in MVP.
   - **b.** Chordal fibrosis and calcification as may occur in rheumatic heart disease.
4. **Papillary muscle abnormalities**
   - **a.** Displacement and hypertrophy of the papillary muscles, contributing to systolic anterior motion in hypertrophic cardiomyopathy.
   - **b.** Rupture as may occur in the setting of myocardial infarction.
   - **c.** Dysfunction, usually from an ischemic insult.

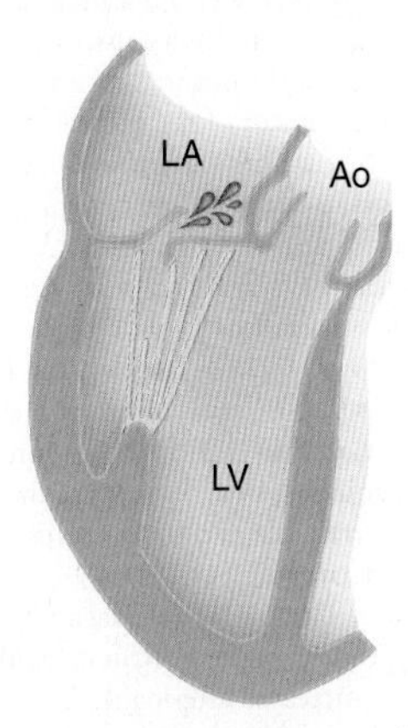

FIGURE 5.3 Pathoanatomy of the mitral valve. Ao, aorta; LA, left atrium, LV, left ventricle.

5. **Left ventricle abnormalities.** The LV can contribute to MR through two major mechanisms:
   - Restricted motion of the posterior leaflet from inferoposterior wall scarring as occurs with myocardial infarction
   - LV spherical remodeling with decreased contractility and geometric alterations of the MV apparatus (tenting and tethering of the leaflets) as occurs with dilated cardiomyopathy (DCM)

B. Cardiac effects of mitral regurgitation

MR burdens the LV with an excessive volume load that leads to a series of compensatory adjustments that vary during the course of the disease. The impact of MR is determined by the magnitude of the regurgitant volume (ReVol) and the time course of development of the regurgitation.

1. **Acute mitral regurgitation.** There is a sudden increase in preload (LV end-diastolic volume) because of the ReVol returning from the LA. The ventricle utilizes its preload reserve, and the Frank–Starling mechanism contributes to an increase in the total stroke volume. The normal LV compliance (the LV did not have time to accommodate) limits the increase in end-diastolic volume to a modest rise. Therefore, a significant increase in LV filling pressures occurs. LV afterload (wall stress) is decreased as most of the blood is ejected into the lower resistance LA. The increase in LV preload and the decrease in afterload result in increases in ejection fraction (EF) and total stroke volume. Forward cardiac output declines, however, because much of the flow is directed to the LA. The major burden and threat is to the pulmonary venous circulation and the lungs, leading to pulmonary edema. Although most patients require urgent surgery, some evolve into a chronic state.
2. **Chronic mitral regurgitation.** The natural history of chronic MR can be divided into three stages: an early compensated stage during which most patients remain free of symptoms, a transitional stage where there is progressive and adverse LV remodeling, and ultimately the decompensated stage marked by the development of symptoms. The progression may be insidious; thus, it is extremely important to identify deleterious LV changes and recommend surgical intervention prior to the development of irreversible LV damage.
   a. Compensated stage. Chronic volume overload leads to progressive LV enlargement. Eccentric hypertrophy develops as new sarcomeres are added "in series." Systolic wall stress is normalized as a consequence of the hypertrophy. During this compensated stage, both contractility and EF are normal, but total stroke volume is increased as a result of the increased end-diastolic volume.
   b. Transitional stage. Structural and functional remodeling of the ventricle occurs and compensatory mechanisms start to fail. There is progressive increase in the ReVol and a decrease in LV contractile function with an increase in wall stress. EF starts declining below 60%, but usually remains above 50%. This phase is difficult to identify clinically because most patients are asymptomatic. In such cases, an elevated B-type natriuretic peptide or abnormal echocardiographic strain pattern may raise the concern for latent ventricular dysfunction. Surgical intervention at this point may lead to a "paradoxical" worsening of the EF because the low-resistance "pathway" to the LA is no longer available and the LV must eject all its blood against the higher resistance normal pathway (aorta).
   c. Decompensated stage. There is substantial and progressive LV dilation leading to a depressed myocardial state (with increased LV diastolic pressures) and increased wall stress (increased afterload). As a consequence, there is a decline in the EF below 50%. At this stage, these deleterious changes often preclude an optimal result after surgical correction of the regurgitation.

III. CLINICAL PRESENTATION

The clinical manifestations of MR, symptoms, physical examination findings, and electrocardiographic or radiographic changes are mainly determined by the rapidity of MR development.

A. Acute mitral regurgitation

1. **Signs and symptoms:** Patients with acute severe MR usually present in cardiogenic shock with the sudden onset and rapid progression of pulmonary edema (leading quickly to dyspnea at rest and marked orthopnea) and hypotension (with signs of poor perfusion: peripheral vasoconstriction, pallor, and diaphoresis). It is frequently a cardiac emergency; patients are severely ill and require urgent medical and surgical treatment. The presentation may be less dramatic if acute MR is superimposed on chronic MR. In this case, patients will note a marked worsening of their symptoms with sudden increase in their shortness of breath, dyspnea on exertion, fatigue, and weakness.
2. **Cardiac exam:** The arterial pulse is usually rapid and of low amplitude (decreased forward output) with a hyperdynamic cardiac impulse. On auscultation, the systolic murmur is often short and soft owing to the rapid equilibration of pressures between the LV and LA. An S_3 is often present.
3. **Electrocardiography:** ECG findings are nonspecific; however, the ECG may reveal the etiology of the acute MR (myocardial infarction, for example).
4. **Chest radiography:** Typically, there is evidence of bilateral pulmonary edema with a normal cardiac silhouette.

B. Chronic mitral regurgitation

1. **Signs and symptoms:** Patients may remain asymptomatic for years despite severe MR. Symptoms will develop with the occurrence of:
   a. LV failure with progressive increments in the ReVol and chamber size. The LV compensatory mechanisms will ultimately fail with further increase in LV size and reduction in LV contractile function with resultant congestive heart failure. Exercise intolerance and dyspnea on exertion usually occur first, then as the MR progresses, further symptoms will manifest.
   b. Atrial fibrillation due to the dilated LA. Paroxysmal or persistent atrial fibrillation is common and may be the initial presentation of chronic MR.
   c. Pulmonary hypertension. The progressive chronic increase in LA pressure may affect the pulmonary circulation leading to secondary pulmonary hypertension with resultant right ventricular (RV) failure, manifesting with elevated jugular venous pressure, peripheral edema, and hepatomegaly.
2. **Cardiac exam**
   a. The apical impulse is displaced to the left secondary to LV enlargement.
   b. Heart sounds: S_1 is diminished (mitral leaflets do not close properly) and an S_3 is usually heard (LV enlargement and/or failure).
   c. Murmur: Most commonly, the murmur is holosystolic, heard best at the apex and radiating to the axilla. Its characteristics (timing, duration, quality, intensity, location, and radiation) vary with the etiology of MR. It may be distinguished from other systolic murmurs by the following:
      - It has little respiratory variation.
      - It is louder with squatting or isometric handgrip (these maneuvers lead to increased afterload and subsequently more regurgitation).

      There is modest correlation between the grade of the murmur and the severity of regurgitation. This correlation is better in primary rather than secondary MR.
3. **Electrocardiography:** Although nonspecific, common features include LA enlargement, atrial fibrillation, LV hypertrophy, and, in the event of secondary RV failure, RV hypertrophy.

4. **Chest radiography:** Cardiomegaly (from LA and LV enlargement) is typically seen. Pulmonary edema may manifest with progressive LV failure.

IV. CLASSIFICATION OF MITRAL REGURGITATION ETIOLOGIES

A practical classification of the etiologies of MR is shown in Figure 5.4.

A. **Acute MR.** There are two major mechanisms of acute MR:

1. **Nonischemic:** affecting the leaflets and/or chordae.
   a. Ruptured mitral chordae leading to a "flail" leaflet. This can occur spontaneously but also can be seen in patients with:
      - MVP
      - Infective endocarditis
      - Trauma
      - Rheumatic heart disease
   b. Leaflet perforation from infective endocarditis.
2. **Ischemic:** mainly affecting the papillary muscles
   a. Papillary muscle rupture due to acute myocardial infarction (MI), with rupture of the posteromedial muscle being more common because of its single

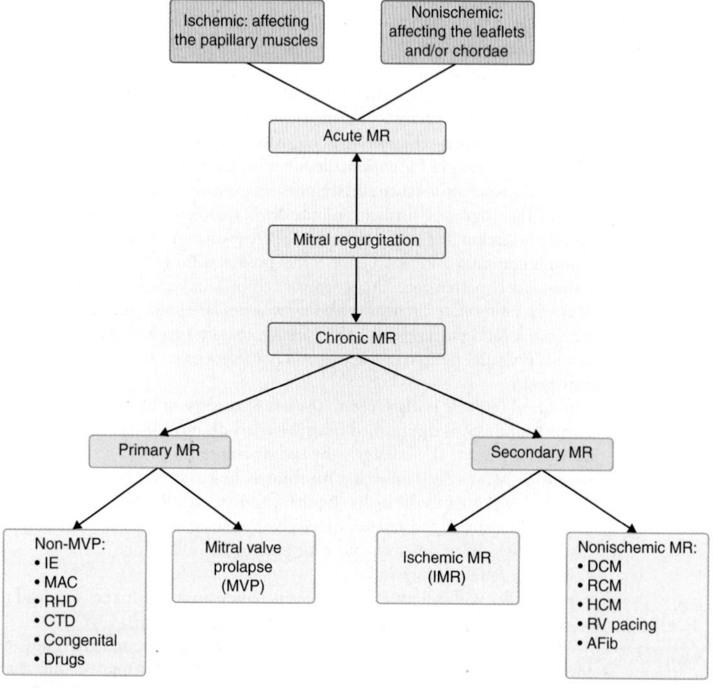

FIGURE 5.4 Practical classification of MR etiologies. AFib, atrial fibrillation; CTD, connective tissue disorder; DCM, dilated cardiomyopathy; HCM, hypertrophic cardiomyopathy; IE, infective endocarditis; MAC, mitral annular calcification; MR, mitral regurgitation; RCM, restrictive cardiomyopathy; RHD, rheumatic heart disease; RV, right ventricle.

blood supply. Of note, acute MI can also lead to chordal rupture, and there are described cases of papillary muscle rupture as a result of cardiac trauma.

b. Papillary muscle infarction in the setting of acute MI (without necessary rupture) can also lead to acute MR.

c. Acute ischemia can cause transient LV dysfunction/dilation with resultant papillary muscle displacement and subsequent MR. This is often termed "reversible IMR" because prompt correction of the ischemic substrate will typically correct the MR.

B. Chronic mitral regurgitation. In chronic MR, it is important to distinguish between primary and secondary MR.

1. Primary mitral regurgitation: Valve incompetence is caused by pathology of at least one of the components of the MV (leaflets, chordae tendineae, papillary muscles, annulus). Etiologies include:

a. Mitral valve prolapse: also called degenerative or myxomatous MV disease. It is recognized as the major cause of MR in developed countries.

b. Infective endocarditis: valvular insufficiency results from infection-induced valvular damage.

c. Mitral annular calcification: common finding in the elderly. Calcification of the mitral annulus increases with age and is often associated with mild-to-moderate MR. It is rarely the cause of severe MR.

d. Rheumatic heart disease: more common in developing countries. While it usually causes mitral stenosis in adults, rheumatic heart disease often causes MR in children.

e. Valvular involvement in connective tissue disorders (e.g., systemic lupus erythematosus). This often progresses over time as acute inflammation of the valve, with disease episodes leading to scarring, leaflet retraction, and impaired coaptation.

f. Congenital MR: due to a cleft valve, for example.

g. Drugs: mainly anorectics (especially the combination of fenfluramine and phentermine called fen/phen) but also ergot derivatives and drugs used in the treatment of Parkinson disease. The mechanism seems related to increased serotoninergic activity with resultant increase in fibrosis at the valvular level.

2. Secondary mitral regurgitation: This is also referred to as functional MR because the MV anatomy is usually grossly normal, though histologic and biochemical abnormalities have been reported. MR in that case is caused by annular enlargement secondary to LV dilation and/or papillary muscle displacement secondary to LV remodeling.

Secondary MR is the most common valve disease, with ischemic heart disease accounting for approximately one-third of cases. It can thus be divided into IMR and nonischemic MR (NIMR).

a. Ischemic mitral regurgitation includes a spectrum of disorders comprising chronic MR post MI, acute MR with acute MI, and reversible MR as a result of myocardial ischemia.

b. Nonischemic mitral regurgitation is the form of MR found in all types of nonischemic cardiomyopathy, including DCM, restrictive cardiomyopathy, and hypertrophic cardiomyopathy. NIMR can also be secondary to RV pacing and atrial fibrillation.

i. Dilated cardiomyopathy: MR is due to annular dilation with displacement of the papillary muscles, which migrate laterally as the LV becomes more spherical with remodeling. The MR will increase the load on the LV and lead to its further dilation, which will worsen the MR—thus the saying "MR begets MR."

ii. Restrictive cardiomyopathy: The mechanism of MR depends on the etiology. For instance, in amyloidosis, the valve itself may be involved by amyloid deposition. In addition, severe LA enlargement (frequent in amyloid heart disease) can lead to annular dilation. In contrast, MR in Loeffler endocarditis (hypereosinophilic syndrome) is due to scarring and fibrosis of the chordae tendineae.

iii. Hypertrophic cardiomyopathy: MR in this case is multifactorial: altered geometry of the LV, systolic anterior motion of the anterior leaflet, and anatomic abnormalities of the leaflets and chordae tendineae.

iv. Right ventricular pacing: RV pacing leads to dyssynchronous contraction of the left and right ventricles. This dyssynchrony may alter the optimal functioning of the papillary muscles and lead to MR that can be severe.

v. Atrial fibrillation: Although the most common scenario is MR leading to atrial enlargement with secondary atrial fibrillation, long-standing atrial fibrillation on its own may lead to MR. The proposed mechanism is the following: long-standing atrial fibrillation results in an enlarged LA with subsequent significant mitral annular dilation. The stretched mitral annulus prevents adequate leaflet coaptation, which results in functional MR. Restoration of sinus rhythm in these patients may lead to a reduction in atrial size and annular dilation with resultant improvement in the degree of regurgitation.

V. MITRAL VALVE PROLAPSE

A. Epidemiology. MVP is the most common cause of chronic primary MR in developed countries, accounting for over 50% of cases. Its prevalence varies among studies depending on the criteria used for diagnosis. Using the currently accepted definition of MVP, the overall prevalence is 2.4%, with equal occurrence in men and women.

B. Definition. Prolapse of the MV is defined as an abnormal systolic displacement (systolic billowing) of one or both leaflets into the LA. Based on the current echocardiographic criteria, MVP is diagnosed when either or both leaflets are displaced 2 mm or more in systole above a line connecting the annular hinge points in a long-axis view (parasternal or apical long axis). A long-axis view is required because even normal leaflets may appear to break the annular plane in other imaging views, owing to the 3-D saddle-shaped anatomy of the MV.

C. Pathology. MVP results from myxomatous degeneration of the MV, which is characterized by abnormal accumulation of mucopolysaccharides, leading to excessive leaflet tissue with elongated chordae prone to rupture. A wide spectrum of pathologic changes are observed with two relatively distinct ends but considerable overlap.

1. **Classic MVP or Barlow disease:** Commonly seen in younger patients, this is characterized by severe myxomatous degeneration. The leaflets are markedly thickened (≥5 mm) and diffusely redundant with prolapse of most of the segments. The chordae are elongated and thickened, and the annulus is typically dilated.
2. **Nonclassic MVP or fibroelastic deficiency:** Typically seen in older patients, this is characterized primarily by chordal rupture (from lack of connective tissue) with resultant leaflet displacement. Usually, only one segment (most commonly P2) is involved. The leaflets are thin and moderately redundant with a mildly enlarged annulus.

Note: There is a pseudo MVP form: Pseudo MVP is seen when there is a disproportion in the size of the valve leaflets to the LV cavity size. Thus, this may occur in conditions where the LV size is relatively small such as in atrial septal defect or may occur in adolescents with morphologic changes in growth. The leaflets are not thickened but may appear to prolapse in some views and often normalize over time.

D. Classification. MVP may be classified into sporadic MVP, familial MVP, and MVP associated with connective tissue disorders.

1. Sporadic: Many cases of MVP are sporadic with no other family member affected and no identifiable connective tissue disorder. It may be accompanied by myxomatous degeneration and prolapse of other valves, particularly the tricuspid valve.
2. Familial: In this form, the inheritance is considered to be autosomal dominant with variable penetrance. Three loci have been identified in extended families with multiple affected members, mapped to chromosomes 11, 13, and 16.
3. Associated with connective tissue disorder: MVP is common in patients with Marfan, Ehlers–Danlos, Loeys–Dietz, and osteogenesis imperfecta syndromes.

E. **Clinical features**

1. **Symptoms:** Most patients are asymptomatic. The diagnosis is usually suspected from cardiac auscultation and then confirmed by echocardiography. When MVP is complicated by significant MR, symptoms due to valve insufficiency are present. Atypical chest pain is common among patients with MVP, the mechanism of which is unknown. A constellation of other symptoms including fatigue, orthostatic hypotension, palpitations, syncope, panic attack, and anxiety were thought to occur more frequently in patients with MVP and were known as the "MVP syndrome." However, newer studies using the current updated definition of MVP have suggested that these symptoms are no more common in true MVP than in the rest of the population.
2. **Physical exam:** The typical auscultatory features of MVP are the nonejection click and the murmur of MR.
   a. The click is thought to result from stretching of the redundant leaflets and chordae. It is mid-systolic to late-systolic and dynamic.
   b. The murmur is absent if prolapse does not lead to regurgitation. When MR is present, the murmur is typically late-systolic early in the course of the disease, and then becomes holosystolic with severe prolapse. Its maximal intensity and radiation vary with the direction of the jet: a posteriorly directed jet from anterior leaflet prolapse may be well appreciated at the back.
   c. Effect of diagnostic maneuvers: Certain maneuvers can produce dynamic changes in the auscultatory findings of MVP.
      i. Maneuvers that reduce venous return and decrease the LV volume, such as standing or the Valsalva maneuver, lead to earlier occurrence of the prolapse, causing the systolic click to occur earlier and the murmur to become longer in duration.
      ii. On the other hand, maneuvers that increase venous return (leg raising or lying down) or afterload (squatting or isometric handgrip) delay the occurrence of the prolapse, causing the click to occur later and the murmur to be shorter in duration.

F. **Complications.** Although commonly a benign condition, MVP is associated with significant complications that are more likely to occur in men. These complications can be grouped into arrhythmic and nonarrhythmic.

1. **Arrhythmic complications**
   a. Sudden cardiac death (SCD): MVP appears to be associated with a low but higher than average rate of SCD. It is presumably attributed to ventricular arrhythmias; however, some studies have suggested that it may be directly related to MR, rather than MVP itself. Risk factors include significant MR, more severe myxomatous changes in the valve tissue, and decreased LV function. Despite this, no specific recommendations for risk stratification have been defined, and the role for electrophysiologic testing in these patients has not been established.
   b. ECG abnormalities: Multiple electrical abnormalities have been reported in MVP: flattening or inversion of the T wave, QT prolongation, and false-positive ST-segment depression in response to exercise. These findings, however, are not supported by all studies.

c. Arrhythmias: While arrhythmias may be more common in MVP patients who develop MR, it is unclear whether their incidence is higher in patients without valvular regurgitation.

2. **Nonarrhythmic complications**

a. Mitral regurgitation: Myxomatous degeneration of the leaflets and chordae leads to loss of MV competence with resultant MR. The majority of MVP patients have mild MR; significant MR occurs in approximately 2% to 7% of cases. However, once regurgitation occurs, it may be progressive over time and needs to be followed closely.

b. Infective endocarditis: Patients with MVP are at higher risk for infected endocarditis; however, the absolute risk is low and the new valvular guidelines no longer recommend antibiotic prophylaxis for patients with MVP either with or without MR unless the patient has suffered a previous bout of endocarditis. Risk factors for infected endocarditis include age (>45 years), male gender, presence of a systolic murmur, and more severe myxomatous changes in the valve tissue.

c. Cerebrovascular accident (CVA): Data are conflicting—it appears that the risk of CVA is increased in patients with complicated MVP (by MR and atrial fibrillation in particular) or those with comorbidities, but the risk is low in young people with uncomplicated MVP.

VI. ISCHEMIC MITRAL REGURGITATION

A. **Definition.** While MR can occur in the acute setting of myocardial ischemia/infarction as previously discussed, the term *ischemic mitral regurgitation* (IMR) is commonly used to describe chronic postinfarction MR. It is the most common form of secondary MR. It is considered secondary, or functional, because the mechanism of MR is largely ventricular rather than valvular.

B. **Mechanism.** Various processes have been implicated in the pathophysiology of IMR (Fig. 5.5) including LV remodeling with resultant papillary muscle displacement and mitral annular dilation, LV dyssynchrony including papillary muscle dyssynchrony, and impaired LV contractility leading to alteration in the forces required for appropriate

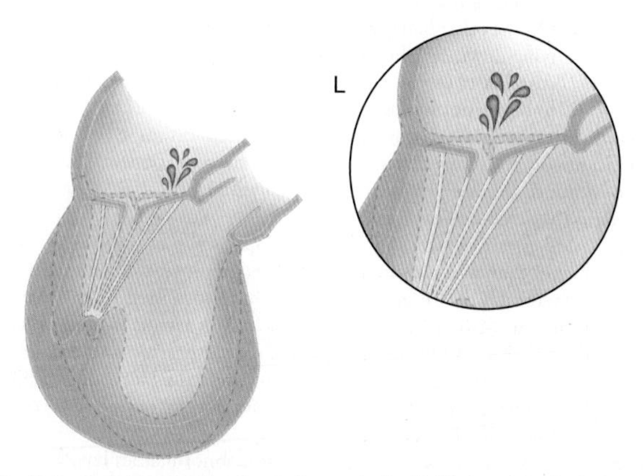

FIGURE 5.5 Pathophysiology of ischemic mitral regurgitation (IMR). As evident in the figure, there is distortion of the left ventricular geometry, with resultant annular dilation and papillary muscle displacement causing tethering of the chordae and restricted leaflet closure. All these changes lead to IMR. L, larger view.

MV closure. The relative importance of each of these processes depends largely on the distribution of coronary artery disease:

1. In the setting of inferior MI, typically caused by right coronary or left circumflex artery disease, the resultant inferobasal wall motion abnormalities lead to tethering of the posteromedial papillary muscle. This causes a restricted motion of the posterior leaflet and subsequently a posteriorly directed jet of MR.
2. In the setting of anterior MI, typically caused by left anterior descending artery disease, alterations in LV geometry—mainly spherical remodeling—and decreased LV contractility lead to papillary muscle displacement and affect the tension exerted on the leaflets. This results in apical tenting of the MV leaflets with failure to close completely.

C. **Dynamic nature of ischemic mitral regurgitation.** The severity of IMR changes with varying loading/hemodynamic conditions: for instance, exercise, hypertensive crisis, and other stressors may induce dynamic changes in LV wall motion contractility and geometry, with resultant worsening of MR. Stress echocardiography may uncover more severe MR in these circumstances. Conversely, the severity of IMR may be underestimated in the operating room: sedation and anesthesia decrease LV afterload and inotropic medications increase LV contractility, both resulting in better mitral coaptation and less MR. Thus, IMR should be evaluated in the preoperative setting under normal loading conditions.

D. **Prognosis.** IMR portends a poor prognosis. It is associated with increased mortality (even a mild degree of MR in the setting of ischemic heart disease affects survival negatively) as well as increased risk of developing heart failure. In fact, studies have shown that patients who develop MR following MI had higher mortality. IMR was also an important predictor of the development of heart failure, even in patients with a normal LV ejection fraction (LVEF) at the time of the MI. It is unclear whether the MR by itself causes the poor outcome, as its surgical correction at the time of coronary artery bypass grafting has little effect on survival.

Outcome studies in IMR have shown poorer prognosis with effective regurgitant orifice (ERO) $\geq$20 mm^2. For this reason, the 2014 valvular guidelines adopted an ERO $\geq$20 mm^2 to define severe secondary MR as opposed to the cutoff of ERO $\geq$40 mm^2 used to define severe primary MR.

VII. NONISCHEMIC MITRAL REGURGITATION IN DILATED CARDIOMYOPATHY

A. **Introduction.** NIMR in DCM is one of the most common forms of functional or secondary MR; some degree of functional MR is almost always present in patients with severe DCM, regardless of the etiology.

B. **Pathophysiology.** In functional MR, a primary ventricular pathology leads to development of regurgitation through an anatomically normal valve. The mechanisms involved are:

Annular dilation secondary to LV enlargement leading to a central area of failed leaflet coaptation.

Tethering and excess tenting of the leaflets because of papillary muscle displacement secondary to LV remodeling. MV tenting has been suggested as the most powerful predictor of functional MR.

The regurgitant flow in functional MR is variable: there is an early systolic peak, a mid-systolic decrease, and a late, smaller late-systolic peak. These variations are closely associated with changes in transmitral pressure and occur in association with parallel changes in regurgitant orifice area.

It is interesting to note that the frequency of LV thrombus is lower in patients with advanced heart failure when functional MR is present, presumably because of higher flow rates.

C. **Prognosis.** Functional MR is associated with a decreased survival in patients with DCM. RV dysfunction may be a predictor of poor outcome among patients with functional MR. In one study, RV systolic function (as assessed by tricuspid annular plane systolic excursion) was an independent predictor of freedom from all-cause mortality or hospitalization.

D. Treatment. There is no proven long-term survival benefit from MV surgery. This is reflected in the 2014 valve guidelines, which give weak recommendations for MV surgery in patients with secondary MR. Treatment of functional MR should emphasize optimal medical therapy of the cardiomyopathy and, in appropriate patients, cardiac resynchronization therapy (CRT).

VIII. RHEUMATIC MITRAL REGURGITATION

A. Introduction. Rheumatic fever is responsible for a wide array of cardiac diseases, and the pathology frequently involves the MV.

B. Acute manifestations. In its acute phase, acute rheumatic fever (ARF) causes valvulitis, of which the most common early manifestation is MR. The MR in ARF is often caused by MVP. In contrast to myxomatous disease, which more commonly involves the posterior leaflet and is associated with prominent leaflet redundancy, the MVP in ARF predominantly involves the anterior leaflet and is associated with minimal leaflet redundancy. Other echocardiographic findings besides MVP include leaflet thickening and verrucous vegetations.

C. Chronic manifestations. In the years following an episode of ARF, progressive valvular disease will commonly develop owing to scarring and eventually calcification of the damaged leaflets.

In rheumatic heart disease, the MV is involved in nearly all cases, but the incidence and pattern of MV pathology will vary according to age and time since last episode of ARF: patients aged less than 30 years will tend to have pure MR, while those who are middle aged will usually develop mitral stenosis. In contrast, older patients often have mixed MV disease.

D. Management. The indications for valve surgery are similar to those with MR of nonrheumatic origin and are discussed separately. However, the particularity of rheumatic heart disease is that it typically leads to progressive fibrotic thickening of the mitral leaflets and the chordal structures.

This scar burden can limit the durability of the valve repair, and reoperation can be required in up to 20% of cases at 10 years. In comparison, MV replacement appears to be associated with similar outcomes, albeit with slightly lower rates of reoperation than MV repair.

IX. CONNECTIVE TISSUE DISORDERS–RELATED MITRAL REGURGITATION

Connective tissue disorders, inherited or autoimmune, can involve the MV, causing MVP. MVP has been described in a wide range of connective tissue disorders, including Ehlers–Danlos syndrome, Marfan syndrome, osteogenesis imperfecta, rheumatoid arthritis (mainly nodular rheumatoid arthritis), and systemic lupus erythematosus.

Particular to SLE is verrucous endocarditis, also known as Libman–Sacks endocarditis, consisting of valvular vegetations ranging from small nodules to large verrucous lesions and forming near the edge of the valve. These vegetations consist of fibrin and platelet thrombi, immune complexes, hematoxylin bodies, and mononuclear cells. SLE patients with antiphospholipids (aPLs) appear to have a significantly higher involvement of valvular defects than those without aPLs.

Verrucous endocarditis is typically asymptomatic. If the lesions are extensive, the healing process of the valve would lead to fibrosis and distortion, and subsequently dysfunction and regurgitation of the MV. The verrucous lesions can also fragment and produce systemic emboli. In addition, infective endocarditis can develop on the damaged valves.

X. CONGENITAL MITRAL REGURGITATION

Congenital malformations of the MV may be found to be either isolated or associated with other congenital heart defects, such as isolated cleft of the MV and DOMV.

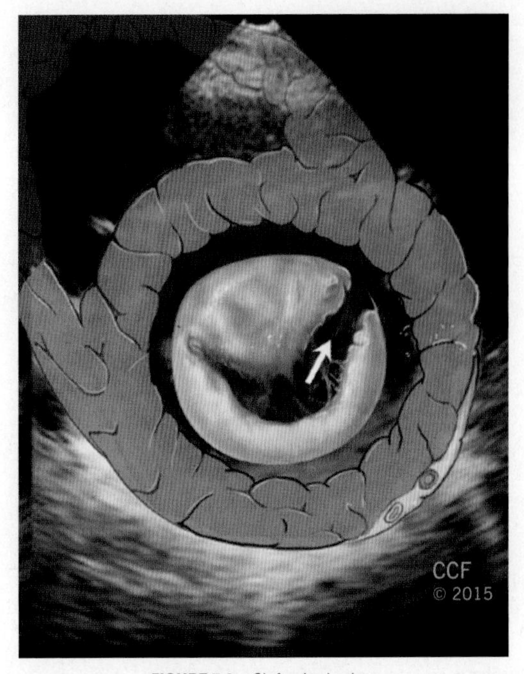

FIGURE 5.6 Cleft mitral valve.

A. **Isolated cleft of the mitral valve (Fig. 5.6, *arrow* points to cleft).** The cleft is a separation in the MV leaflet. The anterior leaflet of the MV is almost always involved, although a cleft of the posterior leaflet has been described. Congenital clefts of the MV are frequently associated with an atrioventricular septal defect, and an isolated cleft in the anterior mitral leaflet is an infrequent finding. Isolated MV cleft can cause severe MR but has good surgical outcomes. Its repair consists of a direct suture of the cleft and is preferred over MV replacement. If the cleft is not repaired early on, the leaflet edges will get thicker and retracted, making repair by direct suture more complicated; in this case, the insertion of an autologous pericardial patch on the MV is preferred.

B. **Double orifice mitral valve (Fig. 5.7).** DOMV is a very rare malformation consisting of two orifices in the left atrioventricular valve zone. Each of those orifices has its own chordal attachment to the papillary muscle. Most commonly, DOMV is associated with other congenital malformations. The clinical presentation and surgical repair or replacement depend on the associated cardiac abnormality and the degree of the resulting MR and/or stenosis. When DOMV is isolated, it is usually asymptomatic and requires no repair.

XI. ECHOCARDIOGRAPHY

Echocardiography plays a central role in the evaluation of MR: it is essential to determination of the mechanism, the presumed underlying cause, the severity, and, where appropriate, the feasibility of various interventions to reduce MR severity such as surgery or percutaneous catheter technologies. Echocardiographic data are pivotal for follow-up, clinical decision-making, and surgical planning.

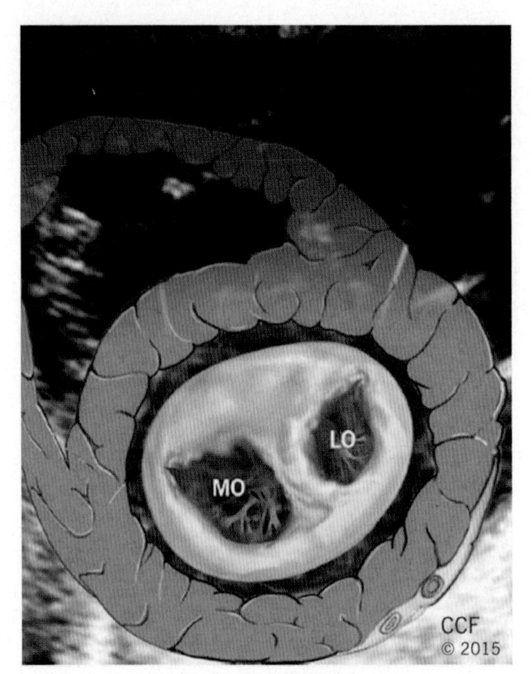

FIGURE 5.7 Double orifice mitral valve. LO, lateral orifice; MO, medial orifice.

A. **Diagnosis and etiology of mitral regurgitation.** Visualization of a regurgitant jet (or multiple jets) entering the LA during systole by color Doppler echocardiography makes the diagnosis of MR. The etiology of MR can also be determined by echocardiography. The findings associated with the most common causes of MR are given below:

1. **Mitral valve prolapse:** Displacement of one or both leaflets, 2 mm or more in systole, above a line connecting the annular hinge points in a long-axis view (parasternal or apical)—Figure 5.8. It is important to note that the direction of the jet in MVP depends on the prolapsed leaflet, being usually directed away from the affected leaflet, that is, anteriorly directed jet in posterior leaflet prolapse and posteriorly directed jet in anterior leaflet prolapse. With bileaflet prolapse, a central jet or a combination of two jets (one anterior and one posterior) may arise. Assessment of the precise origin of the jet and the location of the prolapse often allows determination of the anatomic abnormality or abnormalities. Thus, prolapse with MR originating at P2 is the most common and most easily repaired lesion, whereas MR arising from the anterior leaflet, especially when there is chordal rupture involving this leaflet, is the most difficult to repair surgically. TEE with 3D capability usually allows the precise localization of the lesion and is indicated when TTE is suboptimal in this regard, especially if surgical or catheter-based repair is planned.
2. **Flail mitral valve:** One leaflet (or a segment of it) extends into the LA in systole, with a portion of the chordae attached at its tip. As with prolapse, the jet is usually directed away from the affected leaflet.
3. **Endocarditis:** A vegetation is identified on the valve or there is other evidence of leaflet destruction such as perforation. Perforation is often diagnosed by an

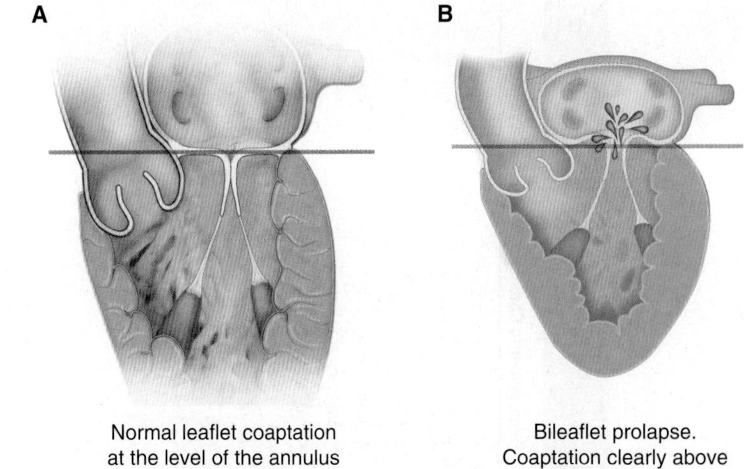

FIGURE 5.8 Normal leaflet coaptation at the level of the annulus (*straight line*) **(A)** and bileaflet prolapse (coaptation clearly above the annulus) **(B)**.

eccentric jet arising at a distance from the coaptation surface. A perforation is often difficult to visualize on echocardiography, though TEE imaging with 3D capability is most likely to ensure appropriate diagnosis.

4. **Ischemic mitral regurgitation:** Stigmata of coronary disease are identified (wall motion abnormalities, scar). There is restricted motion of the posterior leaflet in inferoposterior wall MI. In anterior MI, there is evidence of LV spherical remodeling with decreased contractility and geometric alterations of the MV apparatus:
   a. Apical tenting of the mitral leaflet: the valvular tenting area may be measured as the area enclosed between the annular plane and mitral leaflets from the parasternal long-axis view. The tenting area has been shown to be an independent predictor of annuloplasty failure.
   b. A more concave shape of the MV (as opposed to the normal convex shape).
   c. Tethering of the anterior leaflet.
   d. Annular dilation.
5. **Secondary nonischemic mitral regurgitation:** The underlying LV pathology is identified (dilated or hypertrophic cardiomyopathy, for example). Echocardiography also demonstrates associated LV remodeling and MV apparatus changes found in functional MR.

B. **Determining the severity of mitral regurgitation.** The 2014 Valvular Heart Disease Guidelines define four stages of severity for primary (Table 5.1) and secondary MR (Table 5.2): stage A (at risk of MR), stage B (progressive MR), stage C (asymptomatic severe MR), and stage D (symptomatic severe MR). Based on this classification, the severity of MR is determined by assessing the valve itself (anatomy and hemodynamics) and its consequences on the heart (LV function, LA size, and pulmonary pressures) and on the patient (symptoms).

Multiple echocardiographic parameters are helpful in determining the severity of MR (Tables 5.1 and 5.2):

1. **Color Doppler measurements**

TABLE 5.1 Stages of Primary MR—According to the 2014 AHA/ACC Valvular Guidelines

Grade	Definition	Valve Anatomy	Valve Hemodynamics	Hemodynamic Consequences	Symptoms
A	At risk of MR	• Mild mitral valve prolapse with normal coaptation • Mild valve thickening and leaflet restriction	• No MR jet or small central jet area <20% LA on Doppler • Small vena contracta <0.3 cm	• None	• None
B	Progressive MR	• Severe mitral valve prolapse with normal coaptation • Rheumatic valve changes with leaflet restriction and loss of central coaptation • Prior IE	• Central jet MR 20–40% LA or late-systolic eccentric jet MR • Vena contracta <0.7 cm • Regurgitant volume <60 mL • Regurgitant fraction <50% • ERO <0.40 cm^2 • Angiographic grade 1–2+	• Mild LA enlargement • No LV enlargement • Normal pulmonary pressure	• None

C	Asymptomatic severe MR	• Severe mitral valve prolapse with loss of coaptation or flail leaflet • Rheumatic valve changes with leaflet restriction and loss of central coaptation • Prior IE • Thickening of leaflets with radiation heart disease	• Central jet MR >40% LA or holosystolic eccentric jet MR • Vena contracta ≥0.7 cm • Regurgitant volume ≥60 mL • Regurgitant fraction ≥50% • ERO ≥0.40 cm^2 • Angiographic grade 3–4+	• Moderate or severe LA enlargement • LV enlargement • Pulmonary hypertension may be present at rest or with exercise • C1: LVEF >60% and LVESD <40 mm • C2: LVEF ≤60% and LVESD ≥40 mm	• None
D	Symptomatic severe MR	• Severe mitral valve prolapse with loss of coaptation or flail leaflet • Rheumatic valve changes with leaflet restriction and loss of central coaptation • Prior IE • Thickening of leaflets with radiation heart disease	• Central jet MR >40% LA or holosystolic eccentric jet MR • Vena contracta ≥0.7 cm • Regurgitant volume ≥60 mL • Regurgitant fraction ≥50% • ERO ≥0.40 cm^2 • Angiographic grade 3–4+	• Moderate or severe LA enlargement • LV enlargement • Pulmonary hypertension present	• Decreased exercise tolerance • Exertional dyspnea

MR, mitral regurgitation; LA, left atrium; IE, infective endocarditis; ERO, effective regurgitant orifice; C1, compensated stage; C2, decompensated stage; LVEF, left ventricular ejection fraction; LVESD, left ventricular end-diastolic diameter.

TABLE 5.2 Stages of Secondary MR—According to the 2014 AHA/ACC Valvular Guidelines

Grade	Definition	Valve Anatomy	Valve Hemodynamics	Hemodynamic Consequences	Symptoms
A	At risk of MR	• Normal valve leaflets, chords, and annulus in a patient with coronary disease or cardiomyopathy	• No MR jet or small central jet area $<20\%$ LA on Doppler • Small vena contracta <0.3 cm	• Normal or mildly dilated LV size with fixed (infarction) or inducible (ischemia) regional wall motion abnormalities • Primary myocardial disease with LV dilation and systolic dysfunction	• Symptoms because of coronary ischemia or HF may be present that respond to revascularization and appropriate medical therapy
B	Progressive MR	• Regional wall motion abnormalities with mild tethering of mitral leaflet • Annular dilation with mild loss of central coaptation of the mitral leaflets	• ERO <20 cm^2 • Regurgitant volume <30 mL • Regurgitant fraction $<50\%$	• Regional wall motion abnormalities with reduced LV systolic function • LV dilation and systolic dysfunction because of primary myocardial disease	• Symptoms because of coronary ischemia or HF may be present that respond to revascularization and appropriate medical therapy
C	Asymptomatic severe MR	• Regional wall motion abnormalities with severe tethering of mitral leaflet • Annular dilation with severe loss of central coaptation of the mitral leaflets	• ERO >20 cm^2 • Regurgitant volume ≥30 mL • Regurgitant fraction $\geq50\%$	• Regional wall motion abnormalities with reduced LV systolic function • LV dilation and systolic dysfunction because of primary myocardial disease	• Symptoms because of coronary ischemia or HF may be present that respond to revascularization and appropriate medical therapy
D	Symptomatic severe MR	• Regional wall motion abnormalities and/or LV dilation with severe tethering of mitral leaflet • Annular dilation with severe loss of central coaptation of the mitral leaflets	• ERO >20 cm^2 • Regurgitant volume ≥30 mL • Regurgitant fraction $\geq50\%$	• Regional wall motion abnormalities with reduced LV systolic function • LV dilation and systolic dysfunction because of primary myocardial disease	• HF symptoms because of MR persist even after revascularization and optimization of medical therapy • Decreased exercise tolerance • Exertional dyspnea

MR, mitral regurgitation; LA, left atrium; LV, left ventricle; HF, heart failure; ERO, effective regurgitant orifice.

a. Jet area: a small jet is defined as occupying <20% of the LA area, whereas a large jet occupies >40% of the LA area and extends into the pulmonary veins.

Caveats: While this measurement is reliable with central jets, underestimation of MR may occur in eccentric jets. In case of low blood pressure (sedation, shock), the decrease in afterload will make the MR appear less severe. In cases where the jet is not optimally visualized, use of other modalities (TEE, cardiac magnetic resonance [CMR]) may be required.

b. Vena contracta: this is defined as the narrowest portion of the regurgitant jet across the valve. The wider it is, the more severe the MR. A vena contracta of <0.3 cm usually denotes mild MR, whereas the cutoff for severe MR is 0.7 cm.

Caveat: There is tendency to overestimate the width of the vena contracta because of limited lateral resolution.

2. **Pulsed wave Doppler**

a. Interrogation of the pulmonary veins: MR also affects pulmonary venous flow. Normal pulmonary venous flow is antegrade during both ventricular systole and diastole, with slight retrograde flow during atrial systole. With increasing MR, there is a progressive blunting of the systolic component. With severe MR, systolic flow reversal occurs (Fig. 5.9).

Caveat: Atrial fibrillation and severe LV dysfunction cause systolic blunting of pulmonary venous flow and thus make it a less reliable indicator of severe MR.

b. Interrogation of the mitral inflow: In severe MR, mitral inflow pattern often shows an increased peak E wave velocity >1.2 m/s. An inflow pattern with E/A <1 can exclude severe MR.

3. **Continuous wave (CW) Doppler**

a. Jet density and contour are useful adjuncts in MR severity determination. A triangular jet contour with early peaking indicates elevated LA pressures, most often seen in acute severe MR. Also, more severe MR causes the density of the signal to increase and approach that of antegrade flow.

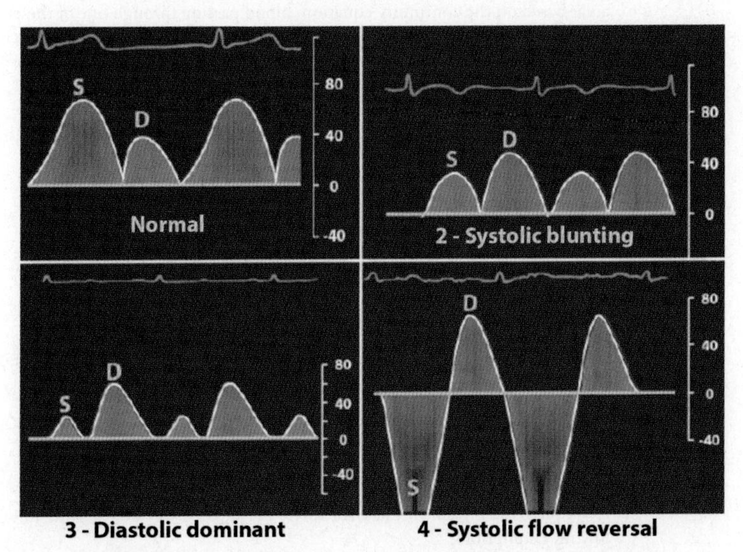

FIGURE 5.9 Pulsed wave Doppler of the pulmonary veins. S, systole; D, diastole.

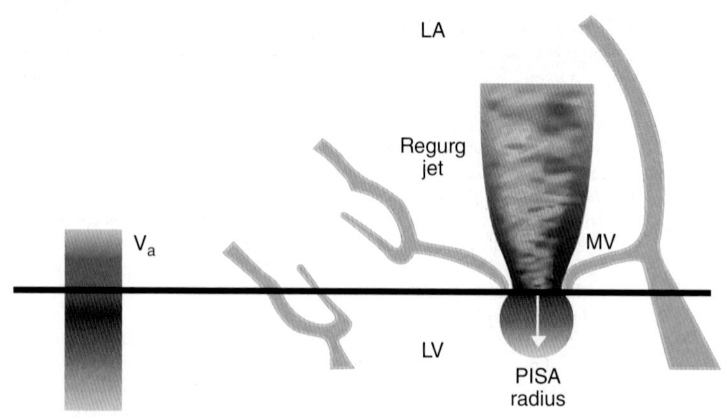

FIGURE 5.10 Proximal isovelocity surface area (PISA). V_a, aliasing velocity; Regurg jet, regurgitation jet; LA, left atrium; LV, left ventricle; MV, mitral valve.

Caveat: Jet duration: if the regurgitation appears severe but the jet is of short duration, its "volume effect" (i.e., hemodynamic consequence) is limited and the MR jet should not be qualified as severe. The duration of the MR is best assessed by either CW Doppler tracing or color M-mode.

4. **Proximal isovelocity surface area (PISA) or flow convergence (Fig. 5.10)**
   a. The region proximal to the regurgitant orifice displays smoothly accelerating flow as blood rushes into the regurgitant orifice forming hemispherically shaped isovelocity contours of increasing velocity and decreasing surface area. Based on the continuity equation, blood passing through one of these isovelocity contours is ultimately destined to pass through the regurgitant orifice. Therefore, flow can be calculated by multiplying the area of the hemispheric proximal convergence zone ($2\pi r^2$ is the cross-sectional area of a hemisphere, where r = radial distance from the regurgitant orifice) by the velocity of that contour (v):

$$Q = 2\pi r^2 v$$

   In routine application, this contour is most easily identified as the one where there is aliasing in the Doppler velocity (V_a = aliasing velocity).

   Caveat: Applying the PISA method is limited in the following situations: (1) multiple jets are present; (2) nonspherical orifice of regurgitation; and (3) eccentric jets (accuracy may be improved by using angle-correction formulas).

5. **Volumetric method:** Various quantitative measures can be calculated by echocardiography, which help in determining the severity of MR. The parameters used are the following:
   a. ERO area: Dividing the flow rate (Q) by the peak velocity through the regurgitant orifice (V_{peak}) yields an estimation of the regurgitant orifice area, the size of the actual hole in the valve.

$$ERO = Q/V_{peak}$$

   b. A simplified approach to calculate ERO: Formulated by adopting the following assumptions:
      - The peak velocity of the mitral regurgitant jet is 5 m/s (i.e., the pressure between the LV and the LA is 100 mm Hg)

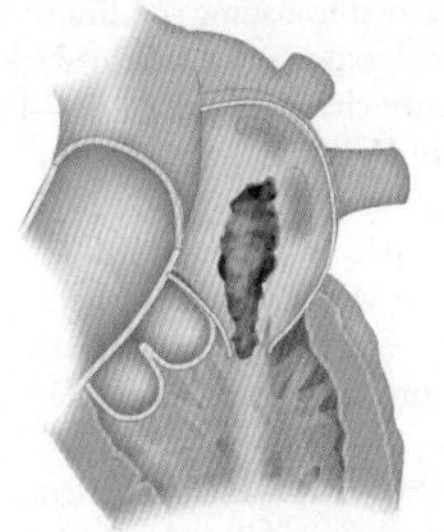
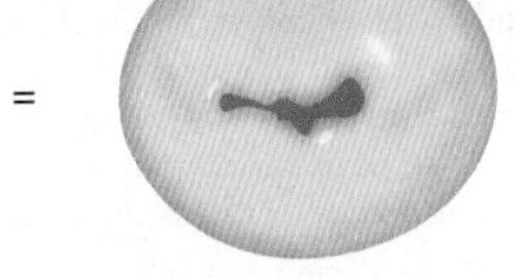
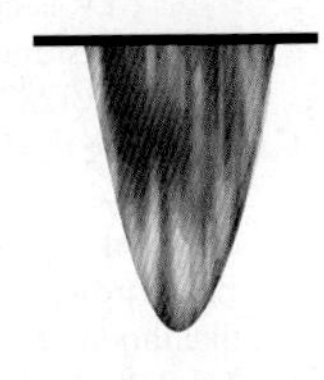

FIGURE 5.11 Regurgitant volume.

- The aliasing velocity is set to 40 cm/s (0.4 m/s)
- ERO = 2 × 3.14 × r^2 × 40/500 ≈ 250r^2/500

$$ERO = r^2/2$$

For primary MR, an ERO ≥0.40 cm^2 usually denotes severe MR, while for secondary MR, an ERO ≥0.20 cm^2 is severe.

c. Regurgitant volume (ReVol): multiplying the ERO by the regurgitant jet velocity-time integral (VTI) yields ReVol (Fig. 5.11):

$$ReVol = ERO \times VTI$$

The ReVol can also be calculated as the difference in the flow across the MV and the LV outflow tract (LVOT) (in the absence of aortic regurgitation):

$$ReVol = MV\ flow - LVOT\ flow$$

A ReVol ≥60 mL/beat corresponds to severe primary MR, while a ReVol ≥30 mL/beat corresponds to severe secondary MR.

d. Regurgitant fraction (RF): Obtained by dividing the ReVol by the mitral inflow stroke volume:

$$RF = (RV/MV\ flow) \times 100$$

An RF ≥50% is indicative of severe primary MR.

Why are the ERO and ReVol cutoffs different for primary versus secondary MR? In patients with secondary MR, and according to the 2014 Valvular Heart Disease Guidelines, the ReVol and ERO cutoffs for severe MR are smaller (ReVol ≥30 mL and ERO ≥0.2 cm^2) compared to primary MR for the following reasons: (1) Adverse outcomes occur at smaller ReVol and ERO cutoffs because of the associated LV dysfunction and adverse remodeling; (2) the LV is already compromised, so smaller amounts of regurgitation are sufficient to lead to a "decompensated" state; and (3) there is an underestimation of the ERO by echocardiographic measurement due to the crescentic shape of the regurgitant orifice in secondary MR.

Echocardiography also helps assess the hemodynamic consequences of the MR, that is, its effects on the heart, which include LA enlargement leading to atrial fibrillation, pulmonary hypertension, and ventricular dilation with latent LV dysfunction.

It is important to note that because MR has favorable loading conditions—that is, increased preload (from ReVol) and normal to decreased afterload (the LV is ejecting blood in part into a lower pressure chamber—the LA)—LV dysfunction in patients with MR is assessed as an LVEF below 60% or by an LVESD (LV end-systolic diameter) more than 40 mm.

C. **Assessing the likelihood of repair in mitral valve prolapse.** In patients with MVP, MV repair at experienced surgical centers is preferred to MV replacement because of the short-term and long-term benefits in terms of morbidity and mortality. Echocardiography (and, if needed, TEE) is the main modality used to define the likelihood of repair.

1. Posterior leaflet prolapse is repairable in more than 90% of cases in experienced centers (Heart Valve Center of Excellence). Triangular or quadrangular resection is the technique most frequently used. In experienced centers, extensive calcification of the leaflet is usually the commonest reason why repair is not possible.
2. Anterior leaflet prolapse is more difficult to repair because of the size of the leaflet (significantly larger than the posterior leaflet), its configuration (sail-like), and the absence of true segmentation. Repair techniques in this case include using artificial chordae or transfer of chordae from the posterior leaflet to support the prolapsing area. Success rates vary among centers, with Cleveland Clinic reporting a repair rate of >80% for anterior repair.
3. Repair of bileaflet prolapse is feasible but somewhat more technically challenging than posterior leaflet repair. In most instances, repairing the posterior leaflet suffices, but if the chordae to the anterior leaflet are elongated or ruptured, then artificial chordae may be needed.

D. **Transesophageal echocardiography** plays an important role in the evaluation of MR because of the proximity of the TEE transducer to the LA, thus providing an unobstructed view. It is a valuable adjunct when more detailed visualization of the MV morphology and of the LA (e.g., to exclude an atrial thrombus) is needed and is particularly helpful in situations that impede TTE (acoustic shadowing from annular calcium or a mitral prosthesis). With the recent incorporation of 3D reconstruction, TEE can provide enhanced views of the MV, allowing detailed information about the nature of the underlying pathology. The 2014 American Heart Association guidelines give a class I indication for the use of TEE in the evaluation of MR in the following situations:

1. Intraoperative TEE to establish the anatomic basis for MR and to guide repair.
2. For evaluation of MR patients in whom TTE provides nondiagnostic images regarding severity of MR, mechanism of MR, and/or status of LV function.

E. **Exercise echocardiography.** This is very helpful when there is a discrepancy between symptom status, especially when symptoms occur during exercise, and severity of MR at rest. In such instances, exercise may induce an increase in the severity of MR and/or pulmonary artery pressures, explaining the patient's complaints. Other potential values of exercise echocardiography lie in determining the following parameters of interest:

1. LV response to exercise, that is, contractile reserve: when there is a failure of LV function to improve with exercise, or of the LV end-systolic volume to decrease, patients tend to demonstrate progressive LV dysfunction when treated medically, which persists after corrective surgery in approximately 20% of patients.
2. Functional capacity: a poor functional capacity (<85% age- and gender-matched capacity) indicates a more severe and limiting MR, is associated with worse outcomes, and may be an indication of the need for early intervention in patients with severe MR who claim they are asymptomatic.
3. Exercise EF and exercise end-systolic volume index are more sensitive predictors of postoperative ventricular function than any resting index of ventricular performance.

F. **Three-dimensional echocardiography.** The main advantage of 3D echo is its ability to better display the valve anatomically, allowing for a more accurate detection of the mechanism of MR in cases where two-dimensional echo is inconclusive. For instance, the site(s) of prolapse may be better identified with 3D echo, especially in cases of multiple or complex regurgitant jets. It has become a standard test in evaluating MR prior to surgery in many experienced institutions. The use of 3D echo may increase the chances of MV repair by providing the surgeon with a more accurate understanding of the MV pathology.

XII. OTHER MODALITIES USED IN THE ASSESSMENT OF MITRAL REGURGITATION

A. **Exercise treadmill testing** can be useful to establish symptom status, determine exercise tolerance, and form a baseline for future follow-up.

B. **Cardiac catheterization** can be useful when the echocardiographic data are nondiagnostic or when there is a discrepancy between the echocardiographic findings and the clinical presentation; further evaluation with invasive pressure measurements is needed.

1. Acute mitral regurgitation. A very tall "v" wave is the hallmark of acute MR—the LA has not had the time to adapt to the ReVol, and as a result the LA pressure rises abruptly with the onset of systole. The LV end-diastolic pressure (LVEDP) also increases because the LV is now suddenly subjected to increased filling volumes. It is important to note that large "v" waves are sensitive but not specific of MR. Other conditions associated with diminished LA compliance can also produce prominent v waves, for instance rheumatic heart disease, postinfarction ventricular septal defect, and the postoperative state.
2. Chronic mitral regurgitation. With chronic MR, the LA and LV have had time to dilate and have increased compliance, resulting in slightly elevated LA pressure and LVEDP despite larger volumes of blood in these chambers.

C. **Coronary angiography** is often needed before valve surgery to detect associated coronary disease and assess the need for concomitant bypass surgery.

D. **Left ventriculography** can be used to quantify MR in the catheterization laboratory using a semiquantitative scale (Table 5.3).

E. **Cardiac magnetic resonance imaging** can be used in equivocal cases where echocardiography is not definitive. The turbulence created by MR can be visualized on cine gradient echo CMR. In addition, CMR can provide accurate measurements of the EF and ventricular volumes, which are important in determining the optimal timing of mitral surgery.

TABLE 5.3 Left Ventriculography Grading of MR Severity

Severity of MR	Finding on Left Ventriculography
1+ (mild)	Contrast clears with each beat, never opacifying the LA
2+(moderate)	Contrast faintly fills the LA and does not clear with each beat
3+ (moderate to severe)	Contrast completely fills the LA over 2 or 3 beats and opacifies it as densely as the LV
4+ (severe)	Contrast completely opacifies the LA in 1 beat and there is reflux of contrast into the pulmonary veins

LA, left article; LV, left ventricle; MR, mitral regurgitation.

XIII. MANAGEMENT OF MITRAL REGURGITATION

A. Acute mitral regurgitation

1. **Medical therapy:** Afterload reduction is a temporizing measure to stabilize the patient before surgery. By decreasing afterload, forward output increases, while ReVol decreases. If blood pressure permits, this is usually accomplished with intravenous vasodilator therapy. In hypotensive patients, an intra-aortic balloon pump (or a more advanced percutaneous circulatory assist device) is required.
2. **Intervention:** Prompt MV surgery is recommended in symptomatic patients with hemodynamic compromise. Mitral repair is usually preferred over replacement if this is technically feasible, but in IMR, recent studies suggest that the results of repair and replacement are relatively equivalent in terms of survival but that replacement may have better durability, as repair failure is common in the first 2 years (as many as 30%).

B. Chronic primary mitral regurgitation

1. **Medical therapy**
   a. Asymptomatic patients. There are no published studies that support the use of vasodilator therapy in asymptomatic patients with chronic MR. Conversely, by decreasing the LV size, vasodilators may increase the degree of prolapse and, therefore, the severity of MR. However, treatment of hypertension, if present, is important not only because of its well-known morbidity and mortality but also because hypertension worsens the MR (by increasing the LV afterload).
   b. Symptomatic patients. These patients are ideally referred for surgery. However, in patients in whom surgery is not contemplated (delayed or not candidates because of comorbidities), standard treatment for LV dysfunction is indicated: β-blockers, angiotensin-converting enzyme (ACE) inhibitors or angiotensin receptor blockers (ARBs), and aldosterone antagonists.
2. **Periodic monitoring:** Because MR is a progressive disease, periodic monitoring with echocardiography is indicated in patients with less-than-severe MR to assess for changes in its severity and to monitor LV size and function and pulmonary pressures:
   a. Mild MR: follow-up every 3 to 5 years
   b. Moderate MR: follow-up every 1 to 2 years
   c. Severe MR: at least every 6 months with consideration of stress echocardiography every year. Onset of pulmonary hypertension, LVEF $<60\%$, LVESD >40 mm, atrial fibrillation, or symptoms may suggest need for surgical consultation, especially if MV repair is feasible and an accomplished repair surgeon is available (Table 5.4).
   d. Any change in clinical status during these time periods suggesting worsening of MR severity necessitates prompt assessment.
3. **Intervention:** Surgical options include valve repair and valve replacement. The choice depends on the cause of the MR, the anatomy of the MV, and the functional status of the LV. If a successful and durable repair can be achieved, MV repair is preferable to replacement for the following reasons: lower operative risk, improved LV function and survival, avoidance of the risks associated with prosthetic valves, and excellent durability.

C. Mitral valve repair.

C. Mitral valve repair. This almost always involves placement of an undersized annuloplasty ring. Additional repair techniques depend on the etiology: while triangular resection is the technique most frequently adopted for posterior prolapse, repair of anterior prolapse is more complex and requires creation of new chords or chordal transfer. In case of leaflet perforation, a pericardial patch may be used to close the defect.

Minimally invasive approaches may be options in experienced centers. These include a partial sternal split (lower J hemisternotomy) or a limited right thoracotomy incision (single or alternatively smaller multiple incisions for a robotic approach). They

TABLE 5.4 Summary of 2014 American Stroke Association/American Heart Association Guideline Recommendations for MV Surgery

Recommendations	COR	LOE
MV surgery is recommended for symptomatic patients with chronic severe primary MR (stage D) and LVEF >30%	I	B
MV surgery is recommended for asymptomatic patients with chronic severe primary MR and LV dysfunction (LVEF 30%–60% and/or LVESD ≥40 mm, stage C2)	I	B
MV repair is recommended in preference to mitral valve replacement (MVR) when surgical treatment is indicated for patients with chronic severe primary MR limited to the posterior leaflet	I	B
MV repair is recommended in preference to MVR when surgical treatment is indicated for patients with chronic severe primary MR involving the anterior leaflet or both leaflets when a successful and durable repair can be accomplished	I	B
Concomitant MV repair or replacement is indicated in patients with chronic severe primary MR undergoing cardiac surgery for other indications	I	B
MV repair is reasonable in asymptomatic patients with chronic severe primary MR (stage C1) with preserved LV function (LVEF >60% and LVESD <40 mm) in whom the likelihood of a successful and durable repair without residual MR is >95% with an expected mortality rate of <1% when performed at a Heart Valve Center of Excellence	IIa	B
MV repair is reasonable for asymptomatic patients with chronic severe nonrheumatic primary MR (stage C1) and preserved LV function in whom there is a high likelihood of a successful and durable repair with (1) new onset of AF or (2) resting pulmonary hypertension (PA systolic arterial pressure >50 mm Hg)	IIa	B
Concomitant MV repair is reasonable in patients with chronic moderate primary MR (stage B) undergoing cardiac surgery for other indications	IIa	C
MV surgery may be considered in symptomatic patients with chronic severe primary MR and LVEF ≤30% (stage D)	IIb	C
MV repair may be considered in patients with rheumatic mitral valve disease when surgical treatment is indicated if a durable and successful repair is likely or if the reliability of long-term anticoagulation management is questionable	IIb	B
Transcatheter MV repair may be considered for severely symptomatic patients (NYHA class III/IV) with chronic severe primary MR (stage D) who have a reasonable life expectancy but a prohibitive surgical risk because of severe comorbidities	IIb	B
MVR should not be performed for treatment of isolated severe primary MR limited to less than one-half of the posterior leaflet unless MV repair has been attempted and was unsuccessful	III: Harm	B

COR, class of recommendation; LOE, level of evidence; MV, mitral valve; MR, mitral regurgitation; LVEF, left ventricular ejection fraction; LVESD, left ventricular end-diastolic diameter; AF, atrial fibrillation; PA, pulmonary artery; NYHA, New York Heart Association.

offer the advantages of faster recovery, less pain, reduced need for blood transfusion, and better cosmetic result. Outcomes of the various types of minimally invasive approaches remain to be determined. Although the results are largely favorable, there are no randomized trials showing their superiority compared to conventional techniques.

The durability of outcomes after MV repair for primary MR is excellent at experienced centers. In a review from the Cleveland Clinic of 1,072 patients who underwent MV repair for MR because of degenerative disease, freedom from reoperation was 93% at 10 years with a low rate of in-hospital mortality (0.3%). In this study, repair durability was greatest in patients with isolated posterior leaflet prolapse who had posterior leaflet resection and annuloplasty. Reoperation was because of progressive degenerative disease in 50% of these cases.

Conversely, outcomes after MV repair for secondary MR (in the setting of underlying cardiomyopathy) are not as good. The rate of late recurrent MR can be as high as 33% in IMR. While ring annuloplasty reduces tethering at the annular level, ventricular remodeling, the main driver of MR, is not addressed, explaining the higher rate of recurrences. Table 5.5 provides the likelihood of mitral repair based on MV pathology.

D. **Mitral valve replacement.** This is mainly indicated when repair is not feasible. Valve replacement with excision has a negative impact on LV function. Therefore, if possible, valve replacement with preservation of the subvalvular apparatus is preferred. The impact of valve replacement on LV function is mitigated by appropriate preservation of the MV apparatus, which conserves the LV structure and reduces considerably the likelihood of subsequent dilation.

Both mechanical and bioprosthetic valves can be used for replacement of an MV. The major issues associated with mechanical valves are thromboembolism and/or bleeding from the chronic anticoagulation required to prevent thromboembolism. The primary problem with bioprosthetic valves is limited durability owing to valve degeneration, which typically affects 20% to 40% of patients at 10 years and over 60% at 15 years.

E. **Transcatheter mitral valve repair.** This is a minimally invasive nonsurgical technique to treat MR. While a number of technologies are in clinical development, an edge-to-edge leaflet repair device (the MitraClip; Evalve, Menlo Park, CA) is currently the only Food and Drug Administration–approved device for commercial use in patients with 3+ to 4+ primary MR. In contrast, both the edge-to-edge leaflet repair and the mitral annuloplasty flexible ring (Carillon; Cardiac Dimensions, Inc., Kirkland, WA) are approved in Europe. According to the 2014 valvular guidelines, percutaneous repair may be considered (class IIb recommendation) in symptomatic patients with severe MR who have a reasonable life expectancy but are not surgical candidates.

1. The edge-to-edge leaflet repair device (MitraClip) is a transcatheter technology based on the surgical Alfieri edge-to-edge repair, which involves approximating the center of the leaflets, thereby creating a "double orifice" MV. Outcomes have been investigated in a number of cohort studies as well as one large randomized trial (the EVEREST II trial), which compared the outcomes of transcatheter repair to surgical intervention among 279 patients with moderate-to-severe or severe (grade 3+ or 4+) MR who were candidates for either procedure.
2. The primary efficacy end point (freedom from death, from surgery for MV dysfunction, and from grade 3+ or 4+ MR at 12 months) was more frequent in the surgery group (73% vs. 55%), owing to the higher rate of subsequent mitral surgery for valve dysfunction in the transcatheter group. Residual severe MR (grade 3+ or 4+ MR) and overall mortality rates were similar in both groups. Major adverse event rates were lower in the transcatheter group (driven by lower transfusion need).
3. Other percutaneous options rely on devices that can be deployed in the coronary sinus and tightened in order to reduce the mitral annulus area. Carillon Mitral Contour system (Cardiac Dimensions, Inc.) is a nitinol device implanted in the coronary sinus that indirectly cinches the mitral annulus. Monrac (Edwards

TABLE 5.5 Likelihood of Successful Mitral Valve Repair Based on Mitral Valve Pathology

Pathology	Feature	Likelihood of Successful Repair
MVP	Anterior leaflet prolapse	Moderate
	Posterior leaflet (most likely P2) prolapse	High
	Bileaflet prolapse	Moderate to high
	Commissural prolapse	High (if recognized)
	Presence of leaflet calcification	Lower
	Ruptured chordae of anterior leaflet	Moderate (with artificial chordae)
	Ruptured chordae of posterior leaflet	High
Congenital	Cleft	High
Endocarditis	Perforation (if single, within body of leaflet)	High
	Chordal rupture	Low
	Extensive fibrosis or calcification	Low
Connective tissue disorder	Restricted thickened leaflet	Low
Ischemic MR	Papillary muscle head involvement	Low
	Extensive tenting	Moderate (with long-term results often poor)
	Inferobasal aneurysm	Low with limited durability of repair
	Annular dilation	Moderate
Rheumatic	No stenosis	Moderate to high but decreased durability
	Stenosis but no calcification	Moderate to high
	Stenosis with calcification	Low (if commissurotomy + ring)
Functional owing to DCM	Annular dilation	Moderate to good

MVP, mitral valve prolapse; MR, mitral regurgitation; DCM, dilated cardiomyopathy.

Lifesciences, Irvine, CA) consists of two stents deployed into the coronary sinus with a connecting coil that is tightened over time. Percutaneous Septal Shortening Systems (Ample Medical, Forester City, CA) is an anchor that is placed in the coronary sinus and attached to the interatrial septum via a cord under tension.

4. **Indications for intervention (Table 5.4 and Fig. 5.12)**
   a. Symptomatic patients
      i. With severe MR and LVEF >30%: MV surgery has a class I indication.

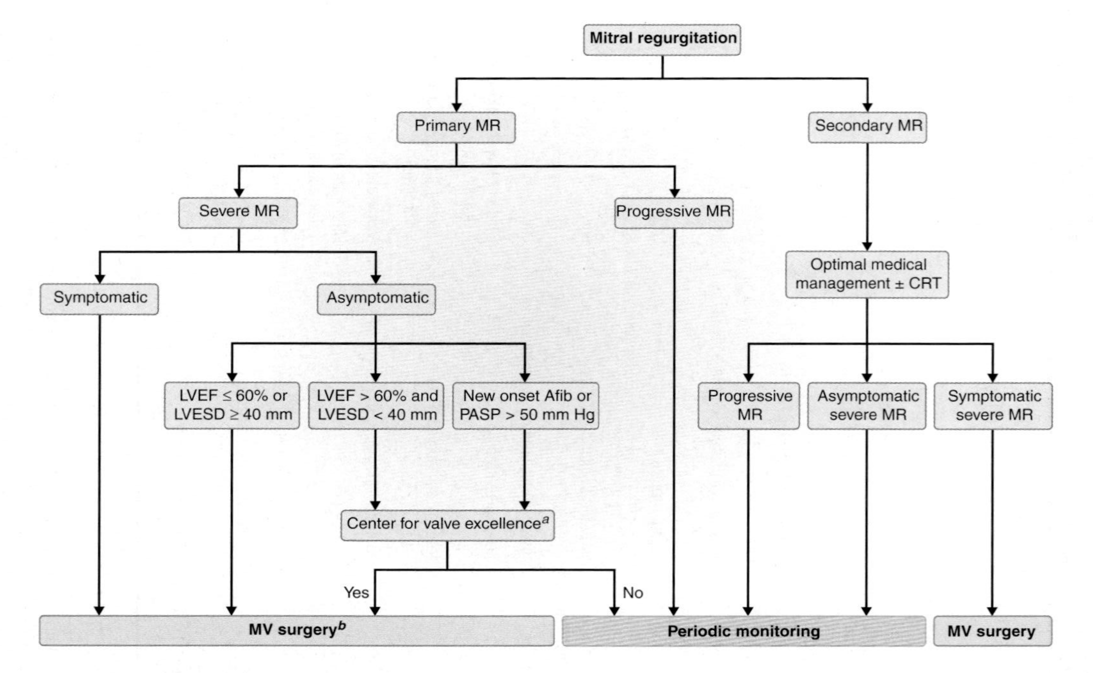

FIGURE 5.12 Management algorithm for mitral regurgitation. [a]Center where likelihood of surgical repair exceeds 95% and expected mortality is less than 1%. [b]Whenever feasible, mitral valve repair is preferred to replacement. Afib, atrial fibrillation; CRT, cardiac resynchronization therapy; LVEF, left ventricular ejection fraction; LVESD, left ventricular end-systolic diameter; MR, mitral regurgitation; MV, mitral valve; PASP, pulmonary artery systolic pressure.

ii. With severe MR and LVEF ≤30%: MV surgery may be considered (class IIb indication) but is not definitely recommended for the following reasons: the LV dysfunction is too advanced (which significantly increases the patient's risk), and there are insufficient data regarding surgery in such patients.

b. Asymptomatic patients

i. With severe MR and LV dysfunction (LVEF 30 to ≤60% and/or LVESD ≥40 mm): MV surgery has a class I indication.

ii. With severe MR and no LV dysfunction (LVEF >60% and LVESD <40 mm): In order to avoid LV deterioration, and to limit further compromise in those who already have other signs of MR complications (new-onset atrial fibrillation or pulmonary hypertension), MV repair is reasonable (class IIa) if the likelihood of success is >95% and the expected mortality is less than 1%. These operations must be performed by experienced surgeons at a Heart Valve Center of Excellence.

F. Chronic secondary mitral regurgitation

1. **Medical therapy:** Patients with secondary MR as a result of LV dysfunction should receive standard treatment for heart failure including diuretics, β-blockers, ACE inhibitors or ARBs, and aldosterone antagonists.
2. **Cardiac resynchronization therapy** is recommended in patients with secondary MR who meet the classic indications for device therapy. CRT, by restoring synchrony and improving LV function, may reduce the severity of MR.
3. **Intervention** (see Fig. 5.12)**:** Secondary MR is a disease of the ventricle, not the valve itself. MR in this context increases the burden on the LV and worsens prognosis; however, there is no evidence that correcting the MR will improve symptoms or prolong survival. Similarly, the benefits of repair over replacement are unclear in this patient population. As a result, there are few recommendations for MV surgery in patients with secondary MR:

a. It may be considered for severely (New York Heart Association class III/IV) symptomatic patients with severe MR (class IIb recommendation).

b. It is reasonable in patients with severe MR undergoing coronary bypass surgery or aortic valve replacement (class IIa recommendation): Even though there is no clear evidence that it is effective, it seems logical to address the MV during these surgeries. However, a recent National Institutes of Health–sponsored study showed no benefit of concomitant MV repair for moderate IMR when coronary artery bypass graft is being performed.

KEY PEARLS

- The mitral valve apparatus consists of two leaflets, the mitral annulus, the chordae tendineae, and two papillary muscles. Integrity of each of the components is necessary for normal mitral valve function.
- Mitral regurgitation (MR) may be primary, because of an abnormality of the valve apparatus, or secondary (referred to as functional) when it is due to left ventricular dysfunction.
- MR imposes a volume overload on the left ventricle (LV). In its acute severe form, there is an abrupt increase in preload, leading to significant pulmonary congestion and patient's distress. When chronic compensatory mechanisms including left atrial (LA) and LV dilation develop, the presentation is more insidious.
- Mitral valve prolapse (MVP) is defined as systolic billowing of the leaflet(s) into the LA and results from myxomatous degeneration of the mitral valve. It typically affects the posterior leaflet and has a characteristic systolic dynamic click on exam. It is the most common cause of primary chronic MR in developed countries. Surgical repair (rather than replacement) is preferred when feasible.

- Ischemic mitral regurgitation (IMR) is the most common cause of secondary MR and mainly results from ventricular rather than valvular mechanisms (LV remodeling, papillary muscle displacement, and mitral annular dilation). It portends a poor prognosis, and surgical intervention on the valve has not been proven beneficial.
- Other less common causes of MR include rheumatic diseases (especially in developing countries), infective endocarditis, connective tissue disorders, drugs, and congenital defects.
- Echocardiography plays a key role in the evaluation of MR. It is essential to establish the diagnosis and to determine the severity, the mechanism, and the underlying etiology. It is also vital in guiding management and timing of intervention.
- Other modalities of testing, including exercise echocardiography, transesophageal echocardiography, cardiac magnetic resonance, and cardiac catheterization, have an important adjunctive role, especially in asymptomatic severe cases, when there is discrepancy between the clinical presentation and the echocardiographic findings, and for surgical planning.
- Acute severe MR is typically a surgical emergency. In its chronic form, surgical intervention is typically recommended when symptoms develop or when there is evidence of LV dysfunction.
- Medical therapy for MR has a limited role. Surgical repair is preferred to replacement when technically feasible. Minimally invasive robotic and nonsurgical catheter-based techniques are emerging.

SUGGESTED READINGS

Bhattacharyya S, Schapira AH, Mikhailidis DP, et al. Drug-induced fibrotic valvular heart disease. *Lancet.* 2009;374:577.

Carpentier A. Cardiac valve surgery—the "French correction". *J Thorac Cardiovasc Surg.* 1983;86:323–337.

Feldman T, Foster E, Glower DD, et al. Percutaneous repair or surgery for mitral regurgitation. *N Engl J Med.* 2011;364:1395.

Freed LA, Levy D, Levine RA, et al. Prevalence and clinical outcome of MVprolapse. *N Engl J Med.* 1999;341:1.

Gaasch WH, Meyer TE. Left ventricular response to mitral regurgitation: implications for management. *Circulation.* 2008;118:2298–2303.

Gertz ZM, Raina A, Saghy L, et al. Evidence of atrial functional mitral regurgitation due to atrial fibrillation: reversal with arrhythmia control. *J Am Coll Cardiol.* 2011;58(14):1474–1481.

Gillinov AM, Cosgrove DM, Blackstone EH, et al. Durability of mitral valve repair for degenerative disease. *J Thorac Cardiovasc Surg.* 1998;116:734.

Grau JB, Pirelli L, Yu PJ, et al. The genetics of mitral valve prolapse. *Clin Genet.* 2007;72:288.

Grigioni F, Detaint D, Avierinos JF, et al. Contribution of ischemic mitral regurgitation to congestive heart failure after myocardial infarction. *J Am Coll Cardiol.* 2005;45:260.

Grigioni F, Enriquez-Sarano M, Zehr KJ, et al. Ischemic mitral regurgitation: long-term outcome and prognostic implications with quantitative Doppler assessment. *Circulation.* 2001;103:1759.

Kim JB, Kim HJ, Moon DH, et al. Long-term outcomes after surgery for rheumatic MV disease: valve repair versus mechanical valve replacement. *Eur J Cardiothorac Surg.* 2010;37:1039.

Leung DY, Griffin BP, Stewart WJ, et al. Left ventricular function after valve repair for chronic mitral regurgitation: predictive value of preoperative assessment of contractile reserve by exercise echocardiography. *J Am Coll Cardiol.* 1996;28:1198–1205.

Marijon E, Ou P, Celermajer DS, et al. Prevalence of rheumatic heart disease detected by echocardiographic screening. *N Engl J Med.* 2007;357:470.

Nishimura RA, Otto CM, Bonow RO, et al. 2014 AHA/ACC guideline for the management of patients with valvular heart disease: a report of the American College of Cardiology/American Heart Association Task Force on Practice Guidelines. *J Am Coll Cardiol.* 2014;63:e99–e100.

Roldan CA, Shively BK, Crawford MH. An echocardiographic study of valvular heart disease associated with systemic lupus erythematosus. *N Engl J Med.* 1996;335(19):1424.

Séguéla P-E, Houyel L, Acar P. Congenital malformations of the mitral valve. *Arch Cardiovasc Dis.* 2011;104(8–9):465–479.

Smith PK, Puskas JD, Ascheim DD, et al. Surgical treatment of moderate ischemic mitral regurgitation. *N Engl J Med.* 2014;371:2178.

Special Writing Group of the Committee on Rheumatic Fever, Endocarditis, and Kawasaki Disease of the Council on Cardiovascular Disease in the Young of the American Heart Association. Guidelines for the diagnosis of rheumatic fever. Jones Criteria, 1992 update. *JAMA.* 1992;268:2069.

Vassileva CM, Mishkel G, McNeely C, et al. Long-term survival of patients undergoing mitral valve repair and replacement: a longitudinal analysis of Medicare fee-for-service beneficiaries. *Circulation.* 2013;127:1870.

Yiu SF, Enriquez-Sarano M, Tribouilloy C, et al. Determinants of the degree of functional mitral regurgitation in patients with systolic left ventricular dysfunction: a quantitative clinical study. *Circulation.* 2000;102:1400.

CHAPTER 6

Balaji Tamarappoo

Tricuspid Valve Disease

I. INTRODUCTION.

I. INTRODUCTION. The tricuspid valve (TV) is a saddle-shaped right-sided heart valve that separates the right atrium (RA) and the right ventricle (RV). The RV is a low-pressure chamber that communicates with a low-resistance pulmonary vascular bed. Hemodynamic abnormalities are often absent until there are significant changes in the pulmonary vascular resistance or tricuspid valvular dysfunction. Disorders of the TV are usually categorized as primary or secondary diseases. This chapter describes the common causes of tricuspid valvular dysfunction, their diagnosis, and current guidelines for treatment.

II. ANATOMY

The highest portion of the TV faces the RA. In anatomic orientation, the TV faces inferiorly and anterolaterally toward the left ventricle. The TV consists of three leaflets, the largest being the anterior leaflet. The septal leaflet is situated in the inferomedial aspect adjacent to the membranous septum, and the posterior leaflet is located in the posterior and inferior aspect of the RV (Fig. 6.1). The tricuspid annulus is an oval-shaped fibrous structure and is larger than the mitral annulus. TV disease affects a large number of patients; however, only a small number of them undergo surgery for correction of valvular regurgitation or stenosis.

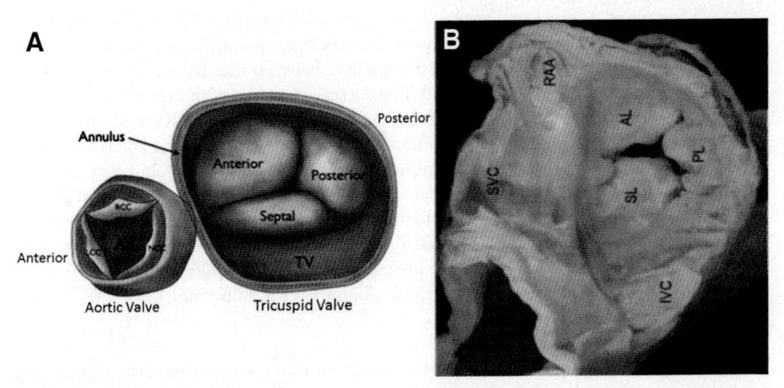

FIGURE 6.1 Tricuspid anatomy relative to the aortic valve **(A)** and pathologic specimen with right atrium removed **(B)**. AL, anterior leaflet; IVC, inferior vena cava; PL, posterior leaflet; RAA, right atrial appendage; SL, septal leaflet; SVC, superior vena cava; PL, posterior leaflet. (Modified from Montealegre-Gallegos et al., 2014; Agarwal et al., 2009.)

III. TRICUSPID STENOSIS

A. Etiology

Tricuspid stenosis (TS) is the least common of the valvular stenoses owing to the low incidence of rheumatic heart disease (RHD). It is also more often seen in association with mitral stenosis (MS).

The causes of TS include:

- RHD
- Carcinoid syndrome
- Valvular endocarditis
- Pacemaker-associated endocarditis
- Lupus valvulitis
- Cardiac or metastatic extracardiac masses
- Congenital malformation
- Prosthetic valve dysfunction

1. Rheumatic heart disease

RHD-induced TS accounts for >90% of cases and is more often seen in association with MS or aortic valve stenosis. Patients often present with a combination of TS and TR (tricuspid regurgitation). Clinically significant TV disease is present in only 5% of patients with RHD. There is thickening and fibrosis of the valve leaflets, with progression to marked leaflet contracture and commissural fusion in advanced disease.

2. Carcinoid heart disease

Carcinoid is a neuroendocrine tumor found in the intestines and does not affect the TV unless there is secondary metastatic spread to the liver. The vasoactive substances (serotonin, histamine, and bradykinin), secreted by the hepatic metastases, fail to be inactivated by the liver, and therefore directly affect the right-sided heart valves. Carcinoid TV disease is characterized by thickened, retracted, shortened, and fixed tricuspid leaflets. Most often, there is significant tricuspid regurgitation associated with carcinoid. The pulmonic valve may also be involved. Mitral and aortic valves are usually spared owing to the clearance of vasoactive substances by the lungs; however, the presence of a significant right-to-left shunt (via an atrial septal defect or patent foramen ovale) may result in left-sided heart valve disease.

B. Pathophysiology

TS results in a persistent diastolic pressure gradient between the RA and RV. Augmentation of blood flow across the TV increases, as occurs with inspiration and exercise and results in an increase in this pressure gradient between the RA and RV. In contrast, the gradient decreases when blood flow decreases, such as with expiration (Fig. 6.2).

As a result of the low pressures normally seen in the RA and RV, a mean pressure gradient as low as 2 mm Hg may signal the presence of TS. A gradient as small as 5 mm Hg may result in elevated mean right atrial pressure (RAP) and may produce systemic venous congestion, jugular venous distention, ascites, and peripheral edema. Right atrial "a" wave is increased and may approach the level of right ventricular systolic pressure (RVSP). Resting cardiac output may be reduced and may fail to increase with exercise owing to the limited RV preload. RV preload may also be limited by atrial fibrillation owing to disorganized and suboptimal RA emptying.

C. Clinical manifestations

1. Signs and symptoms

Presenting signs and symptoms depend on the severity of stenosis. Fatigue and exercise-induced dyspnea related to low and relatively fixed cardiac output may occur. Severe TS may mask pulmonary venous congestion, paroxysmal nocturnal dyspnea (PND), and orthopnea associated with other valvular lesions, such as MS. Right upper quadrant pain and abdominal distention due to hepatic congestion, hepatomegaly, and ascites may be seen.

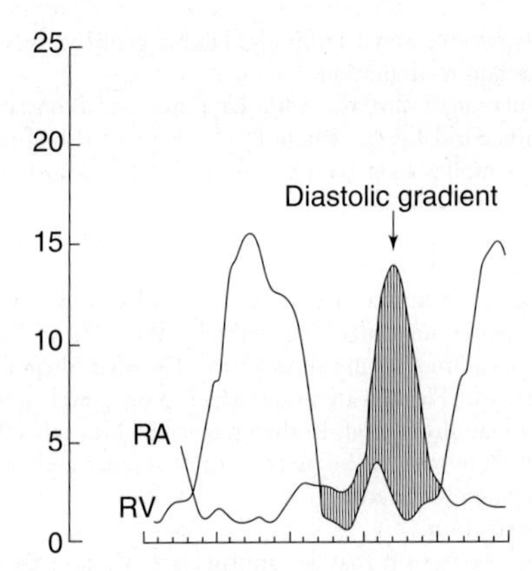

FIGURE 6.2 Pressure tracing from the right atrium (RA) and right ventricle (RV) in a patient with isolated tricuspid stenosis is shown. The *shaded area* represents the pressure gradient between the RA and the RV during diastole. (Modified from Killip T III, Lukas DS. Tricuspid stenosis: physiologic criteria for diagnosis and hemodynamic abnormalities. *Circulation.* 1957;16[1]:3–13.)

2. **Physical diagnosis**

Physical exam findings include an elevated jugular venous pressure, hepatomegaly, ascites, and peripheral edema. A low-pitched diastolic murmur heard best along the left sternal border in the third-to-fourth intercostal space or over the xiphoid process is characteristic. The murmur is prominent at end diastole (if the patient is in sinus rhythm). The murmur may be obscured if there is concomitant MS. The intensity of the murmur in TS is usually accentuated by inspiration (Rivero–Carvallo sign) or other maneuvers such as leg raising and squatting, which augment the preload.

An opening snap (OS) may be heard at the left lower sternal border; however, this may be masked by the OS of coexisting MS. A giant *a* wave in the jugular venous pulse as a result of impaired right atrial diastolic filling.

Owing to the absence of pulmonary venous congestion, there is absence of PND and orthopnea. The discrepancy between the severity of peripheral edema and the absence of pulmonary congestion may help discriminate TS from other valvular lesions.

Respiratory variation in splitting of the second heart sound (S_2) may be absent in TS as a result of the inability to augment diastolic filling of the RV despite increase in venous return with inspiration.

In patients with TS induced by carcinoid syndrome, flushing and diarrhea may be present.

D. Diagnostic testing

1. **Chest X-ray** is most notable for right atrial enlargement.
2. **Echocardiography**

Imaging features of TS include valve thickening and/or calcification, restricted leaflet-to-leaflet separation at peak opening and diastolic doming, leaflet immobility (seen in carcinoid syndrome), and right atrial enlargement.

An increase in transvalvular velocity is recorded by continuous wave Doppler (CWD), which is normally accentuated during inspiration; mean pressure gradient may range between 2 and 10 mm Hg. Higher gradients may be seen in patients with stenosis and regurgitation.

For calculation of valve area, some have proposed a constant of 190, with valve area determined as $190/T_{1/2}$, where $T_{1/2}$ is the pressure half-time in milliseconds. A longer $T_{1/2}$ implies a greater TS severity, and $T_{1/2} > 190$ may represent hemodynamically significant stenosis.

Valve area may also be calculated using the continuity equation, stroke volume/velocity time interval (VTI_{TV}): Stroke volume may be obtained from either left or right ventricular outflow, and VTI_{TV} is the TV inflow recorded by CWD. The main limitation of the method is obtaining an accurate measurement of the inflow volume passing through the TV when there is combined TS and TR. As severity of TR increases, valve area is progressively underestimated by the continuity equation method. In the presence of TR, transvalvular gradient may be clinically more relevant for assessment of severity and decision-making than the actual stenotic valve area.

E. Cardiac catheterization

Right heart catheterization may be appropriate when clinical and noninvasive data are discordant. Invasive hemodynamic assessment is performed with two catheters or one double-lumen catheter, and simultaneous recordings of atrial and ventricular pressure are made in at least 8 to 10 cardiac cycles. The hallmark is an increased pressure gradient from the RA to the RV during diastole. Diastolic pressure gradients may range from 2 to 6 mm Hg, and gradients rarely exceed 10 mm Hg.

F. Treatment

1. Medical treatment

Loop diuretics along with sodium and fluid restriction may be helpful to relieve systemic and hepatic congestion; however, this may be complicated by a low-flow state.

2. Surgical treatment

Patients with severe stenosis and signs and symptoms of systemic venous congestion should be considered for percutaneous balloon valvotomy or valve surgery; however, TV surgery may be preferred in patients with TS because of coexisting tricuspid regurgitation. Masses, vegetations, and thrombi associated with TS are contraindications to valvotomy. TV surgery is also appropriate for patients with severe TS at the time of surgery for left-sided heart valve disease.

IV. TRICUSPID REGURGITATION

A. Etiology

Any disease that causes damage to the TV (annulus, leaflets, chordae, and papillary muscles) may precipitate TR. TR may be associated with anatomic abnormalities from congenital heart disease (e.g., Ebstein anomaly, atrioventricular canal defects, and ventricular septal defect) or from myocardial and valvular disease including myxomatous degeneration, carcinoid heart disease, radiation, and hypereosinophilic syndrome, which may cause scarring and thickening of the TV apparatus, resulting in poor leaflet coaptation and TR.

Primary disorders associated with tricuspid regurgitation include:

- Rheumatic disease
- Tricuspid prolapse
- Ebstein anomaly
- Infective endocarditis
- Carcinoid
- Trauma (pacemaker or implantable cardioverter-defibrillator leads, chest trauma, or RV endomyocardial biopsy)

About 80% of cases of TR are the result of dilation of the RV, causing secondary (functional) TR. TR secondary to left or right heart disease (pulmonary arterial or venous hypertension, ventricular dysfunction, and leaflet tethering) in the face of normal TV leaflet morphology is referred to as functional TR. RV pressure and volume overload distorts the saddle-shaped tricuspid annulus, causing it to dilate in a septal–lateral direction and become planar and circular. This results in poor coaptation and tricuspid regurgitation.

B. Clinical manifestation

1. Signs and symptoms

Although isolated TR may be well tolerated, TR may often be associated with a reduced cardiac output, which may result in symptoms of right heart failure. Common findings are fatigue, hepatic congestion, bowel edema, and peripheral edema.

2. Physical diagnosis

The neck veins exhibit a prominent systolic *cv* wave, followed by a rapid *y* descent.

The *cv* wave has maximal height at S_2, and the rapid *y* descent is most prominent on inspiration.

A venous systolic thrill and murmur in the neck may be present in severe TR. The right ventricular impulse may be hyperdynamic. A pansystolic murmur may be heard at the third-to-fourth intercostal space along the left sternal border, and the intensity of the murmur increases with inspiration (Carvallo sign).

TR that results from a primary etiology (from endocarditis or trauma) is associated with a short and low-pitched murmur, whereas TR that develops owing to pulmonary hypertension may be detected as a high-pitched pansystolic murmur. P_2 may be accentuated. A short and low-pitched early diastolic rumble may be heard by auscultation along the left sternal border as the result of an increase in diastolic flow across the TV. In severe, long-standing TR, the murmur may not be audible owing to the ventricularization of the RA and minimization of the pressure gradient across the TV.

C. Diagnostic testing

Electrocardiography may show an incomplete right bundle branch block. Rhythm abnormalities may include atrial fibrillation.

1. Electrocardiography

2. Echocardiography

TR can be detected in the parasternal right ventricular inflow, basal short-axis, and apical four-chamber views. A small degree of TR may be observed in about 70% of patients with structurally normal hearts. Physiologic TR is characterized by a jet that extends <1 cm into the RA (Table 6.1).

a. Structural characteristics

In TR due to rheumatic or carcinoid disease, the leaflets are shortened and leaflet motion is restricted (Fig. 6.3). In contrast, in functional TR, the leaflets are usually normal. Tricuspid prolapse may be present in myxomatous valve disease. In Ebstein anomaly, the septal leaflet of the TV is displaced toward the apex. Vegetations may be seen with endocarditis, and a flail leaflet may be seen when there has been trauma after endomyocardial biopsy or following papillary muscle rupture with right ventricular infarction. With increasing severity of TR, the right ventricular volume overload manifests as right ventricular enlargement, septal flattening, or a shift to the left in diastole. Dilation of the RA and inferior vena cava (IVC) are also seen.

b. Doppler analysis

Assessment of TR involves incorporation of the size of the color jet, presence or absence of a proximal convergence zone, vena contracta width, and velocity profile. Eccentric, wall-hugging jets may not be visualized fully by echocardiography and may need to be upgraded by one grade when severity is assessed. Grading of TR severity depends on:

- Jet area, which is dependent on the pulse repetition frequency, and the direction and eccentricity of the jet.
- Vena contracta width, which is the narrowest portion of the jet, just downstream from the valve orifice, which gives a rough estimate of the effective orifice area. A jet width of >0.7 cm suggests severe TR.

TABLE 6.1 Echocardiographic Criteria for Classification of Tricuspid Regurgitation (TR)

Mild TR	Moderate TR	Severe TR
Central jet area <5.0 cm^2	Central jet area 5–10 cm^2	Central jet area >10 cm^2
Vena contracta width not defined	Vena contracta <0.70 cm	Vena contracta width >0.70 cm
Continuous wave (CW) jet density and contour: soft and parabolic	CW jet density and contour: dense, variable contour	CW jet density and contour: dense, triangular with early peak
Hepatic vein flow: systolic dominance	Hepatic vein flow: systolic blunting	Hepatic vein flow: systolic reversal

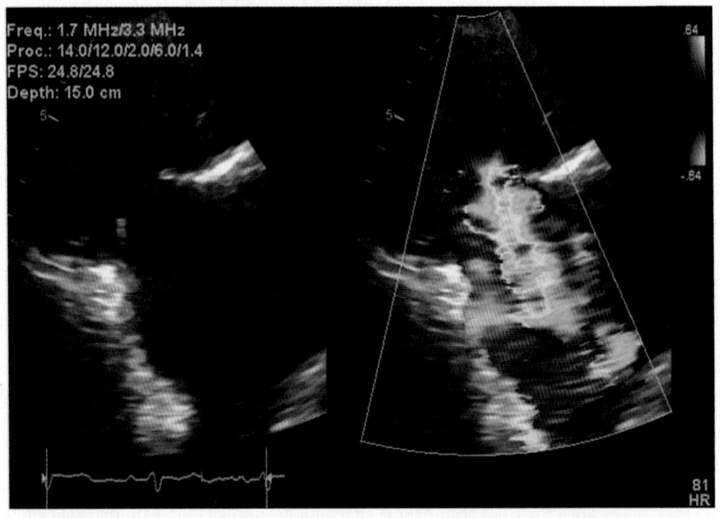

FIGURE 6.3 Tricuspid regurgitation in a patient with carcinoid disease. The panel on the left shows the retracted tricuspid leaflets with poor coaptation. The panel on the right shows the regurgitant jet.

- The intensity and contour of the TR jet on CW Doppler reflect the severity of TR, with severe TR characterized by a dense triangular Doppler profile with an early peaking velocity (Fig. 6.4).
- Hepatic vein flow where systolic flow reversal in the IVC or hepatic veins is characteristic of severe TR.

Echocardiographic measurements also include RVSP, which is quantified using the modified Bernoulli equation from the peak TR jet velocity by CW Doppler. In the absence of pulmonic stenosis, pulmonary artery systolic pressure (PASP) can be estimated as PASP = RVSP + RAP.

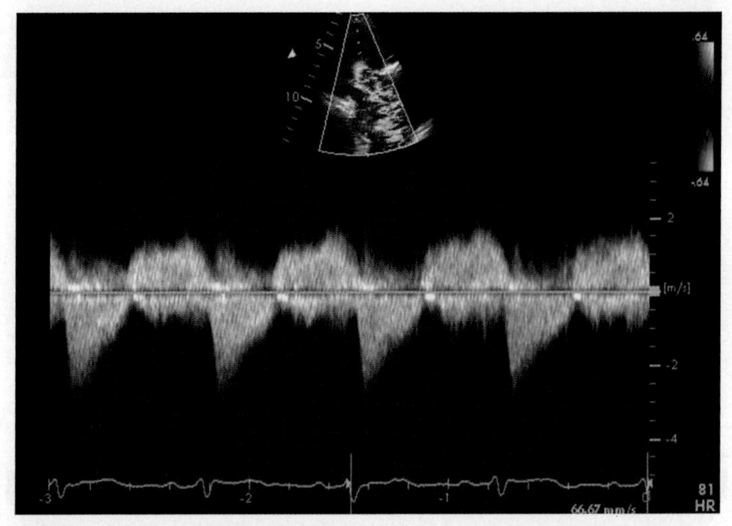

FIGURE 6.4 Continuous wave Doppler of severe tricuspid regurgitation in a patient with carcinoid-induced tricuspid valve disease. There is rapid equalization of pressures between the RV and the RA with a triangular profile of the regurgitant jet.

D. Cardiac catheterization

In the presence of moderate-to-severe TR, right heart catheterization may exhibit a dominant *v* wave in the RAP curve, and, with ventricularization of the RA, the RAP curve may resemble that of the RV. The increase in RV preload may be detected by an increased right ventricular end-diastolic pressure. Cardiac output by thermodilution and Fick techniques may be low.

E. Treatment

1. Medical therapy

In the absence of pulmonary hypertension, mild-to-moderate degrees of TR may be well tolerated for many years. Medical therapy is focused on diuresis for preload reduction and the use of afterload-reducing medications as in other heart failure states. Aldosterone antagonists may be of additive benefit, especially in the setting of hepatic congestion, which may promote secondary hyperaldosteronism. Surgical intervention is not recommended for mild and moderate TR (American College of Cardiology/American Heart Association [ACC/AHA] class III).

2. Surgical therapy

When moderate-to-severe TR results from leaflet destruction or damage, surgical repair or replacement may alleviate the symptoms; however, there is no consensus regarding indications for surgical repair for mild-to-moderate functional TR.

In the case of severe TR in combination with multivalvular lesions, concomitant tricuspid repair should be considered at the time of mitral or aortic valve surgery (class I, level of evidence: C). Several studies have documented a significant improvement in functional status among individuals undergoing concomitant TV repair with mitral valve or aortic valve surgery in comparison to those undergoing left heart valvular surgery. For patients with mild, moderate, or greater functional TR with either tricuspid annular dilation or history of right heart failure, TV repair may be appropriate at the time of left-sided valve surgery (class IIa, level of evidence: B). In symptomatic patients with severe TR, TV surgery is appropriate, especially when they are unresponsive to medical therapy (class IIa, level of evidence: C). Quality and duration of long-term survival are related to residual RV function. Among asymptomatic or minimally symptomatic patients with severe TR and moderate or greater RV dilation and RV dysfunction, TV surgery may be considered to prevent further progression of the disease (class IIb, level of evidence: C). For symptomatic patients with severe TR who have undergone previous left-sided valve surgery and who do not have severe pulmonary hypertension or significant RV systolic dysfunction, TV repair or replacement may be appropriate (class IIb, level of evidence: C).

Usually, tricuspid repair or annuloplasty is favored over prosthetic implantation when this is feasible. The other situations when TV repair may be considered include severe TR with deteriorating exercise capacity (ACC/AHA class I), severe TR with atrial fibrillation (ACC/AHA class IIa), and progressive enlargement of an already dilated RV (ACC/AHA class IIb).

KEY PEARLS

- The tricuspid valve apparatus consists of three leaflets: the tricuspid annulus, which is oval and saddle-shaped and larger in circumference than the mitral annulus; the chordae tendinae; and three papillary muscles.
- Tricuspid stenosis (TS) is an uncommon disorder with the most prevalent etiology of rheumatic heart disease. When present, there is usually associated mitral and/or aortic stenosis.
- The pathophysiology of TS may cause fatigue and dyspnea owing to fixed cardiac output and with progressively severe signs and symptoms of right heart failure.
- The diagnostic evaluation of TS includes echocardiography assessment of valve gradients and valve area using the pressure half-time method (some use $190/T_{1/2}$, instead of the 220 constant used for mitral stenosis) and cardiac catheterization if clinical and diagnostic data are discordant or equivocal.
- Medical treatment of TS is with diuretics, sodium, and fluid restriction. However, surgical tricuspid valve repair or replacement may be needed for medically refractory symptoms.
- Tricuspid regurgitation (TR) may be primary owing to an abnormality of the tricuspid apparatus or more commonly secondary owing to right ventricular dilation. Secondary TR is also referred to as functional TR, if the tricuspid valve leaflets are normal.
- TR may lead to reduced cardiac output and right heart failure with or without associated pulmonary hypertension.
- Echocardiography is vital for the assessment of TR severity and depends on color Doppler and continuous wave Doppler of the TR jet, right atrial and ventricular size, inferior vena cava size, and hepatic vein Doppler flow profile.
- Indications for tricuspid valve repair include many considerations including refractory symptoms or right heart failure despite medical therapy, tricuspid annular dilation, pulmonary hypertension, progressive right ventricular dilation or dysfunction, and concomitant left heart surgical procedures.

SUGGESTED READINGS

Agarwal S, Tuzcu EM, Rodriguez ER, et al. Interventional cardiology perspective of functional tricuspid regurgitation. *Circ Cardiovasc Interv.* 2009;2(6):565–573.

Baumgartner H, Hung J, Bermejo J, et al. Echocardiographic assessment of valve stenosis: EAE/ASE recommendations for clinical practice. *J Am Soc Echocardiogr.* 2009;22(1):1–23; quiz 101–102.

Gustafsson BI, Hauso O, Drozdov I, et al. Carcinoid heart disease. *Int J Cardiol.* 2008;129(3):318–324.

Killip T III, Lukas DS. Tricuspid stenosis: physiologic criteria for diagnosis and hemodynamic abnormalities. *Circulation.* 1957;16(1):3–13.

Montealegre-Gallegos M, Bergman R, Jiang L, et al. Tricuspid valve: an intraoperative echocardiographic perspective. *J Cardiothorac Vasc Anesth.* 2014;28(3):761–770.

Nishimura RA, Carabello BA. Hemodynamics in the cardiac catheterization laboratory of the 21st century. *Circulation.* 2012;125(17):2138–2150.

Nishimura RA, Otto CM, Bonow RO, et al. 2014 AHA/ACC Guideline for the Management of Patients With Valvular Heart Disease: a report of the American College of Cardiology/American Heart Association Task Force on Practice Guidelines. *Circulation.* 2014;129(23):e521–e643.

Rogers JH, Bolling SF. Surgical approach to functional tricuspid regurgitation: should we be more aggressive? *Curr Opin Cardiol.* 2014;29(2):133–139.

Shah PM, Raney AA. Tricuspid valve disease. *Curr Probl Cardiol.* 2008;33(2):47–84.

Shinn SH, Schaff HV. Evidence-based surgical management of acquired tricuspid valve disease. *Nat Rev Cardiol.* 2013;10(4):190–203.

CHAPTER 7

Serge C. Harb
Deborah H. Kwon

Pulmonary Regurgitation and Stenosis

I. INTRODUCTION.

I. INTRODUCTION. The pulmonary valve is a trileaflet valve that lies anterior and to the left of the aortic valve and separates the right ventricular outflow tract (RVOT) from the pulmonary trunk. The three pulmonary leaflets are semilunar in shape and are thinner than the aortic leaflets.

Primary abnormalities of the pulmonic valve are often congenital and are usually diagnosed in childhood. In adults, pulmonary valve disease is more commonly due to pulmonary hypertension from left-sided heart disease.

II. ETIOLOGY

A. **Pulmonary regurgitation (PR).** A mild degree of PR is a common finding in healthy adults. In adults, the most common cause of moderate PR is pulmonary hypertension. Severe PR is most commonly a complication of corrective interventions for congenital heart disease.

1. **PR** is the most common complication after repair of tetralogy of Fallot. It has been shown to be associated with the use of a transannular patch to reconstruct the RVOT, and was more liberally utilized in an earlier surgical era. PR is also commonly seen postvalvotomy for pulmonary stenosis (balloon or surgical).
2. **Other causes of PR** are rare and include endocarditis, rheumatic heart disease, carcinoid, pulmonary artery (PA) and annular dilatation as seen in Marfan syndrome, and congenital anomalies (e.g., absent pulmonary valve syndrome, malformed or fenestrated leaflets, and trauma).

B. **Pulmonary stenosis (PS).** Congenital PS is by far the most frequent cause. It is relatively common, with an estimated prevalence of about 10% of children with congenital heart disease. It is most commonly an isolated lesion but may be associated with other conditions: tetralogy of Fallot, congenital rubella syndrome, Noonan syndrome, Williams syndrome, Alagille syndrome, and LEOPARD syndrome. Other rare causes include rheumatic heart disease, carcinoid, and extrinsic obstruction by cardiac tumors or sinus of Valsalva aneurysms.

1. **Pulmonary stenosis can occur at three levels.**
   a. Valvular—seen in >90% of cases, most commonly because of restricted leaflets from fibrous thickening and commissural fusion. A bicuspid valve is seen in less than 20% of cases. A dysplastic valve is commonly encountered in patients with Noonan syndrome, often associated with hypoplastic annulus and proximal PA.
   b. Subvalvular—PS is extremely rare and results from narrowing of the RVOT as seen in double-chambered RV or from septal malalignment.
   c. Supravalvular—PS is related to narrowing of the main PA or its branches, which can occur as part of another congenital abnormality (as seen in Williams syndrome) or as an isolated defect.

III. PATHOPHYSIOLOGY

A. Pulmonary regurgitation. PR causes volume overload on the RV, the severity of which depends on the degree and duration of the regurgitant flow. The low pulmonary vascular resistance allows blood to easily pass through the lungs despite severe PR, thus limiting significant RV volume overload and allowing this lesion to be tolerated for longer periods. Ultimately, severe chronic RV volume overload leads to RV dilatation and dysfunction with resultant right-sided heart failure symptoms. The RV volume overload when severe manifests as "paradoxical" septal motion during diastole on echocardiography. After intervention and correction of the PR, the RV typically improves; however, an irreversible decline in contractility may occur.

B. Pulmonary stenosis. The RV initial response to the pressure overload created by PS is an increase in its wall thickness with resultant RV hypertrophy. RV pressure overload is associated with paradoxical septal motion during systole, evidenced by echocardiography. If left uncorrected, depending on the severity and chronicity of the pressure overload, RV dilatation and dysfunction may occur. After correction of the pulmonic stenosis with relief of the increased RV afterload, an improvement in RV hypertrophy and function is expected.

IV. PATHOLOGY

A. Pulmonary regurgitation. From a pathology perspective, PR can be divided into two major categories.

1. Conditions associated with anatomically abnormal valve cusps as seen in:
   - **a.** Congenital etiologies such as absent, hypoplastic, bicuspid, malformed tricuspid, or quadricuspid valves.
   - **b.** Rheumatic disease leading to morphologic alterations of the valve leaflets.
   - **c.** Carcinoid syndrome.
   - **d.** Trauma, which may result from external blunt/injury or iatrogenic causes (PA catheters).
   - **e.** Infective endocarditis.
2. Conditions associated with anatomically normal valve cusps as a result of:
   - **a.** PA hypertension with subsequent dilatation of the pulmonary trunk.
   - **b.** Idiopathic dilated pulmonary trunk.
   - **c.** Marfan syndrome with resultant dilatation of the pulmonary annulus.

B. Pulmonary stenosis. Congenital causes of pulmonic stenosis constitute well over 95% of these conditions.

1. Congenital types of pulmonic stenosis include (Fig. 7.1):
   - **a.** Acommissural: usually dome-shaped valve with a central aperture. Ridges mark sites of apparently malformed commissures.
   - **b.** Unicommissural: with a single asymmetric commissure.
   - **c.** Bicuspid: associated with tetralogy of Fallot.
   - **d.** Dysplastic: all three cusps are greatly thickened and rubbery. There is no commissural fusion, but the valve annulus is small.

V. GENETICS

A. Pulmonary regurgitation. Congenitally malformed valves producing isolated pure PR are exceedingly rare. Of the 116 operatively excised pulmonic valves reported by Altrichter and colleagues, 5 (~4%) had pure pulmonary regurgitation. The majority of patients had pure pulmonary stenosis.

B. Pulmonary stenosis. Congenital PS is far more common than the acquired form. It is frequently an isolated lesion. In a minority of cases, it is associated with other congenital conditions including the following:

1. **Noonan syndrome:** This is an autosomal dominant disorder with an estimated incidence of 1 in 1,000 to 2,500 live births. Approximately 50% of cases have a

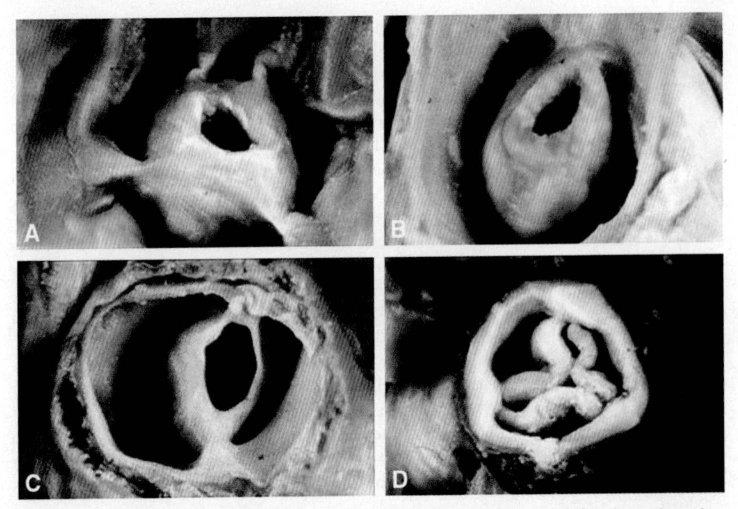

FIGURE 7.1 The abnormal pulmonic valve may be classified as acommissural **(A)**, unicommissural **(B)**, bicuspid **(C)**, or dysplastic **(D)**. (Pathology image courtesy of Dr. William D. Edwards, Department of Pathology, Mayo Clinic, Rochester, Minnesota.)

mutation in the *PTPN11* gene on chromosome 12, which encodes the nonreceptor protein tyrosine phosphatase SHP2. Noonan syndrome is characterized by facial dysmorphism (downward eye slant and low-set ears), proportionate short stature, and heart disease, most often pulmonic stenosis. In a report of 118 patients with Noonan syndrome, a dysplastic pulmonary valve was found in approximately 7% and significant PS in approximately 24% of cases.

2. **Williams syndrome:** Also known as Williams–Beuren syndrome, this is a multisystem genetic disorder caused by hemizygous deletion on chromosome 7, encompassing about 28 genes including the elastin gene *ELN*. Affected patients present with variable phenotypic expression of the following manifestations: "elfin" facies, supravalvular aortic stenosis, branch PA stenosis or other vascular anomalies, hypertension, cognitive impairment, short stature, and endocrine, genitourinary, and other systemic abnormalities.
3. **Congenital rubella syndrome:** Approximately half of children infected during the first 2 months of gestation have congenital heart disease, with the most common lesions being branch PA stenosis and patent ductus arteriosus. Other lesions, including pulmonary valvular stenosis, aortic valve stenosis, tetralogy of Fallot, coarctation of the aorta, and ventricular septal defect, have also been reported.

VI. NATURAL HISTORY

A. **Pulmonary regurgitation.** The clinical course of pulmonic regurgitation is related to its severity and to the underlying etiology. Mild PR is generally benign, and progression to more severe forms is uncommon. Chronic severe PR is usually well tolerated for years until marked RV dilatation from chronic volume overload occurs, with resultant RV dysfunction and right-sided heart failure symptoms (dyspnea on exertion, fatigue, lower extremity swelling). RV failure is associated with increased morbidity and mortality.

B. Pulmonary stenosis. The natural course of patients with PS varies with the severity of the disease, with event-free survival inversely related to the pressure gradient (PG) across the valve—that is, the higher the gradient, the higher the incidence of events.

1. **For mild PS (PG <30 mm Hg):** The course of the disease is generally benign and unlikely to progress to more serious disease. Patients with mild PS are asymptomatic. In the Natural History Study of Congenital Heart Defects, among patients with valve gradient <25 mm Hg, 96% were free of operation at 10-year follow-up.
2. **For moderate PS (PG 30 to 50 mm Hg):** Patients are frequently symptomatic. Most of these patients are detected in childhood and treated with valvotomy (either surgical or percutaneous). The probability of their survival is similar to that of the general population, and only 5% will require reoperation. Asymptomatic, medically treated patients also fare well into adulthood, although some may show evidence of progression of stenosis, and approximately 24% will require intervention.
3. **For severe PS (PG >50 mm Hg):** Most patients commonly present in early childhood with RV failure. If left untreated, it may result in irreversible RV dysfunction from marked RV pressure overload. Most patients are treated with valvotomy (surgical or balloon) early in childhood, regardless of symptoms. Their prognosis continues to be favorable into adulthood.

VII. CLINICAL MANIFESTATIONS

A. Pulmonary regurgitation. The vast majority of patients are asymptomatic. Symptoms develop when RV dilatation and dysfunction occur after many years of RV volume overload from chronic severe PR. In the early stages of RV dysfunction, although asymptomatic, patients may exhibit evidence of exercise intolerance during stress testing. Symptoms and signs of RV failure include dyspnea on exertion, fatigue, lower extremity edema, and rarely ascites.

B. Pulmonary stenosis. The presence of symptoms depends on the severity of obstruction and the degree of RV myocardial compensation. Symptoms thus vary from mild exertional dyspnea to a full picture of right-sided heart failure. Moderate-to-severe obstruction may lead to an inability to augment pulmonary blood flow during exertion, resulting in exercise-induced fatigue, syncope, or chest pain. Patients with syndromic PS (PS associated with other conditions) will also exhibit signs and symptoms related to the condition. For example, patients with Noonan syndrome and PS will have the characteristic features of Noonan including short stature, webbed neck, low-set ears, and chest wall deformities.

VIII. PHYSICAL DIAGNOSIS

A. Pulmonary regurgitation

1. On auscultation, the first heart sound (S_1) is normal. S_2 may be split (owing to a delayed pulmonic component, P_2, because of increased RV stroke volume). An RV S_3 and/or S_4 may be audible.
2. Typically, the murmur of PR is diastolic, decrescendo, best heard in the left upper sternal region, and increases in intensity with inspiration. It is high pitched and "blowing" when PR is associated with pulmonary hypertension (Graham–Steell murmur). In contrast, it is low pitched and soft when pulmonary pressures are normal.
3. When RV dysfunction occurs, the physical examination may reveal elevated jugular venous pressure, distended liver with positive hepatojugular reflux, and varying degrees of peripheral edema.

B. Pulmonary stenosis. Physical signs depend on the severity of stenosis, with often a normal physical exam in mild PS. The typical findings in severe PS include:

1. Prominence of the jugular venous "a" wave.
2. Left parasternal RV lift (owing to RV hypertrophy and prominent systolic impulse).

3. On auscultation, a systolic ejection murmur is heard with maximal intensity at the left upper sternal border with inspiration. With increasing severity of PS, the murmur duration increases, with a peak intensity occurring later in systole.
4. A pulmonary ejection click is usually present in moderate degrees of stenosis and disappears in more severe cases because it occurs earlier and thus becomes "buried" in S_1. Unlike most right-sided heart sounds, the ejection click decreases in intensity with inspiration.
5. Splitting of S_2 (from prolonged ejection and delay in P_2).
6. A right-sided S_4 may be heard over the left sternal border (secondary to RV hypertrophy and diminished compliance).

IX. DIAGNOSTIC TESTING

A. Pulmonary regurgitation

1. **Electrocardiogram (ECG)** findings are nonspecific—QRS widening with an rSr′ morphology in the precordial leads may be observed as a result of RV dilatation from volume overload.
2. **Chest radiography (CXR)** may demonstrate dilatation of the PA and RV dilatation (as evidenced by filling of the retrosternal space in a lateral view) in cases of severe PR.

B. Pulmonary stenosis

1. **ECG:** With moderate-to-severe obstruction, right-axis deviation and RV hypertrophy are evident. Right atrial abnormalities, reflected as peaked P-waves, may also be observed.
2. **CXR:** The most consistent feature is a prominent main PA from poststenotic dilatation. With severe stenosis, RV hypertrophy (as evidenced by filling-in of the retrosternal space in the lateral view) may also be observed.

X. ECHOCARDIOGRAPHY

A. Pulmonary regurgitation

1. **Two-dimensional echocardiography:** The parasternal short-axis view delineates the pulmonary valve anatomy, potentially giving a clue to the etiology of the regurgitant lesion—distorted or absent valves, annular dilatation, leaflet thickening, or vegetations. Echocardiography can also assess the hemodynamic consequences of severe PR including RV volume overload, as evidenced by RV enlargement and paradoxical septal motion.
2. **Color Doppler examination:** The examination of regurgitant flow across the pulmonic valve gives the most information about PR. The severity of PR can be estimated using the following jet characteristics:
   a. Volume of RVOT occupied with the regurgitant jet: According to the 2014 American Heart Association/American College of Cardiology (AHA/ACC) Valvular Heart Disease Guidelines, a jet that fills the RVOT is consistent with severe PR.
   b. The vena contracta (the diameter of the narrowest portion of the PR as it crosses the valve) increases with PR severity.
   c. The density of the jet increases with increasing regurgitation.
   d. Of note, the velocity of flow is not indicative of severity. Higher velocities reflect higher pressure gradients between the PA and the RVOT and are associated with pulmonary hypertension.
3. **Continuous wave Doppler:** Based on the 2014 ACC/AHA guidelines, a dense laminar flow with steep deceleration slope that terminates abruptly is indicative of severe PR. This is due to the rapid equalization of pressures between the PA and the RVOT early in diastole, which results in rapid termination of regurgitant flow around mid-diastole.

B. Pulmonary stenosis

1. **Two-dimensional echocardiography:** Typical severe valvular stenosis is characterized by thickened, distorted, possibly calcified leaflets with systolic doming and/

or reduced excursion. Echocardiography is also useful in depicting the sequelae of PS including RV hypertrophy with possible RV (and sometimes right atrial) enlargement and the poststenotic dilatation of the main PA.

2. **Color Doppler** is useful for identification of the location of obstruction. Flow acceleration proximal to valve level suggests subvalvular pulmonic stenosis (i.e., RVOT obstruction).
3. **Continuous wave Doppler** measurement of peak systolic velocities provides estimates of the transpulmonic gradient. According to the 2014 ACC/AHA guidelines, a velocity >4 m/s or a peak instantaneous gradient >64 mm Hg is indicative of severe PS.

XI. CARDIOVASCULAR MAGNETIC RESONANCE IMAGING

A. Pulmonary regurgitation

1. The pulmonary valve may be difficult to adequately image by echocardiography. In these instances, cardiovascular magnetic resonance (CMR) may be extremely valuable for the diagnosis of PR (the turbulence created can easily be visualized on cine gradient echo CMR) and for the assessment of its severity.
2. While the evaluation of RV function (volumes and ejection fraction) is notoriously difficult with echocardiography, CMR provides more accurate and reproducible determination of the RV function. This can help better define the optimal timing of valvular intervention.

B. Pulmonary stenosis

1. CMR is a vital option to assess the severity of PS and its impact on the RV, especially when image quality is inadequate by echocardiography.
2. It can be very helpful in cases where PS is part of a more complex congenital heart disease because it can better delineate the associated anomalies.
3. Similar to PR, it can help in the decision regarding the optimal timing for intervention because it can more accurately measure RV volume and function.
4. Finally, valvuloplasty may be performed under CMR guidance, reducing the need for radiation exposure.

XII. CARDIAC CATHETERIZATION

A. Pulmonary regurgitation. Nowadays, both hemodynamic assessment and angiography play a minimal role in the diagnosis and management of patients with PR. Patients with severe PR demonstrate the following hemodynamic abnormalities on right heart catheterization:

1. Wide pulse pressure on the PA tracing.
2. Rapid dicrotic collapse of the PA pressure during diastole.
3. Early equilibration of diastolic pressures between the PA and RV.

B. Pulmonary stenosis

1. Cardiac catheterization can be considered when the clinical assessment of PS severity and imaging data is discordant or to facilitate intervention.
2. Obstruction causes a PG across the pulmonic valve, with RV systolic pressure exceeding PA systolic pressure.
3. In mild cases, PG is less than 30 mm Hg, and the cardiac output increases normally with exercise. With severe PS, PG exceeds 50 mm Hg and may reach very high levels causing the RV pressure to equal systemic arterial pressures.

XIII. MANAGEMENT: MEDICAL/SURGICAL/PERCUTANEOUS

A. Pulmonary regurgitation

1. Medical management has not been shown to reduce the degree of PR, slow its progression, or affect its impact on RV function. In adults, intervention for severe PR is most commonly considered in patients with prior repair of tetralogy of

Fallot. In fact, repair with a transannular RVOT patch results in obligate chronic severe PR. Regurgitation may also occur in those who have had repairs with implantation of monocusp valves or a valved conduit from the RV to the PA, as these valves become progressively incompetent over time.

2. The optimal timing of pulmonary valve replacement in patients with severe PR remains uncertain. However, replacement should be strongly considered in the following settings:
   - **a.** Presence of symptoms including a decrease in exercise capacity attributable to PR.
   - **b.** Moderate or severe RV volume overload: based on MRI data, the threshold degree of RV dilatation is an end-diastolic volume of 160 mL/m^2 or an end-systolic volume of 82 mL/m^2. Beyond this threshold, restoration of normal RV volume is unlikely with valve replacement.
   - **c.** RV dysfunction: Studies have shown that while RV volumes decrease with valve replacement, ejection fractions do not significantly increase. This underscores the need to proceed with pulmonary valve replacement before significant RV dysfunction develops.
   - **d.** Moderate-to-severe tricuspid valve regurgitation.
   - **e.** Clinical arrhythmias attributable to the RV enlargement/dysfunction.
3. Survival following pulmonary valve replacement in these patients is excellent, with reported survivals of 97%, 96%, and 92% at 1, 3, and 5 years follow-up, respectively.
4. Percutaneous pulmonary valve implantation is an alternative option to surgical replacement. See Chapter 13 on Pediatric Percutaneous Valve Procedures.

B. Pulmonary stenosis

1. Medical therapy has no proven role in the management of PS. Intervention is in the form of either percutaneous balloon valvotomy or surgery.
2. Balloon valvotomy is the procedure of choice when pulmonary valve anatomy is suitable. The procedure uses an oversized balloon (~1.2 to 1.25 times the measured pulmonary annulus). The balloon is inflated to dilate the pulmonic valve opening. This procedure has an excellent short- and long-term result.

   According to the 2008 ACC/AHA adult congenital heart disease recommendations for intervention in patients with PS, balloon valvotomy is recommended:
   - **a.** For asymptomatic patients with a domed pulmonic valve and peak instantaneous Doppler gradient >60 mm Hg or a mean Doppler gradient >40 mm Hg (in association with less-than-moderate pulmonic valve regurgitation).
   - **b.** For symptomatic patients with a domed pulmonic valve and peak instantaneous Doppler gradient >50 mm Hg or a mean Doppler gradient >30 mm Hg (in association with less-than-moderate pulmonic valve regurgitation).
3. Balloon valvotomy is less effective in patients with a dysplastic valve, so surgery is generally preferred. Surgery is also preferred when severe PS is associated with severe tricuspid regurgitation and when the patient has another indication for cardiac surgery.
4. Surgical therapy is recommended for patients with severe PS and associated hypoplastic pulmonary annulus, severe PR, subvalvular PS, or supravalvular PS.
5. "Suicidal RV," that is, transient severe RVOT obstruction, is a serious complication that has been reported after surgical or percutaneous treatment of pulmonic stenosis. It is related to transient worsening of the RVOT obstruction (as a result of the RVOT muscular hypertrophy from severe PS) after relief of the obstruction. It is treated by volume expansion and β-blocker therapy and tends to regress with time.

KEY PEARLS

- Pulmonic stenosis (PS) is primarily a congenital disease. Pulmonary regurgitation (PR) is most frequently secondary to pulmonary hypertension from left-sided heart disease; however, it is also commonly encountered as a consequence of prior interventions for congenital heart disease (repair of tetralogy of Fallot or valvotomy for relief of PS).
- Pulmonary valve disorders may ultimately lead to right ventricular (RV) failure from chronic volume overload (as seen in PR) or from chronic pressure overload (as seen in PS). Symptoms are related to the occurrence of RV failure rather than to the valve pathology itself.
- On exam, the murmur of PR is diastolic, decrescendo, and increases with inspiration. The systolic ejection murmur of PS increases in duration with increasing severity. Both murmurs are best heard at the left upper sternal border and may be accompanied by RV S_3 and/or S_4 sounds.
- Mild PR is common and generally benign. Severe PR is usually well tolerated for many years. PS severity depends on the gradient across the valve, with severe forms (>50 mm Hg) associated with RV failure if left untreated.
- Echocardiography is the primary tool used not only to diagnose pulmonary valve disorders but also to assess their severity.
- Medical therapy has no known benefit in the management of pulmonary valve disorders. Intervention (either surgical or percutaneous) has favorable short- and long-term outcomes with excellent prognosis.
- Intervention for PR should mainly be considered in the presence of symptoms or when there is evidence of RV volume overload and/or dysfunction.
- Intervention for PS is primarily indicated in patients with high gradients (peak gradient >60 mm Hg or mean gradient >40 mm Hg), even if asymptomatic. Those with symptoms should be intervened upon at lower thresholds (peak gradient >50 mm Hg or mean gradient >30 mm Hg).
- Dysplastic PS, as seen in patients with Noonan syndrome, responds poorly to balloon dilatation. Surgery is generally preferred.

SUGGESTED READINGS

Altrichter PM, Olson LJ, Edwards WD, et al. Surgical pathology of the pulmonic valve: a study of 116 cases spanning 15 years. *Mayo Clin Proc.* 1989;64:1352–1360.

Beatriz B, Philip JK, Michael AG. Pulmonary regurgitation: not a benign lesion. *Eur Heart J.* 2005;26:433–439.

Burch M, Sharland M, Shinebourne E, et al. Cardiologic abnormalities in Noonan syndrome: phenotypic diagnosis and echocardiographic assessment of 118 patients. *J Am Coll Cardiol.* 1993;22:1189.

Carvalho JS, Shinebourne EA, Busst C, et al. Exercise capacity after complete repair of tetralogy of Fallot: deleterious effects of residual pulmonary regurgitation. *Br Heart J.* 1992;67:470–473.

Hayes CJ, Gersony WM, Driscoll DJ, et al. Second natural history study of congenital heart defects: results of treatment of patients with pulmonary valvar stenosis. *Circulation.* 1993;87:I28.

Keith JD, Rowe RD, Vlad P. *Heart Disease in Infancy and Childhood.* 3rd ed. New York, NY: Macmillan; 1978.

Klein A, Burstow D, Tajik A, et al. Age-related prevalence of valvular regurgitation in normal subjects: a comprehensive color flow examination of 118 volunteers. *J Am Soc Echocardiogr.* 1990;3:54–63.

Murphy JG, Gersh BJ, Mair DD, et al. Long-term outcome in patients undergoing surgical repair of tetralogy of Fallot. *N Engl J Med.* 1993;329:593–599.

Nishimura RA, Otto CM, Bonow RO, et al. 2014 AHA/ACC guideline for the management of patients with valvular heart disease: a report of the American College of Cardiology/American Heart Association Task Force on Practice Guidelines. *J Am Coll Cardiol.* 2014;63:e57–185.

Nollert G, Fischlein T, Bouterwek S, et al. Long-term survival in patients with repair of tetralogy of Fallot: 36-year follow-up of 490 survivors of the first year after surgical repair. *J Am Coll Cardiol.* 1997;30:1374–1383.

Oosterhof T, van Straten A, Vliegen HW, et al. Preoperative thresholds for pulmonary valve replacement in patients with corrected tetralogy of Fallot using cardiovascular magnetic resonance. *Circulation.* 2007;116:545.

Rao PS. Percutaneous balloon pulmonary valvuloplasty: state of the art. *Catheter Cardiovasc Interv.* 2007;69:747.

Rocchini AP, Emmanouilides GC. In: Emmanouilides GC, Riemenschneider TA, Allen HD, et al., eds. *Moss and Adams Heart Disease in Infants, Children, and Adolescents.* 5th ed. Baltimore, MD: Lippincott Williams & Wilkins; 1995.

Snellen HA, Hartman H, Buis-Liem TN, et al. Pulmonic stenosis. *Circulation.* 1968;38:93.

Waller BF, Howard J, Fess S. Pathology of pulmonic valve stenosis and pure regurgitation. *Clin Cardiol.* 1995;18(1):45–50.

CHAPTER 8

Maran Thamilarasan

Prosthetic Valves

I. INTRODUCTION.

The development of prosthetic cardiac valves has greatly altered the natural history of patients with valvular heart disease. There have been many advancements in this technology, from the first valve placed in the descending aorta to treat aortic regurgitation by Hufnagel in 1952 to the current percutaneous options for valve placement and even repair. In this chapter, the valve options, the management and follow-up of patients who have undergone valve replacement, as well as procedural indications and complications will be reviewed.

II. TYPES OF VALVES

Broadly, prosthetic valves are divided into those made of biologic tissue (human cadaveric, porcine, bovine, even equine) and those that are mechanical. Whereas the latter require anticoagulation with warfarin, the former have more finite durability.

A. Bioprosthetic valves (Fig. 8.1)

1. **Surgically placed:** A variety of commonly used bioprosthetic valves are currently in use.
   - **a.** Stented
     - i. Carpentier-Edwards Perimount valves (bovine pericardium mounted on flexible frame; Edwards Lifesciences, Irvine, CA).
     - ii. Carpentier-Edwards Magna, which allows for supra-annular placement (Edwards Lifesciences, Irvine, CA).
     - iii. St. Jude Biocor (porcine leaflets with a pericardial shield; St. Jude Medical, St. Paul, MN).
     - iv. St. Jude Trifecta—pericardial supra-annular valve.
     - v. Medtronic Mosaic and Hancock (porcine; Medtronic, Minneapolis, MN).
     - vi. Sorin Mitroflow (Sorin Group USA, Inc., Arvada, CO).
   - **b.** Stentless: These valves do not have the same frame as the stented valves; this can allow for potentially a larger effective orifice area (EOA).
     - i. Medtronic Freestyle (porcine).
     - ii. St. Jude SPV.
     - iii. Sorin Freedom SOLO.
   - **c.** Homografts: Cryopreserved human cadaveric valve. Often the valve choice for operations performed in the setting of acute/subacute endocarditis.
   - **d.** Ross procedure: A native pulmonary valve is placed in the aortic position, and a homograft is then placed in the pulmonary position.
2. Nonsurgically placed
   - **a.** Transcatheter placement: Valves can be delivered via transfemoral, transapical, transaortic access.
     - i. Edwards SAPIEN XT and SAPIEN 3.
     - ii. Medtronic CoreValve.
     - iii. Direct Flow (Direct Flow Medical Inc., Santa Rosa, CA).

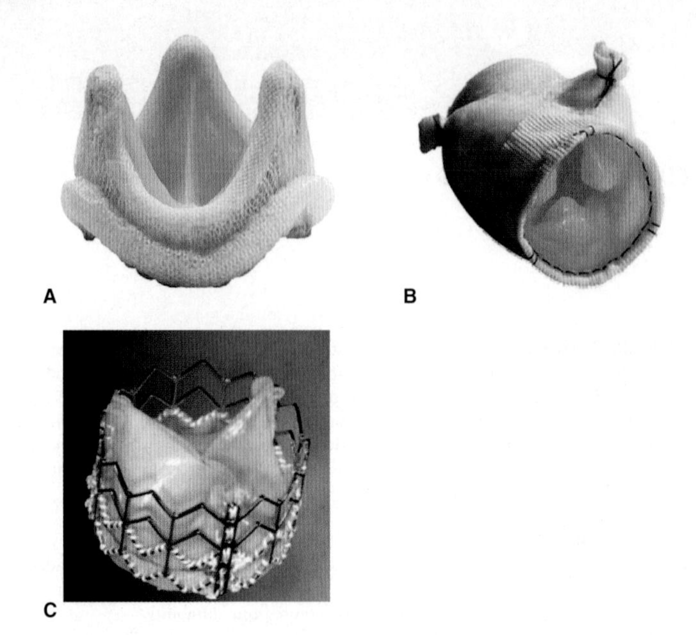

FIGURE 8.1 Bioprosthetic valves. **A:** Stented bioprosthesis; **B:** Stentless bioprosthesis; **C:** Percutaneous bioprosthetic valve. (From Zoghbi WA, Chambers JB, Dumesnil JG, et al. Recommendations for evaluation of prosthetic valves with echocardiography and Doppler ultrasound. *J Am Soc Echocardiogr.* 2009;22(9):976, with permission.)

B. Mechanical valves (Fig. 8.2)

1. Older valves (seldom in use at present)
   a. Caged-ball valves (Starr-Edwards).
   b. Single tilting disk (Björk-Shiley, Medtronic-Hall, and Omniscience).
2. Current generation valves (bileaflet disk)
   a. St. Jude (Masters, Regent).
   b. Sorin Carbomedics.
   c. Medtronic (Open Pivot).
   d. On-X (CryoLife, Kennesaw, GA).

III. CHOICE OF VALVES

The biggest question when it comes to valve replacement is whether to proceed with a biologic or mechanical prosthesis. Issues that affect this decision include expected shorter durability with biologic valves (which is inversely related to age at implantation—Fig. 8.3) and the need for lifelong anticoagulation with warfarin with mechanical valves (the newer-generation anticoagulation agents are not approved for this indication). The decision must take into account patient preferences as well as surgical risks for the original and potentially subsequent procedures. Survival rates and infection rates appear to be comparable between the two valve types, as does the risk of stroke.

Both the American College of Cardiology/American Heart Association (ACC/AHA) and the European Society of Cardiology/European Association for Cardio-Thoracic Surgery (ESC/EACTS) valve disease guidelines have made recommendations with regard to valve choices (Tables 8.1 and 8.2).

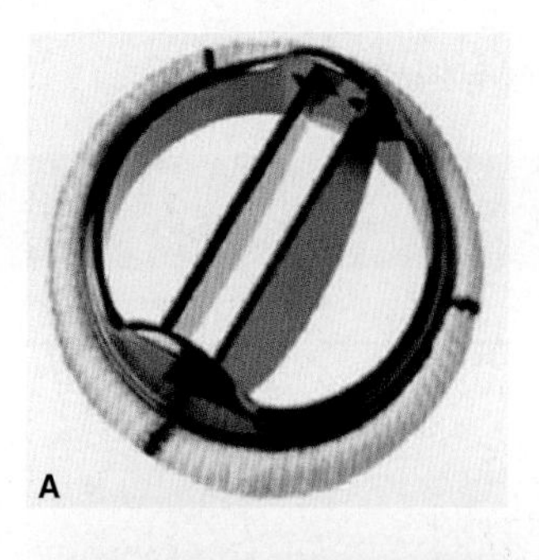

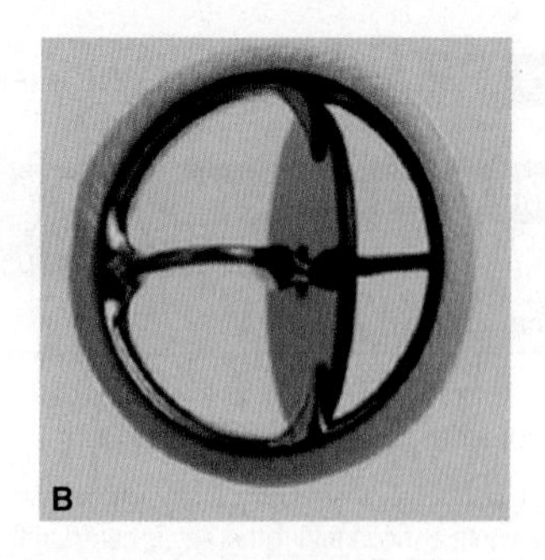

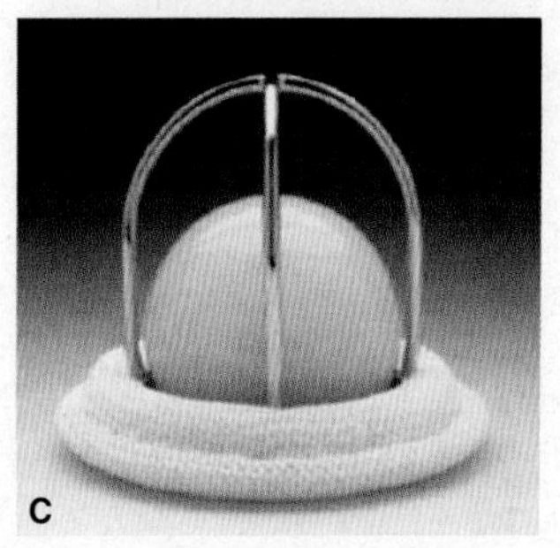

FIGURE 8.2 Mechanical valves. **A:** Bileaflet mechanical; **B:** Single leaflet mechanical; **C:** Ball and Cage Valve. (From Zoghbi WA, Chambers JB, Dumesnil JG, et al. Recommendations for evaluation of prosthetic valves with echocardiography and Doppler ultrasound. *J Am Soc Echocardiogr.* 2009;22(9):976, with permission.)

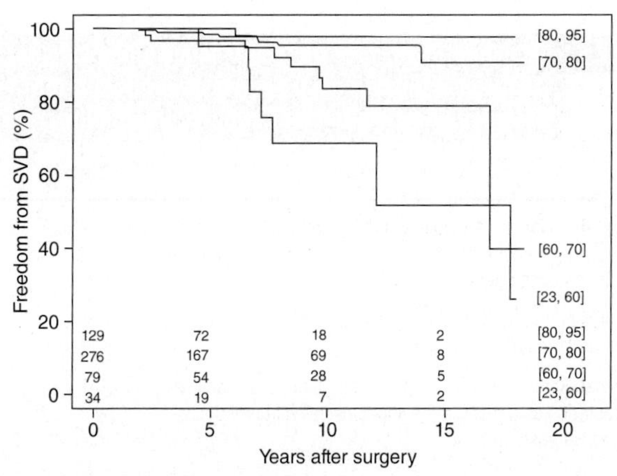

FIGURE 8.3 Durability of Carpentier-Edwards (CE) valves, as a function of age at implantation. This is from a series comparing the CE porcine and pericardial valves in the aortic position, indicating the percentage that were free from structural valve deterioration (SVD) depending on age at implantation (80–95 years, 70–80 years, 60–70 years, and less than 60 years). In the age group less than 60 years, there was greater than 30% deterioration at less than 10 years. (Reprinted with permission from Gao G, Wu Y, Grunkemeier GL, et al. Durability of pericardial versus porcine aortic valves. *J Am Coll Cardiol.* 2004;44[2]:384–388.)

TABLE 8.1 Prosthetic Valve Choice

Recommendations	COR	LOE
Choice of valve intervention and prosthetic valve type should be a shared decision process.	I	C
A bioprosthesis is recommended in patients of any age for whom anticoagulant therapy is contraindicated, cannot be managed appropriately, or is not desired.	I	C
A mechanical prosthesis is reasonable for AVR or MVR in patients <60 yr of age who do not have a contraindication to anticoagulation.	IIa	B
A bioprosthesis is reasonable in patients >70 yr of age.	IIa	B
Either a bioprosthetic or mechanical valve is reasonable in patients between 60 and 70 yr of age.	IIa	B
Replacement of the aortic valve by a pulmonary autograft (the Ross procedure), when performed by an experienced surgeon, may be considered in young patients when VKA anticoagulation is contraindicated or undesirable.	IIb	C

AVR, aortic valve replacement; COR, class of recommendation; LOE, level of evidence; MVR, mitral valve replacement; N/A, not applicable; VKA, vitamin K antagonist.
Nishimura RA, Otto CM, Bonow RO, et al. 2014 AHA/ACC guideline for the management of patients with valvular heart disease. *J Am Coll Cardiol.* 2014.

TABLE 8.2 The Joint Task Force on the Management of Valvular Heart Disease of the European Society of Cardiology (ESC) and the European Association for Cardio-Thoracic Surgery (EACTS)

	Class	Level
A mechanical prosthesis is recommended according to the desire of the informed patient and if there are no contraindications for long-term anticoagulation.	I	C
A mechanical prosthesis is recommended in patients at risk of accelerated structural valve deterioration.	I	C
A mechanical prosthesis is recommended in patients already on anticoagulation as a result of having a mechanical prosthesis in another valve position.	I	C
A mechanical prosthesis should be considered in patients <60 yr for prostheses in the aortic position and <65 yr for prostheses in the mitral position.	IIa	C
A mechanical prosthesis should be considered in patients with a reasonable life expectancy for whom future redo valve surgery would be at high risk.	IIa	C

TABLE 8.2 The Joint Task Force on the Management of Valvular Heart Disease of the European Society of Cardiology (ESC) and the European Association for Cardio-Thoracic Surgery (EACTS) *(continued)*

	Class	Level
A mechanical prosthesis may be considered in patients already on long-term anticoagulation due to high risk of thromboembolism.	IIb	C
A bioprosthesis is recommended according to the desire of the informed patient.	I	C
A bioprosthesis is recommended when good-quality anticoagulation is unlikely (compliance problems: not readily available) or contraindicated because of high bleeding risk (prior major bleed, comorbidities, unwillingness, compliance problems, lifestyle, occupation).	I	C
A bioprosthesis is recommended for reoperation for mechanical valve thrombosis despite good long-term anticoagulant control.	I	C
A bioprosthesis should be considered in patients for whom future redo valve surgery would be at low risk.	IIa	C
A bioprosthesis should be considered in young women contemplating pregnancy.	IIa	C
A bioprosthesis should be considered in patients >65 yr for prosthesis in aortic position or >70 yr in mitral position or those with life expectancy lower than the presumed durability of the bioprosthesis.	IIa	C

Joint Task Force on the Management of Valvular Heart Disease of the European Society of Cardiology (ESC), European Association for Cardio-Thoracic Surgery (EACTS), Vahanian A, et al. Guidelines on the management of valvular heart disease (version 2012). *Eur Heart J.* 2012;33:2451–2496.

The guidelines emphasize that valve choice is a shared decision process. If patients cannot be on or refuse to be on warfarin, then a bioprosthesis must be used. Given longer durability, the older the age at implantation (and potentially greater complications of warfarin use with increasing age), the more reasonable is the choice of bioprosthetic valves for all patients older than 70 years of age (>65 years of age for aortic position by ESC/EACTS guidelines). For younger patients (<60 years old), mechanical valves are considered reasonable, barring any contraindication and willingness of patient for anticoagulation with warfarin. ESC/EACTS guidelines use age less than 65 years for prostheses in the mitral position.

If patients are already on long-term anticoagulation with warfarin, a mechanical valve would be reasonable at any age. In patients who have had mechanical valve thrombosis despite appropriate anticoagulation management, reoperation should be with a bioprosthetic valve.

For patients with a small annular size (and not a small body surface area [BSA]), a stentless valve may be considered. These have more optimal hemodynamics and lower gradients. This may help in avoiding patient–prosthesis mismatch (discussed further later in the chapter). There are no definitive data yet suggesting better outcomes with the stentless valves, but hemodynamics are better.

A. **Transcatheter valves.** At present, these valves can be considered for patients who are at least at intermediate risk for traditional surgical aortic valve replacement (AVR). It is a class I recommendation to proceed with transcatheter aortic valve replacement (TAVR) if surgical risk is deemed prohibitive. For those considered high risk, it is a class IIa recommendation. More recent trial data would suggest TAVR may be extended to intermediate-risk patients. Decisions are best made with a Heart Team approach, with evaluation by both cardiac surgery and interventional cardiology.

B. **Ross procedure.** Guidelines suggest that this procedure can be considered in young patients in whom anticoagulation is undesirable, provided it is performed by a surgeon with considerable experience/expertise with this technique.

IV. ANTICOAGULATION MANAGEMENT (FIG. 8.4)

A. All patients with mechanical valves require therapy with warfarin. ACC/AHA guidelines recommend an international normalized ratio (INR) goal of 3.0 (±0.5) for mechanical mitral valves, along with aspirin (75 to 100 mg).

B. For mechanical aortic valves in the context of atrial fibrillation, prior thromboembolic events, left ventricular (LV) dysfunction, or hypercoagulable condition (or older-generation ball-cage valves or older-generation single tilting disk valves), the INR goal is the same as above. For mechanical aortic valves without the above risk factors, the INR goal is 2.5 (±0.5) along with a daily aspirin (acetylsalicylic acid [ASA]). The above are all class I indications.

C. For bioprosthetic valves in the mitral position, warfarin is considered reasonable for the first 3 months with an INR goal of 2.5 (±0.5), with long-term daily ASA use (75 to 100 mg). These are listed as class IIa indications. For bioprosthetic valves in the aortic position, warfarin may also be reasonable for the first 3 months with an INR goal of 2.5 (±0.5), this being a class IIb recommendation. Long-term ASA use (75 to 100 mg) is a class IIa indication.

D. Following the placement of a transcatheter valve, clopidogrel 75 mg is recommended for the first 6 months along with long-term ASA (75 to 100 mg).

V. PROSTHETIC VALVE PHYSICAL EXAMINATION

Normally functioning bioprosthetic and mechanical valves can produce murmurs related to the mild physiologic transvalvular gradients. An early-peaking systolic ejection murmur can be expected across most aortic valves (may be absent in homograft valves or stentless valves). Likewise, a brief and low-grade apical diastolic rumble can be heard with normally functioning mitral valves. With development of stenosis, the murmurs do become more prominent and consistent with the examination in native valve stenosis. Bioprosthetic valves should result in normal S_1, S_2 sounds. The older-generation caged-ball mechanical valves do produce prominent opening and closing clicks. The newer-generation valves have prominent closing clicks. The physiologic regurgitation present on mechanical valves is usually not audible, and any audible regurgitation on a bioprosthetic valve is abnormal. Severity can be assessed as in native valve regurgitation.

VI. ECHOCARDIOGRAPHY

A. Echocardiography remains the primary method by which routine prosthetic valvular assessment is performed. Two-dimensional imaging (whether transthoracic echocardiography [TTE] or transesophageal echocardiography [TEE]) can identify structural abnormalities of the valves (such as thickening/calcification of bioprosthetic leaflets; mobile lesions, which could represent endocarditis; thrombus; and impaired mechanical leaflet motion). Excessive motion of the prosthesis can be identified. Assessment of chamber sizes and function may also provide clues to occult valvular dysfunction.

B. Doppler measurements of transvalvular gradients are paramount in the assessment of prosthetic valve function. What is considered a normal or acceptable gradient depends on valve size, valve type, and position. Cardiac output and heart rate also

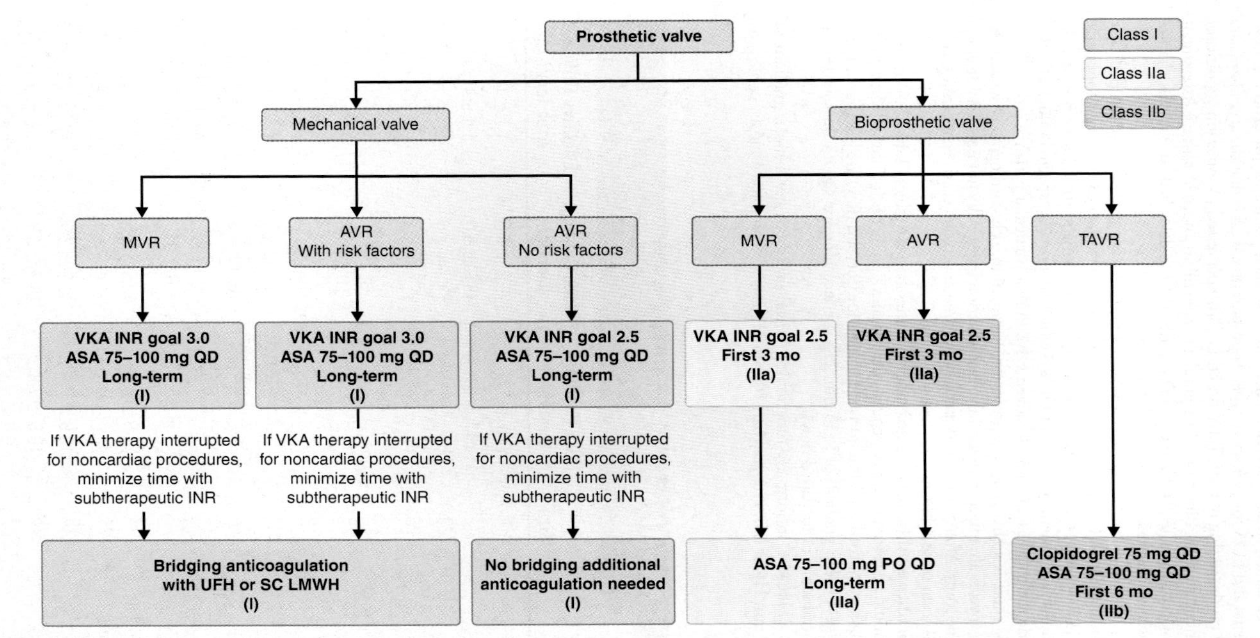

FIGURE 8.4 Anticoagulation management. ASA, acetylsalicylic acid; AVR, aortic valve replacement; INR, international normalized ratio; LMWH, low-molecular-weight heparin; MVR, mitral valve replacement; PO, by mouth; QD, daily; SC, subcutaneous; TAVR, transcatheter aortic valve replacement; UFH, unfractionated heparin; VKA, vitamin K antagonist; VR, transcatheter aortic valve replacement.
Nishimura RA, Otto CM, Bonow RO, et al. 2014 AHA/ACC guideline for the management of patients with valvular heart disease. *J Am Coll Cardiol*. 2014.

influence transvalvular gradients. There are published guidelines for expected valve gradients and EOA for each valve type. An important caveat is that these gradients are based on the setting of normal LV function. With depressed LV function, significant prosthetic stenosis can exist when gradients are still in "normal range." Assessment of flow profile, EOA, and dimensionless index (DI) as described later in this chapter will help to diagnose valvular dysfunction.

C. It is important to have a baseline echocardiographic assessment of any prosthetic valve after implantation (generally performed at the 4- to 6-week point, when postoperative anemia has resolved). This will then serve as a comparison for follow-up studies in any individual patient (whereas published tables can provide expected values, this will provide the true baseline for any given valve in that particular patient).

D. Unless there is a change in symptoms or examination, echocardiography within the first few years after bioprosthetic valve implantation is generally not necessary after the baseline study. After 5-10 years (especially in younger people), yearly echocardiography would seem reasonable.

1. **Gradients:** Although expected range of values as in the tables (Tables 8.3 and 8.4) should be referenced, as a general rule the mean gradients for normally functioning aortic prosthesis (and normal LV function/forward flow) are less than 20 mm Hg. A mean gradient of >35 mm Hg is concerning for significant stenosis (in the absence of increased flow).

   Likewise, a normally functioning mitral prosthesis has a mean gradient of 5 mm Hg or less. Greater than 10 mm Hg is concerning for stenosis.

TABLE 8.3 Normal Prosthetic Aortic Valve Gradients

Valve	Size	Peak Gradient (mm Hg)	Mean Gradient (mm Hg)	Effective Orifice Area (cm^2)
ATS	19	47.0 ± 12.6	25.3 ± 8.0	1.1 ± 0.3
Bileaflet	21	23.7 ± 6.8	15.9 ± 5.0	1.4 ± 0.5
	23		14.4 ± 4.9	1.7 ± 0.5
	25		11.3 ± 3.7	2.1 ± 0.7
	27		8.4 ± 3.7	2.5 ± 0.1
	29		8.0 ± 3.0	3.1 ± 0.8
ATS AP	18		21.0 ± 1.8	1.2 ± 0.3
Bileaflet	20	21.4 ± 4.2	11.1 ± 3.5	1.3 ± 0.3
	22	18.7 ± 8.3	10.5 ± 4.5	1.7 ± 0.4
	24	15.1 ± 5.6	7.5 ± 3.1	2.0 ± 0.6
	26		6.0 ± 2.0	2.1 ± 0.4
Baxter Perimount	19	32.5 ± 8.5	19.5 ± 5.5	1.3 ± 0.2
Stented bovine pericardial	21	24.9 ± 7.7	13.8 ± 4.0	1.3 ± 0.3
	23	19.9 ± 7.4	11.5 ± 3.9	1.6 ± 0.3
	25	16.5 ± 7.8	10.7 ± 3.8	1.6 ± 0.4
	27	12.8 ± 5.4	4.8 ± 2.2	2.0 ± 0.4

TABLE 8.3 Normal Prosthetic Aortic Valve Gradients *(continued)*

Valve	Size	Peak Gradient (mm Hg)	Mean Gradient (mm Hg)	Effective Orifice Area (cm^2)
Biocor	23	30.0 ± 10.7	20 ± 6.6	1.3 ± 0.3
Stented porcine	25	23.0 ± 7.9	16 ± 5.1	1.7 ± 0.4
	27	22.0 ± 6.5	15.0 ± 3.7	2.2 ± 0.4
Extended Biocor	19–21	17.5 ± 6.5	9.6 ± 3.6	1.4 ± 0.4
Stentless	23	14.7 ± 7.3	7.7 ± 3.8	1.7 ± 0.4
	25	14.0 ± 4.3	7.4 ± 2.5	1.8 ± 0.4
BioFlo	19	37.2 ± 8.8	26.4 ± 5.5	0.7 ± 0.1
Stented bovine pericardial	21	28.7 ± 6.2	18.7 ± 5.5	1.1 ± 0.1
Björk-Shiley	21	38.9 ± 11.9	21.8 ± 3.4	1.1 ± 0.3
Single tilting disk	23	28.8 ± 11.2	15.7 ± 5.3	1.3 ± 0.3
	25	23.7 ± 8.2	13.0 ± 5.0	1.5 ± 0.4
	27		10.0 ± 2.0	1.6 ± 0.3
Carbomedics Reduced	19	43.4 ± 12	24.4 ± 1.2	1.2 ± 0.1
Bileaflet				
Carbomedics Standard	19	38.0 ± 12.8	18.9 ± 8.3	1.0 ± 0.3
	21	26.8 ± 10.1	12.9 ± 5.4	1.5 ± 0.4
Bileaflet	23	22.5 ± 7.4	11.0 ± 4.6	1.4 ± 0.3
	25	19.6 ± 7.8	9.1 ± 3.5	1.8 ± 0.4
	27	17.5 ± 7.1	7.9 ± 3.2	2.2 ± 0.2
	29	9.1 ± 4.7	5.6 ± 3.0	3.2 ± 1.6
Carbomedics Top Hat	21	30.2 ± 10.9	14.9 ± 5.4	1.2 ± 0.3
	23	24.2 ± 7.6	12.5 ± 4.4	1.4 ± 0.4
Bileaflet	25		9.5 ± 2.9	1.6 ± 0.32
Carpentier-Edwards Pericardial	19	32.1 ± 3.4	24.2 ± 8.6	1.2 ± 0.3
	21	25.7 ± 9.9	20.3 ± 9.1	1.5 ± 0.4
Stented bovine pericardial	23	21.7 ± 8.6	13.0 ± 5.3	1.8 ± 0.3
	25	16.5 ± 5.4	9.0 ± 2.3	
Carpentier-Edwards Standard	19	43.5 ± 12.7	25.6 ± 8.0	0.9 ± 0.2
	21	27.7 ± 7.6	17.3 ± 62	1.5 ± 0.3
Stented porcine	23	28.9 ± 7.5	16.1 ± 6.2	1.7 ± 0.5
	25	24.0 ± 7.1	12.9 ± 4.6	1.9 ± 0.5
	27	22.1 ± 8.2	12.1 ± 5.5	2.3 ± 0.6
	29		9.9 ± 2.9	2.8 ± 0.5

(continued)

TABLE 8.3 Normal Prosthetic Aortic Valve Gradients *(continued)*

Valve	Size	Peak Gradient (mm Hg)	Mean Gradient (mm Hg)	Effective Orifice Area (cm^2)
Carpentier Supra-annular	19	34.1 ± 2.7		1.1 ± 0.1
Stented porcine	21	28.0 ± 10.5	17.5 ± 3.8	1.4 ± 0.9
	23	25.3 ± 10.5	13.4 ± 4.5	1.6 ± 0.6
	25	24.4 ± 7.6	13.2 ± 4.8	1.8 ± 0.4
	27	16.7 ± 4.7	8.8 ± 2.8	1.9 ± 0.7
Cryolife	19		9.0 ± 2.0	1.5 ± 0.3
Stentless	21		6.6 ± 2.9	1.7 ± 0.4
	23		6.0 ± 2.3	2.3 ± 0.2
	25		6.1 ± 2.6	2.6 ± 0.2
	27		4.0 ± 2.4	2.8 ± 0.3
Edwards Duromedics	21	39.0 ± 13		
Bileaflet	23	32.0 ± 8.0		
	25	26.0 ± 10.0		
	27	24.0 ± 10.0		
Edwards Mira	19		18.2 ± 5.3	1.2 ± 0.4
Bileaflet	21		13.3 ± 4.3	1.6 ± 0.4
	23		14.7 ± 2.8	1.6 ± 0.6
	25		13.1 ± 3.8	1.9
Hancock	21	18.0 ± 6.0	12.0 ± 2.0	
Stented porcine	23	16.0 ± 2.0	11.0 ± 2.0	
	25	15.0 ± 3.0	10.0 ± 3.0	
Hancock II	21		14.8 ± 4.1	1.3 ± 0.4
Stented porcine	23	34.0 ± 13.0	16.6 ± 8.5	1.3 ± 0.4
	25	22.0 ± 5.3	10.8 ± 2.8	1.6 ± 0.4
	29	16.2 ± 1.5	8.2 ± 1.7	1.6 ± 0.2
Homograft	17–19		9.7 ± 4.2	4.2 ± 1.8
Homograft valves	19–21			5.4 ± 0.9
	20–21		7.9 ± 4.0	3.6 ± 2.0
	20–22		7.2 ± 3.0	3.5 ± 1.5
	22	1.7 ± 0.3		5.8 ± 3.2
	22–23		5.6 ± 3.1	2.6 ± 1.4
	22–24			5.6 ± 1.7
	24–27		6.2 ± 2.6	2.8 ± 1.1
	26	1.4 ± 0.6		6.8 ± 2.9
	25–28			6.2 ± 2.5

TABLE 8.3 Normal Prosthetic Aortic Valve Gradients *(continued)*

Valve	Size	Peak Gradient (mm Hg)	Mean Gradient (mm Hg)	Effective Orifice Area (cm^2)
Intact	19	40.4 ± 15.4	24.5 ± 9.3	
Stented porcine	21	40.9 ± 15.6	19.6 ± 8.1	1.6 ± 0.4
	23	32.7 ± 9.6	19.0 ± 6.1	1.6 ± 0.4
	25	29.7 ± 15.0	17.7 ± 7.9	1.7 ± 0.3
	27	25.0 ± 7.5	15.0 ± 4.5	
Ionescu-Shiley	17	23.8 ± 3.4		0.9 ± 0.1
Stented bovine pericardial	19	19.7 ± 5.9	13.3 ± 3.9	1.1 ± 0.1
	21	26.6 ± 9.0		
	23		15.6±4.4	
Labcor-Santiago	19	18.6 ± 5.0	11.8 ± 3.3	1.2 ± 0.1
Stented bovine pericardial	21	17.5 ± 6.6	8.2 ± 4.5	1.3 ± 0.1
	23	14.8 ± 5.2	7.8 ± 2.9	1.8 ± 0.2
	25	12.3 ± 3.4	6.8 ± 2.0	2.1 ± 0.3
Labcor Synergy	21	24.3 ± 8.1	13.3 ± 4.2	1.1 ± 0.3
Stented porcine	23	27.3 ± 13.7	15.3 ± 6.9	1.4 ± 0.4
	25	22.5 ± 11.9	13.2 ± 6.4	1.5 ± 0.4
	27	17.8 ± 7.0	10.6 ± 4.6	1.8 ± 0.5
MCRI On-X	19	21.3 ± 10.8	11.8 ± 3.4	1.5 ± 0.2
Bileaflet	21	16.4 ± 5.9	9.9 ± 3.6	1.7 ± 0.4
	23	15.9 ± 6.4	8.6 ± 3.4	1.9 ± 0.6
	25	16.5 ± 10.2	6.9 ± 4.3	2.4 ± 0.6
Medtronic Advantage	23		10.4 ± 3.1	2.2 ± 0.3
Bileaflet	25		9.0 ± 3.7	2.8 ± 0.6
	27		7.6 ± 3.6	3.3 ± 0.7
	29		6.1 ± 3.8	3.9 ± 0.7
Medtronic Freestyle	19		13.0 ± 3.9	
Stentless	21		9.1 ± 5.1	1.4 ± 0.3
	23	11.0 ± 4.0	8.1 ± 4.6	1.7 ± 0.5
	25		5.3 ± 3.1	2.1 ± 0.5
	27		4.6 ± 3.1	2.5 ± 0.1
Medtronic-Hall	20	34.4 ± 13.1	17.1 ± 5.3	1.2 ± 0.5
Single tilting disk	21	26.9 ± 10.5	14.1 ± 5.9	1.1 ± 0.2
	23	26.9 ± 8.9	13.5 ± 4.8	1.4 ± 0.4
	25	17.1 ± 7.0	9.5 ± 4.3	1.5 ± 0.5
	27	18.9 ± 9.7	8.7 ± 5.6	1.9 ± 0.2

(continued)

TABLE 8.3 Normal Prosthetic Aortic Valve Gradients *(continued)*

Valve	Size	Peak Gradient (mm Hg)	Mean Gradient (mm Hg)	Effective Orifice Area (cm²)
Medtronic Mosaic	21		14.2 ± 5.0	1.4 ± 0.4
Stented porcine	23	23.8 ± 11.0	13.7 ± 4.8	1.5 ± 0.4
	25	22.5 ± 10.0	11.7 ± 5.1	1.8 ± 0.5
	27		10.4 ± 4.3	1.9 ± 0.1
	29		11.1 ± 4.3	2.1 ± 0.2
Mitroflow *Stented bovine pericardial*	19	18.6 ± 5.3	13.1 ± 3.3	1.1 ± 0.2
Monostrut Bjork-Shiley	19		27.4 ± 8.8	
	21	27.5 ± 3.1	20.5 ± 6.2	
Single tilting disk	23	20.3 ± 0.7	17.4 ± 6.4	
	25		16.1 ± 4.9	
	27		11.4 ± 3.8	
Prima	21	28.8 ± 6.0	13.7 ± 1.9	1.4 ± 0.7
Stentless	23	21.5 ± 7.5	11.5 ± 4.9	1.5 ± 0.3
	25	22.1 ± 12.5	11.6 ± 7.2	1.8 ± 0.5
Omnicarbon	21	37.4 ± 12.8	20.4 ± 5.4	1.3 ± 0.5
Single tilting disk	23	28.8 ± 9.1	17.4 ± 4.9	1.5 ± 0.3
	25	23.7 ± 8.1	13.2 ± 4.6	1.9 ± 0.5
	27	20.1 ± 4.2	12.4 ± 2.9	2.1 ± 0.4
Omniscience	21	50.8 ± 2.8	28.2 ± 2.2	0.9 ± 0.1
Single tilting disk	23	39.8 ± 8.7	20.1 ± 5.1	1.0 ± 0.1
Starr-Edwards	23	32.6 ± 12.8	22.0 ± 9.0	1.1 ± 0.2
Caged ball	24	34.1 ± 10.3	22.1 ± 7.5	1.1 ± 0.3
	26	31.8 ± 9.0	19.7 ± 6.1	
	27	30.8 ± 6.3	18.5 ± 3.7	
	29	29.0 ± 9.3	16.3 ± 5.5	
Sorin Bicarbon	19	30.1 ± 4.5	16.7 ± 2.0	1.4 ± 0.1
Bileaflet	21	22.0 ± 7.1	10.0 ± 3.3	1.2 ± 0.4
	23	16.8 ± 6.1	7.7 ± 3.3	1.5 ± 0.2
	25	11.2 ± 3.1	5.6 ± 1.6	2.4 ± 0.3
Sorin Pericarbon	19	36.5 ± 9.0	28.9 ± 7.3	1.2 ± 0.5
Stentless	21	28.0 ± 13.3	23.8 ± 11.1	1.3 ± 0.6
	23	27.5 ± 11.5	23.2 ± 7.6	1.5 ± 0.5

TABLE 8.3 Normal Prosthetic Aortic Valve Gradients *(continued)*

Valve	Size	Peak Gradient (mm Hg)	Mean Gradient (mm Hg)	Effective Orifice Area (cm^2)
St. Jude Medical Haem Plus *Bileaflet*	19	28.5 ± 10.7	17.0 ± 7.8	1.9 ± 0.1
	21	16.3 ± 17.0	10.6 ± 5.1	1.8 ± 0.5
	23	16.8 ± 7.3	12.1 ± 4.2	1.7 ± 0.5
St. Jude Medical Regent *Bileaflet*	19	20.6 ± 12	11.0 ± 4.9	1.6 ± 0.4
	21	15.6 ± 9.4	8.0 ± 4.8	2.0 ± 0.7
	23	12.8 ± 6.8	6.9 ± 3.5	2.3 ± 0.9
	25	11.7 ± 6.8	5.6 ± 3.2	2.5 ± 0.8
	27	7.9 ± 5.5	3.5 ± 1.7	3.6 ± 0.5
St. Jude Medical Standard *Bileaflet*	19	42.0 ± 10.0	24.5 ± 5.8	1.5 ± 0.1
	21	25.7 ± 9.5	15.2 ± 5.0	1.4 ± 0.4
	23	21.8 ± 7.5	13.4 ± 5.6	1.6 ± 0.4
	25	18.9 ± 7.3	11.0 ± 5.3	1.9 ± 0.5
	27	13.7 ± 4.2	8.4 ± 3.4	2.5 ± 0.4
	29	13.5 ± 5.8	7.0 ± 1.7	2.8 ± 0.5
St. Jude Medical *Stentless*	21	22.6 ± 14.5	10.7 ± 7.2	1.3 ± 0.6
	23	16.2 ± 9.0	8.2 ± 4.7	1.6 ± 0.6
	25	12.7 ± 8.2	6.3 ± 4.1	1.8 ± 0.5
	27	10.1 ± 5.8	5.0 ± 2.9	2.0 ± 0.3
	29	7.7 ± 4.4	4.1 ± 2.4	2.4 ± 0.6

Zoghbi WA, Chambers JB, Dumesnil JG, et al. Recommendations for evaluation of prosthetic valves with echocardiography and Doppler ultrasound: a report from the American Society of Echocardiography's Guidelines and Standards Committee and the Task Force on Prosthetic Valves. *J Am Soc Echocardiogr.* 2009;22:975–1014.

TABLE 8.4 Normal Prosthetic Mitral Gradients

Valve	Size	Peak Gradient (mm Hg)	Mean Gradient (mm Hg)	Peak Velocity (m/sec)	Pressure Half-Time (ms)	Effective Orifice Area (cm^2)
Biocor *Stentless bioprosthesis*	27	13 ± 1				
	29	14 ± 2.5				
	31	11.5 ± 0.5				
	33	12 ± 0.5				

(continued)

TABLE 8.4 Normal Prosthetic Mitral Gradients *(continued)*

Valve	Size	Peak Gradient (mm Hg)	Mean Gradient (mm Hg)	Peak Velocity (m/sec)	Pressure Half-Time (ms)	Effective Orifice Area (cm^2)
Bioflo pericardial *Stented bioprosthesis*	25	10 ± 2	6.3 ± 1.5			2 ± 0.1
	27	9.5 ± 2.6	5.4 ± 1.2			2 ± 0.3
	29	5 ± 2.8	3.6 ± 1			2.4 ± 0.2
	31	4.0	2.0			2.3
Bjork-Shiley *Tilting disk*	23			1.7	115	
	25	12 ± 4	6 ± 2	1.75 ± 0.38	99 ± 27	1.72 ± 0.6
	27	10 ± 4	5 ± 2	1.6 ± 0.49	89 ± 28	1.81 ± 0.54
	29	7.83 ± 2.93	2.83 ± 1.27	1.37 ± 0.25	79 ± 17	2.1 ± 0.43
	31	6 ± 3	2 ± 1.9	1.41 ± 0.26	70 ± 14	2.2 ± 0.3
Bjork-Shiley monostrut *Tilting disk*	23		5.0	1.9		
	25	13 ± 2.5	5.57 ± 2.3	1.8 ± 0.3		
	27	12 ± 2.5	4.53 ± 2.2	1.7 ± 0.4		
	29	13 ± 3	4.26 ± 1.6	1.6 ± 0.3		
	31	14 ± 4.5	4.9 ± 1.6	1.7 ± 0.3		
Carbomedics *Bileaflet*	23			1.9 ± 0.1	126 ± 7	
	25	10.3 ± 2.3	3.6 ± 0.6	1.3 ± 0.1	93 ± 8	2.9 ± 0.8
	27	8.79 ± 3.46	3.46 ± 1.03	1.61 ± 0.3	89 ± 20	2.9 ± 0.75
	29	8.78 ± 2.9	3.39 ± 0.97	1.52 ± 0.3	88 ± 17	2.3 ± 0.4
	31	8.87 ± 2.34	3.32 ± 0.87	1.61 ± 0.29	92 ± 24	2.8 ± 1.14
	33	8.8 ± 2.2	4.8 ± 2.5	1.5 ± 0.2	93 ± 12	
Carpentier-Edwards *Stented bioprosthesis*	27		6 ± 2	1.7 ± 0.3	98 ± 28	
	29		4.7 ± 2	1.76 ± 0.27	92 ± 14	
	31		4.4 ± 2	1.54 ± 0.15	92 ± 19	
	33		6 ± 3		93 ± 12	
Carpentier-Edwards pericardial *Stented bioprosthesis*	27		3.6	1.6	100	
	29		5.25 ± 2.36	1.67 ± 0.3	110 ± 15	
	31		4.05 ± 0.83	1.53 ± 0.1	90 ± 11	
	33		1.0	0.8	80	
Duromedics *Bileaflet*	27	13 ± 6	5 ± 3	1.61 ± 0.4	75 ± 12	
	29	10 ± 4	3 ± 1	1.40 ± 0.25	85 ± 22	
	31	10.5 ± 4.33	3.3 ± 1.36	1.38 ± 0.27	81 ± 12	
	33	11.2	2.5		85	

TABLE 8.4 Normal Prosthetic Mitral Gradients *(continued)*

Valve	Size	Peak Gradient (mm Hg)	Mean Gradient (mm Hg)	Peak Velocity (m/sec)	Pressure Half-Time (ms)	Effective Orifice Area (cm²)
Hancock I or not specified *Stented bioprosthesis*	27	10 ± 4	5 ± 2			1.3 ± 0.8
	29	7 ± 3	2.46 ± 0.79		115 ± 20	1.5 ± 0.2
	31	4 ± 0.86	4.86 ± 1.69		95 ± 17	1.6 ± 0.2
	33	3 ± 2	3.87 ± 2		90 ± 12	1.9 ± 0.2
Hancock II *Stented bioprosthesis*	27					2.21 ± 0.14
	29					2.77 ± 0.11
	31					2.84 ± 0.1
	33					3.15 ± 0.22
Hancock pericardial *Stented bioprosthesis*	29		2.61 ± 1.39	1.42 ± 0.14	105 ± 36	
	31		3.57 ± 1.02	1.51 ± 0.27	81 ± 23	
Ionescu-Shiley *Stented bioprosthesis*	25		4.87 ± 1.08	1.43 ± 0.15	93 ± 11	
	27		3.21 ± 0.82	1.31 ± 0.24	100 ± 28	
	29		3.22 ± 0.57	1.38 ± 0.2	85 ± 8	
	31		3.63 ± 0.9	1.45 ± 0.06	100 ± 36	
Ionescu-Shiley low profile *Stented bioprosthesis*	29		3.31 ± 0.96	1.36 ± 0.25	80 ± 30	
	31		2.74 ± 0.37	1.33 ± 0.14	79 ± 15	
Labcor-Santiago pericardial *Stented bioprosthesis*	25	8.7	4.5		97	2.2
	27	5.6 ± 2.3	4.8 ± 1.5		85 ± 18	2.12 ± 0.48
	29	6.2 ± 2.1	3 ± 1.3		80 ± 34	2.11 ± 0.73
Lillehei-Kaster *Tilting disk*	18			1.7	140	
	20			1.7	67	
	22			1.56 ± 0.009	94 ± 22	
	25			1.38 ± 0.27	124 ± 46	
Medtronic-Hall *Tilting disk*	27			1.4	78	
	29			1.57 ± 0.1	69 ± 15	
	31			1.45 ± 0.12	77 ± 17	

(continued)

TABLE 8.4 Normal Prosthetic Mitral Gradients *(continued)*

Valve	Size	Peak Gradient (mm Hg)	Mean Gradient (mm Hg)	Peak Velocity (m/sec)	Pressure Half-Time (ms)	Effective Orifice Area (cm^2)
Medtronic Intact Porcine	29		3.5 ± 0.51	1.6 ± 0.22		
	31		4.2 ± 1.44	1.6 ± 0.26		
Stented bioprosthesis	33		4 ± 1.3	1.4 ± 0.24		
	35		3.2 ± 1.77	1.3 ± 0.5		
Mitroflow	25		6.9	2.0	90	
Stented bioprosthesis	27		3.07 ± 0.91	1.5	90 ± 20	
	29		3.5 ± 1.65	1.43 ± 0.29	102 ± 21	
	31		3.85 ± 0.81	1.32 ± 0.26	91 ± 22	
Omnicarbon	23		8.0			
Tilting disk	25		6.05 ± 1.81	1.77 ± 0.24	102 ± 16	
	27		4.89 ± 2.05	1.63 ± 0.36	105 ± 33	
	29		4.93 ± 2.16	1.56 ± 0.27	120 ± 40	
	31		4.81 ± 1.4	1.3 ± 0.23	134 ± 31	
	33		4 ± 2			
On-X	25	11.5 ± 3.2	5.3 ± 2.1			1.9 ± 1.1
Bileaflet	27–29	10.3 ± 4.5	4.5 ± 1.6			2.2 ± 0.5
	31–33	9.8 ± 3.8	4.8 ± 2.4			2.5 ± 1.1
Sorin Allcarbon	25	15 ± 3	5 ± 1	2 ± 0.2	105 ± 29	2.2 ± 0.6
	27	13 ± 2	4 ± 1	1.8 ± 0.1	89 ± 14	2.5 ± 0.5
Tilting disk	29	10 ± 2	4 ± 1	1.6 ± 0.2	85 ± 23	2.8 ± 0.7
	31	9 ± 1	4 ± 1	1.6 ± 0.1	88 ± 27	2.8 ± 0.9
Sorin Bicarbon	25	15 ± 0.25	4 ± 0.5	1.95 ± 0.02	70 ± 1	
	27	11 ± 2.75	4 ± 0.5	1.65 ± 0.21	82 ± 20	
Bileaflet	29	12 ± 3	4 ± 1.25	1.73 ± 0.22	80 ± 14	
	31	10 ± 1.5	4 ± 1	1.66 ± 0.11	83 ± 14	
St. Jude Medical	23		4.0	1.5	160	1.0
	25		2.5 ± 1	1.34 ± 1.12	75 ± 4	1.35 ± 0.17
Bileaflet	27	11 ± 4	5 ± 1.82	1.61 ± 0.29	75 ± 10	1.67 ± 0.17
	29	10 ± 3	4.15 ± 1.18	1.57 ± 0.29	85 ± 10	1.75 ± 0.24
	31	12 ± 6	4.46 ± 2.22	1.59 ± 0.33	74 ± 13	2.03 ± 0.32
Starr-Edwards	26		10.0			1.4
Caged ball	28		7 ± 2.75			1.9 ± 0.57
	30	12.2 ± 4.6	6.99 ± 2.5	1.7 ± 0.3	125 ± 25	1.65 ± 0.4
	32	11.5 ± 4.2	5.08 ± 2.5	1.7 ± 0.3	110 ± 25	1.98 ± 0.4
	34		5.0			2.6

TABLE 8.4	Normal Prosthetic Mitral Gradients *(continued)*					
Valve	**Size**	**Peak Gradient (mm Hg)**	**Mean Gradient (mm Hg)**	**Peak Velocity (m/sec)**	**Pressure Half-Time (ms)**	**Effective Orifice Area (cm²)**
Stentless quadrileaflet	26		2.2 ± 1.7	1.6	103 ± 31	1.7
	28			1.58 ± 0.25		1.7 ± 0.6
Bovine pericardial	30			1.42 ± 0.32		2.3 ± 0.4
Stented bioprosthesis						
Wessex	29		3.69 ± 0.61	1.66 ± 0.17	83 ± 19	
Stented bioprosthesis	31		3.31 ± 0.83	1.41 ± 0.25	80 ± 21	

Zoghbi WA, Chambers JB, Dumesnil JG, et al. Recommendations for evaluation of prosthetic valves with echocardiography and Doppler ultrasound: a report from the American Society of Echocardiography's Guidelines and Standards Committee and the Task Force on Prosthetic Valves. *J Am Soc Echocardiogr.* 2009;22:975–1014.

2. **Effective orifice area (EOA)**
   a. **Aortic valves**

$$\text{EOA} = \text{Cross-sectional area of LVOT} \times \frac{\text{Time velocity integral LVOT}}{\text{Time velocity integral prosthetic aortic valve}}$$

where LVOT is the left ventricular outflow tract. The cross-sectional area is derived from the diameter measurement just underneath the prosthesis from the parasternal long-axis view. Generally, the labeled prosthesis size should not be used in the measurement, as it will likely overestimate the EOA.

   b. **Mitral valves**
      i. The stroke volume across the aortic or pulmonic valves can be used, provided there is no significant insufficiency.
      ii. The calculated EOA can be compared with what is expected for the valve type/size as per the tables. If the calculated value is 1 to 2 standard deviations below what is reported for that particular valve, prosthetic stenosis should be suspected.
      iii. In general, for a normally functioning aortic valve prostheses, the EOA is >1.2 cm^2. Less than 0.8 cm^2 is abnormal and suggestive of stenosis. Intermediate values could represent stenosis, a smaller size valve, or some degree of mismatch.
      iv. For normally functioning mitral prostheses, the EOA is ≥ 2 cm^2. Less than 1 cm^2 is generally indicative of severe stenosis. Intermediate values could represent stenosis, a smaller size valve, or some degree of mismatch.

   c. **Dimensionless index:** This looks only at the ratio of the LVOT velocity time integral (VTI) and atrioventricular VTI. Thus, any error imposed by uncertainty of LVOT diameter is eliminated. A normally functioning valve will typically have a DI of ≥ 0.30. A ratio of <0.25 usually suggests significant stenosis.

   d. **Pressure half-time:** Estimated valve area from the pressure half-time method is not valid for prosthetic mitral valves. However, in an individual patient, an increase in the pressure half-time over serial studies could be indicative of development of stenosis. Also, a pressure half-time greater than 200 ms is often suggestive of significant stenosis. A normally functioning valve typically has a pressure half-time of less than 130 ms.

e. **Aortic velocity profile:** In a normally functioning aortic prosthesis, the continuous-wave Doppler velocity profile is early peaking. The acceleration time is typically <100 ms. As stenosis develops, the contour becomes more rounded and later peaking.

f. **Causes of increased gradients**
   i. Prosthetic stenosis (EOA will be low, DI will be low, pressure half-time may be prolonged for mitral prostheses).
   ii. Patient–prosthesis mismatch (normally functioning valve, but EOA too small for patient's BSA cardiac output requirements, resulting in increased flow and gradients). This is discussed further under complications. This is usually evident from the initial postoperative echocardiogram.
   iii. High-flow states where the DI is typically preserved as both LVOT and aortic valve gradients are increased. In the setting of mitral prosthesis, elevated velocities may be noted across the LVOT/aortic valve, giving a clue to increased output.
   iv. Prosthetic regurgitation often will have a greater elevation in peak gradient than mean gradient. TEE may be needed to assess the degree of regurgitation.
   v. Pressure recovery when the velocity through the smaller central orifice of a mechanical bileaflet tilting disk valve is sampled. This smaller central orifice gives rise to a higher velocity jet, creating a localized pressure drop. This is largely recovered once the flows from the two lateral orifices coalesce with the central jet and hence are not reflective of the true pressure gradient across the valve. The normal values usually account for this.

g. **Prosthetic valve regurgitation (Fig. 8.5):** Mechanical prostheses do have a built-in or physiologic regurgitation. For the bileaflet tilting disks, these occur laterally (at the disk/housing interface) as well as centrally. For mitral valves,

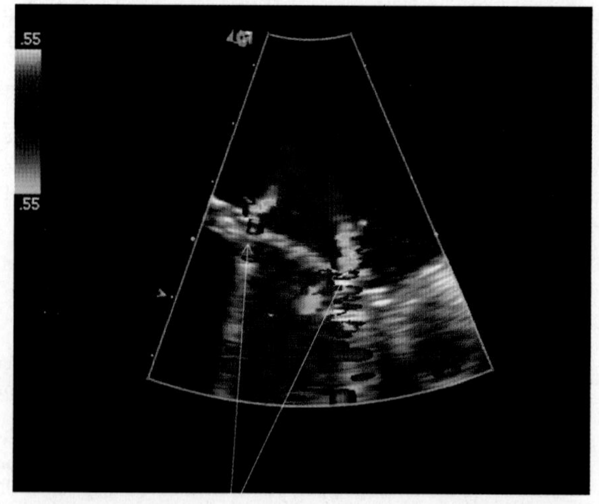

FIGURE 8.5 Normal physiologic regurgitation. Normal physiologic regurgitant washing jets with a mechanical valve *(arrows)*.

these are assessed with TEE (as the left atrium is shadowed from the prosthesis on TTE). The lateral jets are seen to either converge or diverge (depending on the transducer angle). The jets are usually narrow at the origin and often do not have much aliasing as the jets proceed into the left atrium. It is important to distinguish these jets from perivalvular jets, which originate outside the sewing ring. Although bioprosthetic valves do not have any built-in regurgitation, trivial valvular jets can often be seen.

VII. FLUOROSCOPY/CHEST X-RAY (FIG. 8.6)

Chest X-ray can identify the presence of prosthetic valves. Fluoroscopy can identify excessive motion of prosthetic valves, which indicates presence of partial valve dehiscence. For mechanical prosthesis, fluoroscopy can identify prosthetic leaflet motion, identifying leaflets that do not open or close completely. There are normative values for opening angles for the various valves.

VIII. CARDIAC CATHETERIZATION

Angiography is obviously needed to define concomitant coronary artery disease in patients undergoing valvular intervention. Aortography and left ventriculography

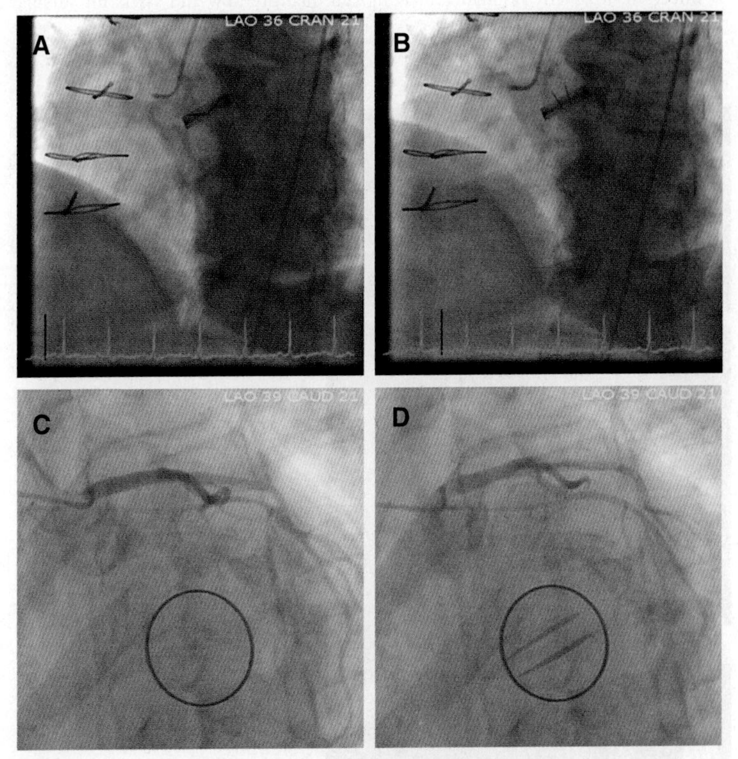

FIGURE 8.6 Fluoroscopic evaluation. **A, B:** Bileaflet valve viewed from the side. **C, D:** Bileaflet valve viewed *en face*. Leaflets are not visible when closed in this imaging plane.

will identify presence of aortic and mitral regurgitation. Although these are rarely needed at the present time given the accuracy of echocardiography and TEE, there are select patients in whom angiography may better identify these jets. Aortography can be useful for eccentric jets, as well as in patients who have both aortic and mitral valve replacements. Assessing aortic regurgitation can be difficult with echocardiography when there is confluence with mitral inflow and shadowing from the mitral prosthesis. In the setting of suspected prosthetic stenosis, invasive assessment of pressure gradients may sometimes be needed, if echocardiographic parameters are equivocal.

IX. COMPUTED TOMOGRAPHY/MAGNETIC RESONANCE IMAGING (FIGS. 8.7 TO 8.9)

Computed tomography (CT) scanning can be used to assess for tissue ingrowth on prosthetic valves, as well as valve thrombosis and vegetations. Abscess cavities can be identified and can complement TEE (especially in regions where there is acoustic shadowing from mechanical prostheses). Four-dimensional CT can allow for dynamic assessment of mechanical leaflet motion. Stuck leaflets and valve dehiscence can be identified. As a bioprosthetic valve degenerates, calcification can occur on the leaflets. This can be visualized by CT imaging. Fluorodeoxyglucose positron emission tomography imaging can be done with CT imaging and may help to identify prosthetic valve infection. Magnetic resonance imaging can quantify flow and assess for valvular regurgitation.

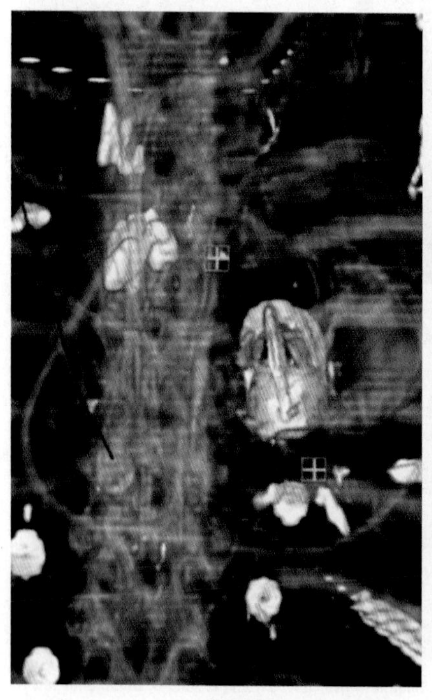

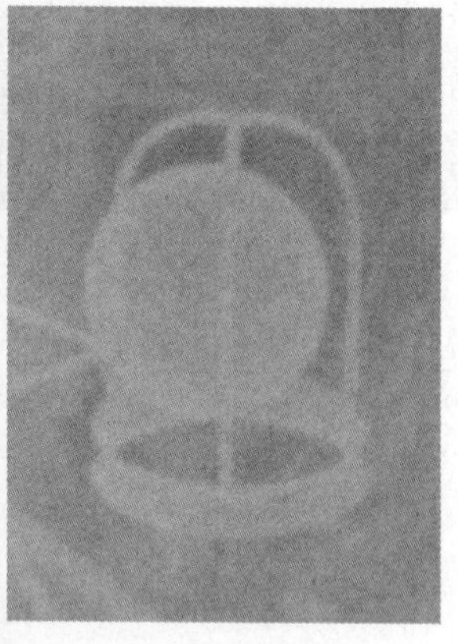

FIGURE 8.7 Ball-cage valve with CT scan.

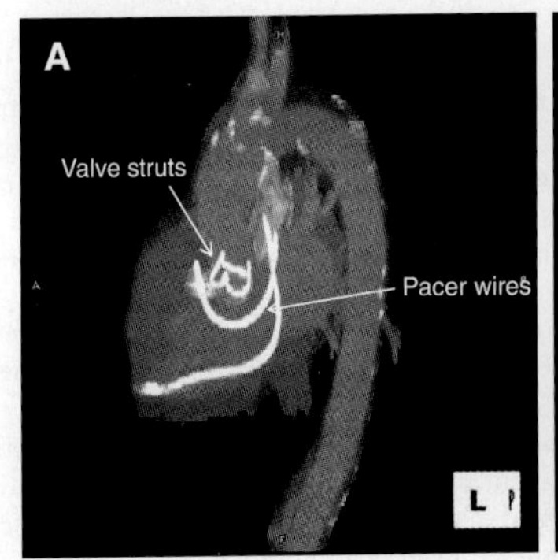

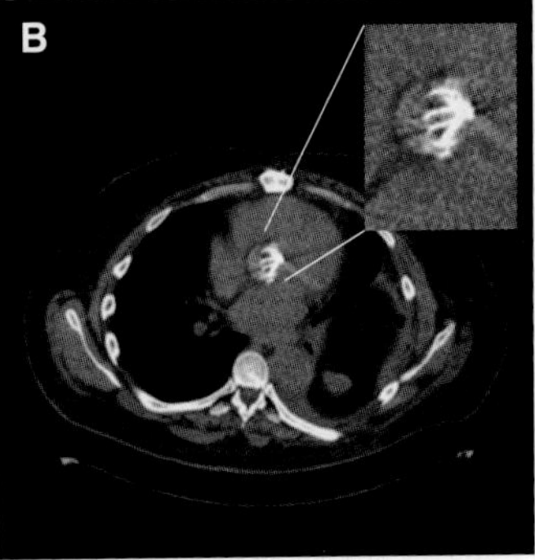

FIGURE 8.8 CT assessment of prosthetic valves. **A:** CT scan maximum intensity projection (MIP) image of bioprosthetic aortic valve struts and pacemaker wires. **B:** CT scan MIP image of mechanical aortic valve with leaflets open.

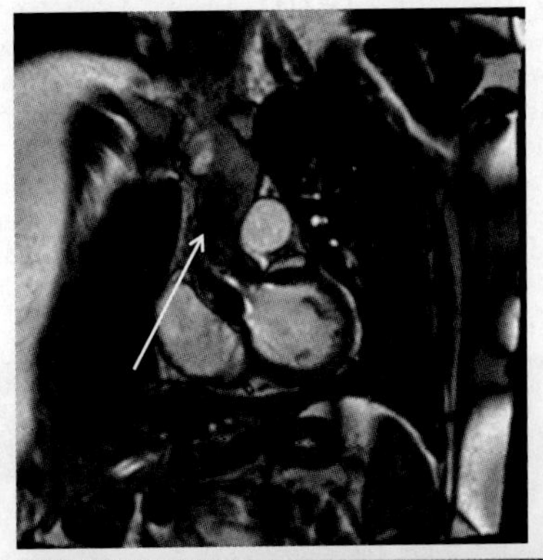

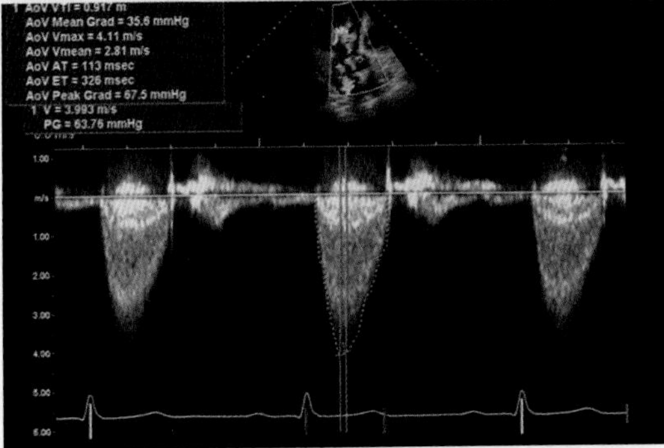

FIGURE 8.9 Magnetic resonance imaging in prosthetic aortic stenosis. Increased flow velocity as evident by the turbulent flow *(black)* in ascending aorta.

X. PROSTHETIC VALVE DYSFUNCTION

A. Patient–prosthesis mismatch

1. Although discussed under dysfunction, this term applies to a valve that performs as expected hemodynamically but is relatively obstructive given the size of the patient and the necessary cardiac output requirements. This phenomenon is generally seen with aortic valve prostheses and occurs when the valve that is placed is small relative to a patient's BSA. This can result in inadequate relief of symptoms for the patient and worse long-term outcomes.
2. This assessment is made by calculating the indexed EOA. An EOA of $\leq 0.85\ cm^2/m^2$ is thought to indicate the presence of moderate mismatch, and $\leq 0.65\ cm^2/m^2$ indicates severe mismatch.
3. Normative tables can provide expected or projected EOA for any given bioprosthetic valve and can be used to see if a patient may be at risk for this outcome. A valve with an effective EOA of 1.2 cm^2 would calculate to result in mismatch if implanted in a patient with a BSA of 2 m^2 (indexed ROA of 1.2/2 or 0.6 cm^2/m^2). If this is the case, a root enlargement procedure (to allow for a larger valve) or a stentless valve should be considered.
4. Mismatch may be evident immediately after valve placement. However, if mismatch is in the mild to moderate range, it may not be apparent for a few years. With superimposed functional degeneration, it can lead to a further increase in gradients.

B. Prosthetic valve stenosis (Figs. 8.10 and 8.11)

1. For bioprosthetic valves, their finite life span culminates in stenosis and/or regurgitation. Degeneration leads to leaflet fibrosis and calcification. When mechanical valves develop stenosis, it is a result of pannus (tissue ingrowth) and/or progressive thrombus accumulation.
2. The indications for reoperation in the setting of prosthetic stenosis are the same as for native valve stenosis. For patients in whom surgical risk is deemed high, a percutaneous transcatheter valve-in-valve approach can be considered. Long-term

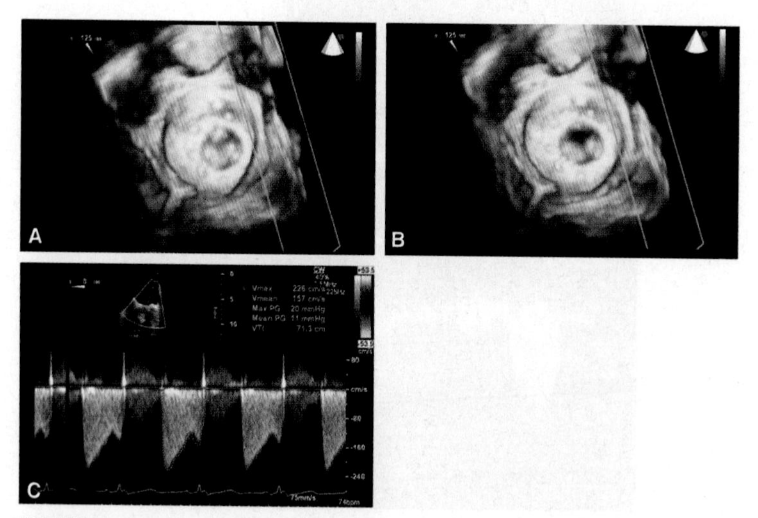

FIGURE 8.10 Prosthetic mitral stenosis. **A:** All three leaflets closed in systole. **B:** Incomplete opening of two leaflets in diastole. **C:** Increased gradients consistent with prosthetic stenosis.

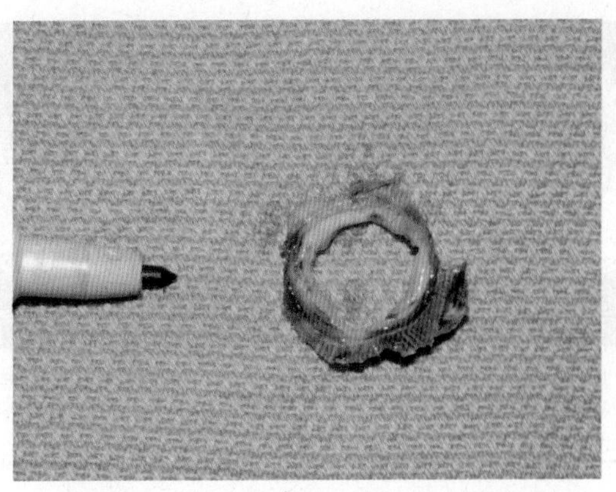

FIGURE 8.11 Pannus on mechanical aortic valve replacement.

efficacy data are still not available, and these devices are not yet approved for this indication. Registry data suggested a 93% initial success rate (however, not taking into account elevated gradients). One-year survival has been reported at 83% (recognizing that this is a subgroup of patients thought to be at high risk for reoperation because of comorbidities). Patients with smaller original valve size and predominant bioprosthetic stenosis fared worse (with lower EOA and higher gradients, and potential mismatch). During the procedure, ostial coronary obstruction and device malposition are complications that must be carefully guarded against.

3. The promise of this technique appears to be resulting in younger patients increasingly opting for a biologic valve instead of a mechanical prosthesis, in the hope that reintervention can be accomplished via these means. Therefore, placing the largest valve at time of the initial surgery would appear to be paramount in this regard.

C. **Prosthetic valve regurgitation**

1. **Valvular regurgitation** of a bioprosthetic valve can result from structural deterioration over time.
2. When regurgitation becomes severe, it is reasonable to proceed with surgery even in the absence of symptoms (class IIa recommendation from ACC/AHA guidelines). This is based on the risk of sudden clinical deterioration if further leaflet degeneration/tearing occurs. As for prosthetic valve stenosis, regurgitant valves have also been approached via valve-in-valve transcatheter approach. In mechanical valves, pannus or thrombus may result in incomplete leaflet closure, resulting in regurgitation (Fig. 8.12).
3. **Perivalvular regurgitation** can result from weakness of the tissues surrounding the prosthesis (leading to disruption of sutures) or as a sequela of endocarditis. Annular calcification at time of the original operation is also a risk factor for this occurrence. Perivalvular regurgitation can be seen with both bioprosthetic valves and mechanical valves. This can result in hemolytic anemia. Mild cases can be managed medically. However, if this is severe and results in need for frequent transfusions, then reoperation should be considered. Likewise, surgery is indicated if regurgitation is significant and results in symptoms.
4. In patients in whom reoperation carries a significant risk, there may be percutaneous options (Fig. 8.13) to address perivalvular regurgitation. Occluder devices can be delivered, which can reduce the severity of the regurgitation. Devices that are used include the Amplatzer devices (atrial and ventricular septal devices, vascular

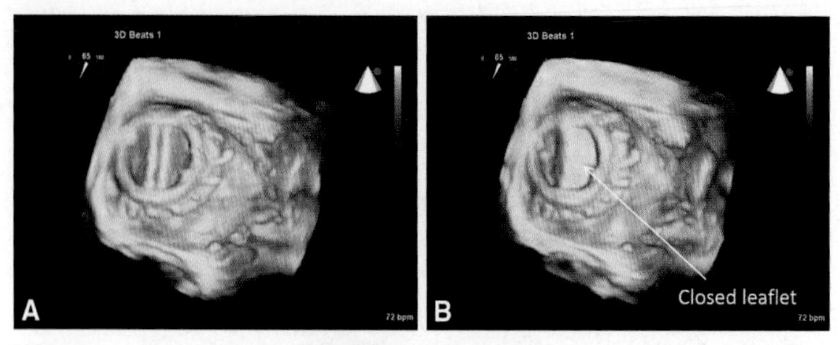

FIGURE 8.12 Incomplete closure of one leaflet of a mechanical mitral valve replacement. **A:** Both leaflets open in diastole. **B:** Incomplete closure of one leaflet in systole *(white arrow)*. Closed leaflet *(black arrow)*.

plugs). The device that best suits the size and shape of the defect is chosen. More than one device may be needed. Care must be taken not to impede prosthetic leaflet motion with the device, and also not to compromise inflow or outflow.

5. These procedures require a highly skilled team of interventionalists, with detailed imaging analysis of these leaks with TTE, TEE, and even CT scan preprocedure.

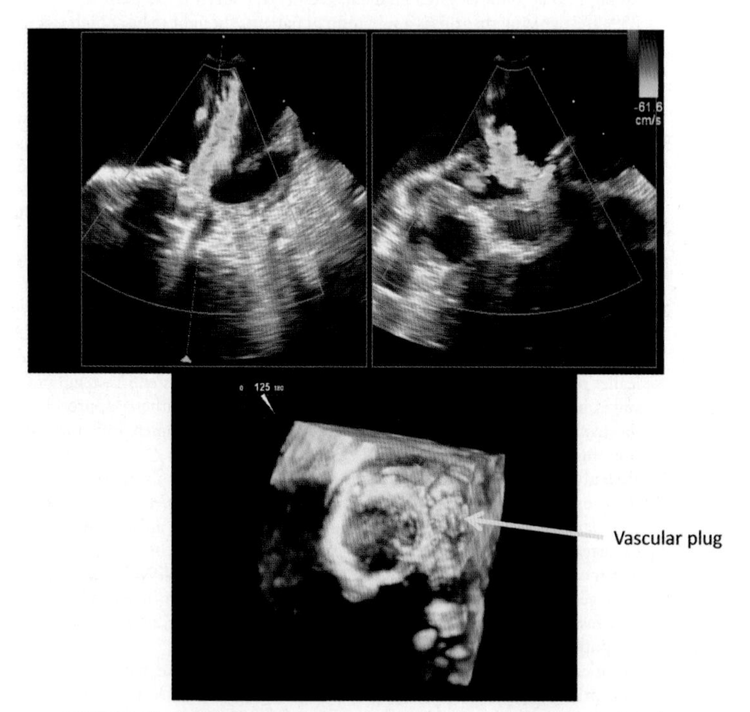

FIGURE 8.13 Perivalvular leak, percutaneous closure. Vascular plug *(arrow, top left)*.

Imaging guidance during the procedure complements fluoroscopy and is important to assess for degree of residual regurgitation, as well as for any compromise to leaflet function or inflow/outflow. Catheter access is obtained via a transseptal approach, transapical approach, or retrograde aortic approach. Improvement in regurgitation will improve symptoms of congestive heart failure (CHF), but near-complete resolution is needed to ameliorate hemolysis.

6. Perivalvular regurgitation in transcatheter valves is more common than with surgically placed valves, as a result of incomplete apposition to the annulus. Severity of perivalvular regurgitation does affect outcomes because the presence of more than mild regurgitation is associated with increased 1-year mortality. Given the eccentric nature of the jets, estimating severity can be difficult at times. Parameters that are used include the extent of diastolic flow reversal in the descending aorta, the circumferential extent of the regurgitation in short-axis view ($<10\%$ considered mild, $\geq 30\%$ severe), and the effective ROA (<0.10 cm^2 is mild, ≥ 30 cm^2 is severe). Regurgitant volume and regurgitant fraction can also be estimated.

XI. COMPLICATIONS

A. Prosthetic valve thrombosis (Fig. 8.14)

1. This complication occurs more with mechanical valves than with bioprosthetic ones, but is possible for both. Differentiation of thrombosis from pannus (tissue ingrowth) can be difficult by imaging. However, a more abrupt presentation and history of inadequate anticoagulation would favor a more thrombotic process than pannus. TEE, fluoroscopy, or CT can all be used to identify impaired leaflet motion and even the presence of a thrombus.
2. Management is guided by the ACC/AHA guidelines. The initial recommendation in suspected cases of prosthetic valve thrombosis is TTE to assess the hemodynamic severity. TEE can then be done to assess thrombus and valve motion. CT/fluoroscopy can also assist with detection of thrombus and valve motion.
3. For thrombosed valves (left-sided) with class III and IV symptoms, emergency surgery is recommended (class I recommendation). If symptoms are less severe, but if there is a large or mobile thrombus (>0.8 cm^2), then surgery is also felt to

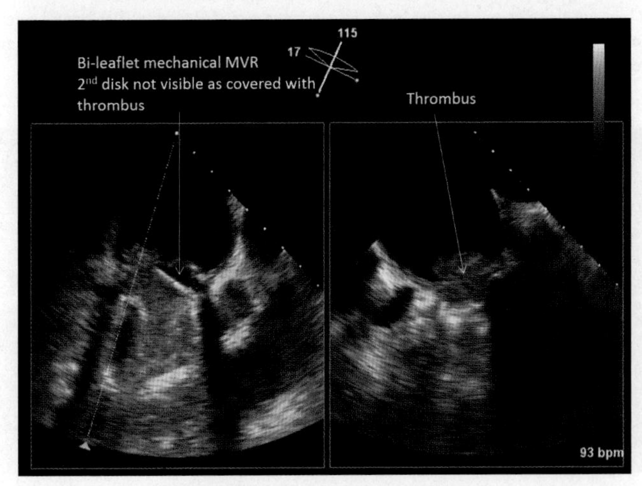

FIGURE 8.14 Prosthetic valve thrombosis.

be reasonable (as a class IIa indication). These larger lesions have more embolic potential and risk of stroke with thrombolysis.

4. If symptoms are recent (<14 days) and mild (class I and II) and the thrombus is small (<0.8 cm^2), then it is reasonable to treat initially with unfractionated heparin. If the thombus persists, then fibrinolytic therapy is reasonable. For right-sided valves, fibrinolytic therapy appears to be a reasonable first-line therapy.

B. Endocarditis (Fig. 8.15)

1. Prosthetic valve endocarditis still results in significant morbidity and mortality. Early identification and treatment are key, along with coordinated efforts from infectious disease specialists, cardiologists, and cardiac surgeons. Endocarditis that occurs within the first 60 days of valve implantation is generally acquired from the hospital setting, and the most common agent is *Staphylococcus aureus*. Endocarditis that develops after 60 days but within the first year of valve implantation (two-thirds of cases occur within the 1st year) represents a mix between health care–acquired infection and community-acquired infection. Coagulase-negative *Staphylococcus* is the most common pathogen. Infection that develops after the first year is typically community acquired, and the pathogens resemble those of native valve endocarditis.
2. Earlier surgery (before completion of the full course of antibiotic therapy) is often needed. This is especially the case if there is valve dysfunction resulting in CHF, the causative agent is *Staphylococcus aureus* or a fungus, or there is an abscess cavity and/or heart block. Large (>1 cm) mobile vegetations, recurrent embolic events, persistent bacteremia despite appropriate therapy, and relapsing infection are also indications for surgery.

C. Struts causing LVOT obstruction (Fig. 8.16)

A rarer immediate complication can occur with a bioprosthetic mitral valve. If the LV cavity is small and the valve is seated with the struts oriented toward the LV outflow tract, then a fixed obstruction can occur to LV outflow. When intraoperative TEE is used, this can usually be identified at the time of surgery and the situation remedied (may require a lower-profile mechanical valve).

XII. INTERVENTIONAL INDICATIONS FOR PROSTHETIC VALVE DISEASE

These are also discussed earlier in the respective sections. However, current and emerging indications include valve-in-valve transcatheter procedures for bioprosthetic stenosis/regurgitation and percutaneous occluder devices for perivalvular regurgitation.

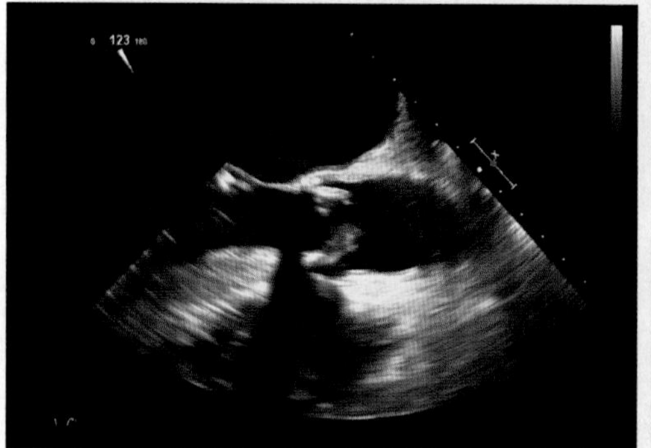
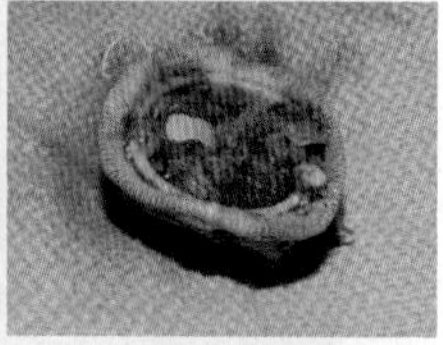
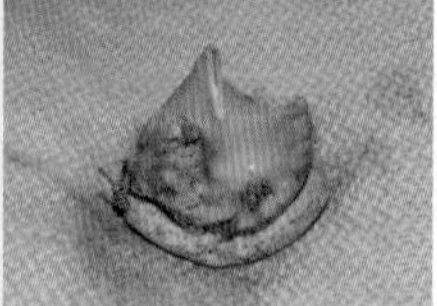

FIGURE 8.15 Infective endocarditis.

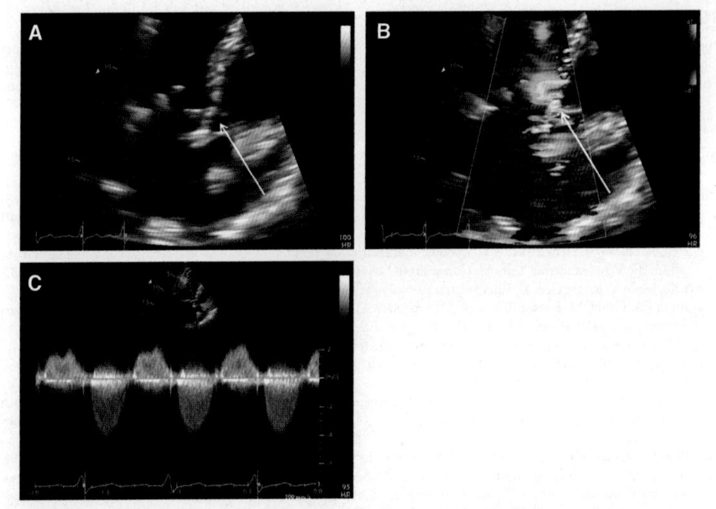

FIGURE 8.16 Bioprosthetic mitral struts causing left ventricular outflow tract (LVOT) obstruction. **A:** Strut oriented toward LVOT *(arrow)*. **B:** Flow accelerations across LVOT *(arrow)*. **C:** Fixed LVOT obstruction.

XIII. SURGICAL INDICATIONS FOR PROSTHETIC VALVE DISEASE

These include prosthetic valve mismatch, prosthetic valve stenosis/regurgitation, valve thrombosis, perivalvular regurgitation, and endocarditis.

KEY PEARLS

- It is important to have echocardiographic assessment of prosthetic valves 4 to 6 weeks after implantation to establish baseline valvular gradients, dimensionless index, and pressure half-time (for mitral prostheses).
- The choice of bioprosthetic versus mechanical valve is a shared decision process, taking into account patient preference, durability of valves, risk for reintervention, and risk of anticoagulation.
- Careful evaluation preoperatively can minimize the likelihood for patient–prosthesis mismatch.
- Aspirin therapy is recommended for all prosthetic valves (along with warfarin for mechanical valves).
- A high index of suspicion and early diagnosis of prosthetic valve endocarditis are important to minimize morbidity and mortality.
- Echocardiography, transesophageal echocardiography, computed tomography, and magnetic resonance imaging can all help in assessment of prosthetic valve dysfunction, and multimodality imaging may be needed at times.
- Transcatheter options are evolving and require skilled operators and a team approach to assess candidates suitable for these approaches, as opposed to surgical intervention.

SUGGESTED READINGS

Binder RK, Webb JG. Percutaneous mitral and aortic paravalvular leak repair: indications, current application, and future directions. *Curr Cardiol Rep*. 2013;15:342.

Chlang YP, Chikwe J, Moskowitz AJ, et al. Survival and long-term outcomes following bioprosthetic vs mechanical aortic valve replacement in patients aged 50 to 69 years. *JAMA*. 2014;312(13):1323–1329. doi:10.1001/jama.2014.12679.

Dvir D, Webb JG, Bleiziffer S, et al. Transcatheter aortic valve implantation in failed bioprosthetic surgical valves. *JAMA*. 2014;312(2):162–170.

Dvir D, Webb J, Brecker S, et al. Transcatheter aortic valve replacement for degenerative bioprosthetic surgical valves: results from the global valve-in-valve registry. *Circulation*. 2012;126:2335–2344.

Joint Task Force on the Management of Valvular Heart Disease of the European Society of Cardiology (ESC), European Association for Cardio-Thoracic Surgery(EACTS), Vahanian A, et al. Guidelines on the management of valvular heart disease (version 2012). *Eur Heart J*. 2012;33:2451–2496.

Kappetein AP, Head SJ, Généreux P, et al. Updated standardized endpoint definitions for transcatheter aortic valve implantation: the Valve Academic Research Consortium-2 consensus document. *J Thorac Cardiovasc Surg*. 2013;145:6–23.

Kumar R, Jelnin V, Kliger C, et al. Percutaneous paravalvular leak closure. *Cardiol Clin*. 2013;31:431–440.

Nishimura RA, Otto CM, Bonow RO, et al. 2014 AHA/ACC guideline for the management of patients with valvular heart disease. *J Am Coll Cardiol*. 2014. doi:10.1016/j.jacc.2014.02.536.

Pibarot P, Demesinil JG. Doppler echocardiographic evaluation of prosthetic valve function. *Heart*. 2012;98:69–78.

Pibarot P, Demesinil JG. Valve prosthesis–patient mismatch, 1978 to 2011: from original concept to compelling evidence. *J Am Coll Cardiol*. 2012;60(12):1136–1139.

Taramasso M, Maisano F, Latib A, et al. Conventional surgery and transcatheter closure via surgical transapical approach for paravalvular leak repair in high-risk patients: results from a single-centre experience. *Eur Heart J Cardiovasc Imaging*. 2014;15:1161–1167.

Zoghbi WA, Chambers JB, Dumesnil JG, et al. Recommendations for evaluation of prosthetic valves with echocardiography and Doppler ultrasound: a report from the American Society of Echocardiography's Guidelines and Standards Committee and the Task Force on Prosthetic Valves, developed in conjunction with the American College of Cardiology Cardiovascular Imaging Committee, Cardiac Imaging Committee of the American Heart Association, the European Association of Echocardiography, a registered branch of the European Society of Cardiology, the Japanese Society of Echocardiography and the Canadian Society of Echocardiography, endorsed by the American College of Cardiology Foundation, American Heart Association, European Association of Echocardiography, a registered branch of the European Society of Cardiology, the Japanese Society of Echocardiography, and Canadian Society of Echocardiography. *J Am Soc Echocardiogr*. 2009;22:975–1014.

CHAPTER 9

Paul C. Cremer

Infective Endocarditis

I. INTRODUCTION

A. **Epidemiology.** The overall incidence of infective endocarditis is 3 to 10 per 100,000 patient-years, and in the United States, approximately 15,000 new cases are diagnosed every year. In developing countries, infective endocarditis is still most often associated with rheumatic heart disease, and patients are more likely to have a subacute or chronic presentation. Despite the decline of rheumatic heart disease in the developed world, the incidence of infective endocarditis has not decreased. Instead, the predominant risk factors have changed. In the developed world, an acute presentation is more common, and patients are more likely to be elderly with degenerative valve disease, prosthetic valves, chronic indwelling devices, or other predisposing medical conditions.

B. **Morbidity and mortality.** In the past few decades, outcomes have improved dramatically in other cardiovascular diseases, but endocarditis still has significant morbidity and mortality. Despite advances in diagnostic and therapeutic procedures, in-hospital mortality is 15% to 20%, and 1-year mortality is approximately 40%. In part, this persistently high morbidity and mortality is related to the shift in the epidemiology of infective endocarditis. More cases are now attributable to highly destructive microorganisms in older patients with prior cardiac disease and other comorbidities.

C. **Heart valve team.** Because of this changing risk profile and the diverse nature of presentation, the diagnosis and treatment of endocarditis remain a challenge. A high index of suspicion is required because delayed or missed diagnoses can lead to complications related to invasive and metastatic disease. Therefore, a heart valve team approach including cardiology, infectious disease, and cardiothoracic surgery is recommended to ensure expeditious diagnosis and treatment. In patients with destructive disease who may require urgent or emergent surgery, care should be provided in a center with immediate access to cardiac surgery. Occasionally, metastatic disease may also require the expertise of neurology, interventional neurology, neurosurgery, and abdominal or vascular surgery.

II. ETIOLOGY

A. **Classification.** Given the variable presentations of infective endocarditis, a systematic approach to the disease is essential. Sir William Osler famously distinguished subacute from acute bacterial endocarditis in 1885. Acute infective endocarditis leads to valve destruction and metastatic complications in days to weeks, whereas subacute disease progresses over weeks to months. This distinction remains a cornerstone in any evaluation of a patient with suspected endocarditis. However, in the current era of cardiac surgery and devices, frequent health care contact, and resistant microorganisms, patients can be further classified according to the structures involved, mode of acquisition, and culpable pathogen.

B. **Structures involved.** Patients are typically classified as having native valve, prosthetic valve, or cardiac device–related endocarditis.

1. Native valve endocarditis is further classified into left- and right-sided disease. The most common predisposing valve lesion for left-sided endocarditis is degenerative mitral valve disease with mitral regurgitation, which has been observed in 40% to 45% of cases. In the developed world, mitral valve prolapse with regurgitation is the most frequent abnormality, but in elderly patients, mitral annular calcification can also serve as a nidus for endocarditis. In 25% to 30% of patients with native left-sided endocarditis, aortic regurgitation is the predisposing lesion, and a bicuspid aortic valve is also a risk factor.
2. Right-sided endocarditis typically involves the tricuspid valve. The pulmonic valve is rarely infected. The most common risk factor for right-sided endocarditis is intravenous drug use. Indwelling lines and cardiac devices are also common risk factors as line-related infection can spread to involve the tricuspid valve. A ventricular septal defect is a risk for endocarditis, often involving the septal leaflet of the tricuspid valve. Other congenital heart defects that increase the risk for endocarditis include a patent ductus arteriosus, coarctation of the aorta, and tetralogy of Fallot. Conversely, secundum atrial septal defects are not associated with an increased risk of infective endocarditis.
3. When compared to the general population, patients with prosthetic valves are 50 times more likely to develop infective endocarditis. Two-thirds of all cases occur within the first year after surgery, and the incidence of infective endocarditis is similar in bioprosthetic and mechanical valves. Given the preponderance of infection within the first year, prosthetic valve endocarditis is categorized as early-onset (within 2 months of surgery), intermediate-onset (2 months to 1 year after surgery), and late-onset (greater than 1 year after surgery) disease. Early-onset prosthetic valve endocarditis is most likely related to surgery or another health care encounter. Intermediate-onset disease is less likely to be related to the index surgery, but health care–related infection is still the most common cause. Risks for early- and intermediate-onset endocarditis include prolonged surgery, reoperation, and sternal wound infections. As intermediate prosthetic valve endocarditis approaches 1 year, infection is more likely to be community acquired, and late-onset disease more closely resembles native valve endocarditis in microbiology. Data on infective endocarditis after transcatheter valve replacement are emerging, but the incidence and epidemiology appear similar to surgical valve replacement, with most cases occurring within the first year after the procedure.
4. Given the rising number of patients with cardiac devices (permanent pacemakers and implantable defibrillators) and the increased risk of infection with an intravenous lead, the incidence of endocarditis is increasing in these patients. Of note, local device infection should be distinguished from device-related endocarditis. A local device infection is restricted to the pocket. In device-related endocarditis, infection can spread along the lead to the endocardium and the electrode tip. The primary cause of cardiac device–related infection is contamination by local bacteriologic flora at the time of device implantation, although hematogenous seeding is also common. In general, risks for device-related endocarditis include diabetes mellitus, heart failure, generator replacement, and renal dysfunction.

C. **Mode of acquisition.** Infective endocarditis is community acquired, health care associated, or related to intravenous drug use. Health care–associated infection is further divided into nosocomial and non-nosocomial acquisition. The latter refers to infection acquired after a recent hospitalization, at a nursing home or long-term care facility, at a hemodialysis center, or at an infusion clinic. The etiologies of infective endocarditis in specific communities can vary widely, and the spectrum of disease is primarily determined by the rates of intravenous drug use and health care–associated infection. Overall, community acquisition is most common (~70%), followed by nosocomial (~15%) and non-nosocomial (~10%) infection. In North America, health care–associated endocarditis is more common (35% to 40%) and is primarily related to non-nosocomial infection; chronic intravenous access is present in approximately 25% of cases of infective endocarditis. In intravenous drug users, concomitant human immunodeficiency virus (HIV) infection is common and increases the risk for infective endocarditis. Finally, with community-acquired disease, the source of infection is usually not identified but may be attributed to a dental procedure or an infected skin lesion.

D. Microbiology

1. When the mode of acquisition and infected cardiac structures are established, the most likely microorganisms can be determined (Table 9.1). Overall, in the developed world, staphylococci (~40%) are now a more common cause of infective endocarditis than streptococci (~30%). In fact, *Staphylococcus aureus* is not only the most common microorganism in intravenous drug users, but also the most frequent pathogen in native valve nonintravenous drug users as well as in patients with prosthetic valves and cardiac devices. Among community-acquired cases of infective endocarditis, staphylococcal infection is most frequent (30% to 35%) and is closely followed by oral streptococci (20% to 25%). In health care–associated infection, staphylococcal infection predominates and is responsible for approximately 70% of nosocomial and 65% of non-nosocomial infections.

TABLE 9.1 Frequency of Infective Endocarditis by Most Common Microorganisms in Patients with Native Valves, Intravenous Drug Use, Prosthetic Valves, and Cardiac Devices

Native Valve Endocarditis		Endocarditis of Intracardiac Material	
No Intravenous Drug Use	**Intravenous Drug Use**	**Prosthetic Valve**	**Cardiac Device**
Staphylococcus aureus (28%)	*S. aureus* (68%)	*S. aureus* (23%)	*S. aureus* (35%)
Oral streptococci (21%)	Oral streptococci (10%)	Coagulase-negative staphylococcus (17%)	Coagulase-negative staphylococcus (26%)
Enterococcus species (11%)	*Enterococcus* species (5%)	Oral streptococci (12%)	Culture negative (11%)
Culture negative (9%)	Culture negative (5%)	*Enterococcus* species (12%)	Oral streptococci (8%)
Coagulase-negative staphylococcus (9%)	Coagulase-negative staphylococcus (3%)	Culture negative (12%)	*Enterococcus* species (6%)
Streptococcus gallolyticus (7%)	*S. gallolyticus* (1%)	*S. gallolyticus* (5%)	*S. gallolyticus* (3%)
HACEK (2%)	Fungi/yeast (1%)	Fungi/yeast (4%)	Fungi/yeast (1%)
Fungi/yeast (1%)	HACEK (0%)	HACEK (2%)	HACEK (0.5%)

Adapted from Murdoch DR, Corey GR, Hoen B, et al. Clinical presentation, etiology, and outcome of infective endocarditis in the 21st century: the international collaboration on endocarditis-prospective cohort study. *Arch Intern Med.* 2009;169:463–473. HACEK, *Haemophilus, Aggregatibacter actinomycetemcomitans, Cardiobacterium hominis, Eikenella corrodens,* and *Kingella* species.

The coagulase-negative *S. epidermidis* is a frequent cause of prosthetic valve and cardiac device–related endocarditis.

2. *Enterococcal* species cause approximately 10% of cases of infective endocarditis, typically related to *Enterococcus faecalis* (85% to 90%). The remaining cases are mostly because of *E. faecium*, with a few cases attributed to *E. durans*. Enterococci typically reside in the gastrointestinal and genitourinary tracts, and endocarditis can be nosocomial, related to manipulation of the colon, urethra, or bladder.
3. Culture-negative endocarditis represents another 10% of cases and is defined by the lack of identification of a causative organism after three blood cultures.
4. The HACEK organisms (*Haemophilus*, *Aggregatibacter actinomycetemcomitans*, *Cardiobacterium hominis*, *Eikenella corrodens*, and *Kingella* species) are now a rare cause of endocarditis (~2%), especially in North America. Other Gram-negative bacteria (Enterobacteriaceae, *Acinetobacter* species, *Pseudomonas aeruginosa*) infrequently cause endocarditis, and risk factors include intravenous drug use, end-stage liver disease, central venous catheters, and older age. *P. aeruginosa* can be highly destructive and poorly responsive to antibiotics.
5. *Coxiella burnetii*, the causative agent of Q fever, can cause endocarditis; herding cattle, sheep, or goats is a risk factor. *Bartonella henselae* (cat scratch disease) and *B. quintana* (trench fever) can also cause endocarditis, most often in homeless or alcoholic patients. Most cases of endocarditis related to *C. burnetii* or *Bartonella* species have been diagnosed in Europe.
6. Fungi are another rare cause of endocarditis (~2%). *Candida albicans* causes approximately 25% of cases of fungal endocarditis, other *Candida* species are responsible for another 25%, and *Aspergillus* species also cause 25% of cases. Fungal endocarditis is most common in patients with prosthetic heart valves. Other risk factors include intravenous drug use and an immunocompromised condition. Often, *Candida* endocarditis is nosocomial.

III. PATHOPHYSIOLOGY

A. **Vegetations.** The primary manifestation of infective endocarditis is a vegetation on an endothelial defect. Normal valve endothelium is resistant to colonization by circulating bacteria. Endothelial damage commonly occurs from inflammation as in rheumatic heart disease, degenerative valve changes in the elderly, and indwelling catheters. These damaged areas often have platelets and fibrin that can promote the growth and adherence of microorganisms. Typical endocarditis pathogens can adhere to damaged valves and promote local procoagulant activity. Bacterial colonies thus attract further fibrin and inflammatory cells and nurture vegetations.

B. **Foreign material.** Microorganisms can also adhere to foreign material. In cardiac device–related infective endocarditis, vegetations can be found from the subclavian vein to the superior vena cava, on the electrode lead, the tricuspid valve, and endocardium of the right atrium and ventricle. In prosthetic valve endocarditis, the sewing ring is often infected, and bioprosthetic cusps seem more resistant to disintegration by bacterial enzymes compared to native valve cusps.

C. **Invasive disease.** Tissue disintegration that involves the valve annulus and spreads to extravascular areas is referred to as invasive disease. Typically, invasive disease develops in stages beginning with cellulitis, then forming an abscess and abscess cavity, and finally resulting in a pseudoaneurysm. Specific consequences of invasive disease include internal fistulas, perforations, and heart block. In general, enzymatic degradation by invasive bacteria prefers connective tissue and fat, and muscle is often preserved. Also, the invasive nature of microorganisms is different, and this distinction relates to acute and subacute presentations of infective endocarditis. Enterococcal infections are often minimally invasive, and fungal infections can have large vegetations with minimal invasion or tissue destruction. Oral streptococci can develop invasive complications, but usually over weeks to months. Conversely, *S.*

aureus can dissolve annular tissue and cause dehiscence of a prosthesis within days to weeks. The coagulase-negative *S. lugdunensis* can also have a rapidly destructive clinical course.

D. Anatomic considerations

1. Vegetations on native valves typically form on leaflets, but can also occur on chordae. In general, vegetations form on the low-pressure side of the valve where blood flow strikes the valve surface. Regurgitation results from a loss of leaflet integrity or chordal rupture. In aortic valve endocarditis, a secondary ("kissing") lesion commonly forms on the anterior mitral valve leaflet and less commonly develops on the aortic wall.
2. The magnitude of invasive disease is defined by the percentage of annulus involved, extent beyond the annulus, and the depth and size of cavities. Invasive disease is more common on the left side of the heart and is more frequent with the aortic valve compared to the mitral valve. In native valve endocarditis, extra-aortic invasion is often localized. The site of subcommissural invasion may be small, effectively hiding an extra-aortic focus of infection. Invasive disease is more common in prosthetic valve endocarditis, and extra-aortic invasion is frequently circumferential. However, cellulitis and abscesses can occur anywhere along the annulus. Heart block is most often associated with aortic valve endocarditis. Typically, bacterial invasion extends from the posterior aortic root into the right atrium and triangle of Koch, resulting in destruction of the atrioventricular node and bundle of His. In mitral valve endocarditis, anterior annular invasion leads to destruction of the aortomitral curtain, and posterior invasion enters the atrioventricular groove and separates the atrium from the ventricle.

IV. CLINICAL MANIFESTATIONS

Infective endocarditis can have a variable presentation depending on the pathogen and preexisting cardiac disease. Nonetheless, the hallmark manifestations of infective endocarditis are fever and a heart murmur.

A. Fever. Most patients (~80% to 90%) will present with a fever and often have chills, poor appetite, or weight loss. Notable exceptions include patients that are pretreated with antibiotics, elderly or immunocompromised patients, and patients with cardiac device–related endocarditis. These patients can have atypical presentation, and a high index of suspicion is essential. In addition, infective endocarditis should be considered in any patient with fever and one of the following: known cardiac lesion, recent procedure associated with bacteremia, congestive heart failure, new stroke or unexplained embolic event, or a peripheral abscess without a known cause. In addition, endocarditis should be suspected in any patient with a catheter-related bloodstream infection and persistently positive blood cultures after catheter removal.

B. Heart murmur. The majority of patients have a heart murmur (~85%). Many patients have preexisting heart murmurs related to valvular stenosis or regurgitation, valve replacement, congenital heart disease, or previous endocarditis.

C. Classic signs. Three-quarters of patients in the developed world present acutely within 30 days of infection. Embolic or vasculitic skin lesions are uncommon in these patients. In addition, patients with health care–associated and cardiac device–related endocarditis are unlikely to have classic features. However, these features are more common in the developing world where oral streptococcal infection still predominates. Examples include subungual hemorrhages, Roth spots (oval retinal hemorrhages), Osler nodes (subcutaneous nodules in the pulp of the digits), and Janeway lesions (hemorrhagic macular nontender lesions on the palms and soles of the feet).

D. Modified Duke criteria (Table 9.2). The modified Duke criteria are the most sensitive and specific criteria available and are divided into definite, probable, and rejected diagnostic groups. These criteria have been well validated in numerous studies in diverse populations including children, elderly, patients with prosthetic valves, and injection

TABLE 9.2 Modified Duke Criteria for the Diagnosis of Infective Endocarditis

Pathologic Criteria

1. Vegetation or intracardiac abscess confirmed by histologic examination
2. Microorganisms on culture or histology of a vegetation, thromboembolism, or intracardiac abscess

Major Clinical Criteria

1. At least two blood cultures positive for an organism typical for infective endocarditis, single blood culture positive or immunoglobulin G antibody titer for *C. burnetii* >1:800
2. Echocardiogram findings consistent with infective endocarditis including vegetation, abscess, partial dehiscence of a prosthetic valve, or new valvular regurgitation

Minor Clinical Criteria

1. Predisposing heart condition or intravenous drug use
2. Fever
3. Vascular phenomena: septic pulmonary infarcts, major arterial emboli, mycotic aneurysm, intracranial hemorrhage, conjunctival hemorrhages, Janeway lesions
4. Immunologic phenomena: glomerulonephritis, Osler nodes, Roth spots, elevated rheumatoid factor
5. Positive blood culture that does not meet major criteria (excludes single-positive culture for coagulase-negative staphylococci and microorganisms that do not cause endocarditis)

Adapted from Li JS, Sexton DJ, Mick N, et al. Proposed modifications to the Duke criteria for the diagnosis of infective endocarditis. *Clin Infect Dis.* 2000;30:633–638.

drug users. However, although still clinically useful, the modified Duke criteria may be less sensitive in these populations.

1. A definite pathologic diagnosis requires one of two criteria. For a definite clinical diagnosis, two major, one major and three minor, or five minor criteria are needed.
2. The possible diagnostic group includes one major and one minor or three minor criteria.
3. With a rejected diagnosis, an alternative diagnosis is evident. A diagnosis is also rejected if clinical manifestations resolve within a few days of antibiotics, or if there is no pathologic evidence of infective endocarditis at surgery or autopsy.

E. **Complications.** Patients with infective endocarditis can have complications related to valve damage, invasive disease, metastatic disease or as a result of treatment.

1. The most common complication of endocarditis is heart failure (30% to 40%), and the most common cause is aortic or mitral regurgitation. Heart failure is less common in right-sided endocarditis.
2. Stroke occurs in 15% to 20% of patients with infective endocarditis. The most common mechanism is ischemic stroke from a septic embolism. Clinically apparent embolic strokes most often involve the middle cerebral artery. Hemorrhagic transformation of an ischemic stroke can also occur and is often devastating. Other mechanisms of stroke include septic erosion of an artery without aneurysm and rupture of a mycotic aneurysm. Cerebral mycotic aneurysms tend to occur at branch points in the distal vessels.

3. Emboli besides stroke affect another 20% of patients. Septic pulmonary emboli or abscesses in right-sided or cardiac device–related endocarditis can present as pleuritic chest pain, cough, or hemoptysis. In addition to the brain, left-sided endocarditis frequently embolizes to the spleen. Vegetations can also embolize to coronary arteries, kidneys, and bowel. In general, embolism is more common with larger vegetations, and the risk of embolism is greatest in the first few days of antibiotic therapy. Fungi in particular may have especially large vegetations that embolize and cause major limb artery occlusion.
4. Periannular complications can frequently present with heart failure or heart block and are associated with *S. aureus* endocarditis. In patients with infective endocarditis, especially involving the aortic valve, the electrocardiogram should be followed closely for PR prolongation and complete heart block. The development of complete heart block in a patient with significant aortic regurgitation can result in rapid hemodynamic decompensation, but it is unclear if patients with a prolonged PR interval benefit from a prophylactic temporary pacemaker.
5. Acute renal failure is a frequent complication (~30%) in patients with infective endocarditis. Common causes include hemodynamic impairment, antibiotic toxicity, contrast nephropathy, renal infarction, and immune complex and vasculitic glomerulonephritis.

V. LABORATORY TESTING

A. **Blood cultures.** In patients with fever for more than 48 hours who have risk factors for endocarditis or newly diagnosed left-sided valvular regurgitation, at least two sets of blood cultures should be drawn. Risk factors include preexisting valvular heart disease, prosthetic valves, certain congenital heart diseases, immunodeficient conditions, injection drug users, or patients with a history of infective endocarditis. In stable patients with a subacute or chronic presentation, three sets of blood cultures should be drawn at peripheral sites at least 6 hours apart before antibiotics are given. Similarly, if a stable patient has suspected subacute or chronic endocarditis and is already on antibiotics, therapy should be stopped and blood cultures repeated. Antibiotic therapy may need to be discontinued for 7 to 10 days until blood cultures return positive. In fact, "culture-negative" endocarditis is often a result of the use of antibiotics before blood cultures are obtained. Furthermore, in endocarditis, bacteremia is constant. Therefore, blood cultures can be drawn when a patient is afebrile, and positive results from only one set of several blood cultures may be a contaminant. Finally, with continuous monitoring of blood cultures and nonculture-based diagnostics, routine incubation for more than 7 days is no longer necessary.

B. **Serologic testing.** Blood cultures are positive in 90% of patients, and serologic testing to identify the culprit should be performed in the other 10%. Serology for *C. burnetii* (Q fever) or *Bartonella* species is considered positive when respective immunoglobulin G serologies are ≥1:800.

C. **Tissue**
   1. In patients with culture-negative endocarditis, surgically removed tissue should be tested for bacterial DNA via polymerase chain reaction (PCR). PCR primers target bacterial DNA that codes for the 16S ribosomal subunit. This sequencing can help to identify rare causes of infective endocarditis, such as *Tropheryma whippelii*. Although PCR results can reliably identify the cause of endocarditis, they do not necessarily indicate ongoing infection. Bacterial DNA may have persisted in the tissue from past infections.
   2. In cardiac device–related endocarditis, generator pocket tissue should undergo Gram stain and culture. The lead tip should also be cultured when the device is explanted.

D. **Other tests.** Nonspecific laboratory findings are also common in infective endocarditis. Examples include an elevated C-reactive protein or erythrocyte sedimentation rate, leukocytosis, anemia, and microscopic hematuria.

VI. ECHOCARDIOGRAPHY

A. Indications (Fig. 9.1)

1. Echocardiography is essential in the evaluation of infective endocarditis, and all patients with suspected endocarditis should have a transthoracic echocardiogram (TTE). In addition to identifying vegetations, TTE assesses the severity of valvular lesions, ventricular function, pulmonary pressures, and complications. In native valve endocarditis, TTE has variably reported sensitivity for vegetations (50% to 90%). In general, sensitivity is modest in native valve endocarditis and poor in prosthetic valve endocarditis (35% to 70%). However, the overall specificity of a TTE is approximately 90%. Transesophageal echocardiogram (TEE) performs extremely well in the evaluation of endocarditis, with sensitivity and specificity greater than 90%, although sensitivity is lower in patients with prosthetic valves. Given the good specificity of TTE, and because TTE is noninvasive and often provides a more complete hemodynamic assessment than TEE, TTE is the first-line imaging test in suspected endocarditis for most patients.
2. TEE is pursued in two general scenarios. First, in a patient with confirmed endocarditis on TTE, TEE is performed for a better assessment of anatomic complications. In addition, TEE is pursued if the index of suspicion for endocarditis remains high after TTE. For example, patients with persistent *S. aureus* bacteremia without a source should have a TEE because approximately 30% will have infective endocarditis. Patients with bacteremia and a prosthetic valve should also have a TEE, and a TEE should be strongly considered in patients with a prosthetic valve and

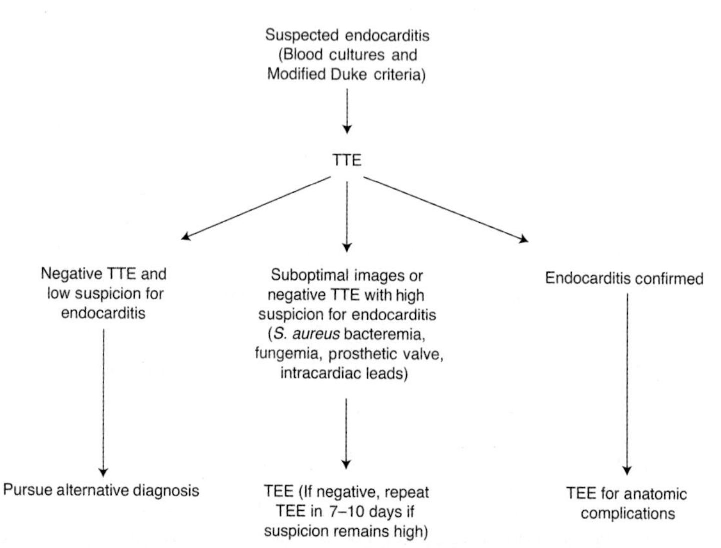

FIGURE 9.1 Echocardiographic evaluation of patients with suspected endocarditis. All patients with suspected endocarditis should have a TTE given the high specificity and comprehensive noninvasive hemodynamic assessment. If the TTE is negative and there is a low clinical suspicion for endocarditis, alternative diagnoses should be pursued. Conversely, if the TTE is negative in a patient with a high clinical suspicion for endocarditis, a TEE should be pursued. Finally, if the TTE confirms endocarditis, a TEE can be performed to further define the extent of valvular involvement and assess for associated anatomic complications. TEE, transesophageal echocardiography; TTE, transthoracic echocardiography.

persistent fever, even in the absence of bacteremia or a new murmur. TEE is also useful to assess for vegetations on intracardiac leads. Intracardiac echocardiography is helpful in this setting as well, though it is usually performed at the time of device extraction. Of note, the distinction between an infected vegetation and thrombus on a lead is not possible with echocardiography alone, and the clinical context must be considered for correct diagnosis. Finally, intraoperative TEE is routine to assess whether a vegetation has changed or embolized, to define the extent of invasive disease, and to evaluate whether other valves have become involved.

3. If the clinical suspicion remains high despite a negative TEE, echocardiography should be repeated in 7 to 10 days. Thickened leaflets may be the only initial evidence of endocarditis. Moreover, patients with prosthetic valves often have vegetations attached to the sewing ring. These vegetations are not always visible because of acoustic shadowing of the prosthesis. Therefore, a negative TEE should not supersede a strong clinical suspicion for prosthetic valve endocarditis. Finally, after therapy for infective endocarditis is completed, a follow-up TTE should be obtained to assess for valvular function and complications. However, echocardiography may not discriminate between active and healed vegetations.

B. **Specific findings** (Figs. 9.2 and 9.3)**.** The major finding of infective endocarditis is a vegetation (85% to 90%). Echocardiographic findings that can have similar appearances to infected vegetations include nonbacterial thrombotic endocarditis (Libman-Sacks and marantic endocarditis), chordal rupture, and fibroelastomas. Less common echocardiographic findings of infective endocarditis include abscess, pseudoaneurysm, perforation, fistula, and dehiscence of a prosthetic valve.

1. On echocardiography, a vegetation is usually an oscillating mass on a valve, other endocardium, or intracardiac material that moves independently from other cardiac structures. Because vegetations tend to adhere to the low-pressure side of the valve, they are typically on the atrial surface of the mitral and tricuspid valves and the ventricular surface of the aortic and pulmonic valves.

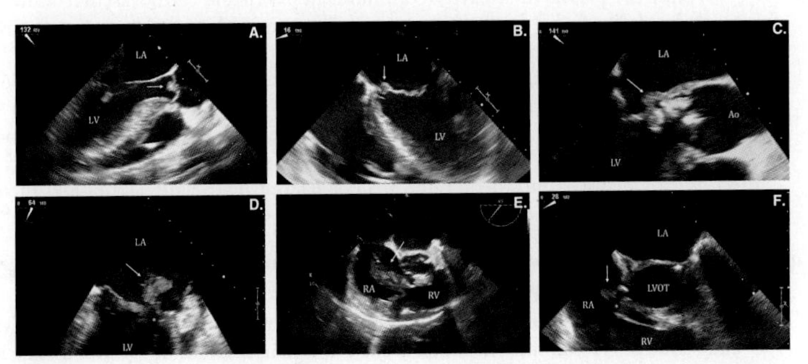

FIGURE 9.2 Echocardiography of native valve infective endocarditis **(A–F)**. **A:** *E. faecalis* aortic valve endocarditis with a vegetation *(arrow)* prolapsing into the LVOT. **B:** The same patient had a "kissing" lesion *(arrow)* on the anterior mitral valve leaflet. **C:** *S. mitis* aortic valve endocarditis with destruction of the aortic–mitral intervalvular fibrosa *(arrow)*. **D:** *S. aureus* mitral valve endocarditis with a vegetation *(arrow)* and destruction of the P1 scallop of the mitral valve *(asterisk)*. **E:** *C. albicans* tricuspid valve endocarditis with a large vegetation *(arrow)*. **F:** *S. aureus* aortic valve and tricuspid valve endocarditis with a vegetation *(arrow)* and a fistula between the LVOT and the RA, termed an acquired Gerbode defect. Ao, aorta; LA, left atrium; LV, left ventricle; LVOT, left ventricular outflow tract; RA, right atrium; RV, right ventricle.

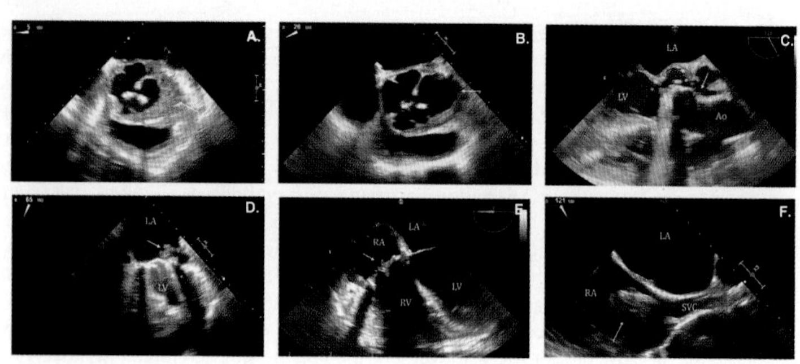

FIGURE 9.3 Echocardiography of prosthetic valve endocarditis **(A–F)**. **A:** *S. aureus* endocarditis of a bioprosthetic aortic valve with an aortic root abscess *(arrow)*. **B:** Intraoperative echocardiogram in the same patient 2 days later shows a developing pseudoaneurysm *(arrow)* and progressive dehiscence of the bioprosthesis. **C:** *S. aureus* endocarditis of a bioprosthetic aortic valve in a patient with previous aortic root and ascending aorta replacement. The bioprosthetic valve is posteriorly dehisced *(asterisk)*, and there is systolic compression of the aortic graft by a pseudoaneurysm *(arrow)*. **D:** *S. epidermidis* endocarditis of a mechanical mitral valve with a vegetation *(arrow)* and partial lateral dehiscence *(asterisk)*. **E:** *E. faecalis* endocarditis with vegetations *(arrow)* on a bioprosthetic tricuspid valve. **F:** *S. epidermidis* endocarditis with a vegetation *(arrow)* on a permanent pacemaker lead. Ao, aorta; LA, left atrium; LV, left ventricle; RA, right atrium; RV, right ventricle; SVC, superior vena cava.

2. A perivalvular abscess has necrosis and purulent material that is not communicating with the cardiovascular lumen. On echocardiography, the perivalvular area is nonhomogeneously thickened with an echodense or echolucent appearance.
3. A pseudoaneurysm is often confused with an abscess. With a pseudoaneurysm, the perivalvular cavity communicates with the cardiovascular lumen. Echocardiography demonstrates a pulsatile perivalvular echolucent space with detectable color flow.
4. A perforation is the interruption of endocardial continuity and is seen with color flow imaging on echocardiography.
5. A fistula is a perforation with communication between neighboring cavities and is also seen with color flow imaging.
6. With a dehisced prosthetic valve, there is paravalvular regurgitation, and there may be a rocking motion of the prosthesis.

VII. COMPUTED TOMOGRAPHY (CT), MAGNETIC RESONANCE IMAGING (MRI), AND INVASIVE ANGIOGRAPHY

A. **Computed tomography** (Fig. 9.4). CT imaging has two general functions in infective endocarditis. CT can further delineate anatomic complications of invasive disease if questions remain after echocardiography, and CT can evaluate for metastatic disease when clinical suspicion arises.

1. With invasive disease, CT can assess for suspected myocardial or pericardial extension of infection. In aortic valve endocarditis, thickening of the aortic root on CT often suggests an abscess. CT also outlines the anatomic consequences of a pseudoaneurysm and can assess for coronary involvement. In prosthetic valve endocarditis, CT can evaluate the motion of mechanical valve leaflets and may visualize thrombosis or infection. With experienced operators, valve fluoroscopy is often a useful adjunct to detect mechanical valve obstruction because of reduced

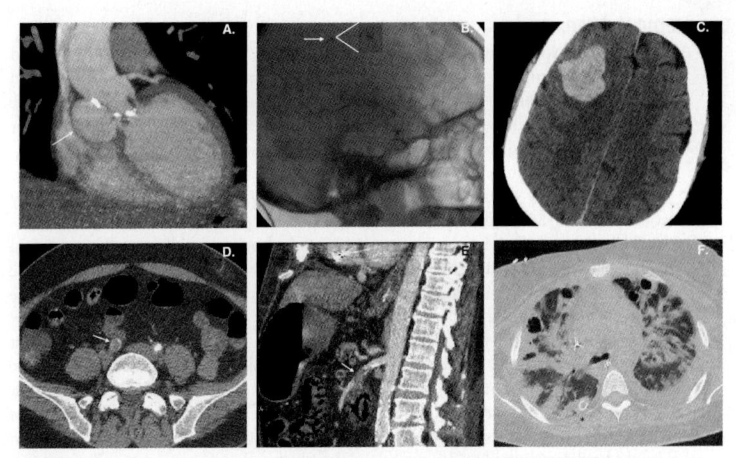

FIGURE 9.4 Invasive **(A)** and metastatic **(B–F)** complications of infective endocarditis, viewed with CT and invasive angiography. **A:** CT angiogram of the thoracic aorta in a patient with *S. mitis* endocarditis of a native aortic valve. There is a large pseudoaneurysm *(arrow)* that was causing dynamic compression of the right coronary artery. **B:** Cerebral angiogram in a patient with *S. aureus* aortic valve endocarditis complicated by a 2.3 by 2.4 mm mycotic aneurysm *(arrow and inset)* in a distal branch of the right middle cerebral artery. **C:** Head CT in a patient with *S. aureus* endocarditis of a bioprosthetic aortic valve complicated by hemorrhagic conversion of a right frontal embolic stroke. **D:** CT angiogram of the abdomen in a patient with *C. albicans* endocarditis of a bioprosthetic aortic valve. There is near-occlusive septic thromboembolism of the right common iliac artery *(arrow)*. **E:** CT angiogram of the abdomen in a patient with *S. epidermidis* endocarditis of a bioprosthetic aortic valve. There is septic thromboembolism to the proximal superior mesenteric artery *(arrow)*. **F:** Chest CT in an intravenous drug user with *S. aureus* endocarditis of a native tricuspid valve. There are numerous septic pulmonary abscesses, and a chest tube has been placed for a right-sided pneumothorax. CT, computed tomography.

excursion or fixed leaflets. Fluoroscopy may also demonstrate a rocking motion of a biologic or mechanical valve, consistent with dehiscence.

2. In right-sided endocarditis, CT may demonstrate septic pulmonary emboli, infarcts, and abscesses. CT can also demonstrate splenic abscesses, though splenic infarcts are a more common finding. If major limb artery occlusion from embolism is suspected, CT angiography can be useful, though direct invasive angiography in a hybrid operating room may be more appropriate in an acute presentation with a high index of suspicion. In patients with neurologic symptoms, CT or MR angiography should be performed to assess for intracranial aneurysm. If clinical suspicion is high, cerebral angiography can be pursued.

B. Invasive coronary angiography. Prior to cardiac surgery, coronary angiography is typically performed in men older than 40 years, postmenopausal women, and patients with at least one cardiovascular risk factor. The approach is generally similar in stable patients with infective endocarditis that need cardiac surgery. Notable exceptions include patients with large aortic valve vegetations that could be dislodged during coronary angiography and patients that need emergency surgery. In certain situations, high-resolution coronary CT can be considered.

VIII. MEDICAL THERAPY

A. General principles. Given the varied clinical presentations and different antimicrobial susceptibility profiles, management of patients with infective endocarditis should include an infectious disease specialist. In general, vegetations are difficult to eradicate because they exist in an area of impaired host defense, and tolerant microorganisms may escape drug-induced killing and resume growth after treatment discontinuation. Therefore, long courses of intravenous therapy are usually necessary. Appropriate antibiotic therapy should be guided by susceptibility, and the minimum inhibitory concentration (MIC) should be established.

B. Empiric therapy. Patients who present with septic shock, a rapidly progressive clinical course, or a highly destructive infection should receive empiric antibiotics. Empiric regimens in patients with suspected infective endocarditis should be based upon the severity of infection and risk factors for atypical or resistant microorganisms. For example, vancomycin will treat most staphylococci, and ceftriaxone will treat most streptococci. After the causative microorganism is identified, antibiotics should be narrowed. Of note, antibiotics reduce emboli and prevent further bacterial growth, but cannot improve valve function. After 2 weeks of antibiotics, embolic events are infrequent. In patients who have had an embolic stroke, heparin anticoagulation should be discontinued to decrease the risk of hemorrhagic conversion. The optimal time to wait before restarting anticoagulation is unclear and should be based upon the risk for thrombotic complications.

C. Stable patients. In hemodynamically stable patients with subacute endocarditis, early antibiotics do not prevent complications and may delay identifying the etiologic agent. Also, patients with masses on cardiac leads seen on TEE without positive blood cultures or other features of infection are likely to have thrombus alone. They warrant close observation, but do not need empiric antibiotics or lead removal. Finally, if a patient with native valve endocarditis needs valve replacement, the postoperative regimen should be for native valve endocarditis. A new full course of treatment should only be given if the valve culture is positive because bacterial DNA with PCR does not indicate active infection.

D. Recurrent disease. Recurrent endocarditis can be relapse or reinfection. Recurrence of endocarditis with the same microorganisms within 6 months is typically a relapse. Relapses can occur because of a suboptimal antibiotic, an inadequate course of antibiotics, or a persistent focus of infection. Reinfection is more frequent with intravenous drug use (1.3% per patient-year), prosthetic valve endocarditis, and chronic dialysis.

E. Specific microorganisms

1. The only coagulase-positive staphylococcus is *S. aureus* (Table 9.3). Methicillin-resistant staphylococci produce low-affinity plasma binding protein 2A that confers cross-resistance to most β-lactams. Overall, 25% to 30% of *S. aureus* endocarditis is resistant to methicillin, though rates of resistance are higher in health care–associated infections. In native valve endocarditis because of *S. aureus*, at least 4 weeks of intravenous antibiotics is recommended, and at least 6 weeks is needed in patients with lung abscesses or osteomyelitis. Gentamicin should not be routinely used in native valve staphylococcal endocarditis given an increased incidence of renal dysfunction. The clinical benefit of gentamicin in prosthetic valve endocarditis has also not been demonstrated. Similarly, the evidence is poor for rifampin, but it can be added in staphylococcal prosthetic valve endocarditis. However, rifampin must be used with another antistaphylococcal drug to decrease the risk of resistant mutant selection. Often, another antistaphylococcal drug is used for several days to reduce the number of staphylococci before rifampin is introduced.
2. Unlike the typically destructive nature of *S. aureus*, coagulase-negative staphylococcus is usually indolent, though *S. lugdunensis* and some cases of *S. capitis* are notable exceptions that can be destructive and often require surgery. The antimicrobial regimens for coagulase-negative staphylococcal endocarditis are similar to those of *S. aureus* (Table 9.3).

TABLE 9.3 Therapy for Infective Endocarditis Caused by Staphylococci

	Agent	Dose[a]	Duration[b]
Native Valve			
Methicillin sensitive	Nafcillin or oxacillin	12 g IV per 24 hr in 4–6 divided doses	At least 4–6 wk
	+/− Gentamicin[c]	3 mg/kg IV per 24 hr in 3 divided doses	3–5 d
Methicillin resistant	Vancomycin	30 mg/kg IV in 24 hr in 2 divided doses	At least 4–6 wk
Prosthetic Valve			
Methicillin sensitive	Nafcillin or oxacillin	12 g IV per 24 hr in 4–6 divided doses	At least 6 wk
	+/− Rifampin	900 mg per 24 hr IV/PO in 3 divided doses	At least 6 wk
	+/− Gentamicin[c]	3 mg/kg IV in 3 divided doses	2 wk
Methicillin resistant	Vancomycin	30 mg/kg IV per 24 hr in 2 divided doses	At least 6 wk
	+/− Rifampin	900 mg per 24 hr IV/PO in 3 divided doses	At least 6 wk
	+/− Gentamicin[c]	3 mg/kg IV in 3 divided doses	2 wk
Cardiac Device			
Methicillin susceptible	Nafcillin or oxacillin	12 g IV per 24 hr in 4–6 divided doses	At least 2 wk after device removal
Methicillin resistant	Vancomycin	30 mg/kg IV per 24 hr in 2 divided doses	At least 2 wk after device removal

[a]Doses assume normal renal function.
[b]Suggested durations should be extended if a patient has osteomyelitis, abscess, valvular involvement in cardiac device endocarditis, or foreign material has not been removed.
[c]Given nephrotoxicity, gentamicin is not routinely used.
Adapted from Baddour LM, Wilson WR, Bayer AS, et al. Infective endocarditis: diagnosis, antimicrobial therapy, and management of complications. *Circulation.* 2005;111:e394–e433; Baddour LM, Epstein AE, Erickson CC, et al. Update on cardiovascular implantable electronic device infections and their management. *Circulation.* 2010;121:458–477; Gould FK, Denning DW, Elliott TS, et al. Guidelines for the diagnosis and antibiotic treatment of endocarditis in adults: a report of the working party of the British society for antimicrobial chemotherapy. *J Antimicrob Chemother.* 2012;67:269–289.

3. Oral streptococci (*S. sanguis, S. mitis, S. salivarius, S. mutans*, and *Gemella morbillorum*) are often fully susceptible to penicillin. In addition, oral streptococci are killed synergistically with penicillin plus gentamicin. Aminoglycosides therefore can be used to shorten the duration of therapy in infection with oral streptococci (Table 9.4). Penicillin-resistant oral streptococci are classified as relatively resistant (MIC 0.125 to 2 mg/L) and fully resistant (MIC > 2 mg/L), though some consider

TABLE 9.4 Therapy for Infective Endocarditis Caused by Streptococci

Agent	Dose[a]	Duration
Strains Susceptible to Penicillin		
1. Penicillin G or	24 million units per 24 hr continuously IV or in 4–6 divided doses	At least 4–6 wk
Ceftriaxone	2 g per 24 hr	At least 4–6 wk
2. Penicillin G or Ceftriaxone and Gentamicin	3 mg/kg IV per 24 hr	2 wk[b]
Strains Relatively or Fully Resistant to Penicillin		
1. Penicillin G or	24 million units per 24 hr continuously IV or in 4–6 divided doses	At least 4–6 wk
Ceftriaxone	2 g per 24 hr	At least 4–6 wk
and Gentamicin	3 mg/kg IV per 24 hr	At least 2 wk
2. Vancomycin	30 mg/kg IV per 24 hr in 2 divided doses	At least 4–6 wk
Treatment of Nutritionally Variant Streptococci		
1. Penicillin G	24 million units per 24 hr continuously IV or in 4–6 divided doses	At least 4–6 wk
and Gentamicin	2 mg/kg IV per day in 2 divided doses	At least 4–6 wk

[a]Doses assume normal renal function.
[b]The 2-week regimen is not advised for patients with prosthetic valves, extracardiac foci of infection, or an indication for surgery.
Adapted from Baddour LM, Wilson WR, Bayer AS, et al. Infective endocarditis: diagnosis, antimicrobial therapy, and management of complications. *Circulation.* 2005;111:e394–e433; Gould FK, Denning DW, Elliott TS, et al. Guidelines for the diagnosis and antibiotic treatment of endocarditis in adults: a report of the working party of the British society for antimicrobial chemotherapy. *J Antimicrob Chemother.* 2012;67:269–289.

an MIC > 0.5 mg/L as fully resistant. In these infections, antibiotic regimens are similar, but aminoglycoside treatment may be longer, and short-term regimens are not recommended.

4. *Streptococcus gallolyticus* (formerly known as *S. bovis*) is highly penicillin susceptible and is frequently associated with polyps or malignant disease of the colon. Colonoscopy is indicated in these patients. Streptococcal infections are generally less invasive than infections with *S. aureus*, but infections with *S. anginosus* can cause destructive infections with intracardiac complications. *S. anginosus* and *S. milleri* also tend to form abscesses and may require a longer duration of antibiotics. Endocarditis from *S. pneumoniae* is now rare but is associated with meningitis. Penicillin poorly penetrates the central nervous system barrier and should be avoided in these patients. Finally, nutritionally variant streptococci (*Abiotrophia* and *Granulicatella*) are often tolerant to penicillin. Endocarditis has a protracted course with higher rates of complications and treatment failures.

TABLE 9.5 Therapy for Infective Endocarditis Caused by Enterococci

Agent	Dose[a]	Duration
Strains Susceptible to Penicillin		
Ampicillin	12 g per 24 hr in 6 divided doses	At least 4–6 wk (6 wk for prosthetic valves)
and Gentamicin	3 mg/kg per 24 hr in 3 divided doses	At least 4–6 wk (6 wk for prosthetic valves)
Strains Resistant to Penicillin		
Vancomycin	30 mg/kg IV per 24 hr in 2 divided doses	At least 6 wk
and Gentamicin	3 mg/kg per 24 hr in 3 divided doses	At least 6 wk

[a]Doses assume normal renal function.
Adapted from Baddour LM, Wilson WR, Bayer AS, et al. Infective endocarditis: diagnosis, antimicrobial therapy, and management of complications. *Circulation.* 2005;111:e394–e433; Gould FK, Denning DW, Elliott TS, et al. Guidelines for the diagnosis and antibiotic treatment of endocarditis in adults: a report of the working party of the British society for antimicrobial chemotherapy. *J Antimicrob Chemother.* 2012;67:269–289.

5. Enterococci are highly tolerant, and effective treatment for endocarditis requires prolonged administration of synergistic combinations of β-lactams or glycopeptides with aminoglycosides (Table 9.5). Furthermore, enterococci may be resistant to multiple drugs. β-Lactam and vancomycin resistance is rare and is predominantly seen in *E. faecium.* Fully penicillin-susceptible enterococcal strains are treated with ampicillin combined with gentamicin.
6. HACEK Gram-negative bacilli are fastidious organisms that grow slowly, so standard MIC tests may be difficult to interpret. Some HACEK group bacilli now produce β-lactamase. Ceftriaxone may therefore be the first choice, but ampicillin can be used if the isolate is susceptible. In penicillin-allergic patients, ciprofloxacin is an acceptable alternative. Gentamicin can be used for the first 2 weeks of therapy. Native valve endocarditis is typically treated for 4 weeks, and prosthetic valve endocarditis is treated for 6 weeks.
7. *C. burnetii* (Q fever) is typically treated with doxycycline and hydroxychloroquine for more than 18 months. Antibody titers should be checked every 6 months while on treatment and every 3 months for at least 2 years after treatment has stopped. *Bartonella* endocarditis is treated with gentamicin in combination with a β-lactam or doxycycline for a minimum of 4 weeks.
8. The initial treatment for *Candida* endocarditis is with an echinocandin or amphotericin B. Echinocandin therapy is preferred for *C. krusei*, and amphotericin B is preferred for *C. parapsilosis*, *C. guilliermondii*, and *C. famata*. If the strain is susceptible, long-term oral fluconazole therapy should be given after prolonged intravenous therapy. For *Aspergillus* endocarditis, initial treatment is with voriconazole.

F. **Antibiotic prophylaxis.** Identifying patients that may benefit from antibiotics to prevent infective endocarditis is difficult and controversial. Although certain conditions and procedures are associated with infective endocarditis, the extent to which this risk is modified with prophylactic antibiotics is unclear. Current guidelines recommend good oral hygiene and improved access to dental care. Antibiotics are restricted to the highest risk patients undergoing the highest risk procedures. High-risk patients include those with a prosthetic valve, patients with previous endocarditis, patients with unrepaired cyanotic heart disease or residual defects (including patients with palliative shunts or conduits), patients with congenital heart disease and complete repair with prosthetic material for up to 6 months after surgery, patients with a residual defect at the site of prosthetic material, and transplant patients with valvular disease.

Prophylaxis is not recommended for patients with a bicuspid aortic valve, mitral valve prolapse and regurgitation, rheumatic heart disease, and atrial septal or ventricular septal defects.

High-risk procedures include dental manipulation of gingival or periapical regions of the teeth as well as perforation of the oral mucosa. Prophylaxis is not indicated for respiratory tract, gastrointestinal, or urogenital procedures.

Typically, prophylactic antibiotics are administered 30 to 60 minutes before the procedure. A single dose of 2 g of amoxicillin can be given, and 600 mg of clindamycin is given to penicillin allergic patients.

IX. SURGERY

A. Indications

The goal of surgery for infective endocarditis is removal of infected tissue and reconstruction of anatomy. Overall, surgery is necessary in approximately 50% of patients with infective endocarditis.

1. Heart failure is the most frequent indication for surgery. In observational studies, surgery in patients with heart failure has been associated with decreased mortality compared to medical therapy alone.
2. Uncontrolled infection is the second most common reason for surgery and is most often because of local destruction or resistant microorganisms. Early surgery is recommended in patients with heart block, annular or aortic abscesses, and destructive penetrating lesions. Patients with left-sided endocarditis related to *S. aureus*, resistant *P. aeruginosa* or enterococcus, and fungal infections often benefit from early surgery. Few patients with endocarditis from *Aspergillus* species have survived without surgery. When possible, a primary focus of infection should be addressed prior to cardiac surgery to decrease the chance of recurrent endocarditis. In patients with persistent fever without another focus of infection, surgery should be undertaken. However, other causes of fever, such as from antibiotics, should be excluded. Patients with prosthetic valves and persistent bacteremia without another source should also have surgery.
3. Early surgery can be considered in patients with large vegetations to prevent embolic events, and surgery should be pursued in patients with recurrent emboli and persistent vegetations despite antibiotic treatment. After an ischemic stroke, the optimal timing of surgery is unclear. The risk of hemorrhagic transformation with heparin for cardiopulmonary bypass must be balanced against the risk of further embolic events. Patients with a mycotic aneurysm should undergo embolization before cardiac surgery. In the setting of an intracranial hemorrhage, surgery is ideally postponed for at least 1 month. If urgent surgery is needed, management with neurology and neurosurgery is essential.
4. Surgery for right-sided native valve endocarditis is less common, in part because invasive disease involving the tricuspid valve is infrequent. However, surgery may be necessary in patients with right heart failure secondary to severe tricuspid regurgitation with poor response to diuretic therapy or in patients with microorganisms that are difficult to eradicate.

B. Approach to specific valves

1. In general, all infected and necrotic tissue should be debrided, and foreign material should be minimized. For this reason, an aortic allograft is often preferred for aortic valve endocarditis.
2. The mitral valve should be repaired when possible. Often, "kissing" lesions with perforation of the anterior mitral valve leaflet are amenable to autologous pericardial patch repair.
3. In tricuspid valve endocarditis, the infected area is debrided, and the valve is repaired whenever possible.

C. Approach to cardiac devices

1. In a patient undergoing valve surgery for endocarditis, a cardiac device can serve as a nidus for recurrent infection and should be removed. If a new device is required after valve surgery, an epicardial system should be considered.
2. In definite device-related endocarditis, medical therapy alone has been associated with high mortality and risk of recurrence. Percutaneous extraction is possible in the majority of patients. However, surgical backup to manage complications is essential. Because overall risks are higher with surgery, percutaneous extraction is still preferred for large vegetations. Pulmonary embolism as a result of vegetation displacement during extraction occurs frequently, but these episodes are frequently asymptomatic. Surgery should be performed in patients where percutaneous extraction is not possible or in patients who also have severe tricuspid valve endocarditis.
3. Patients with occult staphylococcal bacteremia should have complete device and lead removal. In addition, patients with persistent occult Gram-negative bacteremia despite appropriate antibiotics should have complete device and lead removal.
4. After removal, a careful assessment is needed to assess whether a new device is needed, and replacement should not be ipsilateral to extraction. If blood cultures were positive before extraction, repeat blood cultures after extraction should be negative for 72 hours before a new device is implanted. When there is valvular infection, new lead placement should be delayed for 14 days.

X. PROGNOSIS

The prognosis in endocarditis is influenced by the interplay of patient characteristics, infecting microorganism, and the presence of complications.

A. Patient characteristics. Mortality is increased in older patients, in patients with prosthetic valve endocarditis, and in patients with diabetes mellitus or renal failure. Patients that receive a transcatheter valve often have multiple comorbidities and may not be operative candidates. Accordingly, mortality is high in infective endocarditis of transcatheter aortic valves. Mitral valve vegetations are also associated with increased mortality, and right-sided native valve endocarditis in intravenous drug users has a better prognosis with an in-hospital mortality of $<10\%$. However, mortality is increased in patients with HIV infection and a low CD4 count.

B. Microorganisms. Patients with infective endocarditis from *S. aureus*, fungi, or Gram-negative bacilli have increased mortality. This increased mortality relates in part to patient characteristics. Patients with fungal or Gram-negative endocarditis are more likely to be immunocompromised. *S. aureus* is highly destructive, and when it infects prosthetic valves, in-hospital mortality is approximately 45%. In patients with heart failure, periannular complications, and *S. aureus* endocarditis, mortality is very high ($\sim$70% to 80%).

C. Complications. Heart failure, stroke, acute renal failure, and persistent infection also predict poor outcomes.

KEY PEARLS

- In the developed world, major risk factors for endocarditis include degenerative valve disease, prosthetic valves, intravenous drug use, and chronic indwelling devices.
- Infective endocarditis still carries a high mortality: 15% to 20% in-hospital and approximately 40% at 1 year.
- Predisposing abnormalities for left-sided native valve endocarditis include mitral valve prolapse, mitral annular calcification, and a bicuspid aortic valve.
- Early- and intermediate-onset endocarditis is most likely related to the index surgery or health care–related infection, whereas late-onset disease is most likely community acquired.
- Most patients with infective endocarditis present acutely within 30 days of infection.
- TEE should be performed to assess for anatomic complications in patients with known endocarditis and when clinical suspicion remains high for endocarditis after a negative TTE.
- In the developed world, staphylococci are the most common cause of infective endocarditis.
- Tissue disintegration that involves the valve annulus with extravascular spread is termed invasive disease, with specific complications including internal fistulas, perforations, and heart block.
- The most common complication of endocarditis is heart failure related to aortic or mitral regurgitation.
- In patients with endocarditis, the most common indications for surgery include heart failure, uncontrolled infection, and the need to prevent embolic events.

SUGGESTED READINGS

Amat-Santos IJ, Ribeiro HB, Urena M, et al. Prosthetic valve endocarditis after transcatheter valve replacement. *JACC Cardiovasc Interv*. 2015;8:334–346.

Cosgrove SE, Vigliani GA, Fowler VG Jr, et al. Initial low-dose gentamicin for *Staphylococcus aureus* bacteremia and endocarditis is nephrotoxic. *Clin Infect Dis*. 2009;48:713–721.

Gaca JG, Sheng S, Daneshmand MA, et al. Outcomes for endocarditis surgery in North America: a simplified risk scoring system. *J Thorac Cardiovasc Surg*. 2011;141:98–106.

Kang DH, Kim YJ, Kim SH, et al. Early surgery versus conventional treatment for infective endocarditis. *N Engl J Med*. 2012;366:2466–2473.

Kiefer T, Park L, Tribouilloy C, et al. Association between valvular surgery and mortality among patients with infective endocarditis complicated by heart failure. *JAMA*. 2011;306:2239–2247.

Li JS, Sexton DJ, Mick N, et al. Proposed modifications to the Duke criteria for the diagnosis of infective endocarditis. *Clin Infect Dis*. 2000;30:633–638.

Murdoch DR, Corey GR, Hoen B, et al. Clinical presentation, etiology, and outcome of infective endocarditis in the 21st century. *Arch Intern Med*. 2009;169:463–473.

Pettersson GB, Hussain ST, Shrestha NK, et al. Infective endocarditis: an atlas of disease progression for describing, staging, coding, and understanding the pathology. *J Thorac Cardiovasc Surg*. 2014;147:1142–1149.

Wang A, Athan E, Pappas PA, et al. Contemporary clinical profile and outcome of prosthetic valve endocarditis. *JAMA*. 2007;297:1354–1361.

KEY GUIDELINES

Baddour LM, Epstein AE, Erickson CC, et al. Update of cardiovascular implantable electronic device infections and their management. *Circulation*. 2010;121:458–477.

Baddour LM, Wilson WR, Bayer AS, et al. Infective endocarditis: diagnosis, antimicrobial therapy, and management of complications. *Circulation*. 2005;111:e394–e433.

Gould FK, Denning DW, Elliot TS, et al. Guidelines for the diagnosis and antibiotic treatment of endocarditis in adults: a report of the working party of the British society for antimicrobial chemotherapy. *J Antimicrob Chemother*. 2012;67:269–289.

Habib G, Hoen B, Tornos T, et al. Guidelines on the prevention, diagnosis, and treatment of infective endocarditis. *Eur Heart J*. 2009;30:2369–2413.

Nishimura RA, Otto CM, Bonow RO, et al. 2014 ACC/AHA Guidelines for the management of patients with valvular heart disease. *Circulation*. 2014;129:1–235.

Sandoe JAT, Barlow G, Chambers JB, et al. Guidelines for the diagnosis, prevention, and management of implantable cardiac electronic device infection. *J Antimicrob Chemother*. 2015;70:325–359.

RELEVANT BOOK CHAPTERS

Fuster V, Alexander RW, O'Rourke RA, eds. *Hurst's the Heart*. 13th ed. New York, NY: McGraw-Hill; 2011:chap 86.

Karchmer AW. Infectious endocarditis. In: Braunwald E, ed. *Heart Disease: A Textbook of Cardiovascular Medicine*. 8th ed. Philadelphia, PA: WB Saunders; 2008:1713–1734.

Sabe MA, Griffin BP. Infective endocarditis In: Griffin, BP, ed. *Manual of Cardiovascular Medicine*. 4th ed. Philadelphia, PA: Lippincott Williams & Williams; 2013:327–347.

SECTION II

Special Conditions

CHAPTER 10

Ellen Mayer Sabik

Special Considerations (Drugs, Pregnancy, Noncardiac Surgery, Anticoagulation, Valve-related Tumors)

I. DRUG-INDUCED VALVE DISEASE

The concept of drug-induced valvular heart disease first surfaced in the mid-1960s when patients taking ergot alkaloids for migraine prophylaxis developed valvular regurgitation. This idea was later strengthened in the late 1990s by the development of valvular disease in patients taking the appetite suppressants fenfluramine and dexfenfluramine. More recent medications shown to cause valvular heart disease include ergot-derived dopamine agonists used for the treatment of Parkinson disease (pergolide) and those used to treat hyperprolactinemic patients (cabergoline). The most recent additions to the list include MDMA (3,4-methylenedioxymethamphetamine), otherwise known as the recreational drug ecstasy, and benfluorex, used to treat overweight diabetics. All of these drugs (see Table 10.1) share a common pharmacologic action on the 5-hydroxytryptamine 2B (5-HT2B) receptor (a specific serotonin receptor), which is responsible for the development of valvular disease. It is important to note that this "off-target effect" results in pathologic changes on the valves because the 5-HT2B receptors are expressed in high concentrations on the valve leaflets.

A. Histopathology of drug-induced valve disease. To understand the development of valvular disease caused by the above agents, one must first look at the structure and functional histology of the cardiac valves. The cardiac valves and their supporting structures serve to maintain unidirectional blood flow throughout the cardiac chambers.

1. Human semilunar valves are lined with endothelium and have three well-defined tissue layers, each with its own role or function: (1) ventricularis—provides elasticity when leaflet changes shape (made of collagen and elastic fibers), (2) spongiosa—cushions for physical forces (made of loose collagen and proteoglycans), and (3) fibrosa—provides strength (made of collagen).
2. Atrioventricular valves have analogous layers with similar components: (1) atrialis, (2) spongiosa fibrosa, and (3) ventricularis.
3. There are two types of cells present in heart valves, including valvular endothelial cells covering the leaflet surfaces and valvular interstitial cells. The valvular interstitial cells are the most prevalent cells within the valves and are responsible for maintaining the integrity of the valve tissue and regular repair following valve injury. These cells maintain the integrity of the valve by maintaining the extracellular matrix, which is composed of proteoglycans, collagens, and elastin. Heart valve pathology arises when there are changes to the extracellular matrix. This occurs in myxomatous valve disease in addition to drug-induced valvulopathies.

   There are several different 5-HT receptors; however, only 5-HT2B receptor has been implicated in the development of valvular disease because of its high concentration in human heart valves and pulmonary arteries (PAs). Agonists of the

TABLE 10.1 Medications That Cause Valvular Heart Disease

Drug Class	Specific Agents	Therapeutic Use	Valvular Involvement
Anorexigans	Fenfluramine Dexfenfluramine	Appetite suppressants	Aortic regurgitation > restrictive mitral regurgitation, PAHTN
Dopamine agonists	Pergolide Cabergoline	Parkinson disease Parkinson disease and hyperprolactinemia	Mitral > aortic or tricuspid regurgitation
Ergot alkaloids	Methylsergide Ergotamine	Migraine prophylaxis	PAHTN, mitral and/or aortic regurgitation
Recreational drug	MDMA (Ecstasy)	Psychoactive stimulant	Valvular regurgitation

MDMA, 3,4-methylenedioxymethamphetamine; PAHTN, pulmonary artery hypertension.

5-HT2B receptor appear to have direct mitogenic effects on the vascular interstitial cells, causing proliferation of fibroblasts and smooth muscle cells and upregulation of transforming growth factor β, stimulating glucosaminoglycan production. The pathologic findings in these patients are similar to those found in patients with carcinoid heart disease in which the enterochromaffin cells produce high levels of serotonin, with tissue thickening caused by excess extracellular matrix, made up of glycosaminoglycans and collagen, but no significant inflammation and little calcium. It is clear from all of these drugs that have been shown to cause a valvulopathy that the mechanism of this process is 5-HT2B receptor agonism, and future drugs (and metabolites) being developed should be tested for this activity before being used in large clinical trials.

B. Echocardiographic features of drug-induced valvular disease

1. In order to screen a patient for the development of drug-induced valvulopathy, there must be a high clinical index of suspicion for the clinician ordering a transthoracic echocardiogram. It is often difficult to prove a causal relationship in an individual patient because typically there is no pretreatment baseline echocardiogram.
2. Typical features include mild or moderate leaflet thickening without calcification or commissural fusion (a hallmark of rheumatic valve disease). The leaflets appear "furled" or restricted, with the restricted leaflet closure causing the regurgitant lesions. The shortening and thickening of the subvalvular apparatus (especially chordae) appear to be out of proportion to the thickening of the leaflets, and the posterior leaflet is typically more affected than the anterior. When the aortic valve is involved, there is typically centrally originating aortic regurgitation (AR) due to restricted leaflet closure with only mild leaflet thickening. The tricuspid valve appears to be less commonly involved than the mitral and aortic valves.

C. Valvular heart disease associated with specific drugs

1. **Migraine drugs.** These are the oldest drugs recognized to have a potential link with valvular disease. Both are still in use, but only for short-term treatment.
   a. Methylsergide—induces fibrotic tissue changes, causing PA hypertension and retroperitoneal fibrosis
   b. Ergotamine—causes fibrotic valve lesions

2. **Appetite suppressants: fenfluramine and dexfenfluramine**
   a. These drugs cause valve regurgitation involving both right- and left-sided valves. Histopathology showed the characteristic plaques of myofibroblasts with excessive extracellular matrix.
   b. Meta-analysis of nine case–control studies showed evidence that regurgitation was due to the drug, not obesity, and that AR was more common than mitral regurgitation (MR).
   c. Aortic insufficiency (AI) occurred more often if drug was taken >3 to 6 months. Pulmonary hypertension could result from short-term treatment. Furthermore, regurgitation may decrease or stabilize when drug is discontinued.
3. **Benfluorex.** Used for overweight diabetics or for hypertriglyceridemia. Several case reports found unexplained MR. Later, a multicenter registry showed consistent presentation of middle-aged obese women with or without diabetes treated with benfluorex presenting with MR and congestive heart failure (CHF). Leaflet thickening and retraction with involvement of the subvalvular apparatus were found. Stenosis was uncommonly seen, and multivalvular involvement was often present. One study in diabetics showed that regurgitant lesions were more common in patients treated with benfluorex compared with controls (odds ratio 2 to 3:1 depending on which valve was involved).
4. **Ergot-derived Dopaminergic Agonists**
   a. Pergolide used for Parkinson disease (improves bradykinesia and rigidity)
   b. Cabergoline used for Parkinson disease or hyperprolactinemic disorders
   c. When these drugs were used to treat Parkinson disease, there was a significant increase in the incidence of valvular disease compared with patients treated with other (non–ergot-derived) dopamine agonists, with a sevenfold increase in regurgitant lesions with pergolide and a fivefold increase with cabergoline.
      i. With pergolide, valvular heart disease is generally plurivalvular although mitral valve involvement was greater than aortic or tricuspid. The agent was withdrawn in the United States, whereas use in Europe was limited to patients with Parkinson disease resistant to other dopaminergic agonists and with very careful echocardiographic follow-up.
      ii. Cabergoline used for treating hyperprolactinemic patients (first-line agent for this indication) restores normal prolactin levels and gonadal function at low doses. At low dose, the risk of valvular regurgitation is unconfirmed.
5. **MDMA (Ecstasy)**

   There are reports of significant valvular regurgitation with long-term use (3 to 6 tablets/wk for 6 years) with the severity of regurgitation correlated to the dose.

D. **Future research to evaluate drug safety**

An animal model of drug-induced valvular heart disease has been developed (with Wistar rats). These animals developed valvular pathology with similar echocardiographic features and histopathology when exposed to pergolide. Use of a 5-HT2B antagonist blocked the development of these valvular lesions when the rats were exposed to pergolide. New drugs should be analyzed for 5-HT2B agonist activity to predict possible valvulopathy before large clinical trials.

II. PREGNANCY AND VALVULAR HEART DISEASE

Pregnancy in patients with valvular heart disease can cause maternal and offspring morbidity and mortality. Cardiovascular disease is responsible for 10% to 15% of maternal mortality. The valvular disease can be acquired or congenital. The most common causes in pregnant patients include congenital (Marfan syndrome) and acquired (rheumatic) valvular disease.

The relative rates at which these etiologies are encountered depend on whether the woman is from a lower- to middle-income nation (rheumatic heart disease predominates) or a higher-income nation (congenital heart disease predominates). While rheumatic heart disease is declining in the developed world, overall it accounts for 90% of heart disease in women of child-bearing age in nonindustrialized nations. To minimize the morbidity and mortality in these patients with valvular disease, a preconception evaluation is recommended.

A. Risk assessment tools for patients with valvular heart disease

1. **CARPEG (Cardiac Disease in Pregnancy):** Four predictors of maternal cardiac events during pregnancy:
   - **a.** Prior cardiac event or arrhythmia
   - **b.** New York Heart Association (NYHA) functional class >2 or cyanosis
   - **c.** Left heart obstruction
   - **d.** Systemic ventricular dysfunction
2. **ZAHARA (translates to Pregnancy in Women with Congenital Heart Disease):** Eight predictors of risk:
   - **a.** History of arrhythmic event
   - **b.** Baseline NYHA functional class >2
   - **c.** Left heart obstruction (peak aortic valve gradient >50 mm Hg)
   - **d.** Mechanical valve prosthesis
   - **e.** Moderate/severe systemic atrioventricular valve regurgitation (possibly from ventricular dysfunction)
   - **f.** Use of cardiac medication prepregnancy
   - **g.** Repaired or unrepaired cyanotic heart disease
   - **h.** Severe pulmonary arterioventricular valve regurgitation
3. **Modified World Health Organization (WHO) classification:** There are a variety of models that predict risk; however, the modified WHO classification appears to be the most useful. See Tables 10.2 and 10.3 illustrating the WHO risk principles and WHO risk by cardiac disease.

B. Elements of preconception assessment and counseling

1. Careful history, family history, physical exam (including screening for connective tissue disorders)
2. 12-lead electrocardiogram (ECG)

TABLE 10.2 Modified WHO Classification of Maternal Cardiovascular Risk: Principles

Risk Class	Risk of Pregnancy
I	No detectable increased risk of maternal mortality and no/mild risk of morbidity
II	Small increased risk of maternal mortality or moderate increase in morbidity
III	Significantly increased risk of maternal mortality or severe morbidity. Expert counseling required. If pregnancy is chosen, intensive specialist cardiac and obstetric monitoring needed throughout pregnancy, childbirth, and puerperium.
IV	Extremely high risk of maternal mortality or severe morbidity; pregnancy contraindicated. If pregnancy occurs, termination should be discussed. If pregnancy continues, care as for class III.

WHO, World Health Organization. From Regitz-Zagrosek V, Lundqvist CB, Borghi C, et al. ESC guidelines on the management of cardiovascular diseases during pregnancy: the Task Force on the Management of Cardiovascular Diseases during Pregnancy of the European Society of Cardiology. *Eur Heart J.* 2011;32(24):3147–3197.

TABLE 10.3 Modified WHO Maternal Cardiovascular Risk Classification by Cardiac Diagnosis

WHO Category of Risk	Conditions in Pregnancy with WHO Risk Level
I	1. Uncomplicated, small, or mild: • Pulmonary stenosis • Patent ductus arteriosus (PDA) • Mitral valve prolapse 2. Successfully repaired simple lesions (ASD or VSD, PDA, anomalous pulmonary venous drainage) 3. APCs or PVCs
II (if otherwise well and uncomplicated)	1. Unoperated ASD or VSD 2. Repaired tetralogy of Fallot 3. Most arrhythmias
II–III (depending on individual)	1. Mild LV impairment 2. Hypertrophic cardiomyopathy 3. Native or tissue valvular heart disease not considered WHO I or WHO IV 4. Marfan syndrome without aortic dilatation 5. Aorta <45 mm in aortic disease associated with bicuspid AV 6. Repaired coarctation
III	1. Mechanical valve 2. Systemic right ventricle 3. Fontan circulation 4. Cyanotic heart disease (unrepaired) 5. Other complex congenital heart disease 6. Aortic dilatation 40–45 mm in Marfan syndrome 7. Aortic dilatation 45–50 mm in bicuspid AV
IV	1. PA hypertension (any cause) 2. Severe systemic ventricular dysfunction (LVEF <30%, NYHA III–IV) 3. Previous peripartum cardiomyopathy with any residual impairment of LV function 4. Severe MS, severe AS 5. Marfan syndrome with aorta dilated >45 mm 6. Aortic dilatation >50 mm in aortic disease associated with bicuspid AV

APC, atrial premature contraction; AS, aortic stenosis; ASD, atrial septal defect; AV, aortic valve; LV, left ventricle; LVEF, left ventricular ejection fraction; MS; mitral stenosis; NYHA, New York Heart Association; PVC, premature ventricular contraction; VSD, ventricular septal defect; WHO, World Health Organization. From Regitz-Zagrosek, Lundqvist CB, Borghi C, et al. ESC guidelines on the management of cardiovascular diseases during pregnancy. *Eur Heart J.* 2011;32(24):3147–3197.

3. Transthoracic echocardiogram—valve assessment and aortic size
4. In certain patients, functional capacity and symptoms should be assessed using stress testing. Prepregnancy symptoms often predict adverse outcomes during pregnancy or labor and delivery. One study found that women who achieve prepregnancy heart rate (HR) ≥150 bpm and/or peak oxygen uptake >25 mL/mg/min may be considered to have safer or better pregnancy outcomes.
5. Counseling on the basis of risk assessment to discuss maternal and fetal risks for complications and mortality. Discuss risks of therapy, including risk of miscarriage, early delivery, growth retardation resulting in small for gestational age infant, and possible fetal congenital defects. On the basis of risk, a discussion regarding contraception method should be included. These discussions are best approached by a multidisciplinary group including an obstetrician/gynecologist and a cardiologist.

   Women considered at high risk owing to valvular lesions should be considered for definitive treatment of the lesion before pregnancy. If valve surgery is needed, repair is preferable to replacement, and if replacement is needed, a careful discussion should occur regarding choice of prosthesis. Although a bioprosthesis is preferable because it does not require anticoagulation, it is not as durable as a mechanical prosthesis and will require reoperation sooner owing to degeneration. A bioprosthesis would allow a patient to go through her pregnancy without the risks of anticoagulation (bleeding risks, valve thrombosis, or even fetal teratogenesis in the first trimester).

C. Patients at prohibitively high risk are those in WHO classification IV, who should be counseled against pregnancy. These include:
   1. Severe symptomatic aortic stenosis (AS) or mitral stenosis (MS)
   2. Cardiomyopathy with left ventricular ejection fraction (LVEF) ≤30%
   3. Marfan syndrome with aortic root ≥45 mm
   4. Advanced pulmonary hypertension (two-thirds systemic pressures)
   5. Eisenmenger syndrome
   6. History of peripartum cardiomyopathy with LVEF not fully recovered

D. Cardiac considerations for contraception
   1. Contraceptive options include combined hormonal contraceptives, progestin-only contraceptives, intrauterine devices (IUDs), barrier methods, and sterilization/permanent forms of contraception.
   2. Specific issues include the increased risk of thromboembolic events and hypertension with estrogens. Thus, combined hormonal contraceptives (pills, patches, or vaginal rings) are not recommended for the following:
      a. Mechanical prostheses because of risk of valve thrombosis
      b. Eisenmenger syndrome because of risk of pulmonary embolism
      c. Intracardiac shunts because of risk of paradoxical embolus
   3. Monthly injections with medroxyprogesterone are contraindicated in patients with CHF owing to risk of fluid retention. Barrier methods and IUDs releasing levonorgestrel are safest in patients with cardiomyopathy with decreased left ventricular (LV) function, pulmonary hypertension, and cyanotic heart disease. Patients with prohibitively high-risk pathology may wish to consider permanent forms of contraception.
   4. In general, stenotic lesions are poorly tolerated, whereas regurgitant lesions are better tolerated. Although individual lesions will be discussed, including management, in further detail to understand the pathophysiology that occurs with valvular disease in pregnancy, one must first consider the normal physiologic/hemodynamic changes that occur with pregnancy.

E. Physiologic and hemodynamic changes in pregnancy
   1. Cardiac output increases 30% to 50% (increased HR and stroke volume).
   2. Blood volume increases (beginning at 6 weeks, may continue until at least second trimester, although may continue throughout pregnancy); average increase 50% above baseline.

3. Systemic vascular resistance falls, causing systolic and diastolic blood pressure to drop by 10 mm Hg at the end of the second trimester, rising to or above prepregnancy level at term.

F. **Hemodynamic changes associated with labor and delivery**

1. Cardiac output rises with contractions (80% above levels seen at the end of the third trimester) as a result of increased sympathetic tone, increasing blood pressure (BP) and HR, and central blood volume increased by autotransfusion from uterine contractions.
2. Postdelivery preload increases further as the inferior vena cava (IVC) compression is relieved because the gravid uterus is no longer resting on the IVC.

G. **Treatment of specific valve lesions during pregnancy**

1. **Mitral stenosis**
   a. The etiology of MS is usually rheumatic heart disease. Gradients are increased by the increased blood volume of pregnancy as well as by tachycardia. Mitral valve area is most reliably measured by direct planimetry during pregnancy. Functional mitral MS is more closely related to mean gradient across the valve.
   b. If symptomatic, β-blockers are the first-line drugs to decrease HR, improve left atrial emptying, and decompress the left atrium. Pulmonary edema is treated with diuretics. Heart failure is frequent with mitral valve area <1.5 cm^2. Atrial arrhythmias are common, and β-blockers or digoxin can be used for rate control. Early electrical cardioversion for atrial fibrillation or flutter should be considered. Anticoagulation at the onset of atrial fibrillation should also be considered and should be continued for at least 4 weeks.
   c. If one is unable to control symptoms with medical therapy, percutaneous balloon mitral valvuloplasty (PMV) should be considered if anatomy is suitable. However, it should be delayed until after the first trimester given the risks of radiation to fetal development. Abdominal shielding should be used to decrease radiation exposure.
   d. If anatomy is unsuitable for PMV, surgical intervention with mitral valve replacement (MVR) should be considered. There is no increased risk for the mother over surgical MVR in nonpregnant women. However, cardiopulmonary bypass poses significant risk to the fetus (fetal mortality 19% to 29%).
   e. Overall fetal risks in patients with MS include prematurity, low birth weight, and rarely fetal or neonatal death. Risks are higher in offspring with maternal NYHA class >II.
   f. Vaginal delivery is recommended for mild MS or moderate MS with NYHA class I or II without pulmonary hypertension. Cesarean section (C-section) should be considered for moderate or severe MS with class III or IV symptoms or if pulmonary hypertension is present despite medical management.
2. **Aortic stenosis**
   a. The etiology of AS is most commonly congenital (unicuspid or bicuspid aortic valve) or rheumatic disease.
   b. Mild or moderate AS is usually well tolerated (aortic valve area [AVA] >1.0 cm^2).
   c. If AS is severe, it is preferable to replace the valve before pregnancy. High-risk features include a reduced LVEF and a drop in BP with exercise testing.
   d. Fetal risks with AS include prematurity, low birth weights, and intrauterine growth restriction.
   e. For symptomatic patients despite medical therapy, options include balloon valvuloplasty or surgical aortic valve replacement (AVR). Valvuloplasty is preferred owing to a smaller risk of fetal loss (no cardiopulmonary bypass required).
   f. Patients with bicuspid aortic valves and a dilated ascending aorta (>4.5 cm) should be considered for aortic surgery before pregnancy. However, for patients who are already pregnant, close attention to blood pressure control and monitoring for symptoms are warranted owing to increased risk for aortic dissection and rupture.

3. Mitral regurgitation and aortic regurgitation

a. MR etiologies include mitral valve prolapse due to myxomatous disease and rheumatic MR.

b. AR is most commonly due to a bicuspid aortic valve, but other etiologies include a history of endocarditis, rheumatic disease, and aortic dilatation.

c. These regurgitant lesions typically are well tolerated because systemic vascular resistance is reduced (i.e., reduced afterload) owing to the placental circulation. However, because of increased blood volume, patients can develop pulmonary congestion, which is best treated with diuretics, if needed, and with restriction of activities and decreased sodium intake. Standard heart failure medications including β-blockers and vasodilators can be used. In particular, hydralazine and nitrates are safe for use during pregnancy but should be used with caution to avoid uteroplacental hypoperfusion. Importantly, angiotensin-converting enzyme inhibitors and angiotensin receptor blockers are contraindicated in pregnant women. Vaginal delivery is preferred with severe regurgitant lesions, with epidural anesthesia and a shortened second phase of labor.

4. Right-sided valvular lesions

a. Tricuspid regurgitation is usually well tolerated in pregnancy. The exception is Ebstein anomaly associated with an atrial septal defect and Wolff–Parkinson–White syndrome. In this setting, cyanosis may develop owing to shunt reversal, and atrial arrhythmias may occur.

b. Pulmonary stenosis (PS) is most often congenital in etiology. It is usually well tolerated in pregnancy, especially when mild or moderate in severity. Balloon valvuloplasty is preferably performed before pregnancy if peak gradient >64 mm Hg. Vaginal delivery is preferred for mild or moderate PS and severe PS with class I or II symptoms. For severe PS with class III or IV symptoms in which percutaneous intervention has failed or could not be done, C-section is preferred.

c. Pulmonary regurgitation when severe is an independent predictor of maternal complications, especially if associated with reduced right ventricular function.

5. Mechanical valve prostheses

a. Pregnancy is a hypercoagulable state, which increases the risk of thromboembolic events, including valve thrombosis. This risk depends on valve type, position, function, and arrhythmias (atrial fibrillation). Therapeutic anticoagulation during pregnancy is essential for all prostheses, and there are a variety of anticoagulation regimens, which must be individualized for a given patient. These include warfarin, unfractionated heparin, or low-molecular-weight heparin (LMWH). See Table 10.4 for anticoagulant options recommended by the American College of Chest Physicians.

b. Warfarin provides the greatest protection against maternal valve thrombosis, thromboembolism, and death when international normalized ratio (INR) is 2.5 to 3.5 throughout pregnancy. Continuous warfarin results in fewer thromboembolic events than heparin in the first trimester followed by warfarin.

c. The risks of warfarin are well established and include increased fetal wastage, congenital fetal anomalies and higher rates of fetal intraventricular hemorrhage, and, most concerning, fetal embryopathy. The risk of fetal embryopathy is dose related, with the greatest risk occurring when warfarin is used at doses >5 mg daily during weeks 6 to 12 of fetal development.

d. American and European recommendations regarding anticoagulation in pregnant women with mechanical prostheses are not in agreement. The European Society of Cardiology recommends continued use of warfarin throughout the pregnancy, especially if the dose is <5 mg daily, rather than using LMWH owing to concerns of increased risk of thrombotic events with LMWH.

TABLE 10.4 American College of Chest Physicians Recommendations for Anticoagulant Regimens in Pregnant Women with Mechanical Heart Valves

Adjusted-dose low-molecular-weight heparin (LMWH) throughout pregnancy, with doses adjusted to achieve the manufacturer's peak anti-Xa LMWH 4 hr after subcutaneous injection (grade 1A)
Adjusted-dose unfractionated heparin (UFH) throughout the pregnancy administered subcutaneously every 12 hr in doses adjusted to keep the midinterval activated partial thromboplastin time at least twice control or to attain an anti-Xa heparin level of 0.35–0.70 units/mL (grade 1A)
UFH or LMWH (as above) until the 13th week with substitution by vitamin K agonists until close to delivery when UFH or LMWH is resumed (grade 1A)
For women judged to be at very high risk of thromboembolism in whom concerns exist about the efficacy and safety of UFH or LMWH as dosed above (e.g., older-generation prosthesis in the mitral position or history of thromboembolism), vitamin K antagonists throughout the pregnancy with replacement by UFH or LMWH (as above) close to delivery (grade 2C)

Bates SM, Greer IA, Middeldorp S, et al. VTE, thrombophilia, antithrombotic therapy, and pregnancy: antithrombotic therapy and prevention of thrombosis, 9th edition: American College of Chest Physicians Evidence-based Clinical Practice Guidelines. *Chest*. 2012;141(2, suppl):e691S–e736S.

e. Any change in symptoms in patients with mechanical prosthesis should be evaluated by a complete transthoracic and possibly transesophageal echocardiogram to exclude valve thrombosis.

H. Principles of medication use in pregnancy and postpartum period

It is important to ascertain if a medication crosses the placenta or if it is transferred to breast milk. This can be accomplished by determining the Food and Drug Administration (FDA) designation for a drug based on research regarding fetal risk.

1. **Category A:** Safest to use in pregnancy
2. **Category B:** Either animal reproduction studies have not demonstrated a fetal risk but there are no controlled studies in pregnant women, or animal studies have shown an adverse effect that was not confirmed in controlled studies in women
3. **Category C:** Either studies in animals have revealed adverse effects on the fetus and there are no controlled studies in women, or studies in women and animals are not available. Drugs should be given only if potential benefits justify the potential risk to the fetus.
4. **Category D:** There is evidence of human fetal risk, but the benefits from use in pregnant women may be acceptable despite the risk (e.g., treatment of life-threatening conditions).
5. **Category X:** Studies in animals or human beings have demonstrated fetal abnormalities or there is evidence of fetal risk based on human experience, or both, and the risk of the use of the drug in pregnant women clearly outweighs any possible benefit. The drug is contraindicated in women who are or may become pregnant.

   See Table 10.5 for several medications used to treat valvular heart disease and their FDA categorization and fetal risks. Note that several medications are designated as class D (angiotensin-converting enzyme inhibitors and angiotensin receptor blockers, or warfarin in the first trimester unless low dose), although they may be used in the case of life-threatening conditions. However, they are generally contraindicated for use in pregnancy given their teratogenicity.

TABLE 10.5 The FDA Classification of Medications for Use in Pregnancy and Breastfeeding

Medication	Drug Class	FDA Category	Placenta Permeable	Transfers to Breast Milk	Adverse Effect to Fetus
Acetylsalicylic acid (low dose)	Antiplatelet agent	B	Yes	Yes (well tolerated)	No teratogenic effects known
Amiodarone	Antiarrhythmic (class III)	D	Yes	Yes	Thyroid insufficiency, hyperthyroidism, goiter, bradycardia, growth retardation, premature birth
Atenolol	β-Blocker (class II)	D	Yes	Yes	Hypospadias (first trimester), birth defects, low birth weight, bradycardia, and hypoglycemic fetus (second and third trimester)
Benazepril	ACE inhibitor	D	Yes	Yes (breastfeeding tolerated)	Renal or tubular dysplasia, oligohydramnios, growth retardation, ossification disorders of skull, lung hypoplasia, contractures, large joints, anemia, and intrauterine fetal death
Bisoprolol	β-Blocker (class II)	C	Yes	Yes	Bradycardia and hypoglycemia in fetus
Candesartan	ARB	D	Unknown	Unknown, not recommended	Renal or tubular dysplasia, oligohydramnios, growth retardation, ossification disorders of skull, lung hypoplasia, contractures, large joints, anemia, and intrauterine fetal death
Captopril	ACE inhibitor	D	Yes	Yes (breastfeeding tolerated)	Renal or tubular dysplasia, oligohydramnios, growth retardation, ossification disorders of skull, lung hypoplasia, contractures, large joints, anemia, and intrauterine fetal death

Digoxin	Cardiac glycoside	C	Yes	Yes	Serum levels unreliable, safe
Furosemide	Diuretic	C	Yes	Yes (well tolerated) can reduce breast milk production	Oligohydramnios
Heparin (LMW)	Anticoagulant	B	No	No	Long-term application: seldom osteoporosis and markedly less thrombocytopenia than unfractionated heparin
Heparin (unfractionated)	Anticoagulant	B	No	No	Long-term application: osteoporosis and thrombocytopenia
Hydralazine	Vasodilator	C	Yes	Yes (breastfeeding tolerated)	Maternal side effects: lupus-like symptoms, fetal tachyarrhythmias
Hydrochlorothiazide	Diuretic	B	Yes	Yes (milk production may be reduced)	Oligohydramnios
Metoprolol	β-Blocker (class II)	C	Yes	Yes	Bradycardia and hypoglycemia in fetus
Spironolactone	Aldosterone antagonist	D	Yes	Yes (milk production may be reduced)	Antiandrogenic effects, oral clefts (first trimester)
Warfarin	Vitamin K antagonist	D	Yes	Yes (maximum 10%) well tolerated as inactive metabolite	Warfarin embryopathy, bleeding

ACE, angiotensin-converting enzyme; ARB, angiotensin II receptor blocker; FDA, Food and Drug Administration; LMW, low-molecular-weight.
Adapted and modified from Bonow RO, Carabello BA, Chatterjee K, et al. 2008 focused update incorporated into the ACC/AHA 2006 Guidelines for the Management of Patients with Valvular Heart Disease. *Circulation.* 2008;118:e523–e661.

III. MANAGEMENT OF ANTICOAGULATION IN PATIENTS WITH PROSTHETIC VALVES

Antithrombotic therapy following placement of prosthetic valves varies depending on type of prosthesis, valve position, and concomitant factors increasing risk of thromboembolic event (including presence of atrial fibrillation, hypercoagulable state, or prior embolic event). When selecting the type of prosthesis to place in an individual patient, there is a trade-off between long-term durability of mechanical valves and the lack of need for lifelong systemic anticoagulation for bioprosthetic valves. The Society of Thoracic Surgeons' Adult Cardiac Database has reported an increase in the proportion of patients choosing bioprosthetic valves due to the burden of lifelong oral anticoagulation, and the hope that potential transcatheter valves will be available for valve procedures when the bioprosthesis degenerates.

A. Mechanical prostheses

1. Lifelong anticoagulation is necessary for mechanical prostheses. Observational studies have shown that antiplatelet drugs without anticoagulation are associated with unacceptably high rates of thromboembolic events. In the 1990s, the target INR was 3.0 to 4.5. Subsequently, three randomized trials showed that in selected patients a target INR of 2 to 3 was associated with lower bleeding risk without a significant increase in thromboembolic risk. Some studies have shown that with even lower target INRs (1.5 to 2 or 1.8 to 2.5), there is a further reduction in bleeding risks without an increase in the thromboembolic risk. However, not all of these trials have found consistent results.
2. The addition of low-dose aspirin with vitamin K antagonists has been shown to be beneficial in a randomized trial including patients with mechanical prostheses and atheromatous disease. The mortality reduction, however, was due to a decrease in death from CHF, MI, and sudden cardiac death, not from stroke. Therefore, to decide whether or not to add aspirin to oral anticoagulants, one must weigh the increased risks of bleeding and thromboembolism.
3. **American and European Guidelines Recommendations**
   - **a.** Aortic mechanical prosthesis: Target INR 2.5 (if no additional risk factors for thromboembolism)
   - **b.** Mitral mechanical prosthesis: Target INR 3.0 (American Heart Association/American College of Cardiology [AHA/ACC] or American College of Clinical Pharmacy [ACCP] consensus) or 3.0 or 3.5 (European Society of Cardiology/European Association for Cardio-Thoracic Surgery [ESC/EACTS] guidelines)
4. The addition of aspirin to warfarin differs between the AHA/ACC guidelines, which recommend low-dose aspirin as a class I indication for any type of valve in any position, and the ESC/EACTS guidelines, which are more restrictive.
5. INR variability is associated with all-cause mortality. Anticoagulation clinics serve to improve monitoring as well as adjust dosing for individual patients and thus minimize INR variability and improve outcomes. Self-monitoring of INR may also serve to improve INR stability through more frequent checks and adjustments.
6. Direct inhibitors of factor II or factor Xa are contraindicated in patients with mechanical prostheses. One study using dabigatran with mechanical prostheses was stopped early owing to an excess of thromboembolism and bleeding.
7. Recommendations for anticoagulation for noncardiac surgery in patients with mechanical valves:
   - **a.** For intervention with low risk of bleeding: continue anticoagulation uninterrupted (e.g., dental, ophthalmologic, and dermatologic surgery).
   - **b.** For patients undergoing major surgery that requires an INR <1.5 and interruption of warfarin: ESC/EACTS guidelines require bridging heparin; however, the AHA/ACC guidelines allow short interruptions (≤ 5 days) in patients with low-risk prostheses. If heparin bridging is required, intravenous unfractionated heparin is preferred immediately before and after surgery because it allows more rapid dose changes and also can be reversed with protamine sulfate.

B. Bioprostheses. Long-term anticoagulation is not required. However, long-term aspirin is recommended by AHA/ACC guidelines (IIa). In contrast, the ESC/EACTS guidelines do not recommend aspirin after 3 months. Postoperative antithrombotic therapy with warfarin is recommended for the first 3 months after surgery, allowing for the sewing ring to endothelialize. The ESC/EACTS and AHA/ACC guidelines recommend use of aspirin alone and not with warfarin during the postoperative period after aortic valve replacement with bioprosthesis. Nevertheless, warfarin is recommended for the first 3 months following mitral valve bioprosthesis surgery (especially considering the higher rates of postoperative atrial fibrillation and thromboembolic events).

C. **Transcatheter AVR (TAVR).** Long-term low-dose aspirin is recommended following TAVR. The majority of patients who have TAVR also have coronary artery disease, peripheral vascular disease, or prior stroke. Overall, the atrial fibrillation burden of TAVR patients is about 50% (30% with a history of prior atrial fibrillation and 10% to 15% following the procedure). There are no clear recommendations regarding aspirin therapy on top of the anticoagulant therapy for atrial fibrillation in these patients. Immediately post TAVR, the current recommendation is for clopidogrel 75 mg daily with low-dose aspirin for the first 1 to 6 months following the procedure. After that low-dose aspirin is continued for long-term therapy.

D. **Management of acute coronary syndromes and stenting in patients with mechanical prostheses.** Dual antiplatelet therapy is recommended for treatment of acute coronary syndromes and following stenting. However, there is a threefold increase in bleeding risk with vitamin K antagonists used together with dual antiplatelet therapy. Optional strategies are to limit to 3 to 6 months of triple therapy, or use a combination of clopidogrel with warfarin without aspirin.

See Figure 8.4 for anticoagulation for prosthetic valves from 2014 AHA/ACC Guidelines for Management of Patients with Valvular Heart Disease.

IV. NONCARDIAC SURGERY IN PATIENTS WITH VALVULAR HEART DISEASE

A. **Risk assessment models in noncardiac surgery.** Perioperative risk is procedure related. Eagle et al. categorized surgical procedures into groupings of similar risk. Procedures were categorized as low risk, intermediate risk, or high risk (Table 10.6). High-risk procedures included:
   1. Emergent major operations (especially in the elderly)
   2. Aortic and other major vascular surgery
   3. Peripheral vascular surgery
   4. Anticipated prolonged surgical procedures associated with large fluid shifts and/or blood loss

B. **Other risk classifications**
   1. American Society of Anesthesiologists (ASA) classification: good predictor of perioperative death
      a. NYHA classification designed for chronic heart failure—useful in assessing risk in preoperative patients with heart failure
      b. The Revised Cardiac Risk Index (Lee et al., 1999)—six predictors of major cardiac complications:
         i. High-risk type of surgery
         ii. Ischemic heart disease
         iii. History of CHF, defined as pulmonary edema, paroxysmal nocturnal dyspnea, an S_3 on physical exam, or chest X-ray with pulmonary vascular redistribution
         iv. History of cerebrovascular disease
         v. Insulin treatment for diabetes
         vi. Preoperative serum creatinine >2.0 mg/dL
   2. Hulselmans et al. proposed a risk classification for patients with valve disease undergoing noncardiac surgery that is broken down by valve lesion.
      a. **Aortic stenosis:** Moderate to severe AS is associated with worse outcomes including higher risk of myocardial infarction and death following noncardiac surgery. High-risk variables include LV dysfunction, abnormal response to

TABLE 10.6 Cardiac Risk Stratification for Noncardiac Surgical Procedures

High (cardiac risk >5%)	Intermediate (cardiac risk <5%)	Low (cardiac risk <1%)
Emergent major operations, especially in the elderly	Carotid endarterectomy	Endoscopic procedures
Aortic and other major vascular surgery	Head and neck surgery	Superficial procedures
Peripheral vascular surgery	Intraperitoneal and intrathoracic surgery	Cataract surgery
Anticipated prolonged surgical procedure associated with large fluid shifts and/or blood loss	Orthopedic surgery Prostate surgery	Breast surgery

From Hulselmans M, Vandermeulen E, Herregods MC. Risk assessment in patients with heart valve disease facing non-cardiac surgery. *Acta Cardiol.* 2009;62(2):151–155.

exercise testing, ventricular tachycardia, LV hypertrophy (>1.5 cm), and critical stenosis (AVA <0.6 cm^2). The AHA/ACC guidelines recommend preoperative correction for severe symptomatic AS (surgery or balloon valvuloplasty).

b. **Aortic insufficiency:** Severe symptomatic AI patients are at high risk. Asymptomatic severe AI patients with impaired LV function (ejection fraction [EF] <50%), LV dilatation (>55 mm), or enlarged aortic diameter (>50 mm) are also at high risk. Goals for treating patients with severe AI in the perioperative period include maintaining adequate preload, low-normal systemic blood pressure, and a high-normal HR to decrease the proportion of time spent in diastole (to decrease the regurgitant volume).

c. **Mitral stenosis:** Severe MS patients (mitral valve area [MVA] <1.0 cm^2) are at high risk. In addition, those with symptomatic MS (MVA 1.0–1.5 cm^2) with PA systolic pressure >50 mm Hg are also at high risk. Asymptomatic patients with moderate MS and PA systolic pressure <50 mm Hg are at moderate risk of cardiac events. Asymptomatic patients with mild MS are at low risk. Goals for managing patients with MS include maintenance of sinus rhythm and euvolemic loading conditions. AHA/ACC guidelines recommend preoperative correction of severe MS before undergoing high-risk surgery.

d. **Mitral regurgitation:** The 2002 ACC/AHA guidelines on perioperative care recommended preoperative correction of severe MR or MR associated with reduced LV systolic function. More recent guidelines from the American and European Societies only discuss optimal medical therapy. Symptomatic patients with severe MR and patients with impaired LV function, atrial fibrillation, or pulmonary hypertension are considered high risk. Symptomatic patients with severe MR and preserved LV systolic function are considered intermediate risk.

For 2014 AHA/ACC recommendations regarding noncardiac surgery in patients with valvular heart disease, see Table 10.7.

V. VALVE-RELATED TUMORS

A. **Papillary fibroelastoma.** This is a non-neoplastic tumor in adult hearts known for its embolic potential. It is a benign endocardial papillary growth found anywhere along the endocardial surface of a valve. The histology is similar to that of Lambl excrescences. Grossly, the tumors are soft, rounded nodules that expand when placed in fluid. The

TABLE 10.7 AHA/ACC Recommendations for Noncardiac Surgery in Patients with VHD

Class IIa	Class IIb
Moderate-risk elective noncardiac surgery with appropriate intraoperative and postoperative hemodynamic monitoring is reasonable to perform in patients with asymptomatic severe AS (level of evidence B)	Moderate-risk elective noncardiac surgery with appropriate intraoperative and postoperative hemodynamic monitoring may be reasonable to perform in asymptomatic patients with severe MS if the valve morphology is not favorable for percutaneous balloon mitral commissurotomy (level of evidence C)
Moderate-risk elective noncardiac surgery with appropriate intraoperative and postoperative hemodynamic monitoring is reasonable to perform in patients with severe MR (level of evidence C)	
Moderate-risk elective noncardiac surgery in patients with appropriate intraoperative and postoperative hemodynamic monitoring is reasonable to perform in patients with asymptomatic severe AR and a normal LVEF (level of evidence C)	

AHA/ACC, American Heart Association/American College of Cardiology; AR, aortic regurgitation; AS, aortic stenosis; LVEF, left ventricular ejection fraction; MR, mitral regurgitation; MS, mitral stenosis; VHD, valvular heart disease. From Nishimura RA, Otto CM, Bonow RO, et al. 2014 AHA/ACC Guideline for the Management of Patients with Valvular Heart Disease: a report of the American College of Cardiology/American Heart Association Task Force on Practice Guidelines. *Circulation.* 2014;129(23):e521–e643.

most common locations are the aortic valve > mitral valve > LV endocardium and tricuspid valve. Often diagnosed incidentally during transthoracic echocardiography (TTE), it may present with syncope, stroke, or chest pain from prolapse of the tumor into a coronary artery. Although seen with TTE, computed tomography (CT), or magnetic resonance imaging, transesophageal echocardiography (TEE) is the most sensitive modality. Most fibroelastomas do not interfere with valvular function. A TEE performed as part of an evaluation for source of embolus following a stroke may show a fibroelastoma, or on occasion only a remnant stalk may be visualized. Fibroelastomas are usually small (<1 cm), well-outlined lesions showing soft tissue attenuation on CT scan and hypointense or intermediate signals in T1-weighted sequences or intermediate signals in T2-weighted sequences. They do not enhance with contrast. Note that when a small mobile echodensity is found in association with a valve, although it may be characteristic of a fibroelastoma, other potential entities such as endocarditis, lupus, or antiphospholipid antibody syndrome should be considered. Indications for surgery include left-sided fibroelastomas with prior embolic events or for those >1 cm or those that are mobile with low surgical risk. Surgical resection of tumors typically does not require resection of leaflet tissue (Figs. 10.1 and 10.2).

B. Cardiac myxomas. All myxomas are endocardial based and project into the heart chamber cavity. The majority arise from the left atrial septum (85%); however, they can arise from the right atrial septum (11%) or from a variety of other sites, rarely including a valve. Usually myxomas are single; however, they can be multiple. Myxomas may indirectly affect valvular function by distortion of the supporting apparatus of the valves.

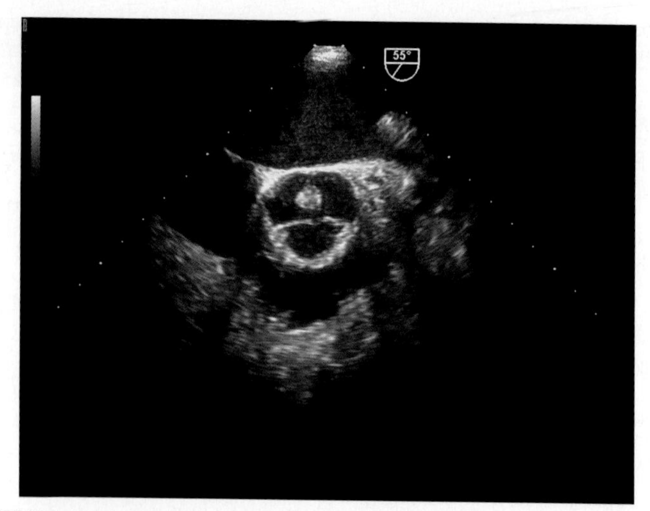

FIGURE 10.1 This is an example of a fibroelastoma on the aortic valve seen by transesophageal echocardiography in the short-axis view. Notice its well-circumscribed appearance, and on moving images it was highly mobile and was attached to the valve by a stalk.

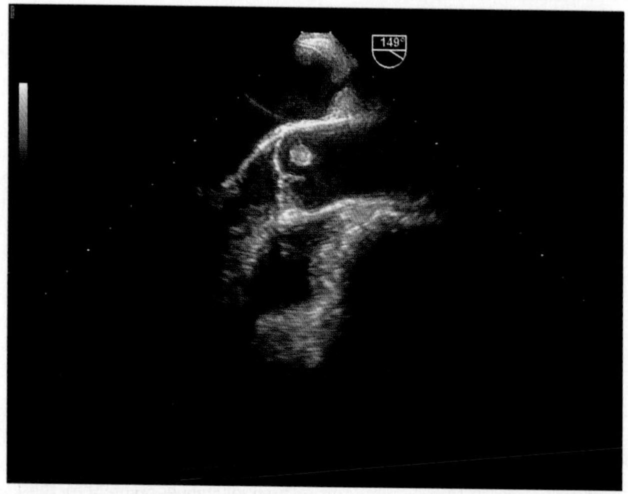

FIGURE 10.2 An example of the same fibroelastoma on the aortic valve seen by transesophageal echocardiography in the midesophageal long-axis view.

KEY PEARLS

- Five categories of drugs cause valvular heart disease through activation of the 5-hydroxytryptamine 2B serotonin receptor, causing proliferation of myofibroblasts and production of excessive extracellular matrix on valve leaflets. Those classes include migraine drugs (methylsergide and ergotamine), appetite suppressants (fenfluramine and dexfenfluramine), benfluorex, ergot-derived dopaminergic agonists (pergolide and cabergoline), and MDMA (3,4-methylenedioxymethamphetamine).
- Patients with valvular heart disease should have a preconception consultation/evaluation regarding risk assessment before becoming pregnant. This assessment should include a careful history and physical, 12-lead ECG, transthoracic echocardiography, and possible stress testing. A level of risk is determined, and discussions regarding risks of therapy and possible complications (maternal and fetal) should be performed by a multidisciplinary team including a cardiologist and an obstetrician/gynecologist.
- In general, stenotic lesions are poorly tolerated, whereas regurgitant lesions are better tolerated. This can be explained by the physiologic and hemodynamic changes that occur with pregnancy, labor, and delivery.
- Patients at prohibitively high risk (who should be counseled against pregnancy) include those with severe symptomatic aortic stenosis or mitral stenosis, cardiomyopathy with left ventricular ejection fraction ≤30%, Marfan syndrome with aortic root ≥45 mm, or advanced pulmonary hypertension (two-thirds systemic pressures).
- Medications used to treat valvular disease in pregnancy (and postdelivery) must be selected with careful attention to their Food and Drug Administration classification regarding fetal risk (i.e., teratogenicity and more) and whether or not the medication crosses the placenta or passes into breast milk in the postpartum period.
- The management of anticoagulation for mechanical valve prostheses in pregnant patients needs to weigh the risks of thromboembolic events in this hypercoagulable state with the risks of teratogenicity and bleeding complications. The exact antithrombotic regimen is tailored to the specific patient's needs (depending on type and position of prosthesis, any high thrombotic risk features, and dose of anticoagulant needed).
- The risk of noncardiac surgery in patients with valvular heart disease is best predicted by the revised cardiac risk index with additional considerations for specific types of valve lesions. High-risk features include high-risk surgery, ischemic heart disease, history of congestive heart failure, history of cerebrovascular disease, insulin treatment for diabetes, and a preoperative creatinine of >2 mg/dL, as well as severe symptomatic aortic stenosis (AS); severe asymptomatic AS with left ventricular (LV) dysfunction or an abnormal response to exercise; severe symptomatic aortic insufficiency (AI) or asymptomatic AI with impaired LV function or dilated LV (LV end-systolic diameter >55 mm); severe mitral stenosis (MS) or symptomatic moderate MS, or asymptomatic moderate MS with right ventricular systolic pressure >50 mm Hg; or severe symptomatic mitral regurgitation.

SUGGESTED READINGS

Andrejak M, Tribouilloy C. Drug induced valvular heart disease: an update. *Arch Cardiovasc Dis.* 2013;106(5):333–339.

Bates SM, Greer IA, Middeldorp S, et al. VTE, thrombophilia, antithrombotic therapy, and pregnancy: antithrombotic therapy and prevention of thrombosis, 9th ed: American College of Chest Physicians Evidence-based Clinical Practice Guidelines. *Chest.* 2012;141(2, suppl):e691S–e736S.

Burke A, Tavora F. The 2015 WHO classification of tumors of the heart and pericardium. *J Thorac Oncol.* 2016;11(4):441–452.

Diaz Angulo C, Diaz CM, Garcia ER, et al. Imaging findings in cardiac masses: Part I: study protocol and benign tumors. *Radiologia.* 2015;57(6):480–488.

Eagle KA, Brundage BH, Chaitman BR, et al. Guidelines for Perioperative Cardiovascular Evaluation for Noncardiac Surgery. Report of the American College of Cardiology/American Heart Association task force on Practice Guidelines. *Circulation.* 1996;93(6):1278–1317.

Elangbam CS. Drug induced valvulopathy: an update. *Toxicol Pathol.* 2010;38(6):837–848.
Freeman WK, Gibbons RJ. Perioperative cardiovascular assessment of patients undergoing noncardiac surgery. *Mayo Clin Proc.* 2009;84(1):79–90.
Hulselmans M, Vandermeulen E, Herregods MC. Risk assessment in patients with heart valve disease facing non-cardiac surgery. *Acta Cardiol.* 2009;62(2):151–155.
Lee TH, Marcantonio ER, Mangione CM, et al. Derivation and prospective validation of a simple index for prediction of cardiac risk of major noncardiac surgery. *Circulation,* 1999;100:1043–1049.
Lung B, Rodes-Cabau J. The optimal management of anti-thrombotic therapy after valve replacement: certainties and uncertainties. *Eur Heart J.* 2014;(35):2942–2949.
Nanna M, Stergiopoulos K. Pregnancy complicated by valvular heart disease: an update. *J Am Heart Assoc.* 2014;3(3):e000712.
Nishimura RA, Otto CM, Bonow RO, et al. 2014 AHA/ACC Guideline for the Management of Patients with Valvular Heart Disease: a report of the American College of Cardiology/American Heart Association Task Force on Practice Guidelines. *Circulation.* 2014;129(23):e521–e643.
Regitz-Zagrosek V, Lundqvist CB, Borghi C, et al. ESC guidelines on the management of cardiovascular diseases during pregnancy: the Task Force on the Management of Cardiovascular Diseases during Pregnancy of the European Society of Cardiology. *Eur Heart J.* 2011;32(24):3147–3197.
Sliwa K, Johnson MR, Zilla P, et al. Management of valvular disease in pregnancy: a global perspective. *Eur Heart J.* 2015;36(18):1078–1089.
Vahanian A, Alfieri O, Andreotti F, et al. Guidelines on the management of valvular heart disease (version 2012). Joint Task Force on the Management of Valvular Heart Disease of the European Society of Cardiology (ESC); European Association for Cardiothoracic Surgery (EACTS). *Eur Heart J.* 2012;33(19):2451–2496.
Windram JD, Colman JM, Wald RM, et al. Valvular heart disease in pregnancy. *Best Pract Res Clin Obstet Gynaecol.* 2014;28(4):507–518.
Whitlock RP, Sun JC, Fremes SE, et al. Antithrombotic and thrombolytic therapy for valvular disease: antithrombotic therapy and prevention of thrombosis, 9th ed: American College of Chest Physicians Evidence-Based Practice Guidelines. *Chest.* 2012;141(2, suppl):e576S–e600S.

SECTION

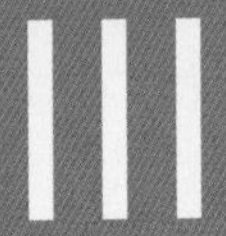

Percutaneous and Surgical Valve Procedures

CHAPTER 11

Jayendrakumar S. Patel
Amar Krishnaswamy

Percutaneous Mitral Valve Procedures

Percutaneous strategies for the treatment of mitral valve (MV) stenosis and MV regurgitation are important therapeutic options for selected patients. In the growing field of structural cardiac interventions, the MV presents a new frontier for technologic innovation and less-invasive patient care. In this chapter, we discuss patient selection, technical aspects, and data supporting percutaneous mitral valvotomy, repair, and valve replacement.

I. PERCUTANEOUS MITRAL BALLOON VALVOTOMY

A. Introduction. First performed in the mid-1980s, percutaneous mitral balloon valvotomy (PMBV) has now become the preferred method of treating symptomatic patients with severe mitral stenosis (MS) of rheumatic etiology and favorable valve morphology. The procedure entails controlled fracture and separation of fused commissures. Hence, there is no role for PMBV in cases of MS without commissural fusion (e.g., congenital MS or MS secondary to mitral annular calcification) or in cases where the valves are not pliable. Several randomized trials have shown that PMBV offers outcomes that are equivalent to or better than surgical closed or open commissurotomy, with added benefits of lower cost and a minimally invasive approach. Optimal outcomes depend upon accurate assessment of valve anatomy, valve hemodynamics, and patient symptoms.

B. Indications

1. The indications for intervention for patients with rheumatic MS are shown in Figure 11.1 and are derived from the 2014 American Heart Association/American College of Cardiology (AHA/ACC) Guidelines for the Management of Patients with Valvular Heart Disease. In general, there is strong evidence supporting PMBV in patients with reduced exercise capacity and exertional dyspnea in the setting of moderate-to-severe MS and with favorable valve characteristics in the absence of contraindications as detailed later. Weak evidence suggests that the procedure is reasonable for asymptomatic patients with very severe MS (mitral valve area [MVA] $\leq$1.0 cm^2) and may be considered in those with severe MS with MVA $\leq$1.5 cm^2 and systolic pulmonary pressure >50 mm Hg, need for major noncardiac surgery, or new-onset atrial fibrillation, as this represents a high risk of thromboembolism.
2. Although the European Society of Cardiology does not recommend intervention in patients with MVA >1.5 cm^2 regardless of the presence of symptoms, the AHA/ACC guidelines state that PMBV may be considered in symptomatic patients with increased transmitral flow velocities, mild-to-moderate left atrial enlargement, and pulmonary capillary wedge pressure >25 mm Hg or mean gradient >15 mm Hg during exercise. Pregnancy also presents unique hemodynamic considerations, and there is a weak level of evidence in support of preconception PMBV for women with asymptomatic MS with MVA $\leq$1.5 cm^2, especially if there is pulmonary hypertension at rest or with exercise. Patients with recurrence of symptomatic MS post-PMBV and with evidence of commissural fusion can also be considered for a repeat intervention if anatomy is favorable.

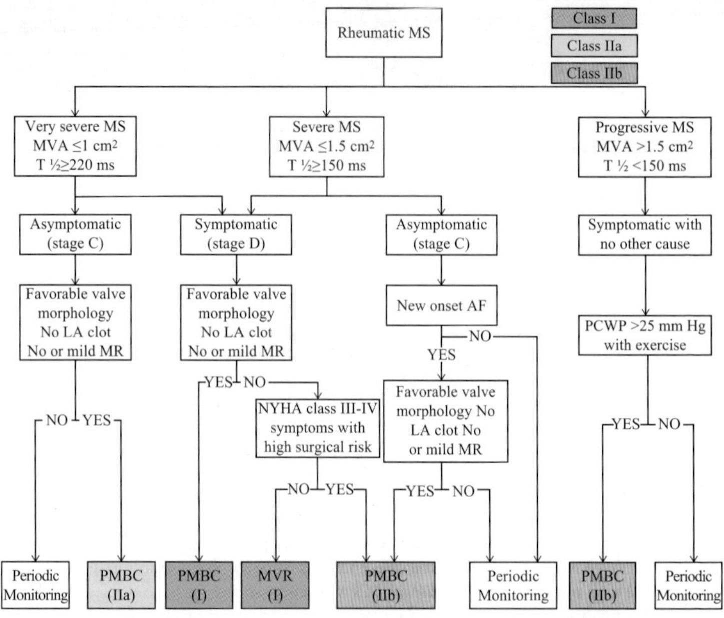

FIGURE 11.1 Indications for intervention in patients with rheumatic mitral stenosis. LA, left atrium; MR, mitral regurgitation; MVA, mitral valve area; MVR, mitral valve replacement; PCWP, pulmonary capillary wedge pressure; PMBC, percutaneous mitral balloon commissurotomy. (Adapted from Figure 3 in Nishimura RA, Otto CM, Bonow RO, et al. 2014 AHA/ACC guideline for the management of patients with valvular heart disease: executive summary: a report of the American College of Cardiology/American Heart Association Task Force on Practice Guidelines. *J Am Coll Cardiol.* 2014;63[22]:2438–2488.)

C. Contraindications to PMBV

1. Transesophageal echocardiography (TEE) must be performed before PMBV to accurately assess valve anatomy and most importantly to ensure the absence of left atrial clot and/or moderate-to-severe mitral regurgitation (MR). If thrombus is present and the need for intervention is not urgent, the patient may undergo a trial of therapeutic anticoagulation for 2 to 6 months followed by reassessment with TEE. If thrombus persists or the need for intervention is urgent, a surgical approach is indicated.
2. Several scoring systems have been developed to assess anatomic suitability for PMBV and are discussed later. In order for PMBV to be successful with sustained durability, the valve leaflets and commissures should be relatively noncalcified and pliable with minimal valvular and subvalvular thickening. Heavy calcification of the commissures (especially both commissures) predicts development of postprocedural severe MR; thus, percutaneous valvotomy should be avoided in such patients. Similarly, asymmetric fusion of only one commissure may provide a greater risk for tearing the valve and creating significant MR. Nevertheless, patients with less-than-ideal valve anatomy may still be considered for PMBV if surgery is contraindicated or considered too high risk. Finally, the concomitant presence of MS and severe aortic valve disease, severe tricuspid stenosis or regurgitation, or severe coronary artery disease requiring bypass should prompt consideration of surgical intervention.

D. Evaluation

1. Evaluation of the patient begins with careful assessment of symptoms and the degree of functional disability (New York Heart Association [NYHA] class). These include dyspnea with exertion or at rest, cough, hoarseness, hemoptysis, atrial fibrillation, thromboembolism, and right-sided heart failure from elevated pulmonary pressures. For asymptomatic patients or patients with symptoms that seem out of proportion to valve severity, exercise or dobutamine echocardiography can help identify patients with hemodynamically significant disease.
2. A thorough assessment of the valve apparatus using either transthoracic echocardiography (TTE) or TEE is imperative to determine suitability and likelihood of success (and complications) of PMBV. This can be accomplished through several scoring systems, the most common of which is shown in Table 11.1 (Wilkins score). Of note, none of the scoring systems are perfectly reproducible and the Wilkins score omits commissural calcification. Thus, even patients deemed to have an ideal Wilkins score may experience suboptimal outcomes, including the development of severe MR. The commissural calcification scoring system shown in Table 11.2 can be used adjunctively to further predict the development of severe MR. In patients with an echo score that is favorable (i.e., ≤8 by Wilkins score),

TABLE 11.1 Wilkins Echocardiographic Scoring System of the Mitral Valve

	Component			
Grade	Leaflet Mobility	Valvular Thickening	Subvalvular Thickening	Valvular Calcification
1	Highly mobile, restricted only at tips	Near normal (4–5 mm)	Minimal thickening of chordae just below valve	Single area of brightness
2	Base and mid-portion have reduced mobility	Mid-leaflet thickening, marked thickening of margins	Thickened chordae up to one-third of length	Scattered areas of brightness restricted to leaflet margins
3	Forward during diastole, mainly at base	Entire leaflets thickened (5–8 mm)	Thickening extending to distal one-third	Brightness extending to mid-portion of leaflets
4	No or minimal forward movement during diastole	Marked leaflet thickening (>8–10 mm)	Extensive thickening and shortening of all chordae down to papillary muscle	Extensive brightness through most of the leaflet tissue

NOTE: Total score is calculated by adding each component score; <8 indicates favorable anatomy for percutaneous mitral balloon valvotomy.

Adapted from Wilkins GT, Weyman AE, Abascal VM, et al. Percutaneous balloon dilatation of the mitral valve: an analysis of echocardiographic variables related to outcome and the mechanism of dilatation. *Br Heart J.* 1988;60(4):299.

TABLE 11.2 Commissural Calcification Scoring System

Grade	Echocardiographic Findings
0	Severe stenosis but no bright echoes across either commissure
1	Bright echoes extending across one-half of a commissure
2	Bright echoes extending throughout entire single commissure or bright echoes across half of each commissure
3	Bright echoes extending throughout entire single commissure AND half of the other commissure
4	Bright echoes extending throughout both commissures

NOTE: Each commissure (anterolateral and posteromedial) is divided into halves, and each half may receive one point. The commissural calcification score can range from 0 to 4. Bright echoes are presumed to represent areas of calcification.
Adapted from Sutaria N, Northridge DB, Shaw TRD. Significance of commissural calcification on outcome of mitral balloon valvotomy. *Heart.* 2000;84:398–402.

a commissural calcification score ≥2 predicts a smaller increase in valve area and reduced success rate of achieving a final valve area >1.5 cm^2 without MR. Cardiac catheterization with direct measurement of valve gradients has largely been supplanted by echocardiography and is only necessary when there is conflicting information derived from noninvasive studies.

E. Technique

1. A transvenous approach (femoral or jugular) is most commonly employed to perform PMBV. Arterial access may be helpful to perform left ventriculography before the start of the PMBV procedure in order to establish the MV plane and also the degree of MR. Transseptal catheterization to gain access to the left atrium and MV is routinely performed using a Brockenbrough needle via a Mullins sheath (Medtronic Inc, Minneapolis, MN). In some labs, this step is performed with intracardiac echocardiography guidance as an adjunct to routine fluoroscopic imaging. Once this step is complete, the operator may choose a single (more common) or double balloon technique to perform commissurotomy (Fig. 11.2).
2. With the single balloon technique, an Inoue balloon (Toray Industries, Tokyo, Japan) is selected according to the patient's height (maximum diameter [mm]: [patient height in cm]/10 + 10). The device is then passed through the atrial septum into the left atrium and the distal portion of the balloon is inflated with a few milliliters of diluted contrast. This action serves to reduce the risk of ventricular perforation. After crossing the valve and entering the left ventricle (LV), the distal portion of the balloon is further inflated and then pulled back into the mitral orifice. The proximal and central portions are then inflated up to 4 mm below the maximum balloon size for the initial balloon procedure.
3. TTE or TEE is then utilized to assess the response to balloon inflation (MV orifice is assessed by planimetry), and if the valve area is inadequate without an increase in MR by more than one grade (based on color Doppler), repeat valvotomy is performed with a 1-mm increase in balloon diameter. Such stepwise dilation ensures that the risk of creating severe MR is minimized. Further balloon dilations are ceased if the MVA is >1 cm^2/m^2 of the body surface area, if there is complete opening of at least one commissure, or if there is worsening of MR by more than one grade. Greater caution is taken in patients older than age 65 or

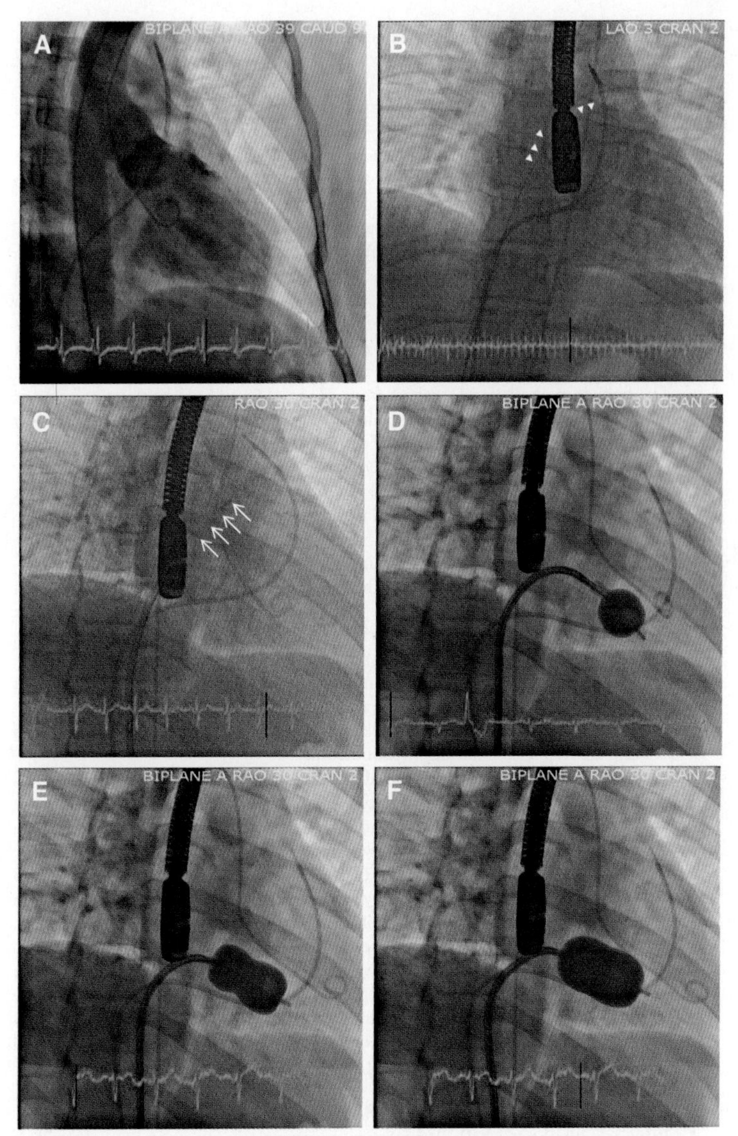

FIGURE 11.2 Key steps in percutaneous mitral balloon valvotomy. A: Left ventriculography is performed to establish the plane of the mitral valve and assess the degree of mitral regurgitation. **B:** Transseptal puncture is then performed *(arrowheads)*. **C:** The deflated Inoue balloon is then passed through the atrial septum into the left atrium *(arrows)*. **D:** The distal portion of the balloon is inflated with a few milliliters of diluted contrast. **E:** The mitral valve is crossed. The distal portion of the balloon is further inflated and then pulled back into the mitral orifice. **F:** The proximal and central portions are finally inflated.

pregnant patients. Good immediate results are defined as final valve area >1.5 cm^2 and an increase of at least 25% of valve area, or final valve area >1.5 cm^2 with less than moderate MR.

F. **Periprocedural management.** All patients who have undergone PMBV should be admitted to the hospital and monitored for complications. Approximately 24 to 48 hours after the procedure, repeat TTE is indicated to assess valve area and the degree of MR. If MR appears to be significantly worsened, TEE can be performed to determine the mechanism and further assess severity and need for valve surgery.

G. **Complications.** Rates of various complications from PMBV are fairly low and are dependent upon a variety of factors including operator experience, technique employed, patient clinical profile, and valve characteristics. In-hospital death is rare (<1%), and embolic events can be seen in up to 1.8% of cases. The most catastrophic complication is left ventricular perforation, with the development of hemopericardium necessitating emergent pericardiocentesis (observed in 1% of cases). Severe MR post-PMBV is not common but is difficult to predict owing to imprecise anatomic prediction scores. The frequency of severe MR ranges from 2% to 19% and can be due to tearing of the leaflets, excessive commissural splitting, or papillary muscle rupture. The most frequent mechanism is MR at the site of successful commissurotomy. Valve replacement is usually necessary in cases of leaflet laceration as valvular and subvalvular anatomy is not ideal for repair. Overall survival rate for those who develop severe MR is not significantly different when compared with those who do not develop severe MR.

H. **Outcomes**

1. The short-term results of PMBV in properly selected patients are usually excellent. Most operators are able to achieve a significant increase in valve area (by at least 100%), and as a result, there is an immediate decline in left atrial pressure and pulmonary artery pressure with improvement in cardiac output. In general, if the immediate results are successful, then long-term survival rates are excellent. Long-term freedom from a combined end point of death, MV surgery, or repeat PMBV ranges from 35% to 70% after 10 to 15 years postprocedure. The wide variation in event rates is largely explained by heterogeneity in patient characteristics that are responsible for long-term outcome.
2. Risk factors predictive of events include advanced age, NYHA class IV, presence of atrial fibrillation, advanced valve deformity (Wilkins score >8), greater valve calcification, higher postprocedural pulmonary artery pressure, preprocedural MR that is ≥2+, postprocedural MR that is ≥3+, severe tricuspid regurgitation, and final valve area. Recurrence of stenosis (loss of more than 50% of the initial gain with an MVA <1.5 cm^2) and the need for repeat intervention after PMBV are time dependent, with around 40% of patients requiring either surgery or repeat PMBV at 10 to 12 years. The mechanism for restenosis is likely progressive scarring and calcification due to turbulent flow through an abnormal valve. For those patients with restenosis after prior commissurotomy, PMBV is safe in properly selected patients and offers reasonable long-lasting favorable outcomes, particularly in those patients who remain in sinus rhythm. However, up to two-thirds of cases may require another repeat intervention over a period of 20 years (with most cases going on to MV replacement).

II. PERCUTANEOUS TRANSCATHETER MITRAL VALVE REPAIR

A. Patients with chronic MR often remain asymptomatic for many years depending upon the severity, etiology, and mechanism of regurgitation. Chronic MR may be either due to a primary abnormality of the valve apparatus (i.e., degenerative MR) or secondary due to another cardiac process (i.e., functional MR). The distinction between these two general categories and even the exact etiology within each category has implications for specific treatment strategies and prognosis. In general, MR is best described by the etiology, the pathologic lesions that follow, and the leaflet motion abnormality (in reference to the annular plane) that results. Leaflet motion in MR can be normal (as seen in patients with atrial fibrillation), increased (i.e., prolapsed), restricted during diastole and systole (as seen in rheumatic MR), or restricted primarily during systole (as seen in ischemic MR).

B. The most common causes of degenerative MR in the United States are Barlow disease (seen in younger patients) and fibroelastic deficiency (seen in older patients), both of which lead to chordae elongation or rupture. Barlow disease is characterized by redundant, large, thick leaflets generally affecting many segments of the valve and with associated annular dilation. Fibroelastic deficiency on the other hand is characterized by thin, normal-sized leaflets. Correction of primary MR is curative. However, many patients are not surgical candidates due to the presence of comorbid conditions, advanced age, or significantly impaired left ventricular function. In such cases, percutaneous MV repair offers the potential for symptomatic improvement, reduction in severity of MR, and possibly reversal of left ventricular remodeling, with advantages of shorter length of hospitalization and improved recovery time. Percutaneous repair technologies can be divided into those that target the leaflets, the annulus, the chordae, and the LV.

III. PERCUTANEOUS EDGE-TO-EDGE LEAFLET REPAIR—MITRACLIP SYSTEM

The only percutaneous technique currently approved by the US Food and Drug Administration is the MitraClip (Abbot Vascular, Santa Clara, CA). The procedure is based on the surgical concept pioneered by Ottavio Alfieri in the late 1990s and involves edge-to-edge coaptation of anterior and posterior leaflets at the site of regurgitation with the use of a percutaneously delivered clip. The clip was first introduced in 2004 and is commercially available in 40 countries. The acute procedural success rate is estimated to be around 75% to 100%, and the procedure is relatively safe and well tolerated. Worldwide, more than 10,000 patients have been treated with the clip, and the predominant indication in the commercial setting is the surgically prohibitive patient with secondary MR. Although the Alfieri stitch has been shown to be effective in both primary and secondary MR, the device is currently only approved in the United States for the treatment of degenerative MR.

A. Indications

1. **Degenerative MR:** Current AHA/ACC guidelines give strong evidence-based recommendations for surgical MV repair over MV replacement in symptomatic patients with severe primary, or degenerative, MR (DMR) and for those without symptoms and with impaired left ventricular systolic function (≤60%) or with cavity dilation (end-systolic dimension ≥40 mm). It is reasonable to consider surgery in asymptomatic patients with severe DMR who have preserved left ventricular dimensions or have new-onset atrial fibrillation or pulmonary artery systolic pressure >50 mm Hg if the likelihood of successful repair is >95% and the expected mortality is <1%. When the risk of surgery is excessively high owing to comorbid conditions, the MitraClip device may be considered for patients with NYHA class III to IV symptoms with ≥3+ DMR, favorable valve anatomy, and reasonable life expectancy (>1 year). Such patients are typically too frail for surgery, are of advanced age (>75), and have an elevated predicted operative mortality risk typically ≥6% to 8%, hostile chest, severe pulmonary hypertension, or extensively calcified ascending aorta.
2. **Functional MR:** All recommendations from major societies regarding surgical intervention for severe secondary, or functional, MR (FMR) are based on limited evidence. Although effectiveness has not been established, isolated MV surgery may be considered in those with severe FMR if symptoms persist despite optimal medical therapy (including resynchronization therapy) or with no options for revascularization. Survival after surgery for FMR is generally poor and recurrence is common, which provides the rationale for a less-invasive percutaneous option. Despite a large worldwide experience in this group of patients, the MitraClip system is not approved for this application in the United States. Two large prospective

trials (COAPT and RESHAPE-HF) are currently underway to assess the utility of the clip in this patient population.

B. Contraindications. Implantation of the MitraClip requires transseptal catheterization to access the left atrium and MV. The presence of left atrial thrombus, vegetation, deep venous thrombus, or a bleeding disorder is a contraindication to the procedure. Additional contraindications include active endocarditis and rheumatic valve disease. The EVEREST trial also excluded patients with acute myocardial infarction in the preceding 12 weeks, ejection fraction <25% and/or end-systolic dimension >55 mm, severe mitral annular calcification, and valvular anatomy that may preclude safe and proper clip deployment. The clip was also not evaluated in patients with a history of prior MV surgery or valvuloplasty.

C. Evaluation. Evaluation of the patient begins with careful assessment of symptoms and the degree of functional disability (NYHA class). In most cases, TTE provides adequate evaluation of left ventricular dimensions, pulmonary pressures, and the mechanism and severity of MR. Operative mortality for surgical MV repair or replacement should be estimated with the Society of Thoracic Surgeons (STS) risk calculator. Additional predictors of poor surgical outcome should be identified (frailty, inability to tolerate cardiopulmonary bypass, hostile chest, advanced cirrhosis), and the decision to defer surgical intervention should be made in conjunction with an experienced surgeon. Optimal results are obtained when the primary regurgitant jet originates from malcoaptation of the A2 and P2 scallops, with a flail width <15 mm and a flail gap <10 mm. If a secondary jet exists, it should be clinically insignificant. In addition, the MVA should be ≥4 cm^2 with minimal calcification and absence of cleft in the grasping area and minimal forward gradient across the valve as placement of one (or more) clip(s) will result in a marginal degree of MS. TEE is usually performed before valve repair to confirm the absence of thrombus and further assess valve suitability for clip implantation as described earlier. When there is discrepancy between symptoms and the severity of MR at rest, it is reasonable to perform exercise stress testing with TTE. Identification of pulmonary artery systolic pressure >60 mm Hg or worsening severity of MR in the setting of exercise warrants consideration for valve repair.

D. Technique. The entire percutaneous repair is usually performed under general anesthesia and with fluoroscopic and TEE guidance. After successful venous access, transseptal catheterization is performed and the patient is given heparin to achieve therapeutic anticoagulation. A steerable #24 French delivery guide sheath (unique to the MitraClip) is then advanced into the left atrium and the clip follows (Fig. 11.3). The arms of the clip are subsequently opened once the clip is aligned with the long axis of the heart. The clip is positioned over the origin of the regurgitant jet and then rotated until the arms are perpendicular to the line of coaptation of the valve leaflets. Three-dimensional TEE can be very useful at this stage to confirm perpendicularity of the clip to the line of coaptation at the area of MR. The open clip is advanced into the LV and retracted during systole to grasp both leaflets. Closure of the device approximates the leaflets and the clip is locked into position. Adequacy of clip placement is assessed with TEE, and immediate procedural success is defined as MR ≤2+. If the outcome is suboptimal, the clip can be reopened, detached from the leaflets, everted, withdrawn to the LA, and repositioned. If necessary, repositioning should be performed with the clip in the LA as entanglement in the subvalvular apparatus may occur with excessive manipulation in the LV. Sometimes, a second device needs to be implanted to achieve procedural success. In the EVEREST II trial, a second clip was required in approximately 40% of cases. Over time, fibrosis and scarring occur at the point of clip attachment. Closure of the venous access site may be achieved using Perclose preclosure technique, a figure-of-eight stitch placed in the overlying soft tissue, or manual compression hemostasis.

E. Postprocedural management. All patients who have undergone MitraClip implantation should be admitted to the hospital and monitored for complications including

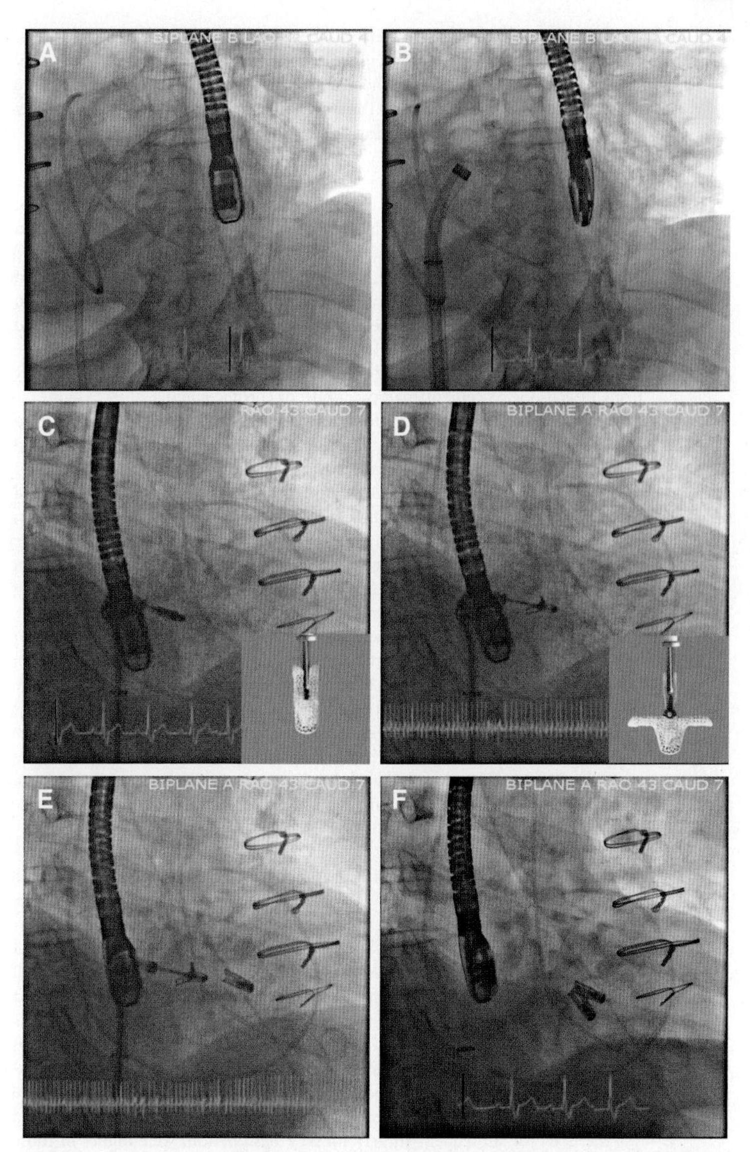

FIGURE 11.3 Key steps in MitraClip implantation. A, B: Trans-septal catheterization is performed and a steerable #24 Fr delivery guide sheath is advanced into the left atrium. **C:** The clip is introduced into the left atrium in the closed position. **D:** The clip is positioned over the origin of the regurgitant jet. The open clip is advanced into the left ventricle and retracted during systole to grasp both leaflets. **E, F:** A second clip may be implanted to achieve procedural success.

clip detachment, stroke, pericardial effusion/tamponade, and access-site concerns. Most patients are started on aspirin daily for 6 months and clopidogrel 75 mg daily for 30 days after the procedure. Prophylactic antibiotics are indicated if patients are undergoing any additional procedures. Patients should limit strenuous physical activity for at least the first month postprocedure.

F. Complications

1. Short-term (30-day) complications related to MitraClip implantation occur at a relatively low rate. These data are derived from a systematic review consisting of 12 prospective observational studies (with patient samples ranging from 16 to 202 and including degenerative and functional MR) on the safety of the device in the United States and Europe. Thirty-day mortality after clip implantation ranges from 0% to 7.8%, with a weighted mean of 3.3%. The most common complication observed was the need for transfusion of ≥2 units of packed red blood cells, ranging from 0% to 17.9% (weighted mean 5.7%). This seems to be primarily due to access site–related complications, gastrointestinal bleed (possibly from TEE probe placement/manipulation), or chronic anemia.
2. The second most common complication was partial clip detachment, occurring at a rate of 0% to 12.5% (weighted mean of all studies 6.2%). Complete clip detachment and embolization appear to be exceedingly rare, and partial clip detachment is often discovered on routine echocardiographic evaluation, with most cases occurring within the first month after implant. In almost all cases, patients are able to undergo elective conventional valve surgery and most are able to undergo MV repair over replacement. Clip-related chordal rupture has been reported in 2% to 6.2% of cases (weighted mean 2.4%), with most developing acute heart failure necessitating emergent surgery.
3. Transseptal complications were observed in 1.2% to 3% (weighted mean 2.17%) and include the development of cardiac tamponade. The rates of myocardial infarction, stroke, tamponade, and the need for urgent surgery for adverse events are each ≤4%. In the EVEREST II trial (discussed later), there were no significant differences in major adverse events excluding transfusion (death, myocardial infarction, stroke, renal failure, urgent cardiac surgery, sepsis, or gastrointestinal bleed) at 30 days among those who received the clip compared with the surgical group. Transfusions were significantly more common in the surgical group.

G. Outcomes

1. **Degenerative MR**
   a. Acute procedural success (defined as clip implantation with MR ≤2+) is estimated to be around 75% to 100%. Most of the North American experience comes from the EVEREST II trial, which was the first prospective, randomized controlled trial in which the MitraClip was compared with conventional surgery in 279 patients eligible for surgery (i.e., not at prohibitive risk). All patients had severe MR and most (73%) had DMR. The study showed that although the clip is safe, it is less effective at reducing MR than surgery. Rates of the primary composite end point (freedom from death, from surgery for MV dysfunction, and from grade 3+ or 4+ MR) were 55% in the percutaneous group and 73% in the surgery group at 1 year. Rates of death were similar in both groups at 1 year (~6%), but the rate and degree of MR, and the need for subsequent surgery for MV dysfunction, were higher in those who received the clip.
   b. At 4 years, mortality continued to remain similar between the two groups, but the surgical group tended to have a more durable result as evidenced by more patients in the clip group requiring MV surgery (24.8% vs. 5.5%). The majority of MV surgeries in the clip group occurred within the first year, and most underwent MV repair. Both groups experienced sustained improvements in left ventricular dimensions, NYHA functional class, and reductions in

hospitalizations for heart failure. Post hoc subgroup analyses at 12 months and 4 years suggested that there was no difference in the primary composite end point between the treatment groups among patients who were ≥70 years of age.

c. Lim and colleagues analyzed the group of patients with DMR and prohibitive surgical risk treated in EVEREST and its continued access registries. The 127 patients demonstrated a 30-day mortality of 6.3%, significantly lower than the 13.2% mortality predicted by the STS score. At 1 year, 85% of patients had maintained a reduction in MR of ≤2+, and mean LV volume was significantly reduced. Clinically, 87% of patients had NYHA I–II symptoms translating into a 73% reduction in hospitalizations for heart failure.

d. Although effective at reducing DMR, the MitraClip does not do so as effectively as traditional surgical MV repair techniques, which often include concomitant ring annuloplasty. Therefore, patients who present as reasonable candidates for open-heart surgery should be considered for the same. On the other hand, the safety and efficacy of the MitraClip as demonstrated by the totality of data validate it as a reasonable treatment option for patients considered at prohibitive risk for open heart surgery, and it is therefore approved by the US Food and Drug Administration for this application.

2. Functional MR

a. As with DMR, clip implantation in patients with FMR is safe. Limited evidence from a post hoc subgroup analysis of the EVEREST II trial suggests that efficacy at 1 and 4 years is similar between those who received the MitraClip versus surgery among patients with FMR.

b. More robust evidence comes from European real-world registries where the clip is most commonly implanted for high-surgical-risk patients with FMR. One-year results from the ACCESS-EU registry demonstrated that most patients who received the clip experienced an improvement in NYHA functional class (71.4% with class I or II symptoms), 6-minute walk, and Minnesota-Living-With-Heart-Failure score and sustained reduction in MR when compared with preimplant. This is rather impressive considering that 85% of patients had class III or IV symptoms preimplant. Mortality benefit could not be determined as this study was a prospective observational registry with no comparison group. The study also did not report changes in ventricular dimensions or other echocardiographic parameters.

c. As clinical experience with the MitraClip has increased, interventionalists have also developed a better understanding of patient selection for this treatment strategy. For instance, although EVEREST II enrolled a majority (73%) of patients with DMR, the high-risk cohort and continued access registries enrolled a majority (71%) of patients with FMR, demonstrating the understanding that this was the group of patients for whom percutaneous intervention may perform better than surgery. Similarly, 77% of patients in the above real-world ACCESS-EU registry had FMR. Results from the ongoing randomized COAPT and RESHAPE trials will hopefully provide the robust evidence needed to approve the use of the MitraClip system for patients with symptomatic FMR in the United States.

IV. OTHER PERCUTANEOUS DEVICES UNDER DEVELOPMENT

Several other percutaneous mitral repair devices are currently under development and based loosely on established surgical techniques. Most of these devices are aimed at the treatment of FMR and are in the preclinical, phase I, or phase II clinical trial stage; none are currently approved for use in the United States. The indirect annuloplasty devices (Carillon [Cardiac Dimensions, Inc., Kirkland, WA], MONARC [Edwards Lifesciences, Irvine, CA], and percutaneous transvenous mitral annuloplasty [PTMA] systems) utilize the anatomic proximity of the coronary sinus to the mitral annulus to favorably modify the annular geometry and bring the anterior and posterior leaflets closer together. The proximity of the coronary sinus to the annulus is variable, and so not all patients are candidates for this approach. In addition, the left circumflex coronary artery passes between the myocardium and coronary sinus in approximately half of patients, increasing the risk of coronary injury. Results thus far are exciting and promising. In the percutaneous direct annuloplasty approach (Mitralign [Boston, MA], Accucinch [Guided Delivery Systems, Inc., Santa Clara, CA], and Cardioband [Valtech, Or Yehuda, Israel] systems), a mitral annuloplasty device is delivered via the retrograde transventricular approach, and the annulus is then plicated using standard suture material or an anchor-based cable cinching system.

In the QuantumCor (Bothell, WA) system, subablative radiofrequency energy is applied in a controlled fashion to shrink the mitral annulus. Finally, cardiac chamber remodeling devices are designed to address the paravalvular geometry in functional and ischemic MR. Preliminary results are encouraging for both of these strategies, but efficacy has been suboptimal and device development has been slow.

V. TRANSCATHETER MITRAL VALVE REPLACEMENT

To date, there have been tens of thousands of successful percutaneous transcatheter aortic valve replacements (TAVRs) with outstanding outcomes. The technology has revolutionized the management of high-risk and inoperable patients with aortic stenosis and has begun to be available to patients with intermediate surgical risk with encouraging data. Thus, it is no surprise that this concept has been extended with great enthusiasm and excitement to patients with severe MV regurgitation and high surgical risk. Proof of concept has been demonstrated in patients with dysfunctional mitral bioprosthetic valves, and the SAPIEN XT (Edwards Lifesciences, Irvine, CA) TAVR prosthetic is currently approved in Europe for mitral valve-in-valve implantation.

In contrast to the relatively straightforward aortic valve, the native MV apparatus is extremely complex and thus represents a greater challenge to the development of percutaneous valve replacement technologies. Some specific challenges regarding transcatheter mitral valve replacement (TMVR) technology include valve location, an asymmetric D-shaped annulus without stable structure for valve anchoring, need for preservation of the subvalvular apparatus, high dislodgement forces due to dynamic changes in mitral annular geometry throughout the cardiac cycle, and the need for large delivery systems due to larger annular size compared with the aortic position. Nevertheless, at this time, nine TMVR systems are under development, with four having undergone first-in-human implants: Tendyne (Tendyne Holding Inc., Roseville, MN), Fortis (Edwards Lifesciences, Irvine, CA), CardiAQ (CardiAQ, Irvine, CA), and Tiara (Neovasc Inc, Richmond, BC). Of these, the Tendyne and Tiara systems are currently enrolling patients for early phase I feasibility clinical studies and are registered at www.clinicaltrials.gov (Fig. 11.4).

Our understanding of which subgroups of patients will benefit the most from TMVR is significantly limited at this stage, and all studies have been conducted on highly selected patients at prohibitive surgical risk. Acute results from first-in-human implants appear quite promising and have in general resulted in instantaneous complete or near-complete resolution of severe MR. Very short-term results from implantation of the self-expanding bioprosthetic Tiara valve (delivered transapically) in two patients were recently published. At 2 months post-TMVR, both patients had normal prosthetic valve function, no evidence of thrombus or paravalvular leak, and low transvalvular gradients. One of the patients died from cardiac failure despite normal MV function. The other experienced significant functional improvements.

Early results with the use of the Fortis valve were also reported in 2014. Five patients underwent transapical implantation on compassionate grounds and achieved good acute procedural success, and three patients survived beyond 30 days. One of the five patients experienced partial displacement of the valve into the left atrium with resultant MR, decompensated heart failure, and ultimately death. This was likely secondary to incomplete capture of the posterior MV leaflet during implant. Another died from progressive heart

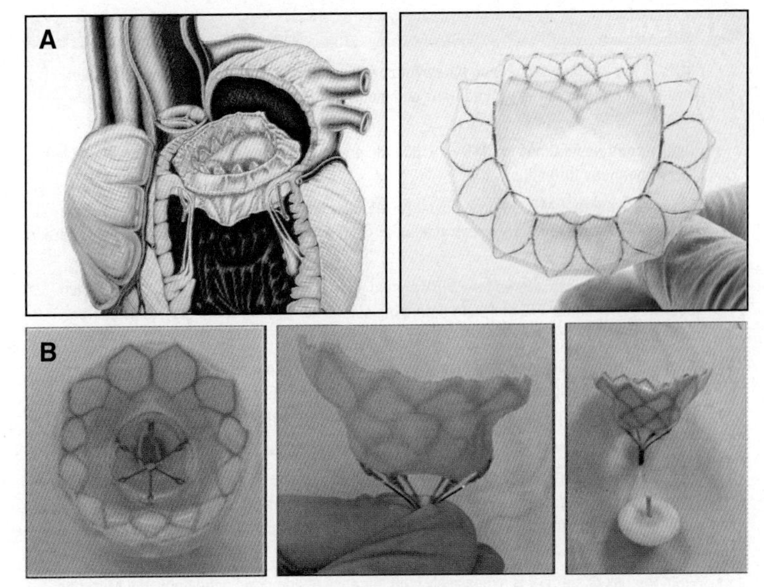

FIGURE 11.4 Prosthetic transcatheter mitral valves. A: Tiara valve. **B:** Tendyne valve. (Reproduced with permission from Neovasc Inc., Richmond, BC, Canada, and Tendyne Holding Inc., Roseville, MN.)

failure despite minimal postprocedural MR. A third died likely from infective endocarditis with possible valve thrombosis despite therapeutic international normalized ratio (INR) and negative blood cultures. Two patients continued to do well with improving symptoms at 30 days post-TMVR.

VI. FUTURE DIRECTIONS

Percutaneous TAVR has paved the way for TMVR, and the field of transcatheter valve therapy in general is growing at an exciting and rapid pace. Early results in the area of percutaneous transcatheter repair in patients at prohibitive surgical risk are promising, but the currently approved technology limits treatment to a very specific patient population with degenerative MR, leaving many patients with debilitating symptoms. The smaller US experience and the larger European experience with MitraClip therapy in patients with FMR is encouraging, and ongoing clinical trials in the United States will hopefully bring the clip treatment to this broader patient population.

Even so, the MV apparatus is the most complex of all the heart's valves, and not all patients with MR have the same anatomic and pathophysiologic basis of disease. As such, a "one-size-fits-all" approach is unlikely to provide durable long-term success and may leave many with residual MR and symptoms. Thus, it will be necessary to study what added benefit (if any) might be realized with the combination of multiple percutaneous techniques targeting the specific pathology in an individual patient (i.e., leaflet, annular, left ventricular geometry) so that we can truly tailor therapy. Ultimately, percutaneous repair and TMVR show great promise, and further refinement of current technologies and innovative new technologies are likely to add to the growing list of percutaneous interventions.

KEY PEARLS

- PMBV is the treatment of choice for symptomatic patients with severe MS and favorable valve characteristics. The procedure is commonly carried out in patients with rheumatic disease.
- Primary contraindications to PMBV include the presence of moderate-to-severe MR and left atrial appendage thrombus.
- There is no role for PMBV in cases of mitral stenosis without commissural fusion (e.g., congenital MS or MS secondary to mitral annular calcification) or in cases where the valves are not pliable.
- All patients being considered for PMBV should undergo anatomic assessment of the valve apparatus with either TTE or TEE to determine suitability. Various scoring systems can be used to predict successful PMBV.
- In patients with recurrence of clinically significant MS after prior commissurotomy, repeat PMBV may be considered if valve morphology is suitable, and success is predicted by the presence of sinus rhythm, minimal symptoms, and Wilkins score ≤8.
- Every effort must be made to understand the exact mechanism and etiology of mitral valve regurgitation. All patients should undergo TTE or TEE.
- Surgery remains the mainstay of therapy for severe symptomatic mitral regurgitation if surgical risk is acceptable. At this time, it is also more efficacious than the percutaneous approach.
- When the risk of surgery is excessively high because of comorbid conditions, the MitraClip device may be considered for patients with NYHA class III to IV symptoms with ≥3+ degenerative MR, favorable valve anatomy, and reasonable life expectancy.
- Our understanding of long-term outcomes with percutaneous mitral valve repair is still limited.
- Transcatheter mitral valve replacement technology is in rapid development, and phase I clinical trials are currently under way.

SUGGESTED READINGS

Bapat V, Buellesfeld L, Peterson MD, et al. Transcatheter mitral valve implantation (TMVI) using the Edwards Fortis device. *EuroIntervention.* 2014;10(suppl U):U120–U128.

Bouleti C, Iung B, Himbert D, et al. Long-term efficacy of percutaneous mitral commissurotomy for restenosis after previous mitral commissurotomy. *Heart.* 2013;99(18):1336–1341.

Bouleti C, Iung B, Himbert D, et al. Reinterventions after percutaneous mitral commissurotomy during long-term follow-up, up to 20 years: the role of repeat percutaneous mitral commissurotomy. *Eur Heart J.* 2013;34(25):1923–1930.

Cheung A, Webb J, Verheye S, et al. Short-term results of transapical transcatheter mitral valve implantation for mitral regurgitation. *J Am Coll Cardiol.* 2014;64(17):1814–1819.

De Backer O, Piazza N, Lutter G, et al. Percutaneous transcatheter mitral valve replacement: an overview of devices in preclinical and early clinical evaluation. *Circ Cardiovasc Interv.* 2014;7(3):400–409.

Feldman T, Foster E, Glower DD, et al. Percutaneous repair or surgery for mitral regurgitation. *N Engl J Med.* 2011;364(15):1395–1406.

Feldman T, Wasserman HS, Herrmann HC, et al. Percutaneous mitral valve repair using the edge-to-edge technique: six-month results of the EVEREST phase I clinical trial. *J Am Coll Cardiol.* 2005;46(11):2134–2140.

Glower DD, Kar S, Trento A, et al. Percutaneous mitral valve repair for mitral regurgitation in high-risk patients: results of the EVEREST II study. *J Am Coll Cardiol.* 2014;64(2):172–181.

Jang I, Block PC, Newell JB, et al. Percutaneous mitral balloon valvotomy for recurrent mitral stenosis after surgical commissurotomy. *Am J Cardiol.* 1995;75(8):601–605.

Krishnaswamy A, Kapadia SR. Percutaneous mitral valve repair. In: Topol EJ, Teirstein PS, eds. *Textbook of Interventional Cardiology.* 6th ed. Philadelphia, PA: Elsevier Saunders; 2012:635–646.

Maisano F, Franzen O, Baldus S, et al. Percutaneous mitral valve interventions in the real world: early and 1-year benefits from the ACCESS-EU, a prospective, multicenter, nonrandomized post-approval study of the MitraClip therapy in Europe. *J Am Coll Cardiol.* 2013;62:1050–1061.

Mauri L, Foster E, Glower DD, et al. 4-year results of a randomized controlled trial of percutaneous repair versus surgery for mitral regurgitation. *J Am Coll Cardiol.* 2013;62(4):317–328.

Munkholm-Larsen S, Wan B, Tian DH, et al. A systematic review on the safety and efficacy of percutaneous edge-to-edge mitral valve repair with the MitraClip system for high surgical risk candidates. *Heart.* 2014;100(6):473–478.

Nishimura RA, Otto CM, Bonow RO, et al. 2014 AHA/ACC guideline for the management of patients with valvular heart disease: executive summary: a report of the American College of Cardiology/American Heart Association Task Force on Practice Guidelines. *J Am Coll Cardiol.* 2014;63(22):2438–2488.

Palacios IF, Sanchez PL, Harrell LC, et al. Which patients benefit from percutaneous mitral balloon valvuloplasty? Prevalvuloplasty and postvalvuloplasty variables that predict long-term outcome. *Circulation.* 2002;105(12):1465.

Sutaria N, Northridge DB, Shaw TRD. Significance of commissural calcification on outcome of mitral balloon valvotomy. *Heart.* 2000;84:398–402.

Vahanian A, Alfieri O, Andreotti F, et al; The Joint Task Force on the Management of Valvular Heart Disease of the European Society of Cardiology (ESC) and the European Association for Cardio-Thoracic Surgery (EACTS). Guidelines on the management of valvular heart disease (version 2012). *Eur Heart J.* 2012;33:2451–2496.

Vahanian A, Himbert D, Brochet E, et al. Mitral valvuloplasty. In: Topol EJ, Teirstein PS, eds. *Textbook of Interventional Cardiology*. 6th ed. Philadelphia, PA: Elsevier Saunders; 2012:635–646.

Whitlow PL, Feldman T, Pedersen WR, et al. Acute and 12-month results with catheter-based mitral valve leaflet repair: the EVEREST II (Endovascular Valve Edge-to-Edge Repair) High Risk Study. *J Am Coll Cardiol.* 2012;59(2):130–139.

Wilkins GT, Weyman AE, Abascal VM, et al. Percutaneous balloon dilatation of the mitral valve: an analysis of echocardiographic variables related to outcome and the mechanism of dilatation. *Br Heart J.* 1988;60(4):299.

CHAPTER 12

Brandon M. Jones
Amar Krishnaswamy
E. Murat Tuzcu
Samir R. Kapadia

Transcatheter Aortic Valve Replacement

I. INTRODUCTION.

Calcific aortic stenosis (AS) is an increasingly common problem in developed countries, with an estimated prevalence of 2% to 4% among adults 65 years or older. Once symptoms develop, severe AS is associated with a median survival of approximately 2 years without intervention. Surgical aortic valve replacement (SAVR) has long been the standard of care for managing severe, symptomatic AS and can be done safely in the majority of patients. Historically, at least 30% of patients do not undergo SAVR owing to risk factors that are thought to put them at prohibitive surgical risk such as old age, prior cardiac surgeries, or other significant comorbidities. Unfortunately, the management of inoperable patients with medical therapy has done little to affect the natural history of the disease. Balloon aortic valvuloplasty (BAV) provides a short-term improvement in symptoms but a high rate of stenosis recurrence and no improvement in long-term survival without definitive valve replacement. In more recent years, transcatheter aortic valve replacement (TAVR) has provided a therapeutic option for many of these inoperable patients and is an alternative to SAVR in patients considered at moderate or high risk for complications with surgery.

II. INDICATIONS

A. TAVR is currently approved by the US Food and Drug Administration (FDA) and was granted the Conformité Européenne (CE) mark for high surgical risk and inoperable patients with severe AS deemed to be symptomatic from their valve disease with New York Heart Association (NYHA) functional class II or greater. For this indication, the US FDA has approved use of the balloon-expandable Edwards SAPIEN, SAPIEN-XT, and SAPIEN-3 (S3) valves (Edwards Life Sciences, Inc., Irvine, CA) and the self-expanding Medtronic CoreValve and CoreValve Evolut R (Medtronic, Inc., Minneapolis, MN). Patients considered at moderate risk for cardiac surgery have undergone TAVR with these valves as part of various clinical trials designed to test the safety and efficacy of this procedure among lower-risk groups. As a result of these trials, the S3 valve is approved for use in patients at intermediate surgical risk. The MCV is also approved for "valve-in-valve" TAVR for patients with severe bioprosthetic valve degeneration who are considered high risk or inoperable; the SAPIEN-XT is currently used for this application as part of a registry for inoperable patients. There are several additional devices that have obtained the CE mark of approval but are not currently FDA approved. These include the self-expandable Portico valve (St. Jude Medical, St. Paul, MN) and the uniquely designed Lotus Valve (Boston Scientific, Natick, MA) and Direct Flow Valve (Direct Flow Medical, Santa Rosa, CA), which is now discontinued and no longer available (Fig. 12.1).

B. The severity of calcific AS and appropriateness for intervention should be determined based on the recently published 2014 American Heart Association/American College of Cardiology Guidelines for the Management of Patients with Valvular Heart Disease. Surgical risk should be determined based on evaluation by a cardiac surgeon experienced in SAVR and should consider many factors including traditional tools such as the Society of Thoracic Surgeons predicted risk of mortality (STS-PROM) calculator or the European System for Cardiac Operative Risk Evaluation (Logistic EuroSCORE).

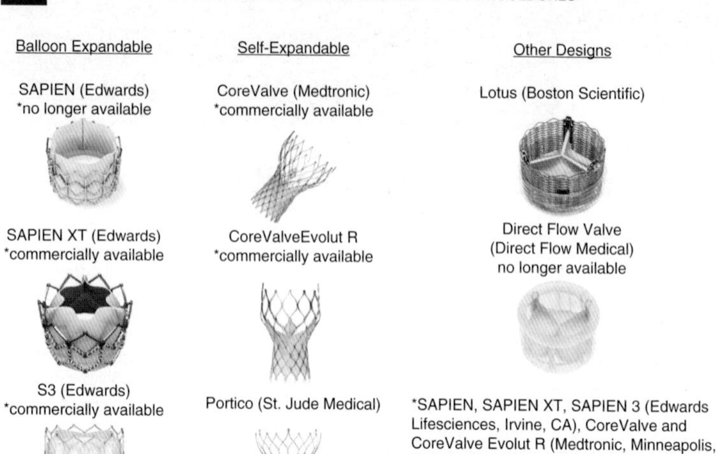

FIGURE 12.1 Commercially available and investigational transcatheter aortic valve replacement devices available in the United States.

Certain factors that are not included in the formal risk calculators but are known to increase the risk for surgical mortality and/or morbidity include cirrhosis, prior radiation to the chest, prior bypass graft anatomy with an unsafe proximity of grafts to the chest wall to accommodate redo sternotomy, significant frailty, or a porcelain aorta.

III. CONTRAINDICATIONS

A. TAVR is contraindicated in patients with a severely limited life expectancy owing to comorbid conditions, severe incapacitating dementia, or clear medical futility. The use of TAVR in patients with pure aortic regurgitation (AR) without stenosis is not currently approved although this indication is under study. Barriers to use in patients with isolated AR include the need to engineer devices that are designed to treat what is typically a dilated and noncalcified annulus. Noncalcified or minimally calcified valves may hold the device less securely and should be approached with caution. Some congenitally malformed valves are also not appropriate for TAVR.

B. TAVR is otherwise limited primarily by device availability and anatomic constraints. A very small or very large annulus may exceed the limits of the currently available devices. The most recently FDA-approved Edwards S3 devices are appropriate for annular sizes between 16 and 27 mm in diameter, and the CoreValve can be used for annular sizes between 18 and 30 mm according to manufacturer-published guidelines (Table 12.1).

C. The next anatomic limitation to TAVR relates to vascular access, and transfemoral (TF) TAVR may not be possible in some patients with small or severely calcified iliofemoral arteries. Generally, a minimal luminal diameter of 6 mm is required for most devices that utilize a #18 French sheath system, although the most recently approved Edwards S3 and Medtronic CoreValve Evolut R may be delivered through iliofemoral vessels as small as 5 mm in diameter depending on the degree of calcification present. Patients without a TF option can be considered for "alternative access," which most often includes transapical (TA) or transaortic (TAo) approaches (Fig. 12.2). Other device delivery options include the carotid artery, subclavian artery, axillary artery, or femoral vein with either a trans-septal or transcaval (inferior vena cava to abdominal aorta) approach.

TABLE 12.1 Commercially Available and Investigational TAVR Devices in the United States

Valve	Available Sizes (Diameter, mm)	Target Annulus Size (mm)	Sheath Size (Inner Diameter)	Minimum Femoral Artery Diameter (mm)[a]	FDA/CE Approval
		Commercially Available			
Edwards SAPIEN-XT	23	18–22	16 Fr	6.0	• CE mark
	26	21–25	18 Fr	6.5	• FDA approved
	29	24–27	20 Fr	7.0	
Edwards S3	20	16–19	14 Fr	5.5	• CE mark
	23	18–22	14 Fr	5.5	• FDA approved
	26	21–25	14 Fr	5.5	• PARTNER II trial (intermediate risk)
	29	24–28	16 Fr	6.0	
Medtronic CoreValve	23	18–20	18 Fr	6.0	• CE mark
	26	20–23	18 Fr	6.0	• FDA approved
	29	23–27	18 Fr	6.0	• SURTAVI trial (intermediate risk)
	31	26–29	18 Fr	6.0	
Medtronic Evolut R	23	18–20	14 Fr equivalent	5.0	• CE mark
	26	20–23		5.0	• FDA approved
	29	23–26		5.0	• Evolut R US clinical study ongoing
	34	26-30	16 Fr	5.5	
		Investigational Devices			
St. Jude Portico	23	19–21	18 Fr	6.0	• CE mark
	25	21–23	18 Fr	6.0	• US trials suspended
Boston Scientific Lotus	23	20–23	18 Fr	6.0	• CE mark
	25	23–25	18 Fr	6.0	• REPRISE III RCT vs. CoreValve (US)
	27	25–27	20 Fr	6.5	
Direct Flow Valve (DF Medical)	23	19–21	18 Fr	6.0	• CE mark
	25	21–24	18 Fr	6.0	• SALUS Trial (US)
	27	24–26	18 Fr	6.0	
	29	26–28	18 Fr	6.0	

[a]Based on manufacturer labeling where available. In practice, most valves that require a #18 French sheath can be placed through a minimal luminal diameter of 6 mm, and with the 14 French S3 sheath, as low as 5 mm, but individual practices may differ.

CE, Conformité Européenne; FDA, Food and Drug Administration; RCT, randomized controlled trial; TAVR, transcatheter aortic valve replacement. Adapted from Jones B, et al. How to choose the right TAVR for the right patient. *Nat Rev Cardiol*. In press.

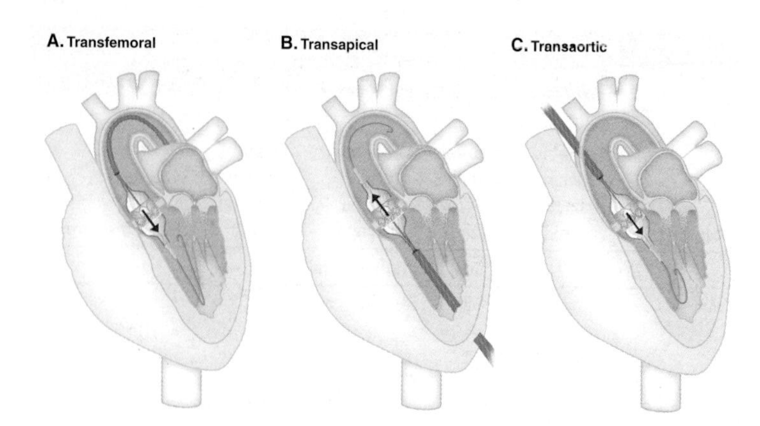

FIGURE 12.2 The most common vascular and surgical access options for transcatheter aortic valve replacement with the balloon-expandable S3 valve (Edwards Life Sciences) from the transfemoral approach **(A)**, transapical approach **(B)**, and transaortic approach **(C)**. Note that the valve must be loaded onto the balloon in the opposite orientation for the transapical approach.

IV. EVALUATION

A. Evaluating the patient for high-risk aortic valve replacement (AVR) is a complex and multidisciplinary process termed the "Heart Team" approach that involves collaboration between experts in interventional cardiology, cardiac surgery, cardiovascular imaging, radiology, anesthesiology, and nursing to collectively determine the most appropriate strategy for each individual patient. It is also important to take into account the goals, expectations, and preferences of the patient. When considering TAVR, the first step is to determine surgical risk, and patients who are at low risk for SAVR should be offered a traditional valve replacement, or can be considered for enrollment in a randomized controlled trial such as the PARTNER III low-risk trial, if appropriate. When surgical risk is thought to be elevated or even prohibitive, further evaluation for transcatheter options is warranted.

B. The overwhelmingly preferred strategy for TAVR is via the TF approach, so the first step is to determine annular size and vascular access options. In patients with normal renal function, both factors can be quickly determined by a contrast-enhanced computed tomography (CT) scan. The CT of the chest should be gated (timed to the ECG so as to capture each image during the same portion of each cardiac cycle) to limit motion artifact and obtain the most accurate annular measurement. The annulus is frequently an elliptical structure, so it is important to determine size based on a three-dimensional imaging analysis that will take this asymmetry into account. Estimates of annular size based on two-dimensional echocardiography may underestimate the true annular size and lead to undersizing of the valve, a risk factor for paravalvular AR. The CT scan can then be continued through the abdomen and upper thigh to evaluate the iliofemoral system. When determining the appropriateness for TF-TAVR, it is important to consider not only the minimal luminal diameter but also the presence and extent of calcification and the tortuosity of the vessels.

C. When the patient's renal function is not appropriate for a contrast-enhanced CT scan, alternative strategies for determining annular size include cardiac magnetic resonance imaging (MRI) and three-dimensional transesophageal echocardiography (TEE). In such cases, iliofemoral anatomy can be assessed by noncontrast CT scan. If further anatomic detail is required, CT of the iliofemoral system may be performed after positioning a pigtail catheter in the distal aorta under fluoroscopy and then transporting the patient to the CT scanner for a direct, arterial contrast-injected CT scan using 10 to 15 mL of dye. Consideration may also be given to intravascular ultrasound evaluation of the pelvic vessels, though operators should be aware of the concern for a nonperpendicular image of the vessel and inaccurate sizing as a result.

D. In patients requiring alternative access, TA-TAVR is performed by puncturing the left ventricle (LV) apex through a small left anterior thoracotomy and crossing the aortic valve (AV) in an antegrade fashion. This technique has been limited to the balloon-expandable (SAPIEN) valves, which can be loaded onto the delivery device to accommodate either antegrade or retrograde implantation (Fig. 12.2). The unsheathing mechanism of the CoreValve, however, does not allow for the TA approach. TAo-TAVR is commonly performed via a partial sternotomy, although some operators prefer a right thoracotomy or manubriotomy. The delivery sheath is placed directly in the ascending aorta, followed by a traditional retrograde crossing of the AV, which can be performed with either balloon-expandable or self-expandable valves. Although both TA and TAo-TAVR require a more extensive surgical approach as compared to the TF approach, they do not require full sternotomy or cardiopulmonary bypass. In our experience, the TAo approach is less desirable in patients with a history of prior open heart surgery in whom mediastinal scarring can complicate the path to reexposing the ascending aorta. Thus, we prefer TA access for patients with prior coronary artery bypass grafting or valve surgery. The TAo approach is preferred, however, for most patients without prior surgery who do not have appropriate femoral access.

E. Alternative vascular access approaches have been extensively studied in hopes of finding safe and feasible options for TAVR in patients who lack appropriate TF access and who are not appropriate for TA or TAo-TAVR. Although these strategies are mostly limited to small series and case reports, operators have successfully completed TAVR from the carotid, subclavian, and axillary artery, as well as the femoral vein. Initial reports suggest that these approaches are both safe and feasible in selected patients. There are two possible approaches for completing TAVR from the femoral vein. The first involves passage of the catheter across the inter atrial septum, across the mitral valve, into the LV, and across the AV in an antegrade fashion. The second involves trans caval passage of the catheter from the inferior vena cava to the descending abdominal aorta, then over the aortic arch, and across the AV in a typical retrograde fashion. In transcaval cases, the arterio venous communication that is formed in the intra-abdominal retroperitoneal space is typically corrected with a closure device at the conclusion of the case.

F. In addition to determining access route, TAVR evaluation requires careful examination and management of other comorbid conditions, both cardiac and noncardiac. Patients with senile, calcific AS have a high incidence of atherosclerosis, and it is important to complete a left heart catheterization to evaluate for coronary artery disease. Pre-TAVR SYNTAX score (or residual SYNTAX score in patients who have undergone revascularization) has been shown to be a risk factor for cardiovascular mortality after TAVR in one prospective registry. Nevertheless, there are no randomized trials guiding the decision for revascularization. Although the initial trials of TAVR required full revascularization, in current clinical practice, usually only patients with a large area of ischemia, typical angina symptoms, or high-grade stenosis in an "important" anatomic location are likely to undergo percutaneous coronary intervention (PCI) prior to TAVR. Anecdotally, conservative medical management of certain asymptomatic but angiographically severe lesions has not compromised the success of TAVR in selected patients at our institution.

G. Carotid artery disease is also important to consider prior to TAVR. Patients with symptomatic, high-grade lesions should likely undergo carotid endarterectomy or stenting prior to TAVR. Intermediate and asymptomatic lesions do not necessitate prophylactic intervention, but special consideration should be given to unprotected carotid artery stenosis (significant stenosis with complete occlusion of the contralateral internal carotid artery), or patients who may be at an especially high risk for prolonged hypotension during TAVR.

H. Conduction system disease must be considered as well, especially as it pertains to device selection. One drawback of the self-expandable valves has been a significantly higher incidence of heart block requiring permanent pacemaker (PPM) implantation as compared to the balloon-expandable valves (~28% vs. 6%, respectively) and may be a deciding factor in valve selection in certain patients. As with SAVR, the left bundle of His is especially vulnerable to disruption after TAVR, so patients with preexisting right bundle branch block (RBBB) or bifascicular block are at especially high risk for post-TAVR complete heart block. If PPM implantation is required, placement of a biventricular pacemaker may be considered in patients with a reduced ejection fraction.

I. Finally, in some patients, despite optimization of volume and respiratory status, it can be difficult to determine if a patient's dyspnea is due primarily to valve disease or to other comorbid conditions such as chronic obstructive pulmonary disease. In such patients, BAV can be a helpful tool in making this distinction. BAV has been shown to reduce AV gradients and improve symptoms in patients with severe AS but has also been associated with a high incidence of stenosis recurrence at 6 months and no survival benefit. Thus, patients whose symptoms improve significantly in the weeks and months after BAV are presumably more likely to derive a symptom benefit from TAVR, whereas patients who show no improvement in symptoms after BAV may be limited by other factors such as their pulmonary disease.

V. TECHNIQUE/EQUIPMENT

A. The heart-team approach that is critical to the preprocedural evaluation remains paramount during the procedure itself, and performing TAVR requires the ongoing collaboration of interventional cardiologist, cardiac surgeons, imaging specialists, anesthesiologists, nurses, and operating room personnel. At our institution, TAVR is performed in a "hybrid" suite, which has the ability to function as both an operating room and a catheterization laboratory, with the participation of both cardiac surgeons and interventional cardiologists in all procedures. As TF-TAVR can be performed entirely from the groin, some institutions have alternatively elected to perform TF-TAVR in a dedicated catheterization suite. Although this approach has been shown to be safe, it is important to be prepared for any potential complications that might require emergency cardiopulmonary bypass or surgical access to the chest, and for this reason we complete a full surgical scrub for all patients. Although the incidence of conversion to an open surgical procedure during TAVR is very low, it can be life-saving when needed, and it is important to be adequately prepared.

B. Although TA- and TAo-TAVR require general anesthesia, a growing number of TF-TAVR cases are being done under conscious sedation with local anesthesia. This can be of particular benefit in patients with complex lung disease for whom weaning from the ventilator may be difficult. General anesthesia may more easily facilitate TEE, though with the significant reductions in paravalvular leak (PVL) that have been demonstrated by the newest-generation TAVR devices, the need for intraprocedural TEE has decreased. Nevertheless, it is important to always have rapid access to both anesthesiologists and TEE if they become necessary during the procedure.

C. For TF-TAVR, the first step is to obtain vascular access. It is very important to access the common femoral artery at the appropriate location, below the inferior epigastric artery but above the bifurcation. This area is typically located at the midfemoral head but can be confirmed by review of the preprocedural contrast CT scan. One strategy is to obtain access with a #4 French micropuncture needle under fluoroscopic guidance and confirm the location with a small contrast injection. Alternatively, ultrasound can be utilized to ensure the correct placement of the sheath. Prior to insertion of the large TAVR sheath, the next step is preclosure of the arteriotomy site. This entails the stepwise placement of two Perclose ProGlide (Abbott Vascular, Minneapolis, MN) suture-mediated closure systems, which are deployed in a 10 o'clock and 2 o'clock position. The suture ends are placed carefully to the side of the drape and will be used to achieve hemostasis of the large arterial sheath site at the conclusion of the case. Less commonly, the ProStar XL preclosure system (Abbott Vascular) is used. Finally, in cases with extreme calcification of the artery or when an aortofemoral graft is accessed, direct surgical exposure and closure may be required. An additional #5 French arterial sheath is usually placed in the contralateral femoral artery, which is used for placement of a pigtail catheter in the noncoronary sinus to provide aortic root angiography for valve positioning. The radial artery can be utilized for this purpose, but we prefer using the contralateral femoral artery when possible to allow immediate endovascular access in the case of iliofemoral vascular complications.

D. The next step for TF-TAVR is placement of the temporary venous pacemaker. Given the high incidence of PPM requirement after self-expandable valve placement, we prefer to place an active fixation lead from the internal jugular vein in patients who receive a self-expanding valve. A similar strategy is used in patients who are at high risk for postprocedural conduction problems regardless of the type of valve that is placed. Otherwise, for the balloon-expandable TAVR, we place a passive fixation lead from the femoral vein, which will be used for rapid right ventricular (RV) pacing during balloon inflation. If desired, a second venous sheath can be placed to facilitate placement of a Swan–Ganz (pulmonary artery) catheter.

E. Once access is obtained and the pacemaker wire is placed, intravenous heparin is administered to achieve a therapeutic activated clotting time (ACT) > 300 seconds. The TAVR sheath should be upsized over a stiff wire; we prefer the Lunderquist (Cook Medical, Bloomington, IN). The AV is then crossed; in our practice, this is most often performed using an Amplatz Left 1 (AL 1) catheter and a 0.035" straight-tip guidewire. Once the valve is crossed, the guidewire of choice for TAVR device delivery is positioned in the LV with the belly of the wire in the LV apex. For wires without a preformed LV loop, care should be taken to create a gentle curve that can be placed in the LV apex. For balloon-expandable devices, we prefer the Amplatz Extra Stiff 0.035" guidewire (Cook Medical, Bloomington, IN), and for self-expandable devices that require slightly more support we use the Amplatz Super Stiff guidewire (Boston Scientific, Natik, MA).

F. The next step prior to placing the new valve is often BAV. This was once thought to be an essential component of all procedures but is now being performed with decreasing frequency prior to balloon-expandable valve implantation and is rarely required for self-expandable valves. In some valves that are very severely calcified, however, it may be difficult to pass the TAVR device without predilation. Furthermore, predilation may assist with the ultimate expansion of the prosthesis and reduce the incidence of PVL. Drawbacks, however, include the added opportunity for liberation of embolic particles that could lead to neurologic events, and the potential for inducing acute severe AR, which may be poorly tolerated during the time interval required to subsequently implant the valve.

G. When ready, the valve is loaded onto the delivery device and advanced into position in the aortic annulus. The correct position can be confirmed by contrast injection through the pigtail catheter in the noncoronary cusp, usually using a right anterior oblique caudal or left anterior oblique cranial projection. The balloon-expandable valves are typically positioned with the lower 20% of the device in the aortic annulus and the remainder of the scaffolding above the valve level (Fig. 12.3). For the self-expandable valves, the distal portion of the device can be partially unsheathed in the LV outflow tract (LVOT) and withdrawn if needed to the appropriate height (Fig. 12.4). When fully expanded, the CoreValve will be anchored in the proximal aorta above the sinus of Valsalva, so the scaffolding will extend beyond the coronary ostia by design, but this does not impede coronary blood flow or prevent subsequent angiography. Rapid pacing at a heart rate of 180 to 220 bpm is initiated prior to inflation of the balloon-expandable valve in order to temporarily reduce cardiac output. Pacing should not be suspended until the balloon is deflated to prevent the balloon from being ejected and

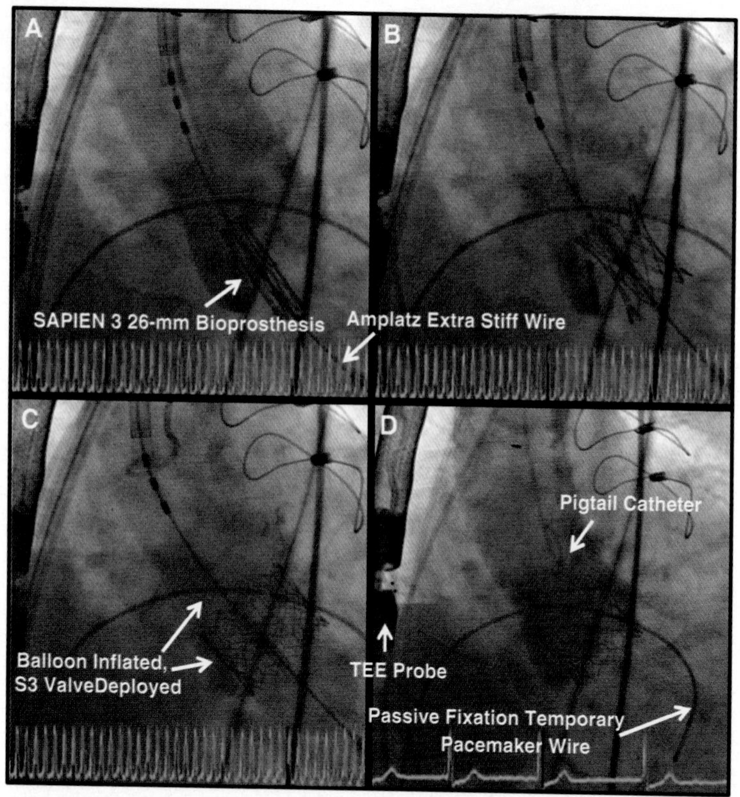

FIGURE 12.3 Deployment of the Edwards SAPIEN 3 valve under rapid pacing **(A, B, C)** and confirmation of appropriate placement and lack of significant aortic regurgitation **(D)**. Images taken at RAO 34 CAUD 31. TEE, transesophageal echocardiography.

dislodging the valve. When placing a self-expanding valve, RV pacing is not required, but sometimes a more modest rate of 100 to 110 bpm is used to reduce cardiac output slightly while the valve is unsheathed.

H. Once the valve is implanted, it should be investigated for appropriate position and function using angiography, hemodynamic measurements, and echocardiography when available. When TEE is not utilized, aortic root angiography or transthoracic echocardiography should be done to exclude AR (Figs. 12.3 and 12.4). A wide pulse pressure and low aortic diastolic pressure can also be clues to significant AR. It is very important to identify AR owing to its association with poor outcomes, and attempts should be made to reduce moderate or severe AR when possible. When regurgitation is paravalvular, subsequent balloon postdilation or placement of a second valve can sometimes reduce the degree of regurgitation, but overexpansion of the scaffolding can at times lead to central regurgitation, which can only be addressed by placement of a second valve. In certain situations, percutaneous PVL closure may be necessary to adequately address the AR.

I. The final step in TF-TAVR is removal of the access sheaths and securing of the preclosure sutures. In the absence of contraindications, protamine can be safely given in

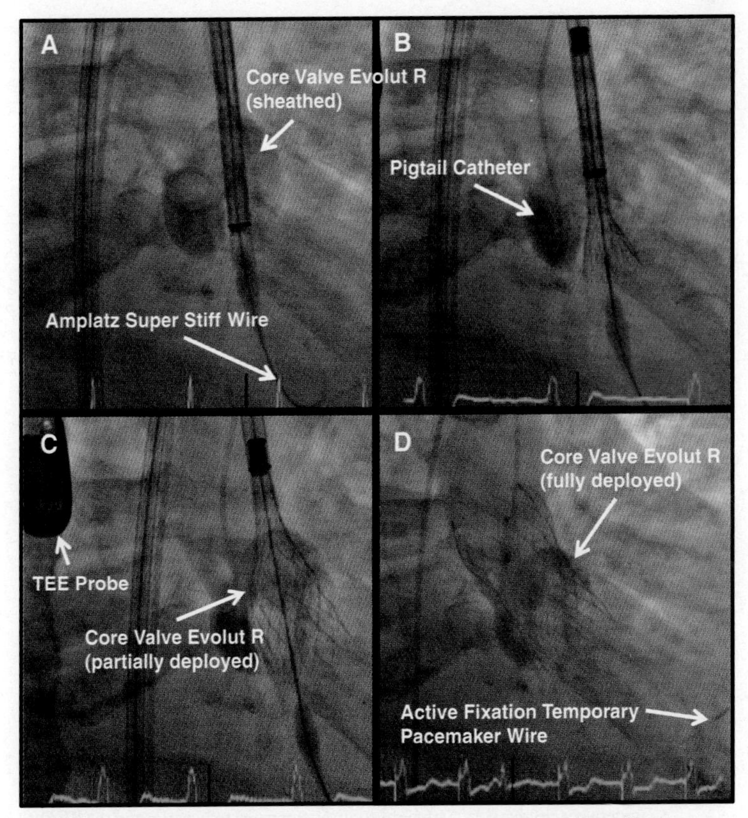

FIGURE 12.4 Deployment of the self-expanding Medtronic CoreValve Evolut R **(A, B, C)** and confirmation of appropriate placement and lack of significant aortic regurgitation **(D)**. Images taken at RAO 28 CAUD 36. TEE, transesophageal echocardiography.

most cases to reverse the effects of heparin prior to sheath removal. It is important to maintain wire access to the femoral artery during this process in the event of a failed suture or a need to reestablish access to manage vascular complications. A final iliac angiogram taken through the contralateral femoral arterial sheath can be helpful to exclude occult hemorrhage or other vessel dissection and, when needed, proximal balloon occlusion/dilation or placement of a stent can be performed from this contralateral access.

VI. ALTERNATIVE ACCESS

When femoral arterial access is not possible, alternative access approaches must be used. TA access can be obtained through a small left anterior intercostal thoracotomy. Pledgeted sutures are secured to a nonfatty portion of the left ventricular apex and needle access, and sheath placement proceeds through the presutured myocardium. We prefer crossing the valve using a balloon-tipped Arrow-Berman catheter (Teleflex, Morrisville, NC) with a 0.035" wire lumen to minimize the risk of passage through the mitral valve chords, and ultimately a stiff wire is advanced to the descending aorta. The valve is then crimped onto the delivery balloon in the opposite orientation, and is advanced through the LV apex to the LVOT. Valve placement proceeds with similar steps including rapid RV pacing, and ultimately the apex and thoracotomy are surgically closed. TAo-TAVR involves a partial sternotomy, right thoracotomy, or manubriotomy to obtain direct visualization of the ascending aorta. This facilitates the placement of the delivery sheath directly into the aorta. The steps for TAVR then follow just as they would for TF-TAVR with retrograde crossing of the AV and delivery of the prosthesis under rapid pacing. TAo-TAVR differs importantly from a mini-AVR in that although the surgical access is similar, it does not require cardiopulmonary bypass and is completed without arresting the heart.

VII. PERIPROCEDURAL/PERIOPERATIVE MANAGEMENT

A. It is important to optimize renal function, respiratory status, and hemodynamic status prior to TAVR. In some patients who are especially tenuous, hospitalization prior to TAVR to ensure optimal volume status can be helpful. Just as with any surgical valve replacement, patients should be free of infection prior to valve implantation, and any active bleeding should be investigated, despite the fact that TAVR does not require the very high levels of heparinization that are typical for surgical procedures that involve cardiopulmonary bypass.

B. After the procedure, it is important to remain vigilant in monitoring for potential complications that may require timely intervention. Special attention should be focused on assessing for bleeding complications, hemodynamic instability, and conduction abnormalities. Although initially all patients at our institution were managed in the cardiovascular intensive care unit for the first evening after TAVR, as the incidence of procedural complications and overall experience with the procedure have improved, we now manage most patients in a postanesthesia care unit prior to transfer to the regular nursing floor.

C. Adjunct therapy

1. Pharmacologic management of patients during TAVR has been largely extrapolated based on the surgical and PCI literature. There are unfortunately no large studies comparing different antiplatelet or anticoagulant strategies for use during TAVR. Generally speaking, intraprocedural anticoagulation is initiated after obtaining arterial access and safely positioning the temporary pacing wire, with a goal of achieving an ACT > 300 seconds. The BRAVO 1 trial showed lower rates of in-hospital major bleeding and similar rates of ischemic stroke in patients who underwent elective BAV with bivalirudin as compared to heparin, and the BRAVO 2/3 trial is a similar trial that is under way for patients undergoing TAVR. However, because of the risk of major bleeding complications during the procedure, we prefer to use heparin as a reversible agent during TAVR.
2. Postprocedurally, there is similarly a lack of evidence to support any specific pharmacologic strategy. Even the surgical literature is controversial regarding the use of warfarin after SAVR with a bioprosthetic valve, and although some surgeons advocate for 3 months of oral vitamin K antagonist therapy, the 2012 American College of Clinical Pharmacology guidelines recommend aspirin alone. The 2012 American College of Cardiology Foundation/American Association for Thoracic Surgery/Society for Cardiovascular Angiography and Interventions/Society of Thoracic Surgeons (ACCF/AATS/SCAI/STS) guidelines for TAVR recommend aspirin (50 to 100 mg daily) plus clopidogrel (75 mg daily) for 3 months after TAVR followed by aspirin alone (grade 2C). The ARTE trial is ongoing and aims to study aspirin alone vs. aspirin plus clopidogrel after TAVR, and the AUREA trial is comparing dual antiplatelet therapy to the oral vitamin K antagonist acenocoumarol. Importantly, post-TAVR atrial fibrillation is associated with higher risk of late neurologic events, and appropriate anticoagulation is necessary in that setting. For those patients, use of therapeutic anticoagulation with a single antiplatelet agent may be reasonable. For patients unable to tolerate anticoagulation, consideration may be given to percutaneous left atrial appendage occlusion.

VIII. COMPLICATIONS

As valve design and delivery sheath technology have advanced, the overall incidence of TAVR-related complications has consistently decreased. Nevertheless, there are several important procedural complications that must be considered in patients undergoing TAVR that can lead to significant morbidity, mortality, and added hospital costs (Table 12.2). Although the early TAVR literature was somewhat inconsistent in the definitions of complications, the Valve Academic Research Consortium (VARC-2) has since outlined standardized criteria that are used in both clinical practice and clinical trials.

A. PVL has been significantly more common in patients who undergo TAVR compared with SAVR. This is not surprising considering that the valve must be expanded inside of a native annulus that is often heavily calcified and asymmetric. What has been surprising though is the strong association between modest degrees of AR and significantly worse outcomes in major clinical trials involving early-generation devices. Even mild PVL has been shown to be a risk factor for mortality after TAVR in some studies. For this reason, many of the technologic advances in newer-generation TAVR

TABLE 12.2 Potential Complications Associated with Transcatheter Aortic Valve Replacement (TAVR)

Complication	Risk Factors	Ways to Mitigate or Manage the Complication
Aortic regurgitation	• Asymmetric or severely calcified annulus. • Device undersizing. • Device malpositioning (too high or too low in the left ventricular outflow tract).	• Annular sizing and valve measurement by computed tomography, cardiac magnetic resonance imaging, or 3D transesophageal echocardiogram rather than single-dimension sizing by 2D transthoracic echocardiogram. • Postdilation or placement of a second valve (must be weighed against risk of stroke or annular rupture). • Central regurgitation usually requires placement of a second valve.
Stroke	• Older age, female, prior cerebrovascular or peripheral vascular disease, diabetes, hypertension, prior cardiac surgery. • Need for balloon postdilation. • No clear differences in TAVR route or device design. • Post-TAVR atrial fibrillation.	• Appropriate heparinization during procedure. • Appropriate pharmacologic treatment postprocedure. • Anticoagulation when needed for atrial fibrillation. • Minimize unnecessary manipulations of the device in the aortic root. • Cerebral embolic protection devices (under investigation). • Alternative antiplatelet and anticoagulant regimens (under investigation).

(continued)

TABLE 12.2 Potential Complications Associated with Transcatheter Aortic Valve Replacement (TAVR) *(continued)*

Complication	Risk Factors	Ways to Mitigate or Manage the Complication
Vascular complications	• Small femoral artery luminal diameter. • Calcified arteries, especially circumferential.	• Careful preprocedural planning and evaluation of arterial access. • Confirm correct femoral artery placement (above bifurcation, below inferior epigastric) prior to large sheath dilation. • Preclosure of the arteriotomy site. • Iliac angiography at conclusion of the case. • Prompt endovascular or surgical repair of vascular injuries.
Conduction system disease	• Preexisting conduction system disease. • Preexisting right bundle branch block. • Valve oversizing. • Low valve implantation. • Self-expandable devices. • Calcified annulus.	• Consider active fixation, temporary pacemaker for high-risk cases and for self-expandable devices. • Carefully monitor patients postprocedure for conduction system disease. • Permanent pacemaker implantation when indicated. • Limit device oversizing (must be weighed against risk of paravalvular regurgitation).
Cardiac tamponade	• Temporary pacemaker perforation. • Guidewire perforation. • Annular rupture during balloon aortic valvuloplasty or valve deployment (more common in oversized valves, calcified annulus, with postdilation, and with balloon-expandable valves).	• Careful wire management. • Limit device oversizing (must be weighed against risk of paravalvular regurgitation). • Prompt diagnosis and management in the setting of hemodynamic instability. • Consider self-expanding device (less risk of annular rupture) for severely calcified annulus.

devices have been focused on reducing PVL. One example is the Direct Flow valve, which is built with two inflatable cuffs on the superior and inferior valve apparatus, designed to create a tight seal between the cylindrical valve and the asymmetric annulus. Another example is the Edwards S3 valve, which is constructed with a skirt on the external portion of the lower portion of the valve stent and is designed to create a seal between the stent and the annulus. With these innovations, more contemporary trials have shown significant reductions in PVL.

B. Given the strong associations between AR and outcomes after TAVR, it is important to evaluate for significant regurgitation at the time of valve placement. This is most commonly done with hemodynamics, TTE, TEE, and/or aortic root angiography. Usually, multiple points of data are taken together to provide a thorough understanding. When significant PVL is identified, valve postdilation can sometimes create a tighter seal and reduce the severity of AR. Another strategy that has been used is to place a second percutaneous valve within the first valve, which is particularly useful if the regurgitation is due to leaflet malfunction or to malpositioning of the initial valve. A valve that is placed too high in the annulus can sometimes leak around the inferior border, and this usually requires a second valve to be placed just inferior to the first. The drawback to postdilation or placement of an additional valve is that it places the patient at slightly higher risk for other complications including embolic stroke, annular rupture, and conduction abnormalities. Finally, in select cases, if AR cannot be reduced by traditional means, percutaneous PVL closure should be performed.

C. Stroke is a dreaded complication of any cardiovascular procedure. Most strokes associated with TAVR are thought to be embolic in nature but may also rarely be related to global hypoperfusion or hemorrhagic complications. The results of the first randomized controlled trial of the Edwards SAPIEN valve (PARTNER IA and IB) raised initial concerns for an increased risk of stroke with TAVR as compared to medical management or SAVR, with rates at 30 days as high as 6.7% in patients at extreme surgical risk. However, recent analyses of this patient group have shown that the rate of stroke with TAVR is significantly lower than initially thought, and that there is no increased risk as compared to surgery over the long term. One large meta-analysis of 10,037 patients undergoing TAVR documented the rate of stroke at 30 days to be 3.3 ± 1.8%. The recently presented results from the PARTNER II trial of the SAPIEN 3 valve showed a 1.5% rate of stroke in the high-risk cohort and 2.6% in the intermediate cohort at 30 days.

1. Despite the declining rates of clinical stroke associated with TAVR, studies utilizing diffusion-weighted MRI have shown a high incidence of subclinical findings in both surgical and transcatheter patients, so there remains an intense focus on reducing the incidence of embolic events during TAVR. There are a number of embolic protection devices that have been studied for use during TF-TAVR, and one filter device that has been used in transaortic TAVR. Thus far, early studies of these devices have shown a reduction in the overall volume of new lesions detected by MRI, but no reduction in clinically apparent events. Several larger trials are ongoing. Finally, several investigations are ongoing to study the optimal anticoagulation and antiplatelet regimen to reduce thromboembolic events during TAVR.

D. Vascular complications are among the most common procedure-related complications during TAVR owing to the relatively large sheaths that are required. Fortunately, as device technology has progressed, the size of the sheaths that are required has improved dramatically from #22 French to #24 French for the first-generation SAPIEN valve, to #16 French to #18 French for the SAPIEN-XT and CoreValve, to #14 French for the SAPIEN3 and Evolut R systems. Thus, although the rate of major vascular complications has been reported to be as high as 16% in some early trials, the incidence was lower than 6% among patients in the PARTNER II trial using the S3 valve.

1. Vascular complications can be as modest as VARC-2 minor bleeding, or as serious as rupture, dissection, or occlusion. Minor bleeding can usually be resolved with simple external pressure, but more serious complications may require urgent endovascular repair. For this reason, it is helpful to maintain contralateral femoral arterial access until hemostasis is achieved and the preclosure sutures have been successfully secured after valve delivery-sheath removal. This facilitates the rapid utilization of endovascular ballooning or even covered stent placement when necessary. Operators should be proficient in peripheral vascular intervention (or have ready access to peripheral vascular specialists) in order to maintain the safety of TAVR procedures.

E. Late bleeding complications are more commonly a result of gastrointestinal complications, neurologic complications, or traumatic falls and are more common in patients with atrial fibrillation requiring systemic anticoagulation. In the PARTNER cohort/registries, late bleeding complications occurred with an incidence of 5.9% at a median of 132 days after TAVR.

F. Conduction system disturbances are another potential complication after TAVR, likely due to mechanical compression of the His bundle fibers as they pass near the septal wall of the LVOT. Patients with a preexisting RBBB are at especially high risk for developing complete heart block after TAVR, as the left-sided fibers are most vulnerable to compression during the procedure. Other risk factors for developing heart block include lower implantation of the prosthesis, a calcified annulus, or a significantly oversized valve. Also, there appears to be a significantly higher risk of requiring a pacemaker after TAVR in patients who receive a self-expanding valve as compared to the balloon-expandable valves. In the GARY registry, the rate of permanent pacemaker implantation after TAVR was 25.2% with the Medtronic CoreValve and 5.0% with the Edwards SAPIEN device. Thus, it is reasonable to maintain an active fixation temporary pacemaker device for 72 hours after placement of the CoreValve to ensure adequate native conduction.

G. Annular rupture and cardiac tamponade are very rare but serious complications associated with TAVR. Annular rupture has been reported in up to 1% of procedures and may occur at any level of the annulus and aortic root. Annular rupture seems to be most closely associated with balloon inflation, so is exceedingly rare with self-expanding devices unless postdilation is needed. Factors that seem to be associated with annular rupture include oversizing of the valve prosthesis by more than 20% and severe LVOT calcification. Annular rupture may range in clinical presentation from asymptomatic and contained to the rapid development of hemopericardium and cardiovascular collapse. The presence of hemopericardium and tamponade should always raise suspicion for annular rupture but can also be a result of trauma from either the temporary pacemaker wire in the right ventricle or the curved support wires in the left ventricular apex. The key to management of cardiac tamponade is rapid identification and treatment. Less severe situations can often be managed conservatively with reversal of procedural anticoagulation or with pericardial drainage alone, though some cases will require emergent cardiopulmonary bypass and surgical correction.

H. Coronary artery obstruction is a rare but potentially avoidable complication of TAVR. In the published literature, it occurs in 0.4% to 1.3% of procedures and should be suspected in the following situations: when the coronary ostia have a low height from the aortic annulus; when there is significant sinotubular effacement; when there is a large septal bulge, which can lead to valve orientation tilted toward the left main ostium; or with a heavily calcified native valve leaflet tip. Of all these factors, the most important may be to understand the relationship between coronary ostium height, coronary sinus depth, and corresponding leaflet length. Patients with a low coronary ostium in the presence of a relatively long leaflet and shallow cusp with sinotubular effacement are at especially high risk for occlusion after valve implantation. The best way to evaluate for this potential complication is by gated cardiac computed tomography angiography (CTA) with contrast. Rarely, this may lead to a decision to avoid TAVR in favor of a surgical valve replacement. There are ways to mitigate the risk of coronary artery obstruction in carefully selected difficult cases. The primary strategy is to protect the coronary ostium by placing a wire, a balloon, or even an undeployed stent into the coronary artery prior to valve implantation. For this reason, we favor a balloon-expandable valve, which allows the operator to maintain access to the coronary artery above the frame of the valve stent. Self-expanding valves by design rest on the proximal ascending aorta covering the sinus, complicating subsequent coronary interventions, which must be completed through the side struts of the valve frame.

IX. OUTCOMES (SHORT TERM, LONG TERM)

There are several pivotal, randomized trials of TAVR that have formed the basis for approval of the technology by the US FDA and serve as the best representation of short- and long-term outcomes after TAVR. The PARTNER trial randomized 699 patients with severe AS who were considered at high surgical risk (cohort A) to TAVR vs. SAVR, and 358 patients with severe AS who were not candidates for surgical AVR (cohort B) to TAVR vs. medical therapy including BAV. Among the inoperable patients, at 1 year, there was 30.7% overall mortality in the TAVR arm as compared to 50.7% mortality in the patients randomized to usual care. In cohort A, there was similar mortality at 1 year with TAVR (24.3%) as compared to SAVR (26.8%), a finding that has now been consistent up to 5 years of follow-up. In this study, which involved the first-generation SAPIEN valve, there was less major bleeding with TAVR but more vascular complications and a higher incidence of paravalvular AR. The initial 1-year outcomes demonstrated a higher risk of the composite of all neurologic events compared to surgical AVR, though subsequent analyses have demonstrated equivalence in the two groups.

Subsequently, the Medtronic CoreValve was studied in the US CoreValve Pivotal trial among 489 patients with severe AS who were deemed to be at extreme surgical risk and demonstrated 24.3% all-cause mortality at 1 year. Among 647 patients at high surgical risk who were randomized to TAVR vs. SAVR, there was 14.2% mortality at 1 year with TAVR vs. 19.1% with SAVR ($p = 0.04$ for superiority of TAVR), and no increased risk of stroke with TAVR. It should be cautioned that because of significant differences in patient characteristics, comparisons cannot be made between the safety and efficacy of the balloon-expandable SAPIEN valves and the self-expanding CoreValve on the basis of these trials.

Most recently presented were the 30-day outcomes from the PARTNER II trial involving high- and intermediate-risk patients treated with the Edwards SAPIEN 3 valve. Among 583 high-risk patients with mean age of 82.6 years and mean STS score of 8.6%, there was 2.2% mortality at 30 days with a 1.5% rate of stroke. Among the 1,076 intermediate-risk patients of mean age 81.9 years and mean STS score of 5.3%, there was 1.1% mortality at 30 days and a 2.6% rate of stroke. Looking at the high- and intermediate-risk patients together, there was only a 3.7% rate of moderate AR and 0.1% rate of severe AR, which had been one of the major issues with the earlier-generation devices. Data at 2 years have now been reported from PARTNER IIA, which randomized 2,032 intermediate-risk patients to TAVR vs. SAVR and showed no difference in all-cause mortality or disabling stroke (HR 0.89 for TAVR; 95% CI 0.73-1.09; $p = 0.25$). The third-generation Edwards S3 valve was also studied in 1,077 intermediate-risk patients, and this trial demonstrated noninferiority as well as superiority for the composite end point of all-cause mortality, stroke, and moderate or severe AR as compared to a contemporary, propensity-matched cohort of patients undergoing SAVR from the PARTNER IIA trial.

Finally, we have data from the Valve-in-Valve (ViV) International Data Registry, which included 459 patients who were enrolled from 55 centers across Europe, North America, Australia, New Zealand, and the Middle East between 2007 and 2013. Patients had a mean age of 77.6 (+/− 9.8) years, were 56% male, had an average STS score of 9.8% (interquartile range, 7.7% to 16.0%), and required a valve procedure owing to isolated bioprosthetic stenosis in 39.4% of cases, isolated regurgitation in 30.3% of cases, and combined degeneration in 30.3%. Overall 30-day mortality was 7.6% with a 1.7% incidence of major stroke, and survival to 1 year was 83.2%. Patients with isolated bioprosthetic stenosis and those with a small bioprosthetic valve size pre-TAVR were at significantly higher risk for 1-year mortality after ViV TAVR. Implanted devices included both balloon-expandable (53.6%) and self-expandable (46.4%) valves.

X. CONCLUSION. In summary, the evidence demonstrates that TAVR is an accepted treatment for patients with severe AS who are at prohibitive surgical risk, and is an effective alternative to surgical AVR for patients at intermediate or high surgical risk. Furthermore, the use of ViV TAVR for degenerated bioprosthetic valves appears to be a promising strategy to avoid reoperation among patients at high risk for surgical complications, and as an only option for appropriately selected patients who are considered inoperable. Randomized trials of TAVR vs. SAVR involving low-risk patients are ongoing.

KEY PEARLS

- Transcatheter aortic valve replacement (TAVR) has become an established therapy for patients with severe aortic valve stenosis who are not candidates for surgery, and is an accepted alternative for patients at intermediate or high surgical risk. Trials in low-risk populations are ongoing.
- TAVR has shown excellent safety and has grown from a technologic standpoint to include multiple valve designs and vascular access approaches.
- Evaluating a patient for TAVR requires a heart-team approach, which is a multidisciplinary assessment of each patient with the collaboration of cardiac surgeons, interventional cardiologists, imaging specialists, other experts from different disciplines, nurses, and other support staff.
- The preferred route for TAVR is via transfemoral access, but in patients without appropriate iliofemoral vessels, alternative access must be considered, the most common of which are the subclavian, transapical, or transaortic approaches.
- Other vascular approaches that have been used include axillary artery, carotid artery, and finally venous options including trans-septal and transcaval access.
- In establishing candidacy for TAVR and planning for appropriate access, it is important to have high-quality imaging of the iliofemoral arteries and the aortic annulus, both of which can typically be evaluated by a gated CT scan with contrast.
- Complications that are particularly important to consider in patients undergoing TAVR include paravalvular AR, stroke, vascular and access site complications, bleeding, conduction system disease, cardiac tamponade, and annular rupture.

SUGGESTED READINGS

Adams DH, Popma JJ, Reardon MJ, et al. Transcatheter aortic-valve replacement with a self-expanding prosthesis. *N Engl J Med.* 2014;370:1790–1798.

Athappan G, Patvardhan E, Tuzcu EM, et al. Incidence, predictors, and outcomes of aortic regurgitation after transcatheter aortic valve replacement: meta-analysis and systematic review of literature. *J Am Coll Cardiol.* 2013;61:1585–1595.

Cribier A, Eltchaninoff H, Bash A, et al. Percutaneous transcatheter implantation of an aortic valve prosthesis for calcific aortic stenosis: first human case description. *Circulation.* 2002;106:3006–3008.

Dvir D, Webb JG, Bleiziffer S, et al. Transcatheter aortic valve implantation in failed bioprosthetic surgical valves. *JAMA.* 2014;312:162–170.

Genereux P, Head SJ, Van Mieghem NM, et al. Clinical outcomes after transcatheter aortic valve replacement using valve academic research consortium definitions: a weighted meta-analysis of 3,519 patients from 16 studies. *J Am Coll Cardiol.* 2012;59:2317–2326.

Holmes DR Jr, Mack MJ, Kaul S, et al. 2012 ACCF/AATS/SCAI/STS expert consensus document on transcatheter aortic valve replacement. *J Am Coll Cardiol.* 2012;59:1200–1254.

Kappetein AP, Head SJ, Genereux P, et al. Updated standardized endpoint definitions for transcatheter aortic valve implantation: the valve academic research consortium-2 consensus document. *J Am Coll Cardiol.* 2012;60:1438–1454.

Leon MB, Smith CR, Mack M, et al. Transcatheter aortic-valve implantation for aortic stenosis in patients who cannot undergo surgery. *N Engl J Med.* 2010;363:1597–1607.

Leon MB, Smith CR, Mack MJ, et al. Transcatheter or surgical aortic-valve replacement in intermediate-risk patients. *N Engl J Med.* 2016;374(17):1609–1620.

Nishimura RA, Otto CM, Bonow RO, et al. 2014 AHA/ACC guideline for the management of patients with valvular heart disease: a report of the American College of Cardiology/American Heart Association Task Force on Practice Guidelines. *Circulation.* 2014;129:e521–e643.

Piazza N, Kalesan B, van Mieghem N, et al. A 3-center comparison of 1-year mortality outcomes between transcatheter aortic valve implantation and surgical aortic valve replacement on the basis of propensity score matching among intermediate-risk surgical patients. *JACC Cardiovasc Interv.* 2013;6:443–451.

Popma JJ, Adams DH, Reardon MJ, et al. Transcatheter aortic valve replacement using a self-expanding bioprosthesis in patients with severe aortic stenosis at extreme risk for surgery. *J Am Coll Cardiol.* 2014;63:1972–1981.

Ross J Jr, Braunwald E. Aortic stenosis. *Circulation.* 1968;38:61–67.

Smith CR, Leon MB, Mack MJ, et al. Transcatheter versus surgical aortic-valve replacement in high-risk patients. *N Engl J Med.* 2011;364:2187–2198.

Thourani VH, Kodali S, Makkar RR, et al. Transcatheter aortic valve replacement versus surgical valve replacement in intermediate-risk patients: a propensity score analysis. *Lancet.* 2016;387(10034):2218–2225.

Whitlock RP, Sun JC, Fremes SE, et al. Antithrombotic and thrombolytic therapy for valvular disease: antithrombotic therapy and prevention of thrombosis, 9th ed: American College of Chest Physicians Evidence-based Clinical Practice Guidelines. *Chest.* 2012;141:e576S–e600S.

CHAPTER 13

Lourdes R. Prieto

Pediatric Percutaneous Valve Procedures

I. INTRODUCTION

The era of percutaneous valve procedures in the pediatric population was ushered in by the first in-man transcatheter implantation of a pulmonary valve in a 12-year-old patient with tetralogy of Fallot (TOF) and a dysfunctional right ventricle (RV) to pulmonary artery (PA) conduit, reported by Bonhoeffer et al. in 2000. The device utilized in that procedure was a bovine jugular venous valve sewn to an expandable stent. After several modifications, the device was marketed as the Melody valve (Medtronic Inc., Minneapolis, MN) (Fig. 13.1), was approved by the Food and Drug Administration (FDA) initially under Humanitarian Device Exemption guidelines in 2010, and received premarket FDA approval in 2015. At the time of this writing, there are two valves approved by the FDA for transcatheter pulmonary valve replacement (percutaneous pulmonary valve replacement [PPVR]), the Melody valve and the Edwards SAPIEN XT valve (Edwards Lifesciences, Irvine, CA), both specifically approved for patients with dysfunctional RV to PA conduits.

Approximately 20% of patients with congenital heart disease have a lesion affecting the RV outflow tract (RVOT), and a subset of these patients require a surgically implanted conduit, often early in childhood. These conduits have a limited life span, either because of somatic growth of the patient or, in fully grown patients, because of acquired stenosis or regurgitation of the valved conduit. The availability of a percutaneous approach will serve to decrease the number of open heart procedures these patients will face over the course of their lifetime, and is one of the most exciting developments in the field of pediatric cardiac intervention in the past decade.

II. INDICATIONS

The majority of patients who undergo PPVR at this time have had surgical placement of an RV to PA conduit to treat their underlying congenital heart disease, most commonly TOF and, in smaller numbers, other conotruncal defects such as truncus arteriosus. Another important group of patients benefiting from this technology includes those who have had a Ross procedure to treat their aortic valve disease and are also at risk of developing RV to PA conduit dysfunction. Although approval of the Melody valve was predicated on placement within an existing RV to PA conduit, its use has been extended to patients with dysfunctional bioprosthetic and also native pulmonary valves, provided the dimensions of the RVOT do not exceed the limit required for stable implantation of the valve. Implantation in a native RVOT requires creation of a "landing zone" by placement of one or more stents ("prestenting"); the valve is then deployed within the stented region. Whether the valve is deployed within a previously existing conduit or a stented native RVOT, the indications for intervention are pulmonary stenosis (PS), pulmonary regurgitation (PR), or a combination of both.

A. **Pulmonary stenosis.** PPVR is recommended when the RV systolic pressure is ≥75 mm Hg, or RV:left ventricular (LV) systolic pressure ratio is >0.7, but may be

FIGURE 13.1 The Melody valve is a bovine jugular venous valve sewn to an expandable platinum–iridium stent. Note the blue sutures on one rim of the valve to ensure it is mounted correctly, with the leaflets opening toward the main pulmonary artery. With permission, Medtronic Inc., Minneapolis, MN.

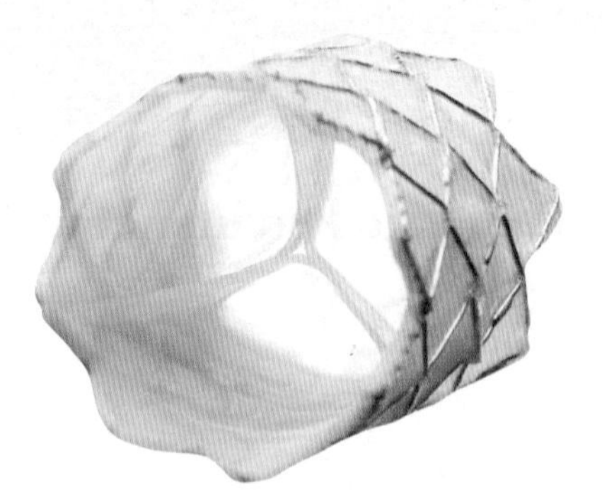

considered at lower pressures if RV function is diminished. Generally, this corresponds to a peak instantaneous gradient of ≥50 to 60 mm Hg, and mean gradient of ≥35 mm Hg by echocardiogram.

B. Pulmonary regurgitation. Indications for PPVR for PR are less well defined than for PS and are in fact evolving in part owing to availability of a less invasive option than surgical replacement. The following considerations have moved the pendulum toward earlier replacement than previously recommended:

1. Using an RV end-diastolic volume of ≥170 mL/m^2, previously the threshold to recommend surgical PVR, RV size does not return to normal following PVR in the majority of patients.
2. RV function is considered normal if RV ejection fraction (RVEF) is ≥45% measured by cardiac MRI. When RV dysfunction is already present at the time of PVR in patients with predominant PR (in contrast to PS) despite evidence of symptomatic improvement and decreased RV volumes after PVR, RVEF frequently remains unchanged.
3. The detrimental effects of chronic PR and irreversible injury to the RV must be weighed against the risk of multiple operations, and the lack of clear evidence to date that PVR improves arrhythmia burden or survival. With a percutaneous alternative, the threshold for intervention might be justifiably lower.
4. Taking the above-mentioned considerations into account, and adapting Geva's recommendations for surgical PVR to percutaneous PVR, PPVR should be recommended when there is moderate to severe PR (≥25% regurgitant fraction) and:
   - **a.** Symptoms, including right heart failure or progressive decrease in exercise tolerance or functional class, or:
   - **b.** No symptoms and at least two of the following:
     - i. RV end-diastolic volume index >150 mL/m^2
     - ii. RV end-systolic volume >80 mL/m^2
     - iii. RVEF <47%
     - iv. LV ejection fraction <55%
     - v. QRS duration > 140 ms
     - vi. Sustained tachyarrhythmia related to right heart volume load (unless a Maze procedure is thought to be indicated, in which case surgical PVR should be performed simultaneously)
     - vii. Increasing tricuspid regurgitation (TR) on serial evaluations
     - viii. RVOT obstruction with RV systolic pressure ≥ 2/3 systemic
     - ix. No associated lesions requiring surgical intervention, such as residual ventricular septal defect (VSD) or severe aortic regurgitation

C. **Mixed PS and PR.** Many patients with RV to PA conduit dysfunction have coexisting stenosis and regurgitation, resulting in both a pressure and a volume load on the RV. The threshold for intervention should be dictated by the predominant lesion, but may be somewhat lower when both present a significant hemodynamic burden.

III. CONTRAINDICATIONS

A. **Patient size too small for PPVR.** The Melody pulmonary valve delivery system is #22 French. The patient's vasculature must be able to accommodate the system. Because of the relatively high profile of the device, maneuverability within a small heart is limited. Generally, the patient's weight must be ≥20 kg, although patients as light as 14 kg have also undergone percutaneous implantation. A perventricular approach has been used in some patients too small to allow the percutaneous route, but generally patients too small for PPVR are better served by surgical PVR.

B. **RVOT dimensions too small or too large for PPVR.** The Melody valve is designed to be expanded to 18, 20, or 22 mm. Expansion to 24 mm is possible, with preliminary data showing good performance of the valve in midterm follow-up. The nominal length of the valve is 28 mm, and it shortens to 26, 24, and 23 mm when expanded to 18, 20, and 22 mm, respectively.

1. **Too small:** The recommended diameter of the surgically implanted conduit receiving the Melody PPV is ≥16 mm. Regardless of the original conduit size, balloon sizing of the conduit must be performed to identify the narrowest diameter, determined by a visible "waist" on the balloon at relatively low inflation pressure. If after adequate preparation of the landing zone, including high-pressure balloon dilation and/or prestenting, the minimal diameter remains <14 mm, the Melody valve should not be implanted.
2. **Too large:** The outer diameter of the Melody valve is approximately 2 mm larger than the diameter it is expanded to. Following strict manufacturer's guidelines, a waist no larger than 20 mm on balloon sizing is required to implant the valve at 22 mm, but in reality it can be implanted up to a waist of 22 mm, particularly after prestenting. Dilating the valve to 24 mm (outer diameter 26 mm) allows implantation in slightly larger RVOTs, up to a waist of 23 to 24 mm. Implantation in larger RVOTs is contraindicated because the valve would not have an anchoring site. The Edwards SAPIEN XT valve can be expanded to 24, 26, and 29 mm, and has allowed implantation up to a minimal diameter of 27 to 28 mm on balloon sizing.

C. **Native RVOT.** The approved indication for the Melody valve is implantation within a surgically implanted RV to PA conduit; however, successful off-label implantation in the native RVOT (most often following TOF repair) has been reported by several investigators and is being commonly performed. Implantation is contraindicated when the native RVOT is too large to meet sizing criteria (as outlined earlier), which occurs in the large majority of postoperative TOF patients.

D. **Coronary artery compression.** In some patients with a surgically implanted RV to PA conduit, the conduit lies above or in close proximity to a coronary artery. One of the most important and potentially life-threatening complications of PPVR is coronary artery compression, which has been found to occur in approximately 5% of patients. The underlying mechanism is a change in the size or geometry of the RV to PA conduit as a result of placement of the stented percutaneous valve, resulting in coronary artery compression. The only foolproof technique to rule out this possibility is aortic root or selective coronary angiography (or both if necessary) while simultaneously inflating a balloon (as much as possible to the same diameter as the intended valve diameter) at the site of intended valve implantation. Patients at highest risk for coronary artery compression are those with coronary artery anomalies, most commonly the left anterior descending (LAD) arising from the right sinus of Valsalva in patients with TOF. Patients with transposition of the great arteries (TGA) are also at increased risk, again with the majority having an anomalous coronary artery congenitally (typically these are patients status post Rastelli procedure for TGA, VSD, and PS).

E. Bacterial endocarditis. Active endocarditis is a contraindication to PPVR.

IV. EVALUATION

Consideration of PPVR in a patient with pulmonary valve dysfunction begins with a thorough history and physical examination to ascertain the presence of symptoms, murmurs of PS and/or regurgitation, and signs of right heart failure if present. Cardiopulmonary stress testing, particularly if performed serially, can be very useful in identifying clinical deterioration. The presence of atrial and/or ventricular arrhythmias should be determined. Echocardiography can identify patients with significant enough RVOT obstruction to render them candidates for PPVR, but to evaluate the RVOT anatomy in detail, cardiac MRI is the gold standard. Cardiac MRI is also the gold standard to measure RV volumes and RVEF in patients with PR as the primary indication. Lastly, the detrimental effect of RV dilation and dysfunction on LV systolic and diastolic function is being increasingly recognized, making evaluation of LV performance also important in this patient population.

A. Signs and symptoms. Symptoms are not always present in patients with significant enough pulmonary valve dysfunction to be considered for PPVR. When present, symptoms in patients with severe PS most often include exertional dyspnea and fatigue, as the RV is not able to increase its output in response to the increased demand. If the stenosis is not relieved, right heart failure may occur. Occasionally, chest pain, syncope, and even sudden death with strenuous exercise may occur in patients with severe PS, likely due to relative myocardial ischemia because of inadequate cardiac output during exercise, resulting in ventricular arrhythmias.

Patients with moderate to severe PR typically remain asymptomatic for long periods of time but ultimately develop progressive fatigue and activity intolerance, and if left untreated right heart failure will occur. Progressive RV enlargement due to PR is a known risk factor for ventricular arrhythmias and sudden cardiac death late after repair of TOF.

B. Physical examination. Increased RV impulse can be felt with significant pressure and/or volume loading of the RV. The typical murmur of PS is a systolic ejection murmur maximal at the upper left sternal border, radiating to the back. A thrill may also be palpable. Generally, the intensity of the murmur increases with the severity of obstruction, but patients with RV to PA conduits that are directly under the chest wall may have relatively loud murmurs with mild obstruction. The length of the murmur increases with increasing stenosis, and the pulmonary closure sound becomes inaudible. The murmur of PR is a low-pitched diastolic murmur also best heard at the left upper sternal border. Even with severe PR, a grade >3 murmur is unusual. Almost always in patients with PR, a "to-and-fro" murmur is heard as the increased flow through the valve causes a murmur of "relative" PS. A fixed and widely split S_2 is common owing to the almost universally present right bundle branch block (RBBB) in repaired TOF and truncus arteriosus patients. Patients with right heart failure have the typical findings of elevated jugular venous pressure, hepatomegaly, and peripheral edema. A right-sided S_4 may be present. In severe cases, splenomegaly from chronic passive congestion and ascites may also be present.

C. Electrocardiography. The majority of patients undergoing PPVR are repaired TOF patients, and characteristically the ECG in these patients has an RBBB pattern. In postoperative TOF patients with PR, a QRS duration ≥180 ms, which correlates with chronic RV volume overload and marked RV enlargement, has been identified as a risk factor for life-threatening ventricular arrhythmias and sudden cardiac death. Symptoms suggestive of ventricular arrhythmias in this subset of patients should be thoroughly evaluated, including electrophysiologic study depending on the clinical scenario, and it is one of the factors taken into account when deciding the timing of PPVR.

D. **Echocardiography**

1. **Pulmonary stenosis:** The echocardiogram is an excellent screening test for patients with RVOT dysfunction, and in the majority, it can give a good estimate of the severity of obstruction by Doppler interrogation of the RVOT. A peak instantaneous gradient ≥50 to 60 mm Hg and mean gradient of ≥35 mm Hg would typically correlate with an RV pressure ≥65% to 75% systemic. RV function can be qualitatively assessed. In the presence of significant dysfunction and low cardiac output, a lower gradient may be measured despite significant stenosis because of inability of the RV to generate a higher pressure and less than normal flow across the pulmonary valve. In patients with a long, tubular stenosis, as can be seen with a diffusely narrow RV to PA conduit, the echo-estimated gradient can overestimate the severity of obstruction. If there is enough TR to obtain a reliable Doppler signal, the RV pressure can be estimated by measuring the TR velocity *(V)* and applying the Bernoulli equation (RV pressure = $4V^2$ + right atrial pressure). In the absence of PA hypertension, which is not typically present in this patient population, a TR velocity of ≥4 m/s would indicate at least moderate to severe obstruction. When using the TR velocity to estimate RV pressure, it must be kept in mind that a subset of patients, particularly those with repaired TOF, may have branch pulmonary artery stenosis (PAS), which if present bilaterally could also result in RV hypertension with or without RVOT obstruction. Similarly, repaired TOF patients with RVOT obstruction who have not undergone prior surgical PVR may have subvalvar PS because of inadequate infundibular resection at the time of their initial repair. Such patients may require surgical RVOT reconstruction instead of PPVR. Detailed understanding of the entire RVOT and PA anatomy is imperative when planning PPVR, and echocardiographic imaging, especially in larger patients, must be complemented by other imaging modalities for adequate visualization of all the relevant structures.
2. **Pulmonary regurgitation:** The degree of PR can be assessed qualitatively by color Doppler interrogation of the pulmonary valve. The width of the PR jet, degree of extension into the RV cavity, and flow pattern in the PAs can differentiate between mild and moderate or severe PR. Flow reversal in the distal PAs indicates severe PR. More important than grading the severity of PR is assessment of the effect of PR-induced volume loading on the RV when evaluating a patient for PPVR. The degree of RV enlargement and RV contractility can be ascertained from multiple views, including parasternal long- and short-axis and apical four-chamber views. Because of the purely qualitative nature of the echocardiogram when imaging the RV, when there appears to be significant enough RV enlargement and/or dysfunction to consider PPVR, cardiac MRI should be performed to quantitate RV volumes and RVEF. In patients unable to undergo MRI owing to the presence of a pacemaker, cardiac CT scan may be considered, although limited data have shown some overestimation of RV volumes and underestimation of PR fraction by CT when compared to MRI in patients with repaired TOF. It is also important to note that progression of TR over time in an individual patient may signal progressive RV dilation and dysfunction. Changes in echocardiographic parameters of LV systolic and diastolic function should also be noted, as ventriculo-ventricular mechanical interactions may affect LV performance.

E. **Cardiac MRI.** Cardiac MRI is the gold standard for quantification of RV volume, RVEF, and PR and TR regurgitant fraction. It also provides excellent visualization of the entire RVOT and supravalvar anatomy, including the subvalvar region and branch PAs. It is important to tailor the study protocol to obtain all the relevant information, the details of which are beyond the scope of this writing, but well outlined by Geva (see Suggested Readings). MRI is subject to significant artifact when metal-containing prosthetic pulmonary valves or PA stents are present. However, quantification of RV volume is not typically compromised by the presence of these prosthetic materials. LV function should also be evaluated. As discussed earlier, the threshold of RV dimensions for recommending PVR has trended downward over the past several years. Indications for PPVR based on MRI quantification of RV volume and regurgitant fraction were detailed earlier.

F. **Cardiopulmonary stress testing.** Functional capacity should be measured serially in patients being followed with PR. With the patient serving as his/her own control, a decrease in exercise capacity would support consideration of PPVR, provided other parameters for PPVR are met.

G. **Biomarkers.** Pro brain-type natriuretic peptide (proBNP) is being increasingly used in patients with congenital heart disease as a marker of deteriorating cardiac status. However, proBNP elevation is not a prerequisite for PPVR. ProBNP elevation in a patient with documented pulmonary valve dysfunction may support intervention, but waiting for this to occur may be intervening at a later than optimal time.

H. **Supravalvar branch PAS.** The majority of patients undergoing PPVR are repaired TOF patients. There is a significant incidence of branch PAS in these patients, either native or as a result of prior surgery. PAS may also be present in patients following repair of truncus arteriosus. Detailed assessment of the PA anatomy prior to PPVR is imperative. As mentioned earlier, RV hypertension can result from obstruction at any level along the RVOT and branch PAs, in addition to PA hypertension, and no patient should arrive in the catheterization laboratory for PPVR without an understanding of the possibility for multilevel obstruction. Cardiac MRI (and also cardiac CT) provides the necessary anatomic detail to exclude significant PAS. When unilateral PAS is present, flow distribution to each lung should be calculated by MRI to help evaluate the severity of the stenosis. Pressure recordings and PA angiography during the catheterization may be necessary for more detailed evaluation. In some cases, intervention for PAS in addition to PPVR is indicated and can sometimes be performed during the same procedure.

I. **Three-dimensional models.** Owing to the extensive variability in RVOT anatomy and size limitations imposed by the current valve technology, patient-specific three-dimensional print models derived from cardiac MRI datasets can be very useful in assessing the candidacy of a patient for PPVR and for planning the procedure. The model can be used to test the RVOT with different-size balloons under fluoroscopy, of course understanding the limitation of the material behaving differently than the actual conduit/tissue. This technology is commercially available, though time consuming, expensive, and not yet widely used in clinical practice, but for a specific patient with complex anatomy it may be considered.

V. TECHNIQUE

Before describing the technical details of the PPVR procedure, it is important to discuss the institutional and operator requirements recommended for a successful transcatheter pulmonary valve program. In addition to the interventional cardiologist, the program requires the collaboration of multiple subspecialists in a "heart team" model, including cardiac surgeons, noninvasive cardiologists, cardiac radiologists, and cardiac anesthesiologists, all of whom actively care for patients with congenital heart disease. The recommended institutional volume of congenital/structural catheterizations is at least 150 cases per year, 100 of which should be therapeutic. The individual performing the procedure should have performed at least 100 catheterizations, 50 of which should have been interventions. He/she should have experience with stent implantation in the RVOT, PAs, removal of embolized foreign bodies, and assessment of the coronary arteries. A biplane catheterization laboratory is preferred. A surgical program with at least 100 open heart surgeries per year in patients with congenital heart disease and extracorporeal membrane oxygenation (ECMO) availability must exist in the same institution. Participation in a national registry (IMPACT) is also recommended.

A. **Technical considerations: Melody valve**

1. **Vascular access:** Implantation of the Melody valve requires a #22 French delivery sheath. The diagnostic portion of the procedure can be performed with a

smaller sheath if placement of the valve is not fairly certain, but from a practical standpoint, starting with a #18 French 30-cm sheath allows easy transition to the #22 French Melody ensemble and enables advancement of other long sheaths for "prestenting" (see later), including long sheaths large enough to deliver a covered stent emergently should a conduit rupture occur. Most operators elect to preclose the vein to minimize the risk of bleeding complications at the groin site. In our experience three ProGlide Perclose devices (Abbott Vascular, Santa Clara, CA) have worked well. If maneuvering large sheaths to the RVOT is difficult, access from the right internal jugular vein (RIJ) may be obtained, and not uncommonly this approach is found to be easier. This is particularly true in smaller hearts where the double curve from the tricuspid valve to the RVOT may be more difficult to negotiate, and advancing from the RIJ may be a smoother route.

2. **Hemodynamics:** A right heart catheterization must be performed with measurement of right-sided pressures in all chambers. A balloon wedge catheter should be utilized and the RV should be entered with the balloon inflated, to ensure that the catheter has not crossed any tricuspid valve chordae that could be injured later when advancing large sheaths. Because many of these patients have had prior closure of a VSD, saturations should also be obtained to exclude any residual shunting, although knowledge of this should nearly always precede the PPVR procedure. In patients with PS, it is important to note exactly where the pressure gradient(s) is so that the site of obstruction is targeted for valve implantation. Careful pullback with an end-hole catheter may be necessary in some instances.
3. **Angiography:** Angiography of the RVOT is performed and measurements of the intended implantation site calculated, ideally in two planes. Typically, best angiographic angles to elongate the RVOT and PA bifurcation are anteroposterior/cranial and straight lateral. For patients with very complex anatomy, rotational angiography may be useful if available to better evaluate the three-dimensional anatomy and select optimal projections for biplane conventional angiography and intervention.
4. **Preparation of the RVOT:** Patients with conduit obstruction may require predilation to achieve a diameter that is suitable for implantation of the Melody valve (≥14 mm), which should be expanded to no less than 18 mm. Generally, if the minimal RVOT diameter is less than 18 mm, but less than the nominal diameter of the conduit at the time of surgical placement, the implantation site should be predilated. The balloon should be no more than 110% of the nominal conduit diameter, and less than 22 mm. Rupture of a stenotic conduit may occur during predilation, particularly with high-pressure balloons, and with waist-to-balloon ratio <0.85. In some cases where the narrowing is close to 18 mm, rather than predilation with a balloon, a stent may be implanted using a balloon of the same diameter as the intended Melody valve. However, coronary compression must be excluded before stent placement.
5. **Balloon sizing:** After preparation of the RVOT, if needed, balloon sizing is performed. The sizing balloon should be at least 4 mm larger than the narrowest diameter to be able to see a waist and should be at least as large as the diameter of the anticipated Melody valve. (Melody ensembles come with 18, 20, and 22 mm balloons, but expansion to 24 mm is also possible.) The minimal waist should be ≥14 mm. For conventional deployment of the valve at the largest diameter of 22 mm, a maximum waist not exceeding 22 mm is required (size of the valve refers to the inner diameter, whereas the outer diameter is about 2 mm larger than the inner diameter). However, the valve mounted on a 24-mm balloon-in-balloon catheter (BIB, NuMED Inc., Hopkinton, NY) can be implanted with a balloon waist up to 23 to 24 mm.
6. **Coronary artery evaluation:** To exclude coronary artery compression, the same balloon used to size the RVOT is again inflated while simultaneously performing an aortic root angiogram (Fig. 13.2). It is important to make sure that the

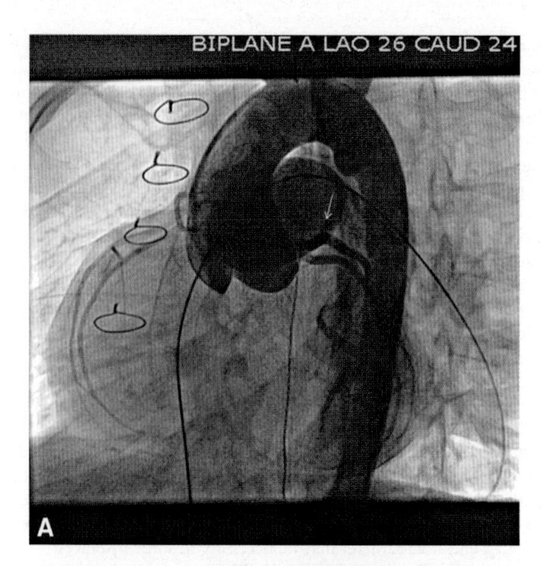

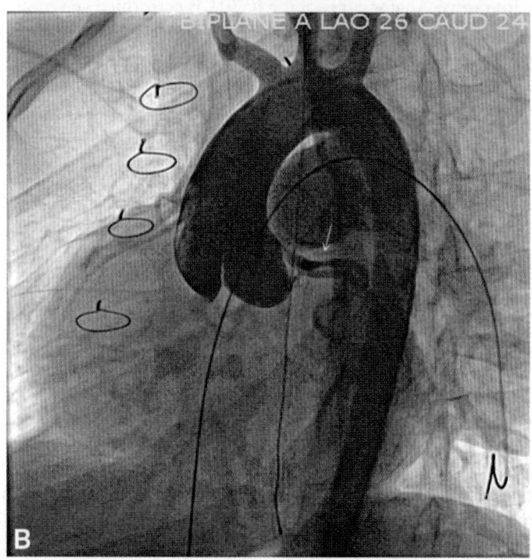

FIGURE 13.2 **A:** Aortic root angiogram with simultaneous balloon inflation in the right ventricular outflow tract in a patient with tetralogy of Fallot. The balloon slips down during inflation, such that it is lower than the site of intended Melody valve implantation. There is no coronary artery compression with balloon inflation at this site. **B:** The balloon is repositioned at the intended landing zone of the valve and the aortic root angiogram repeated. The left anterior descending artery (LAD) is pushed down and compressed by the inflated balloon at this site *(white arrow)*. Note this occurs despite some distance between the balloon and the LAD, but displacement of the intervening tissue by the balloon causes compression. The valve was not implanted.

balloon used mimics the effect of the valve to be implanted. The "balloon water" is diluted more than usual to make it less radiopaque and avoid obscuring the coronary arteries if the balloon is overlapping them. The left coronary artery is at a higher risk of compression, but it is important to assess all the coronary artery branches carefully for their entire length, paying attention to a change in caliber of the vessel and also to any relative decrease in contrast opacification. The most helpful angles tend to be left anterior oblique/caudal and straight lateral, but additional angiograms with different angulation may be needed when in doubt. Selective injection of a coronary artery may also need to be performed if the root injection does not unequivocally exclude compression. Of note, attention should also be paid to any potential distortion of the ascending aorta and aortic valve during balloon testing.

7. **Prestenting:** The most common mechanism of Melody valve dysfunction in midterm follow-up is stenosis resulting from fractures of the valve stent because of fatigue stress. Reinforcing the RVOT by placement of one or more bare metal stents prior to valve implantation has been associated with longer freedom from valve dysfunction and reintervention. Prestenting can also prepare the RVOT by alleviating conduit stenosis more effectively than balloon dilation. It is imperative to exclude coronary artery compression before prestenting, because compression can occur equally with a stent as with a stented valve. The diameter and length of the stent are chosen based on the RVOT anatomy to cover the stenotic segment, and expand to the diameter anticipated for the valve (though not necessarily completely eliminating a small waist) while following the recommendations outlined earlier to decrease the risk of rupture. The length of the expanded Melody valve ranges from 23 to 26 mm, and the expanded stent must be at least as long as the valve. The stent type should be one with high radial strength to overcome the frequently calcified and scarred-down walls of the previously surgically treated RVOT. The Palmaz XL series is generally preferred (Johnson & Johnson, Piscataway, NJ). If the stent shows significant recoil while the balloon is deflated, suggesting it is still subject to significant external forces, one or sometimes more additional stents may be deployed to optimize the "landing zone" environment prior to implantation of the valve.
8. **Preparation of the Melody valve:** The Melody valve is a bovine jugular venous valve sutured to a platinum–iridium stent. The ensemble that accompanies the Melody valve consists of a modified BIB balloon with a tapered "carrot" at its tip to help advance the valve into position. The balloon is prepackaged coaxially inside the #22 French delivery sheath. Once the landing zone is prepared, the Melody valve is mounted on the appropriately sized balloon catheter (18, 20, or 22 mm diameter) and carefully crimped manually (of note, there are currently two Melody valve products, the 16-mm valve designed to expand up to 20 mm and the 18-mm valve designed to expand up to 22 mm). It is imperative that the valve be mounted such that the leaflets will open in the correct direction toward the main pulmonary artery (MPA). To ensure correct positioning, the stent edge that should face the MPA has blue sutures along its circumference, and the "carrot" at the tip of the balloon is also blue (Fig. 13.3). The valve is then covered by the delivery sheath and is ready to be advanced into the body.

FIGURE 13.3 The delivery balloon for the Melody valve has a blue carrot at the tip to help advance the valve into place. The blue sutures on the Melody valve rim should face the blue carrot for proper positioning and opening of the valve in the correct direction. With permission, Medtronic Inc., Minneapolis, MN.

9. **Deployment of the Melody valve:** All of the steps leading to this point, including balloon sizing and prestenting, require a relatively stiff wire across the RVOT with its tip in a distal PA branch. Most often a 0.035″ Amplatz Super Stiff wire (Boston Scientific, Marlborough, MA) works well. This same wire may also work for advancing the Melody valve to the RVOT, but if difficulty is encountered a stiffer wire, such as a Lunderquist wire (Cook Medical, Bloomington, IN), should be used. Although quite stiff this wire has a fairly soft, long tip and can be purchased with a double curve, all nice features when working in branch PAs. Once the valve is positioned within the landing zone, which most often will have been prestented, it is uncovered and implanted by inflating the inner followed by the outer balloon. Because the valve is a covered stent, care should be taken not to protrude beyond the PA bifurcation to avoid occluding a branch PA. After implantation, RV pressure and pressure gradient across the valve are measured. If a significant gradient remains, further dilation with a high-pressure balloon can be performed, aiming to decrease the gradient to less than 20 mm Hg. Angiography in the MPA is then performed to evaluate for PR.
10. **Dilation to 24 mm:** The Melody valve has been shown to work well, at least in the short- to midterm follow-up, when dilated to 24 mm. It must be mounted on a regular 24-mm BIB balloon and backloaded into a long #22 French sheath previously positioned across the RVOT. Alternatively, we have found it easier to use the delivery sheath that accompanies the Melody valve to frontload the valve. To do this, it is necessary to modify a Melody valve ensemble by cutting off the balloon from the coaxial dilation catheter and removing it. A 24-mm BIB balloon is then advanced into the Melody delivery sheath, and the Melody valve is mounted on this balloon and covered by the delivery sheath, leaving about 1 cm of the balloon uncovered to function as the "carrot." The balloon is inflated slightly to create a smoother transition between the uncovered portion and the sheath. Advancement and implantation of the valve are performed as described earlier.
11. **Native RVOT:** The procedure for implantation of the valve in a native RVOT is similar to that for a surgically implanted conduit. Preparation of the RVOT by prestenting should be performed, which essentially creates a "conduit" as well as a landing zone for delivery of the valve. In some cases, particularly those with free PR and larger RVOTs, a two-stage approach may work best, preparing the landing zone with bare metal stents, followed by implantation of the valve a few months later after the stents have undergone endothelialization and are therefore more stable.

B. **Edwards SAPIEN valve.** The main utility of this valve for PPVR is in patients whose RVOTs are too large even for expansion of the Melody valve to 24 mm, meaning a waist ≥25 mm on balloon sizing. The 29-mm Edwards valve can be implanted up to a waist of 27 to 28 mm on balloon sizing. The 30-mm NuCLEUS balloon (NuMED Inc., Hopkington, NY) works well for prestenting in this scenario because of its dog-boning feature, resulting in a 27-mm waist at 30-mm diameter.

1. **Device specifications:** The Edwards SAPIEN XT valve consists of three bovine pericardial leaflets sewn to a cobalt chromium balloon-expandable stent. The valve is shorter than the Melody valve at 14.3-, 17.2-, and 19.1-mm expanded lengths for the 23-, 26-, and 29-mm diameter valves, respectively, and therefore prestenting with a longer bare metal stent is usually performed. The PPVR procedure for this valve is similar to PPVR with the Melody valve. Preparation and delivery of the valve do differ in several respects.
2. **Preparation and delivery of the Edwards SAPIEN XT valve:** This valve is supplied with the Novaflex+ Delivery System (Edwards Lifesciences, Irvine, CA), #20 French Edwards expandable introducer sheath, and Edwards crimper. The valve is crimped to the delivery catheter with the crimper device 2 to 3 mm distal to the

balloon shaft. In order to deploy the valve in the RVOT, it must be loaded on the delivery catheter "upside down" in relationship to the way it would be loaded for TAVR. The delivery ensemble is introduced into the body, and once in the inferior vena cava (IVC) the balloon is pulled back into the valve until it locks into place; further fine-tuning to center it within the valve is accomplished with the valve alignment wheel. The flex wheel enables steering of the ensemble as it is advanced to the RVOT. Once in position the flex catheter is withdrawn to uncover the valve. The balloon is inflated with a specific volume of diluted contrast determined by the diameter of the selected valve—22 mL for the 26-mm valve and 33 mL for the 29-mm valve.

3. **The Edwards SAPIEN 3 valve:** Approved for transcatheter aortic valve replacement in 2016, this has also been used off-label for PPVR. It requires a smaller sheath size, #14 French for the 26-mm valve and #16 French for the 29-mm valve. The covered portion is shorter than that of the Edwards XT valve, which must be kept in mind during placement to avoid paravalvular leaks.

VI. PERIPROCEDURAL MANAGEMENT

PPVR is essentially an outpatient procedure with overnight observation, much like any other interventional cardiac catheterization in children and adults with congenital heart disease. The procedure is performed under general anesthesia, and heparin is administered with a goal-activated clotting time ≥250. An antibiotic dose (cefazolin in most, vancomycin for allergic patients) is administered prior to implantation of any device (stent or valve) and continued for 24 hours. Patients are almost always extubated in the catheterization laboratory, observed overnight, and discharged the following morning. Careful monitoring of the access site is important, but complications are uncommon. Postprocedure bleeding from the large venous sheath may occur, but we have found that preclosing the site is very effective in avoiding this problem.

A. **Adjunct therapy.** Postimplantation aspirin should be administered typically at 81 mg once a day for 6 months. Some data suggest that continuation of aspirin longer, perhaps indefinitely, may offer some protection against bacterial endocarditis (BE) affecting the prosthetic pulmonary valve. Many operators are now recommending aspirin long term.

B. **Postprocedure testing.** Standard testing includes ECG, chest X-ray (CXR), and echocardiogram, performed the morning after the procedure. Stable position of the valve can be easily ascertained by CXR. Echocardiogram serves to assess valve function, namely pulmonary valve gradient and degree of regurgitation. In the vast majority of patients, a $V_{max} < 3$ m/s and no more than trivial or mild regurgitation is observed.

VII. COMPLICATIONS

Procedural mortality from PPVR has been exceedingly low, with no procedure-related deaths reported in the US Multicenter Melody Transcatheter Pulmonary Valve Post-Approval study, including 120 patients (100 implantations) from 10 centers. A handful of deaths have been reported worldwide, most often related to coronary artery compression.

A. **Coronary artery compression.** In a small number of patients, a coronary artery passes behind or in close proximity to the RVOT or a surgically implanted RV to PA conduit. Coronary artery compression may occur by changing the size or geometry of the RVOT and surrounding tissue. The incidence of coronary artery compression on preimplantation testing by simultaneous balloon inflation in the RVOT and coronary angiography has been found to be approximately 5%. Morray et al. found the left coronary artery (main or LAD branch) is compressed most frequently (66%), but the right coronary artery (14%) and other branches (19%) are also at risk. Patients with congenitally abnormal coronary artery anatomy were at highest risk. Patients with TOF and abnormal coronary artery anatomy, particularly those with LAD arising from the right sinus, are at significantly increased risk. However, it can be seen in patients with all types of underlying diagnoses. Compression testing in the catheterization laboratory is the most accurate method of diagnosing this potential complication. Every effort should be made to test the landing zone with a balloon that mimics the effect of the anticipated valve implantation. Assessment of distance alone between the landing zone and coronary artery is not sufficient, because displacement of the surrounding tissue/prosthetic material may also cause compression. Although not 100% foolproof, compression testing, if appropriately performed, appears to minimize this potentially lethal complication to negligible rates.

B. **Conduit tear.** The incidence of conduit disruption, including both contained and uncontained tears, has been reported at about 6% in a series of 251 patients enrolled in the US Melody investigative device exemption (IDE) trial and the post approval study. The type of conduit, including homografts and bioprosthetic valves, does not appear to be a risk factor, and it can also occur in native RVOTs. The original conduit size, minimal diameter, balloon diameter to minimal diameter, and balloon inflation pressure were not risk factors for conduit tear in this series. The pressure gradient across the conduit was higher in patients who had a tear (45 vs. 35 mm Hg). Uncontained tears occurred in only four patients (1.6%), two requiring thoracentesis and chest tube placement. This complication can be treated effectively in the catheterization laboratory with covered stents (Covered Cheatham Platinum stent, NuMED Inc., Hopkinton, NY) in the vast majority of patients, although in rare cases the tear cannot be fully covered and surgical intervention is required.

C. **PA perforation**. Perforation of a branch PA can occur during attempts to advance the valve to the RVOT, but is rare. The carrot at the distal end of the balloon is relatively stiff, and depending on the distance between the landing zone and the PA bifurcation, it may need to advance into one of the branch PAs for the valve to be positioned in the RVOT. Careful manipulation of the wire and advancing catheter to avoid pushing against resistance, trying one or the other PA branch for the smoothest course, and making sure the stiff portion of the wire is coursing through the curvature are all techniques to avoid injury to a branch PA. If a PA tear does occur, it may be treated by placement of a covered stent. Distal perforation due to the tip of the wire may also occur while advancing either a stent or the valve to the RVOT. This can be treated by embolization of the bleeding vessel with either coils or other occlusion devices.

D. **Device dislodgment.** Either a stent or the valve may dislodge during attempted deployment, particularly in large RVOTs with severe PR. However, this is uncommon, with no patient having this complication in the expanded multicenter US Melody valve trial, or the US Melody post approval study. Malposition or forward migration of the valve, which is a covered stent, can result in jailing and occlusion of a branch PA. Depending on the location of the dislodged device, implantation in a site other than the RVOT (e.g., IVC or proximal branch PA) may be possible, but percutaneous retrieval of these large devices is not typically possible and surgery is required. Some operators advocate rapid pacing during deployment, but there are no data showing superiority of this technique to avoid valve dislodgement or malposition.

E. **Other complications.** Other procedural complications include ventricular tachycardia requiring cardioversion, and vascular complications such as bleeding at the access site or deep venous thrombosis postprocedure. A traumatic aortopulmonary communication has occurred in a handful of patients, most after Ross operation, likely related to traumatic distortion of the neoaortic anastomotic site during implantation of the valve.

VIII. OUTCOMES

A. **Short-term outcomes.** Short-term outcomes of PPVR with the Melody valve have been quite favorable. Data from the expanded multicenter US Melody valve trial demonstrated acute reduction in the RV systolic pressure from 69 to 45 mm Hg and RV to PA gradient from 44 to 14 mm Hg in patients with a primary indication of PS or mixed PS/PR. All patients had no or trivial PR on echocardiography after the procedure. Serious procedural adverse events were noted in 8 of 136 patients (6%), including 2 conduit ruptures (1 requiring urgent surgery, 1 contained and treated with covered stent placement) and 1 coronary artery dissection treated with stenting and ECMO. There were no other deaths, and the other seven patients experiencing a serious adverse event were all discharged within 1 week of the procedure. Similar procedural and short-term outcomes were reported in the US post approval study, which included 100 implantations in 120 patients. PPVR was not attempted in 19 patients because of coronary artery compression (n = 6), conduit not suitable for implantation, and other criteria, making PPVR not advisable or not required. Only one patient weighing 19.9 kg had attempted implantation that had to be aborted because of distal PA perforation leading to self-resolving pulmonary hemorrhage, for a procedural success rate of 98%. Serious adverse events occurred in 13.3% of the 120 patients undergoing catheterization. The most common was conduit tear (5%), all of which were contained and successfully treated with covered stent placement. There were no procedural-related deaths. No patient had an RV to PA gradient ≥35 mm Hg and none had more than mild PR.

Recent data on 64 patients from the French registry reported successful implantation in all. RV to PA gradient post-PPVR was <20 mm Hg in 89.5% of the patients, and no patient had more than mild regurgitation. Conduit tears occurred in seven (11%), but were confined in all and treated with covered (n = 4) or bare metal (n = 3) stents. All other complications were relatively minor. There were no procedural-related deaths.

B. Midterm follow-up. Six- and 12-month follow-up for PPVR has been reported from US trials and longer-term follow-up to a median of 4.6 years from European studies. Longer-term follow-up is still being gathered. In the US post approval study including 99 patients, all were alive at 1 year, with only one patient withdrawing from the study and one lost to follow-up after 6 months. The percentage of patients in New York Heart Association (NYHA) functional class I increased from 35% pre-PPVR to 89% at 1 year. Acceptable Melody valve function with mean gradient ≤30 mm Hg and less than moderate regurgitation was documented in 94.3% of patients with evaluable echocardiographic data (>84% had at least moderate PR pre-PPVR). Mean RVOT gradient decreased from 33 mm Hg pre-PPVR to 15 mm Hg at 1 year. No patient required catheter reintervention and two required surgical PVR (one with endocarditis, one with major stent fracture and severe stenosis), for a rate of freedom from Melody valve dysfunction of 96.9% at 1 year. The rate of adverse events on follow-up was 8%, one of the most common being BE. Stent fractures occurred in seven patients, but only one developed severe stenosis requiring surgical PVR.

Similarly good results at a median follow-up of 28 months have been reported from Europe, with freedom from reoperation of 93%, 86%, 84%, and 70% at 10, 30, 50, and 70 months post-PPPVR, respectively, for 155 patients, 59 of whom were implanted with the original design of the device (valve initially not sutured to the entire length of the stent resulting in stenosis from a "hammock" effect in some patients) and before prestenting became standard practice. Survival at 83 months was 97%. Most recent data from the French registry on 64 patients reported 3 deaths (4.7%) over a median follow-up of 4.6 years. Freedom from surgery was 95% at 60 months. A significant decrease in RV end-diastolic volume was observed 6 months post-PPVR (111 to 87 mL/m^2) with no change in RVEF (48% pre- and post-PPVR).

Follow-up on 148 patients from the US Melody valve IDE trial documents equally good outcomes at a median follow-up of 4.5 years and up to 7 years. Five-year freedom from reintervention and explant was 76% and 92%, respectively. Most of the reinterventions (69%) were due to obstruction and occurred in patients with stent fractures. A conduit prestent and lower discharge RVOT gradient were associated with lower freedom from reintervention. In the reintervention-free patients, the gradient at 4.5 years median follow-up was unchanged from early post-PPVR.

Overall, Melody valve dysfunction has been uncommon and has manifested as recurrent obstruction, most often related to stent fractures. The valve has remained remarkably competent in midterm follow-up, with no patient to date reported to require reintervention for Melody valve regurgitation. Preliminary data on prestenting appear favorable, and although recurrent obstruction in the absence of stent fracture occurs, it is rare. In many cases, Melody valve dysfunction can be treated by percutaneous valve-in-valve implantation with another Melody valve, provided the size of the RVOT is not a limiting factor.

C. **Bacterial endocarditis.** All of the series to date have reported cases of BE, with an incidence ranging from 2.5% to 3% per patient-year. The most comprehensive series including 311 patients from three prospective North American and European studies reported an incidence of 2.4% per patient-year, and median duration from implant to diagnosis of 1.3 years. Freedom from BE was 96% at 2 years and 92% at 4 years. Most cases have occurred >6 months postimplantation and do not appear to be procedure related or due to contaminated product. Several different bacteria have been isolated, most often *Staphylococcus* and *Streptococcus* species. Risk factors in this study were found to be higher preimplant RVOT gradient and also higher postimplant RVOT gradient. Additionally about two-thirds of the cases had some extenuating circumstance (prior history of BE, oral laceration, dental cleaning preceding BE episode, IV drug abuse) that may have put the patient at risk. Several other risk factors have been noted in other series, including male sex, multiple RVOT stents, significant RVOT irregularities, and abrupt discontinuation of aspirin. The majority of patients with BE develop increased Melody valve gradient, and that finding, particularly if occurring relatively acutely and not explained by a structural problem such as stent fracture, should be treated as a major criterion. In many cases, direct involvement of the valve is not immediately apparent, and it appears that most patients respond to medical treatment. At this time, valve explant is not recommended during acute therapy with IV antibiotics if there is no severe valve dysfunction or hemodynamic need for intervention. However, some patients present with severe valve obstruction and hemodynamic instability and must undergo surgical PVR. Every effort should be made to decrease the risk of BE, including preimplantation dental clearance, good dental hygiene, and strict adherence to BE prophylaxis for life. Maximizing gradient reduction at time of implant may also be beneficial in protecting against BE. There should be a low threshold for diagnosing and treating BE in these patients, not always guided by strict adherence to Duke criteria. Comparing BE incidence between PPVR and surgical PVR is difficult because of variability of reporting in surgical cases. Most often, cases are reported when they require reoperation. Some data seem to suggest that the Contegra surgical conduit (also a bovine jugular venous valve) may be at increased risk of BE when compared to other conduits, such as homografts, but this has not been reproducible in all series.

D. **Stent fractures.** In the initial experience of Melody valve implantation, stent fractures were found to occur in 20% to 25% of cases, and recurrent RVOT obstruction due to stent fractures has been the most common reason for reintervention. From the European experience, risk factors for stent fractures included implantation into a native RVOT, lack of calcification of the conduit, and recoil of the stented valve following balloon deflation. Follow-up of patients from the US Melody valve IDE trial showed that Melody valve compression and substantial apposition to the anterior chest wall were associated with shorter freedom from stent fractures. That study also demonstrated significantly longer freedom from stent fractures in patients who underwent prestenting, whereas freedom from RVOT reintervention was significantly lower in patients with stent fractures. Since prestenting has become widespread, the incidence of stent fractures has decreased substantially in all series, and when they do occur, stent fractures are more likely to be minor and not lead to valve dysfunction.

E. **Edwards SAPIEN valve.** Outcomes data for this valve are much more limited than for the Melody valve. A multicenter trial using the 23- and 26-mm valves in surgically implanted conduits ≥16 and ≤24 mm in diameter enrolled 70 patients, but only partial early results have been published, and follow-up of implanted patients is ongoing. A single-center series of 25 patients using the 23-, 26-, and 29-mm valves reported an acute technical success rate of 96%, owing to one patient with high residual gradient requiring surgery. At a mean follow-up of 3.5 years, one patient required reintervention for severe PR. There were no stent fractures (all patients were prestented) and no patient developed endocarditis.

IX. UNCONVENTIONAL MELODY VALVE IMPLANTATIONS

In some circumstances, as in high-risk surgical candidates with too large RVOTs not meeting criteria for conventional PPVR, the same physiologic result has been achieved by implanting a Melody valve in each branch PA. Other operators have anchored the valve by implanting bare metal stents into a proximal branch PA and telescoping additional stents all the way to the RVOT. A periventricular hybrid approach via a small subxiphoid incision has been employed in some patients who are not good surgical candidates with arteries that are too small to advance the #22 French delivery system to the RVOT.

X. OTHER PERCUTANEOUS VALVE PROCEDURES IN PEDIATRICS

PPVR is by far the predominant percutaneous valve procedure performed in pediatric and adult patients with congenital heart disease. However, the Melody and less commonly the Edwards SAPIEN valve have been used to replace a failing prosthetic tricuspid valve. Even less commonly, and generally in patients deemed too high a risk to undergo surgery, the Melody valve has been used to replace the mitral or aortic valves.

A. **Tricuspid valve replacement.** Both the Melody and the Edwards SAPIEN valve have been used to replace a failing bioprosthetic tricuspid valve with severe stenosis (TS), regurgitation (TR), or more commonly both. In a few patients with a single ventricle after Fontan operation, the valve has been implanted in a dysfunctional right atrium to RV conduit. Children weighing as little as 13 kg have undergone the procedure. Transesophageal echocardiography and in some instances intracardiac echocardiography are important to guide this procedure along with fluoroscopy. The approach is from either the femoral or the internal jugular vein depending on the orientation of the prosthesis and most direct route, but the femoral vein has been used more frequently. The wire is placed in one of the branch PAs. Balloon sizing is generally performed to identify the location and diameter of the waist and help select an appropriately sized valve. The Melody valve can be implanted at 22 mm if the internal valve diameter is <24 mm. Availability of the 29-mm Edwards SAPIEN XT valve has allowed implantation up to an internal valve diameter of 28 mm. Predilation with high-pressure balloons is not necessary. Prestenting has not been routinely performed by all operators, particularly with the longer Melody valve, but is more commonly done for the shorter Edwards valve, particularly if the bioprosthetic valve is also short. Potential complications include complete heart block because of the proximity of the conduction system (1/15 patients in one series), and endocarditis has also been reported. The longest reported follow-up included 16 patients (17 tricuspid valve replacements [TVRs]), with 12/16 followed for a median of 2.1 years and up to 6.3 years. Acute results were excellent, with mean TS gradient <4 and no to mild TR in all. Only one patient who received a Melody valve at 22 mm required reoperation for significant TR at 22 months and subsequently developed TR of the bioprosthetic valve, for which percutaneous TVR was again performed with a 29-mm SAPIENS XT valve. All other patients continued to have good tricuspid valve (TV) function, with no to mild TR. An international registry of 156 patients with 150 implantations followed for a median of 13.3 months reported high technical and clinical success, and improvement in NYHA class (71% of patients in class III or IV before implantation versus 14% at last follow-up). There was no difference in the performance of the Melody and the Edwards SAPIEN valves. Estimated survival free time from reintervention or TV dysfunction was 83% at 1 year, with several patients developing thrombosis, thickening, or relatively rapid dysfunction, and four cases of endocarditis. Age >60 years and NYHA class IV preimplantation were associated with decreased overall survival.

B. **Mitral valve replacement.** A handful of cases of percutaneous mitral valve replacement (MVR) using the Melody valve have been described in high-risk surgical candidates, but typically outside the pediatric age range.

C. **Aortic valve replacement.** Similarly to percutaneous MVR, percutaneous aortic valve replacement (AVR) with the Melody valve in pediatric and young adults with congenital heart disease has only been performed in a few high-risk patients under extenuating circumstances. Very few of these cases have been truly percutaneous, while most have involved a hybrid approach with surgical exposure of the LV apex, or in one case via innominate artery cutdown. Because of the length of this valve, a portion of the venous wall within the stent has to be resected to avoid coronary artery occlusion. Additionally, as the Melody valve stent expands, the native aortic valve leaflets entrapped by the stent can be distorted and cover a coronary orifice, as did occur in one patient. Partially expanding the valve above the landing zone, and then withdrawing while retracting the native aortic leaflets may avoid this problem. Limited data in a very small number of patients with a median follow-up of 2.9 months have documented preserved Melody valve function with no more than mild regurgitation when implanted in the high-pressure left-sided circulation. At this time percutaneous AVR in the pediatric population can only be considered in extenuating circumstances where all surgical options are deemed untenable.

XI. FUTURE DIRECTIONS

The advent of percutaneous valve technology has been a true game-changer for a subset of patients with congenital heart disease requiring pulmonary valve replacement. Midterm follow-up has demonstrated effectiveness and safety of this technology. However, only a fraction of patients with dysfunctional RVOTs are candidates for PPVR, most having surgically patched RVOTs that are too large for all the currently available valves. New valve designs are needed to overcome size and geometric limitations. A feasibility trial examining the performance of a new device, the Native Outflow Tract Transcatheter Pulmonary Valve (Medtronic Inc., Minneapolis, MN), for patients with PR and native RVOTs >22 mm in diameter, recently completed enrollment of 20 patients. No follow-up information is yet available. The extensive variability in postoperative RVOT size and geometry makes design of a "one-size-fits-all" device challenging. Patient-specific anatomic characteristics may need to be entered into the process of device design and selection in order to extend this valuable technology to the majority of patients requiring pulmonary valve replacement. TAVR is now a well-established intervention in adult patients who are high-risk surgical candidates. FDA approval of the Edwards SAPIEN XT and 3 valves was recently expanded to intermediate-risk patients. Several limitations need to be overcome before this technology can be applied to pediatric and young adult patients with congenital aortic valve disease. These include size of the introducer sheath, stroke risk (albeit currently derived from elderly adults with calcified valves), optimal valve design for bicuspid/unicuspid valves and smaller patients with coronary arteries closer to the annulus, and proven longer-term durability for these younger individuals. Valve-in-valve TAVR for those patients with failing bioprosthetic valves in the aortic position may be closer on the horizon. The rapid advancement of percutaneous valve technology over the past decade holds great promise for this population, which because of their lifelong valve disease necessitating multiple catheter and surgical interventions stands to benefit the most from a less invasive approach.

KEY PEARLS

- About 20% of patients with congenital heart disease have RVOT dysfunction, and a significant number eventually require surgical pulmonary valve replacement. PPVR is intended to decrease the number of open heart surgeries these patients will face over the course of a lifetime.
- Indication for PPVR for patients with predominant PR continues to evolve, with a trend toward earlier intervention. Cardiac MRI is the gold standard for evaluation of RV volumes and EF in patients with PR.

- The current percutaneous pulmonary valve technology can be applied only to a fraction of patients in need of pulmonary valve replacement. Most surgically repaired, often patched RVOTs are too large for the current valves.
- The Melody valve and the Edwards SAPIEN XT valve are the only FDA approved valves for PPVR in surgically implanted RV to PA conduits. Off-label use of both valves has extended PPVR to conduits and native RVOTs as large as 23 to 24 mm (Melody) and 27 to 28 mm (SAPIEN) on balloon sizing.
- The major mechanism of failure of the Melody valve is recurrent obstruction because of stent fractures. Prestenting of the landing zone prior to valve implantation has significantly decreased the incidence of stent fractures, and decreased the failure rate of the valve.
- Coronary artery compression is a life-threatening complication of PPVR. In the vast majority of patients, this can be avoided by compression testing with balloon inflation at the intended landing zone simultaneously with aortic root or selective coronary artery angiography.
- Conduit tears during preparation of the RVOT for PPVR occur in about 6% of patients, and are uncontained in 1% to 2%. There are no clear predictors of this complication, but it can be treated with covered stents in most cases. Some patients, however, require urgent surgery.
- Midterm outcomes for the Melody valve are very favorable, with 5-year freedom from reintervention and explant of 76% and 92%, respectively, in patients from the US IDE trial, including some patients who were not prestented. The valve has remained remarkably competent, with only one patient having more than mild PR at a median follow-up of 4.5 years in this series.
- Endocarditis has occurred in all series, and the incidence appears to be on the order of 2.5% per patient-year. A high index of suspicion should be maintained for this complication. Recurrent stenosis is the typical manifestation along with other typical signs of subacute BE. Medical treatment has been successful in many cases, and explantation of the valve should be decided on a case-by-case basis.
- The Melody valve has been used to replace other valves in the heart in much smaller numbers. Most notably, percutaneous replacement of failed bioprosthetic tricuspid valves has shown excellent acute results, while longer-term follow-up is being gathered.

SUGGESTED READINGS

Armstrong AK, Balzer DT, Cabalka AK, et al. One-year follow-up of the melody transcatheter pulmonary valve multicenter post-approval study. *JACC Cardiovasc Interv.* 2014;7(11):1254–1262.

Bonhoeffer P, Boudjemline Y, Saliba Z, et al. Percutaneous replacement of pulmonary valve in a right-ventricle to pulmonary-artery prosthetic conduit with valve dysfunction. *Lancet.* 2000;356(9239):1403–1405.

Cheatham JP, Hellenbrand WE, Zahn EM, et al. Clinical and hemodynamic outcomes up to 7 years after transcatheter pulmonary valve replacement in the US melody valve investigational device exemption trial. *Circulation.* 2015;131(22):1960–1970.

Fraisse A, Aldebert P, Malekzadeh-Milani S, et al. Melody (R) transcatheter pulmonary valve implantation: results from a French registry. *Arch Cardiovasc Dis.* 2014;107(11):607–614.

Geva T. Repaired Tetralogy of Fallot: the roles of cardiovascular magnetic resonance in evaluating pathophysiology and for pulmonary valve replacement decision support. *J Cardiovasc Magn Reson.* 2011;13:9.

Gillespie MJ, Rome JJ, Levi DS, et al. Melody valve implant within failed bioprosthetic valves in the pulmonary position: a multicenter experience. *Circ Cardiovasc Interv.* 2012;5(6):862–870.

Hijazi ZM, Ruiz CE, Zahn E, et al. SCAI/AATS/ACC/STS operator and institutional requirements for transcatheter valve repair and replacement, Part III: pulmonic valve. *J Am Coll Cardiol.* 2015;65(23):2556–2563.

Kenny D, Hijazi ZM, Kar S, et al. Percutaneous implantation of the Edwards SAPIEN transcatheter heart valve for conduit failure in the pulmonary position: early phase 1 results from an international multicenter clinical trial. *J Am Coll Cardiol.* 2011;58(21):2248–2256.

Lurz P, Coats L, Khambadkone S, et al. Percutaneous pulmonary valve implantation: impact of evolving technology and learning curve on clinical outcome. *Circulation.* 2008;117(15):1964–1972.

McElhinney DB, Benson LN, Eicken A, et al. Infective endocarditis after transcatheter pulmonary valve replacement using the melody valve: combined results of 3 prospective North American and European studies. *Circ Cardiovasc Interv.* 2013;6(3):292–300.

McElhinney DB, Cabalka AK, Aboulhosn JA, et al. Transcatheter tricuspid valve-in-valve implantation for the treatment of dysfunctional surgical bioprosthetic valves: an international, multicenter registry study. *Circulation.* 2016;133(16):1582–1593.

McElhinney DB, Cheatham JP, Jones TK, et al. Stent fracture, valve dysfunction, and right ventricular outflow tract reintervention after transcatheter pulmonary valve implantation: patient-related and procedural risk factors in the US melody valve trial. *Circ Cardiovasc Interv.* 2011;4(6):602–614.

McElhinney DB, Hellenbrand WE, Zahn EM, et al. Short- and medium-term outcomes after transcatheter pulmonary valve placement in the expanded multicenter US melody valve trial. *Circulation.* 2010;122(5):507–516.

Meadows JJ, Moore PM, Berman DP, et al. Use and performance of the melody transcatheter pulmonary valve in native and postsurgical, nonconduit right ventricular outflow tracts. *Circ Cardiovasc Interv.* 2014;7(3):374–380.

Morray BH, McElhinney DB, Cheatham JP, et al. Risk of coronary artery compression among patients referred for transcatheter pulmonary valve implantation: a multicenter experience. *Circ Cardiovasc Interv.* 2013;6(5):535–542.

Nordmeyer J, Khambadkone S, Coats L, et al. Risk stratification, systematic classification, and anticipatory management strategies for stent fracture after percutaneous pulmonary valve implantation. *Circulation.* 2007;115(11):1392–1397.

Roberts PA, Boudjemline Y, Cheatham JP, et al. Percutaneous tricuspid valve replacement in congenital and acquired heart disease. *J Am Coll Cardiol.* 2011;58(2):117–122.

Therrien J, Provost Y, Merchant N, et al. Optimal timing for pulmonary valve replacement in adults after Tetralogy of Fallot repair. *Am J Cardiol.* 2005;95(6):779–782.

Tzifa A, Momenah T, Al Sahari A, et al. Transcatheter valve-in-valve implantation in the tricuspid position. *EuroIntervention.* 2014;10(8):995–999.

Warnes CA, Williams RG, Bashore TM, et al. ACC/AHA 2008 Guidelines for the Management of Adults with Congenital Heart Disease: a report of the American College of Cardiology/American Heart Association Task Force on Practice Guidelines (Writing Committee to Develop Guidelines on the Management of Adults with Congenital Heart Disease): developed in collaboration with the American Society of Echocardiography, Heart Rhythm Society, International Society for Adult Congenital Heart Disease, Society for Cardiovascular Angiography and Interventions, and Society of Thoracic Surgeons. *J Am Coll Cardiol.* 2008;52(23):e143–e263.

Wilson WM, Benson LN, Osten MD, et al. Transcatheter pulmonary valve replacement with the Edwards Sapien system: the Toronto experience. *JACC Cardiovasc Interv.* 2015;8(14):1819–1827.

Yamasaki Y, Nagao M, Yamamura K, et al. Quantitative assessment of right ventricular function and pulmonary regurgitation in surgically repaired Tetralogy of Fallot using 256-slice CT: comparison with 3-tesla MRI. *Eur Radiol.* 2014;24(12):3289–3299.

CHAPTER 14

Patrick R. Vargo
Stephanie L. Mick
A. Marc Gillinov

Surgery of the Mitral and Tricuspid Valves

I. THE MITRAL VALVE

A. Introduction. The mitral valve apparatus is composed of anterior and posterior leaflets, the mitral annulus, chordae tendinae, and papillary muscles. Degenerative, ischemic, rheumatic, and infectious (endocarditis) processes are responsible for the vast majority of mitral valve disease in adults (Table 14.1).

Mitral regurgitation (MR) can occur as a consequence of dysfunction of any one of these components. In primary MR, dysfunction of one or more of the components of the valve itself leads to valve incompetence with systolic regurgitation of blood from the left ventricle to the left atrium. In secondary MR, the valve leaflets and chordae are structurally normal; however, left ventricular dilatation and/or dysfunction (e.g., due to myocardial infarction or nonischemic cardiomyopathy) renders the valve incompetent. This incompetence is the result of displacement of the papillary muscles in the dilated left ventricle, which leads to leaflet tethering; associated annular dilatation may contribute to failure of leaflet coaptation.

Mitral stenosis (MS) is the result of processes (most commonly rheumatic) affecting the leaflets, annulus, and subvalvular apparatus. Thickening and fusion of the leaflets and chordae inhibit normal leaflet excursion during diastole (Table 14.1).

B. Indications for surgery

1. **Acute Mitral Regurgitation:** Patients with acute, severe MR usually require urgent surgical intervention. Leaflet perforation from endocarditis or chordal rupture may be causes of this disorder. However, this presentation is often the result of myocardial infarction resulting in papillary muscle dysfunction or rupture.

   Hemodynamically stable patients benefit from afterload-reducing agents, which help to increase forward flow. In the patient with cardiogenic shock, inotropic and pressor support can often be detrimental, especially in the circumstance of ischemic disease. These agents increase myocardial oxygen demand and can thereby further exacerbate an acute coronary syndrome. If temporization is needed before surgery, intra-aortic balloon pump (IABP) or, occasionally, extracorporeal membranous oxygenation (ECMO) can be used in patients with a competent aortic valve.

2. **Chronic Mitral Regurgitation**

   a. **Symptomatic patients:** The majority of patients with chronic moderately severe to severe primary MR that is symptomatic should be considered for surgery (Table 14.2).

      In the case of chronic moderately severe to severe secondary MR, surgery should be considered for patients with refractory symptoms despite aggressive medical management. For patients with moderate to severe ischemic MR, it is suggested that valve repair or replacement be done concomitantly with coronary artery bypass graft (CABG) (Table 14.3).

   b. **Asymptomatic patients:** In asymptomatic patients, the goal is to identify and monitor patients with severe MR and intervene before permanent left

TABLE 14.1 Causes of Mitral Valve Disease

Regurgitation

- Myxomatous degeneration
- Infective endocarditis
- Rheumatic heart disease
- Congenital heart disease (clefts, hypertrophic obstructive cardiomyopathy)
- Annular dilatation
- Papillary muscle rupture
- Ischemic heart disease

Stenosis

- Rheumatic heart disease
- Infective endocarditis
- Mitral annular calcification
- Carcinoid
- Autoimmune disease
- Congenital heart disease

TABLE 14.2 Summary of AHA/ACC Recommendations in Chronic Primary Mitral Regurgitation

	Level of Evidence
Class I	
Mitral valve surgery is recommended for symptomatic patients with chronic severe primary MR and LVEF greater than 30%.	B
Mitral valve surgery is recommended for asymptomatic patients with chronic severe primary MR and left ventricular dysfunction (LVEF 30–60% and/or LVESD ≥40 mm).	
Mitral valve repair is recommended in preference to mitral valve replacement when surgical treatment is indicated for patients with chronic severe primary MR limited to the posterior leaflet.	
Mitral valve repair is recommended in preference to mitral valve replacement when surgical treatment is indicated for patients with chronic severe primary MR involving the anterior leaflet or both leaflets when a successful and durable repair can be accomplished.	
Concomitant mitral valve repair or replacement is indicated in patients with chronic severe primary MR undergoing cardiac surgery for other indications.	

TABLE 14.2 Summary of AHA/ACC Recommendations in Chronic Primary MR *(continued)*

	Level of Evidence
Class IIa	
Mitral valve repair is reasonable in asymptomatic patients with chronic severe primary MR with preserved left ventricular function (LVEF >60% and LVESD <40 mm) in whom the likelihood of a successful and durable repair without residual MR is >95% with an expected mortality rate of <1% when performed at a Heart Valve Center of Excellence.	B
Mitral valve repair is reasonable for asymptomatic patients with chronic severe nonrheumatic primary MR and preserved left ventricular function in whom there is a high likelihood of a successful and durable repair with (1) new onset of atrial fibrillation or (2) resting pulmonary hypertension (PA systolic arterial pressure >50 mm Hg).	B
Concomitant mitral valve repair is reasonable in patients with chronic moderate primary MR undergoing cardiac surgery for other indications.	C
Class IIb	
Mitral valve surgery may be considered in symptomatic patients with chronic severe primary MR and LVEF ≤30%.	C
Mitral valve repair may be considered in patients with rheumatic mitral valve disease when surgical treatment is indicated if a durable and successful repair is likely or if the reliability of long-term anticoagulation management is questionable.	B
Transcatheter mitral valve repair may be considered for severely symptomatic patients (NYHA class III/IV) with chronic severe primary MR who have a reasonable life expectancy but a prohibitive surgical risk.	B
Class III	
Mitral valve replacement should not be performed for treatment of isolated severe primary MR limited to less than one-half of the posterior leaflet unless mitral valve repair has been attempted and was unsuccessful.	C

AHA/ACC, American Heart Association/American College of Cardiology; LVEF, left ventricular ejection fraction; LVESD, left ventricular end-systolic diameter; MR, mitral regurgitation; NYHA, New York Heart Association; PA, pulmonary artery.

TABLE 14.3 Summary of AHA/ACC Recommendations in Chronic Severe Secondary Mitral Regurgitation

	Level of Evidence
Class IIa	
Mitral valve surgery is reasonable for patients with chronic severe secondary MR who are undergoing CABG or AVR.	C
Class IIb	
Mitral valve surgery may be considered for severely symptomatic patients (NYHA class III/IV) with chronic severe secondary MR.	B
Mitral valve repair may be considered for patients with chronic moderate secondary MR (stage B) who are undergoing other cardiac surgery.	C

AHA/ACC, American Heart Association/American College of Cardiology; AVR, aortic valve replacement; CABG, coronary artery bypass graft; MR, mitral regurgitation; NYHA, New York Heart Association.

ventricular dysfunction or left ventricular dilatation. If a durable repair can be achieved at a center of excellence or there is new-onset atrial fibrillation or resting pulmonary hypertension, then it is reasonable to intervene in asymptomatic severe primary MR.

3. **Mitral stenosis:** Percutaneous mitral balloon commissurotomy (PMBC) is indicated for severe symptomatic MS. Surgical intervention should be considered in patients with severe symptomatic MS who are not candidates for PMBC or who are undergoing surgery for other cardiac lesions. See Chapter 4, Table 4.5 ("Indications for Intervention in Patients with Mitral Stenosis [MS] According to the 2014 ACC/ AHA Guidelines").

C. **Contraindications.** Patients who are too frail to tolerate an operation should not undergo surgical repair. This may be due to advanced age and comorbid conditions. The Society of Thoracic Surgeons (STS) risk score and EuroSCORE are assessment tools that can aid in identifying patients who are too high risk for surgery.

Though not an absolute contraindication, severe mitral annular calcification can make repair and replacement difficult and increase the risk for atrioventricular dissociation. Patients with severe pulmonary hypertension with associated right heart failure are at increased risk for poor outcomes with mitral valve surgery.

D. **Evaluation.** A detailed history and physical examination should first be obtained to identify symptoms and discern comorbidities and patient frailty. The primary modality for interrogation of the mitral valve is echocardiography. A transthoracic echocardiogram should be obtained to determine ventricular function, mitral valve pathophysiology, and the status of the other heart valves. Factors such as severe mitral calcification and extensive damage from endocarditis may prohibit repair. Exercise echocardiography can aid in analyzing left ventricular adaptation to a regurgitant mitral valve. Failure of the left ventricular ejection fraction to increase with exercise is suggestive of diminished reserve.

If the valve is not adequately visualized, transesophageal echocardiography (TEE) should be considered. All patients undergoing PMBC should have preprocedure TEE, and those going for surgical repair should have intraoperative TEE. Sedation may result in decreased afterload and downgrade the degree of MR. Increasingly, cardiac MRI can be used to evaluate chronic MR when echocardiography is insufficient.

E. **Preoperative management.** Mitral valve regurgitation and stenosis both increase the risk for pulmonary edema. Careful diuresis is important to unload the pulmonary vasculature but should not be excessive so as to maintain adequate preload for left ventricular filling. As discussed previously, afterload reduction with vasodilators can improve forward flow and decrease regurgitation through the valve; however, these therapies do not influence the progression of MR. In the unstable patient, IABP and ECMO can be considered.

In the case of MS, patients may require agents to promote sinus rhythm, such as β-blockers or calcium channel blockers.

F. **Surgical intervention.** Open surgical intervention on the mitral valve can be approached through a full sternotomy, partial sternotomy, or right thoracotomy or via the right chest with robotic assistance (Fig. 14.1). The valve can be surgically accessed through a left atrial incision, through a right atrial and trans-septal incision, or rarely via an aortotomy and through the aortic valve (although this can be quite limiting). Concomitant Maze procedure with ligation or clipping of the left atrial appendage is recommended if the patient has atrial fibrillation.

1. **Repair of the mitral valve**
   a. Technique for repair of the mitral valve is dependent on lesion pathology. For degenerative disease resulting in posterior leaflet prolapse or flail, a resection technique can be employed. A portion of the leaflet can be excised (quadrangular or triangular resection) and the remaining leaflet tissue reapproximated and sutured into place.
   b. Another strategy for managing redundant and prolapsing posterior leaflet tissue is suture plication of the diseased portion. Excess leaflet tissue can be folded over itself and secured in place. If the commissure is damaged, it may also be plicated if there is a sufficient valve orifice.

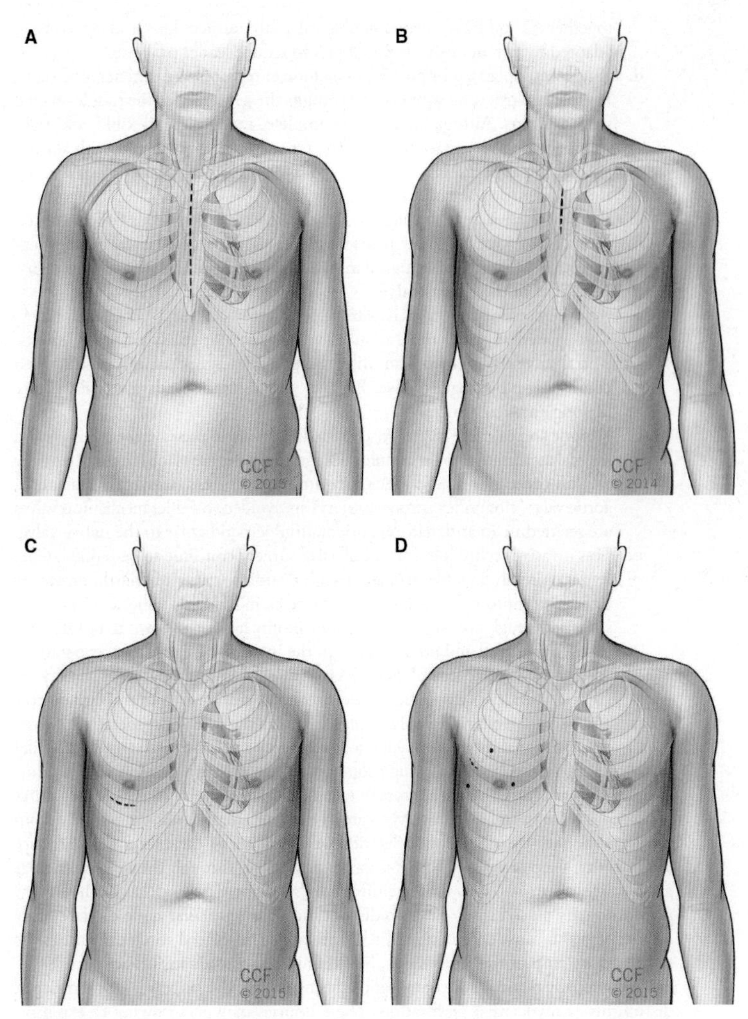

FIGURE 14.1 Incisional approaches for mitral valve surgery. The skin incisions are denoted by the dashed lines. Full sternotomy **(A)**, hemisternotomy **(B)**, right minithoracotomy **(C)**, and thoracoscopic ports **(D)**. (Reprinted with permission, Cleveland Clinic Center for Medical Art & Photography. Copyright 2015. All rights reserved.)

c. Prolapse of the anterior leaflet is far less common and requires use of different techniques for repair. Because of its smaller area, resection is used sparingly to reduce redundant tissue. Instead, chordae are transferred from the posterior to anterior leaflet or artificial chordae are constructed to support areas of prolapse. In another technique, a figure-of-eight (Alfieri) stitch may be placed, suturing together A2 and P2 to create a double-inlet valve orifice. This strategy has been adapted by percutaneous technologies to reduce leaflet prolapse.

d. Ring annuloplasty is important to include in repair of the degenerative valve. It provides structural support and realigns the geometry of the saddle-shaped valve annulus. Although there are complete, incomplete, flexible, and rigid rings, there are few data to favor one type. The ring is secured with sutures around the annulus, taking care not to injure the circumflex coronary artery, the atrioventricular node, or the aortic valve.

e. For mitral valve stenosis, the first-line therapy is percutaneous balloon mitral commissurotomy. When percutaneous therapy is not feasible (severe calcification, combined MS and MR), surgical mitral valve replacement is generally necessary.

2. **Replacement of the mitral valve**

a. Replacement of the valve is warranted when repair or PMBC is not possible, generally when there is subvalvular fusion or thick, calcified leaflets. Mitral valve replacement can utilize bioprosthetic, mechanical, or much less commonly a homograft valve. Patients with a mechanical valve will require lifelong anticoagulation.

b. Fibrotic and calcified tissues are debrided with care to preserve the papillary and chordal attachments to the annulus. Pledgeted sutures are placed circumferentially around the annulus, and previously noted structures (atrioventricular node, aortic valve, circumflex coronary artery) are avoided. Bileaflet mechanical valves are secured in an antianatomic orientation perpendicular to the native valve.

c. Less invasive techniques for mitral valve surgery continue to be refined. Current minimally invasive strategies access cardiac structures via thoracotomy or hemisternotomy. In appropriately selected individuals, robotic mitral valve surgery through port sites or minithoracotomy has been shown to be safe with excellent survival and no difference in the incidence of stroke or reoperation. Alternative interventional therapies for patients not candidates for surgery are currently under investigation. These technologies include mitral clip devices and percutaneous mitral valve replacement. In the case of degenerative disease, interventional modalities will need to continue addressing the leaflet/chordal apparatus and reestablishing proper annulus geometry for a durable repair.

G. **Complications.** Intraoperative errors in technique can result in injuries to structures surrounding the mitral annulus. Myocardial ischemia may develop separately from cardiopulmonary bypass owing to ligation or distortion of the circumflex coronary artery with a deep annular stitch as it passes posteriorly through the atrioventricular groove. Treatment is removal of the offending stitch or CABG distal to the injury. An improperly placed stitch can also disrupt the atrioventricular node directly or by local edema and cause conduction block. Similarly, a misplaced stitch can entrap the noncoronary cusp of the aortic valve, resulting in acute aortic insufficiency.

A potentially catastrophic complication during mitral valve surgery is atrioventricular disruption or myocardial perforation. These injuries may occur owing to extensive annular debridement or strut protrusion as a result of elevation and manipulation of the heart when a prosthetic valve is in place.

Following a mitral valve repair, systolic anterior motion (SAM) of the anterior mitral leaflet may obstruct the left ventricular outflow tract. This is more likely to occur in situations of bileaflet prolapse and when there is excess leaflet tissue. SAM should be detected by intraoperative TEE. Further reduction of the posterior leaflet or larger-ring annuloplasty may be required.

Long-term complications include thromboembolic events and endocarditis. Patients with bioprosthetic valves and those with mechanical valves on therapeutic anticoagulation experience similar risks of thromboembolic events of 1% to 2% per year. Rates of endocarditis are also similar at less than 1% per year.

H. Outcomes. The durability of mitral valve repair is tied to the underlying etiology. For degenerative valve disease, freedom from reoperation is >90% at 10 years compared with 60% for functional or rheumatic disease. Postoperative survival is excellent with 30-day mortality of 1% or less for the treatment of degenerative disease in experienced centers; if the etiology is functional MR, early mortality approaches 5%.

Mortality for isolated mitral valve replacement is slightly increased compared with repair. In-hospital mortality has been reported to range from 5% to 9% in recent analyses of large administrative databases. Bioprosthetic valves degenerate over time, and at 15 years there will be structural failure in approximately 50% of surviving patients. Mechanical valves are resistant to degeneration, but carry with them bleeding risks associated with therapeutic anticoagulation.

II. THE TRICUSPID VALVE

A. Introduction. The tricuspid valve apparatus is composed of the tricuspid annulus, chordae tendinae, and papillary muscles along with three leaflets: the septal, anterior, and posterior leaflets.

The most common cause of tricuspid regurgitation (TR) is dilatation of the right ventricle, producing functional regurgitation with anatomically normal valve leaflets. This can be secondary to pulmonary hypertension from lesions of the mitral and aortic valves, or cor pulmonale. Other etiologies of TR are those that cause structural valve abnormalities. These include congenital malformations, rheumatic disease, degenerative disease, carcinoid disease, infective endocarditis, leaflet entrapment, leaflet scarring due to intracardiac pacemaker leads, or damage to the leaflets from lead extraction and chest radiation (Table 14.4).

TABLE 14.4 Causes of Tricuspid Valve Disease

Regurgitation
Right ventricle dilatation (secondary tricuspid regurgitation)
Infective endocarditis
Rheumatic heart disease
Congenital heart disease (Ebstein anomaly)
Connective tissue disease
Papillary dysfunction
Ischemia/infarction
Radiation
Pacemaker/extraction-related lead injuries
Stenosis
Rheumatic heart disease
Carcinoid
Congenital heart disease
Infective endocarditis

The cause of tricuspid stenosis (TS) is most frequently rheumatic heart disease (>90%). Less common causes include carcinoid heart disease, infective endocarditis, and congenital heart disease (Table 14.4).

B. Indications

1. **Tricuspid regurgitation:** As reflected in current guidelines (Table 14.5), interventions on the tricuspid valve are indicated when concomitant left-sided valve surgery is performed and severe TR or moderate functional TR exists. In the setting of long-standing significant pulmonary hypertension that has developed from mitral disease, it is important to consider that TR will likely not improve with left-sided intervention alone.

   Isolated TR can be well tolerated and medically managed, and as such intervention can often be avoided. Isolated tricuspid surgery may be considered for severe symptomatic TR that is refractory to medical therapy, or minimally symptomatic severe TR with progressive dilatation of the right ventricle (Table 14.5).
2. **Tricuspid stenosis:** Surgery is recommended for patients with severe TS undergoing surgery for left-sided lesions, or in patients with isolated TS that is severely symptomatic (Table 14.6).

C. Contraindications. Patients who are too frail to tolerate an operation should not undergo surgical repair. This may be due to advanced age and comorbid conditions. STS risk score and EuroSCORE are assessment tools that can aid in identifying patients who are too high risk for surgery. The presence of cardiac cirrhosis should be carefully assessed, as this can be an important additional risk factor in these patients.

TABLE 14.5 Summary of AHA/ACC Recommendations in Tricuspid Regurgitation

	Level of Evidence
Class I	
TV surgery is recommended for patients with severe TR undergoing left-sided valve surgery.	C
Class IIa	
TV repair can be beneficial for patients with mild, moderate, or greater functional TR at the time of left-sided valve surgery with tricuspid annular dilatation OR prior evidence of right-sided heart failure.	B
TV surgery can be beneficial for patients with symptoms due to severe primary TR refractory to medical therapy.	C
Class IIb	
TV repair may be considered for patients with moderate functional TR and pulmonary artery hypertension at the time of left-sided valve surgery.	C
TV surgery may be considered for asymptomatic or minimally symptomatic patients with severe primary TR and progressive moderate or greater RV dilatation and/or systolic dysfunction.	C
Reoperation for isolated TV repair or replacement may be considered for persistent symptoms due to severe TR in patients who have undergone previous left-sided valve surgery and who do not have severe pulmonary hypertension or significant RV systolic dysfunction.	C

AHA/ACC, American Heart Association/American College of Cardiology; RV, right ventricular; TR, tricuspid regurgitation; TV, tricuspid valve.

TABLE 14.6 Summary of AHA/ACC Recommendations in Tricuspid Stenosis

	Level of Evidence
Class I	
TV surgery is recommended for patients with severe TS at the time of operation for left-sided valve disease.	C
TV surgery is recommended for patients with isolated, symptomatic severe TS.	C
Class IIb	
PBTC might be considered in patients with isolated, symptomatic severe TS without accompanying TR.	C

AHA/ACC, American Heart Association/American College of Cardiology; PBTC, percutaneous balloon tricuspid commissurotomy; TR, tricuspid regurgitation; TS, tricuspid stenosis; TV, tricuspid valve.

D. Evaluation. A detailed history and physical examination should first be obtained to identify symptoms and discern comorbidities and patient frailty. Transthoracic echocardiography is indicated to evaluate TR and TS. The valve anatomy, lesion severity, and associated defects can be identified.

In the event of discordant or insufficient data, invasive hemodynamic measurements by right heart catheterization should be considered. For patients with severe TR and inadequate transthoracic echocardiograms, cardiac MRI can be an important tool for the assessment of right ventricular characteristics.

E. Preoperative management. Maintaining sinus rhythm that preserves atrial contractions can help to improve cardiac output. Patients with regurgitation may benefit from a faster heart rate, and those with stenosis benefit from a slower rate. Diuresis can help to improve symptoms of right heart failure; however, elevated central venous pressures are necessary to drive forward flow through the right heart.

F. Surgical intervention. Open surgical intervention (generally via full or partial sternotomy) on the tricuspid valve is achieved through a right atrial incision.

1. **Repair of the tricuspid valve:** The primary strategy for surgical repair of TR (which is predominantly functional) is ring annuloplasty. With dilatation of the right ventricle, the annulus is primarily distorted in the anterior–posterior axis because the septal wall and leaflet are more fixed. Annuloplasty rings are sutured in place to restore a normal size and shape and to promote leaflet coaptation. The rings may be complete or incomplete (open). Rings are designed to avoid placing stitches near the atrioventricular node and spare damage to the conduction system. Alternative strategies to repair the tricuspid valve include bicuspidization and annulus suture plication (DeVega technique) of the valve.
2. **Replacement of the tricuspid valve:** If the valve is not amenable to repair, it can be replaced with a prosthesis. Severe TS requires balloon valvuloplasty or replacement. Choices for prosthesis include mechanical, bioprosthetic (intra-annular or supraannular), or more rarely homograft (mitral valve tissue) versions. Mechanical valves do require lifelong anticoagulation, which must be considered. When implanting the valve, care is taken to avoid injuring the atrioventricular node. The leaflets and chordae of the valvular apparatus should be preserved.

G. Complications. Because of the proximity of the atrioventricular node and conduction system to the tricuspid annulus, there is risk for complete heart block postoperatively. In patients with both mitral and tricuspid prosthetic valves, late occurrence of complete heart block is approximately 25% at 10 years. If abnormalities in the conduction system are present preoperatively, an epicardial pacemaker lead can be placed at the time of surgery to avoid later transvenous lead placement through a repaired/replaced tricuspid valve.

There is no difference in overall survival between patients with bioprosthetic and mechanical prosthetic tricuspid valves. However, mechanical valves carry a risk of thrombosis of approximately 1% per year. This complication is generally managed with thrombolysis.

H. Outcomes. Tricuspid repair with annuloplasty rings yields up to 85% freedom from moderate-to-severe recurrent TR at 6 years. Rigid ring annuloplasty has greater freedom from recurrent regurgitation than suture plication or bicuspidization of the valve.

TR most frequently occurs secondary to left-sided valve lesions, and it will often persist even after correction of the left-sided pathologic lesion. Although practice patterns are shifting toward concomitant TV annuloplasty at time of mitral repair, it is uncertain if long-term rates of right heart failure and mortality will decrease. Patients requiring simultaneous mitral and tricuspid valve replacement have operative mortality rates of 5% to 10%, and 55% at 10 years. Reoperations for tricuspid valve repair are associated with both high short- and long-term mortality rates.

KEY PEARLS

- Isolated symptomatic severe MS and TS are treated first with balloon commissurotomy if valve anatomy is favorable.
- Mitral valve posterior leaflet prolapse should be repaired with leaflet resection and annulus support with an annuloplasty ring.
- Outcomes of mitral valve repair are dependent on etiology of the regurgitation.
- TR is most commonly functional owing to right ventricular dilatation.
- Repair of the mitral valve may not improve TR if long-standing pulmonary hypertension has been present.
- During replacement of the mitral and tricuspid valves, care should be taken to maintain papillary or chordal attachments to the annulus.

SUGGESTED READINGS

Cao C, Wolfenden H, Liou K, et al. A meta-analysis of robotic vs. conventional mitral valve surgery. *Ann Cardiothorac Surg.* 2015;4:305–314.

Cohn LH, ed. *Cardiac Surgery in the Adult.* 4th ed. China: McGraw-Hill; 2012.

Cohn LH, Tchantchaleishvili V, Rajab TK. Evolution of the concept and practice of mitral valve repair. *Ann Cardiothorac Surg.* 2015;4:315–321.

Filsoufi F, Anyanwu AC, Salzberg SP, et al. Long-term outcomes of tricuspid valve replacement in the current era. *Ann Thorac Surg.* 2005;80:845–850.

Griffin BP, Callahan TD, Menon V, eds. *Manual of Cardiovascular Medicine.* 4th ed. Philadelphia, PA: Lippincott Williams & Wilkins; 2013.

Johnston DR, Gillinov AM, Blackstone EH, et al. Surgical repair of posterior mitral valve prolapse: implications for guidelines and percutaneous repair. *Ann Thorac Surg.* 2010;89:1385–1394.

Kilic A, Shah AS, Conte JV, et al. Operative outcomes in mitral valve surgery: combined effect of surgeon and hospital volume in a population-based analysis. *J Thorac Cardiovasc Surg.* 2013;146:638–646.

Mick SL, Keshavamurthy S, Gillinov AM. Mitral valve repair versus replacement. *Ann Cardiothorac Surg.* 2015;4:230–237.

Mihaljevic T, Jarrett CM, Gillinov AM, et al. Robotic repair of posterior mitral valve prolapse versus conventional approaches: potential realized. *J Thorac Cardiovasc Surg.* 2011;141:72–80.

Nishimura RA, Otto CM, Bonow RO, et al. 2014 AHA/ACC guideline for the management of patients with valvular heart disease: a report of the American College of Cardiology/American Heart Association Task Force on Practice Guidelines. *J Thorac Cardiovasc Surg.* 2014;148:e1–e132.

Rogers JH, Bolling SF. The tricuspid valve: current perspective and evolving management of tricuspid regurgitation. *Circulation.* 2009;119:2718–2725.

Stout KK, Verrier ED. Acute valvular regurgitation. *Circulation.* 2009;119:3232–3241.

Tang GHL, David TE, Singh SK, et al. Tricuspid valve repair with an annuloplasty ring results in improved long-term outcomes. *Circulation.* 2006;114:I-577–I-581.

Vassileva CM, Mishkel G, McNeely C et al. Long-term survival of patients undergoing mitral valve repair and replacement: a longitudinal analysis of Medicare fee-for-service beneficiaries. *Circulation.* 2013;127:1870–1876.

CHAPTER 15

Douglas R. Johnston

Valve Surgery: Aortic/Pulmonary

I. INTRODUCTION

The aortic and pulmonic valves share similar structure and functional anatomy. Both prevent regurgitation of blood into the ventricle during diastole, and in normal function provide an unimpeded flow of blood from the ventricular outflow tract to the aorta or pulmonary artery (PA). Both are trileaflet in normal configuration, and rely on adequate coaptation of three similarly sized semilunar valve cusps for valve competence. Normal valve function depends on the shape and flexibility of the leaflets, size and orientation of the annulus and sinuses, and the orientation of the commissures between leaflets. Surgical therapy for the aortic and pulmonic valves may be appropriately categorized based on the indication—stenosis versus regurgitation, whether repair or replacement is feasible, whether any adjunctive procedures are required, and the surgical approach. Although the valves share similar anatomy, the pulmonic valve does not share a fibrous skeleton with adjacent valves as does the aortic valve (Fig. 15.1). This has important considerations for evaluation of sizing and concomitant valve procedures.

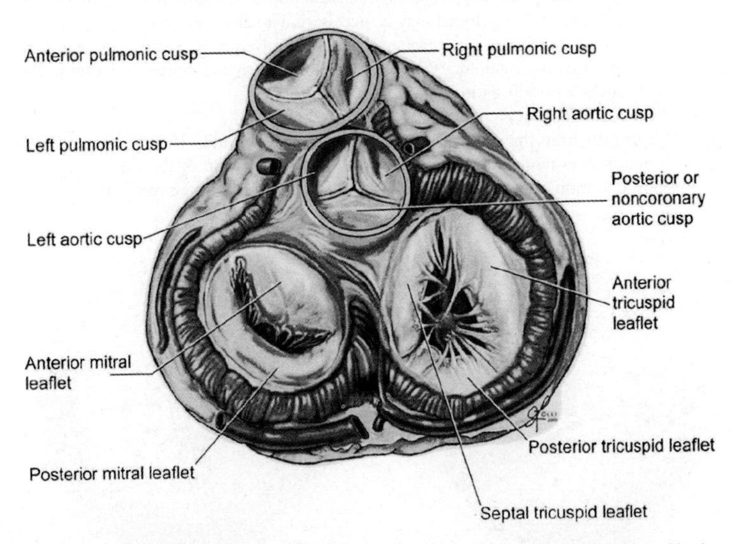

FIGURE 15.1 Relations of the aortic and pulmonic valves. Note the aortic, mitral, and tricuspid valves share a fibrous skeleton, whereas the pulmonic valve annulus shares a muscular connection with the other three valves.

II. AORTIC VALVE INDICATIONS

A. Aortic stenosis

The most common indication for operation on the aortic valve is aortic stenosis (AS), and the most common cause of AS is degenerative valve calcification. Although small amounts of collagen disruption and calcific deposits on aortic valves are common in people without clinically evident aortic valve disease, significant aortic valve calcification is rare before the age of 30 years in patients with tricuspid aortic valves. Accelerated calcification may occur in patients with bicuspid or unicuspid valves. The histopathology of calcific AS is similar to that of atherosclerotic coronary disease, and shares similar risk factors at least in patients with tricuspid valve anatomy. This has prompted research into the potential for lipid-lowering therapy to alter the progression of calcific AS.

Rheumatic disease of the aortic valve is characterized by an early inflammatory phase consisting of edema, lymphocyte infiltration, and neovascularization. This is followed by a proliferative phase in which leaflets become thickened and retracted, with rolled edges and commissural fusion. Valve leaflets may become severely calcified, although annular calcification is rare.

Congenital alteration in the number and orientation of the aortic valve leaflets may result in bicuspid (Fig. 15.2), unicuspid, or quadricuspid morphology. Of these, bicuspid valves are most common, and are present in approximately 2% of the general population, with a male to female ratio of 2:1. They are more common in first-degree relatives with bicuspid valves.

The calcification present in stenotic aortic valves may be limited to the leaflets, or may extend into the annulus, interventricular septum, or anterior leaflet of the mitral valve. Calcium may exist primarily as surface deposits or extend deep into the surrounding tissues. Even mature lamellar bone formation may occur in very calcified aortic valves. Removal of invasive calcium requires care to avoid injuring surrounding structures, and when injury occurs reconstruction of the annulus with autologous pericardium or other material may be necessary. The distribution of calcification has implications for surgical approach and choice of valve prosthesis. Figure 15.3 shows the computed tomographic (CT) appearance of a heavily calcified unicuspid valve, with calcium invading into the ventricular septum.

B. Aortic insufficiency

Derangement in the integrity or morphology of the annulus, leaflets, or sinotubular junction may result in aortic insufficiency (AI). Dilatation of the aortic root is the most common cause of AI in North America. Dilatation of the sinotubular junction,

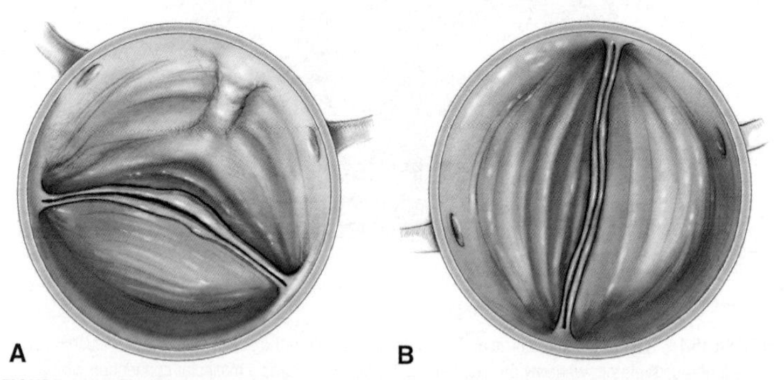

FIGURE 15.2 Bicuspid aortic valve morphology. **A:** The common finding of fusion of the left and right coronary cusps, separated by a raphe. **B:** The uncommon "true" bicuspid valve with equal length cusps and only two commissures.

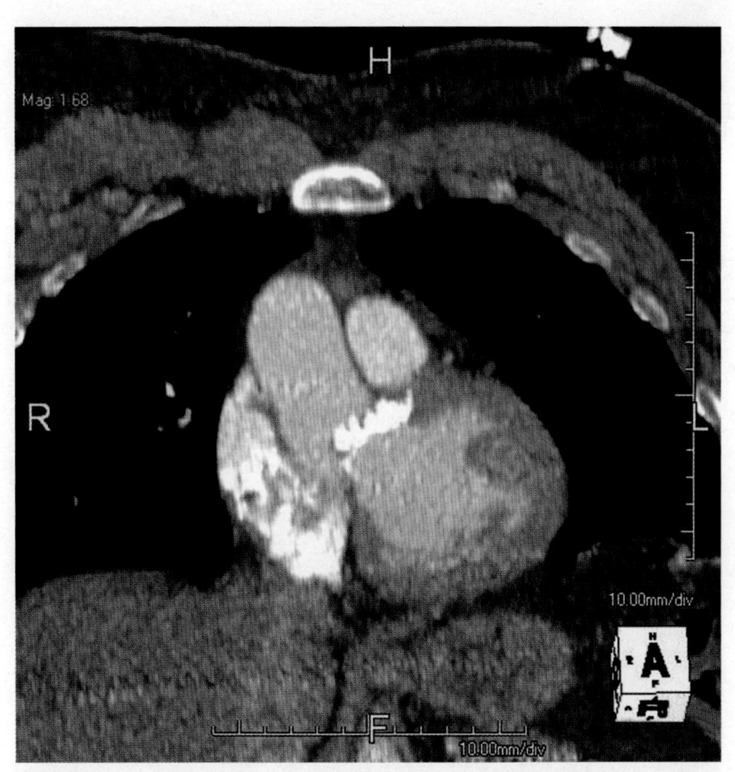

FIGURE 15.3 Computed tomographyic appearance of severe aortic valve calcification, in this case associated with a unicuspid valve, invasive into the ventricular septum.

with relative sparing of the leaflets and annulus, is associated with atherosclerotic ascending aortic aneurysm and AI in older patients.

Patients with degenerative calcific aortic valve disease often have a mixture of AS and AI; as leaflets become stiffened, fixed, and retracted, coaptation is impaired. In a similar fashion, rheumatic heart disease leads to AI through fixation of the leaflets.

Congenital bicuspid valve disease may produce insufficiency via fibrosis and calcification in a manner similar to a degenerated calcified tricuspid valve. In addition, distortion and stretching of the leaflets may result in malcoaptation, in which one leaflet overrides another leading to an eccentrically directed regurgitant jet.

Aortic dissection often produces severe regurgitation in an otherwise anatomically normal valve when the commissures and associated intima are detached from the aortic adventitia and prolapse inward.

Bacterial endocarditis may account for 10% or more of AI. Healed endocarditis lesions may present as an isolated leaflet perforation in an otherwise normal-appearing valve.

Less common etiologies of regurgitation include injury to the valve from blunt or penetrating chest trauma, iatrogenic injury to the leaflets during catheter procedures, and suture injuries during mitral valve surgery.

C. Pulmonic stenosis

Pulmonic stenosis in developed countries occurs most commonly as a result of congenital heart defects, prior surgical or endovascular intervention, or rarely rheumatic disease.

D. Pulmonic insufficiency

Pulmonary insufficiency occurs mostly as a result of annular enlargement, congenital malformations, prior intervention, or pulmonary hypertension.

III. EVALUATION

A. Aortic stenosis

Noninvasive measurement of aortic valve gradients extrapolated from aortic jet velocity on two-dimensional echocardiography has been shown to be the most reproducible and accurate method of grading AS, such that catheter measurement of aortic valve gradients is uncommon except in select cases (see low-gradient AS, later). Recent reports have suggested that gated cardiac CT may provide more precise measurements of aortic valve morphology and area than echocardiography. Evaluation of AS by gated CT may be of particular value in patients being considered for transcatheter aortic valve implantation, because it provides data on the anatomic relationship between leaflet calcification and the coronary ostia (Fig. 15.4). Cardiac CT, cardiac magnetic resonance imaging (MRI), and three-dimensional (3D) echocardiography all have the potential to provide direct (anatomic) measurement of aortic valve area (AVA). However, they may all underestimate the functional severity of AS, which depends on the dynamic interaction between the ejecting ventricle, outflow tract, and aortic

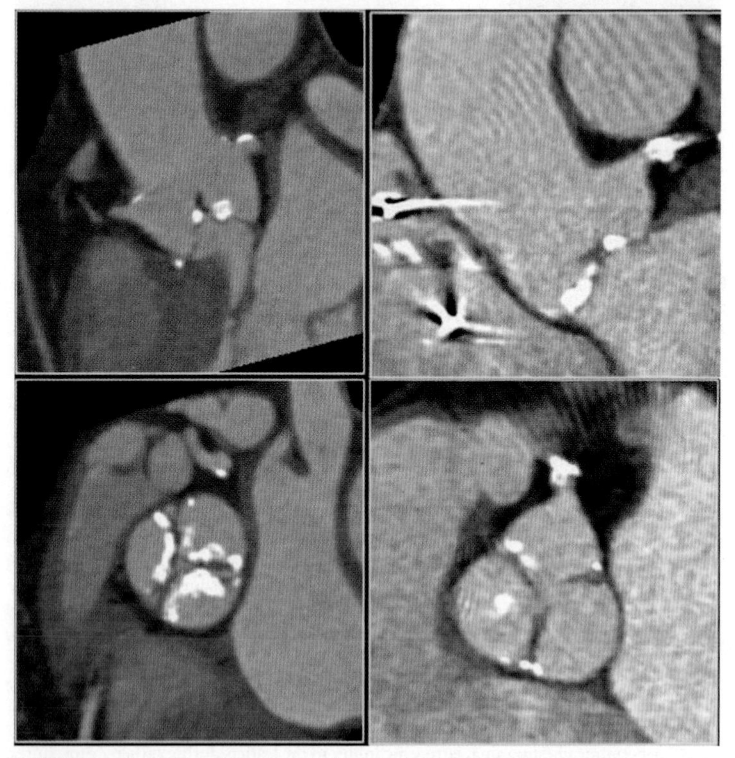

FIGURE 15.4 Computed tomographic evaluation of aortic valve calcium location and extent in relation to coronary ostia.

valve orifice. Thus, a decision on timing for surgery in AS must take into account the etiology, chronicity, the condition of the ventricle, degree of concomitant AI, and the presence of associated valve or coronary lesions.

1. **AS grading table**

Grade	AVA (cm^2)
Mild	>1.5
Moderate	1–1.5
Severe	<1

2. **Natural history**
Much has been learned about the natural history of AS since the landmark study published by Ross and Braunwald in 1968. The classic symptom triad of angina, syncope, and dyspnea has since served as a hallmark for the evaluation of patients with AS. These investigators reported a survival of 3 years with angina and syncope, 2 years with dyspnea, and 1.5 years with heart failure. These dismal survival statistics in untreated symptomatic AS, corroborated by a number of subsequent studies, have since driven recommendations for aggressive operative therapy in patients with symptomatic severe AS. The appropriate treatment of asymptomatic patients is more controversial, however. Estimates of the rate of sudden death in asymptomatic AS are generally in the range of 1% per year. In addition, one-third of asymptomatic patients with severe AS will become symptomatic within 2 years. Two-thirds of patients will proceed to aortic valve replacement (AVR) or cardiac death within 5 years of diagnosis. A significant proportion of "asymptomatic" patients have markers of more advanced disease such as severe left ventricular hypertrophy (LVH) or decreased ejection fraction (EF), and many have a positive stress test. Exercise stress testing is likely underutilized in this population. Asymptomatic patients with a positive stress test have a prognosis similar to that of symptomatic patients and should be offered early surgery.

3. **Medical treatment**
Given the pathologic link between AS and coronary disease, there has been enthusiasm for using lipid-lowering drugs to slow the progression of leaflet disease. Despite high expectations, results have been mixed. The SEAS study, a randomized controlled trial of 1,873 patients with mild–moderate asymptomatic AS receiving simvastatin and ezetimibe or placebo, failed to show any reduction in AS-related events in the lipid-lowering arm. Efforts to find a medical treatment that is effective in reducing severity or progression of AS are ongoing. At present, medical treatment in AS is aimed at hemodynamic stabilization in asymptomatic patients and control of comorbid conditions.

   Hypertension control may help alleviate LVH; however, overmedication raises the risk of decompensation in patients who are dependent on already reduced diastolic pressure for coronary perfusion in a hypertensive ventricle. Angiotensin-converting enzyme inhibitors have been shown to provide short-term benefit in hypertensive patients with AS. Atrial fibrillation may have a significant adverse impact in patients with AS who are particularly dependent on atrial contraction for diastolic filling; therefore, cardioversion and rhythm control are important considerations both before and after AVR. Endocarditis prophylaxis is indicated in all patients with AS.

4. **Timing of intervention for AS**
Published guidelines support AVR in symptomatic patients with severe AS. Patients without clear symptoms, or with symptoms but equivocal echo findings present

a clinical challenge. In these patients, the surgeon must weigh the individual risks of AVR with watchful waiting, which may include a potential for sudden cardiac death, as well as ongoing LV remodeling. LVH as measured on routine electrocardiogram is an independent predictor of symptom development in severe AS, albeit with low sensitivity. Development of symptoms during exercise stress testing is a predictor of symptom development within 12 months. Onset of symptoms in a patient with severe AS who has been previously asymptomatic portends a poor prognosis; however, patients often subconsciously reduce their activity levels and may therefore fail to report "symptoms." Exercise testing may be particularly valuable in these patients.

Iung et al. estimate that at least one-third of patients with symptomatic, severe isolated AS do not undergo surgical repair. These data have been confirmed in multiple studies; however, the number of untreated patients may decrease with wider application of transcatheter aortic valve replacement (TAVR). The fact that even elderly patients benefit from AVR in almost all cases and a large number of "asymptomatic" patients have markers for worse surgical outcome argues for an aggressive approach to early surgery.

5. **Low gradient–low flow AS**

In this subset of patients with anatomic AS who do not demonstrate increased gradients at rest (<40 mm Hg), operative mortality may be as high as 18%, with a 3-year survival of only 57%. Essential to the work-up of these patients is determining whether the etiology of ventricular dysfunction is secondary to ischemic scar or cardiomyopathy, or excessive afterload. Low-dose dobutamine stress echocardiography serves to diagnose those patients with adequate contractile reserve (CR), defined as a ≥20% increase in stroke volume from baseline. Absence of adequate CR is predictive of perioperative mortality. The TOPAS multicenter study of low flow–low gradient AS suggests that patients with this syndrome may benefit from AVR, with AVA as high as 1.2 cm^2, suggesting that even moderate AS may be poorly tolerated in the setting of lower LV CR. Most significant risk factors for poor outcome were impaired functional capacity as measured by Duke activity status index or 6-minute walk test distance, more severe stenosis, and reduced peak stress left ventricular ejection fraction (LVEF). However, both functional status and LVEF improved in patients surviving AVR. Properly selected patients fare better with AVR than with medical therapy.

B. Aortic insufficiency

Evaluation of AI should aim to determine the mechanism, morphology of the leaflets, and concomitant aortic root and ascending aortic disease that guide the pathway for surgical therapy.

Echocardiographic evaluation should focus on leaflet morphology, thickness, mobility, and coaptation. In addition to severity of AI, echocardiographic evaluation is essential to make a preoperative assessment of valve repairability.

With the exception of aortic dissection, trileaflet valves amenable to repair exhibit normal leaflet morphology and mobility, with malcoaptation caused by dilatation of the aortic root and/or sinotubular junction. Bileaflet valves may exhibit eccentric regurgitation related to relative prolapse of the conjoined cusp in addition to dilatation. Thickening, calcification, fenestrations, or other leaflet anomalies suggest a lower probability of successful repair.

Three-dimensional imaging of the aortic root and ascending aorta by CT or MRI is essential in evaluating bicuspid valve patients or those with trileaflet valves with root or ascending aortic enlargement. Wide availability of desktop programs for multiplanar 3D reconstruction has allowed for detailed evaluation of the root and ascending aorta from the surgeon's perspective.

IV. PERIOPERATIVE MANAGEMENT

A. Preoperative work-up

1. **Transthoracic echocardiography.** For aortic valve disease, evaluation of gradients, valve area, degree of regurgitation, valve morphology, ascending aortic dilatation/PA dilatation, concomitant valve disease, and ventricular function is necessary. For pulmonic valve disease, particular attention should be paid to estimation of pulmonary hypertension.
2. **Coronary angiography.** This is done for evaluation of coronary anatomy, presence/absence of coronary anomalies, and coronary disease requiring concomitant bypass.
3. Routine laboratory evaluation includes complete blood count, electrolytes, blood urea nitrogen/creatinine ratio, liver function tests, urinalysis, urine culture, prothrombin time/partial thromboplastin time, and a current blood bank sample.
4. **Chest and abdominal CT angiography.** Chest CT is indicated in patients with aortic dilatation by echocardiography, or for evaluation of ascending and arch calcification, and in the case of TAVR or peripheral cannulation, descending aorta and iliac and femoral vessel diameter and quality. CT is also indicated in patients with prior chest surgery for planning safe reentry, and in patients considered for minimally invasive approaches for planning (Fig. 15.5).
5. **Electrocardiogram.** This is essential for baseline rhythm analysis and important to use for comparison to detect postoperative ischemia.
6. **Ancillary studies for risk stratification.** Pulmonary function testing is indicated in patients with known pulmonary disease or extensive smoking history and in the setting of radiation heart disease. Carotid Doppler studies and lower extremity noninvasive studies may be indicated in patients with relevant history or findings but are not routinely indicated.

B. Contraindications to surgery

1. Absolute contraindications include extreme frailty with poor life expectancy, untreatable malignancy, active cerebral hemorrhage, and Childs C cirrhosis.
2. Relative contraindications are active infection, Childs B cirrhosis, ascending aortic calcification, multiple reoperations, poor ventricular function, patient comorbidities, patient frailty, and patient limitations determined more by comorbidities than aortic valve disease.
3. Perioperative medical management
   a. Long-acting antihypertensives and anticoagulants are held.
   b. Patients with drug-eluting stents may require inpatient admission and bridging with an intravenous group IIa/IIIb inhibitor. Aspirin may be safely continued.
   c. Anesthetic induction is performed with care to avoid hypotension. A short-term fluid load may be required in the case of extreme LVH.

V. POSTOPERATIVE MANAGEMENT

A. **Left ventricular hypertrophy.** Patients with long-standing AS may have severe LVH that may complicate postoperative management. Postoperative atrial fibrillation with rapid heart rates can induce a low cardiac output state, and diuresis should be gentle so that the heart can continue to pump effectively with a small LV cavity. In rare cases, AVR can unmask underlying outflow tract obstruction that has been kept open by the artificially high preoperative LV pressures. Such patients may require concomitant septal myectomy or in rare cases mitral valve replacement to relieve the obstruction related to systolic anterior motion.

B. **Postoperative arrhythmias.** Atrial fibrillation occurs in as many as one-third of patients after valve surgery, and may be a significant hemodynamic issue in patients with severe LVH or low EF. Incidence peaks at 1 to 2 weeks and declines by 6 to 8 weeks. Early cardioversion may be attempted for hemodynamically unstable patients; however, most patients are best managed with rate or rhythm control and short-term anticoagulation with coumadin.

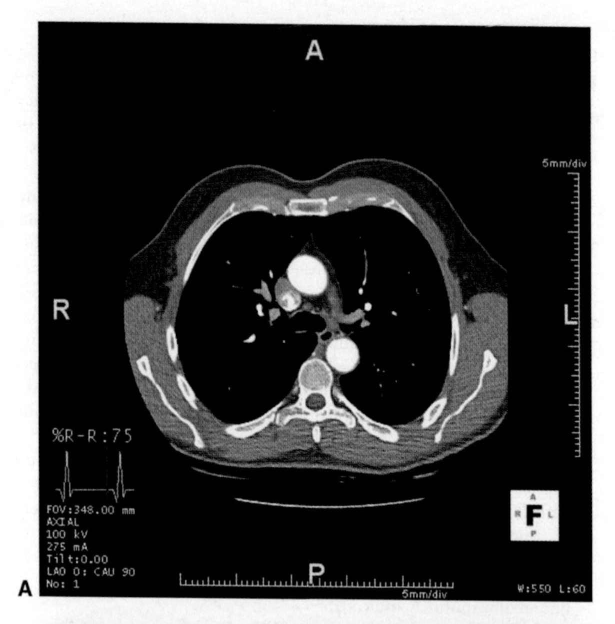

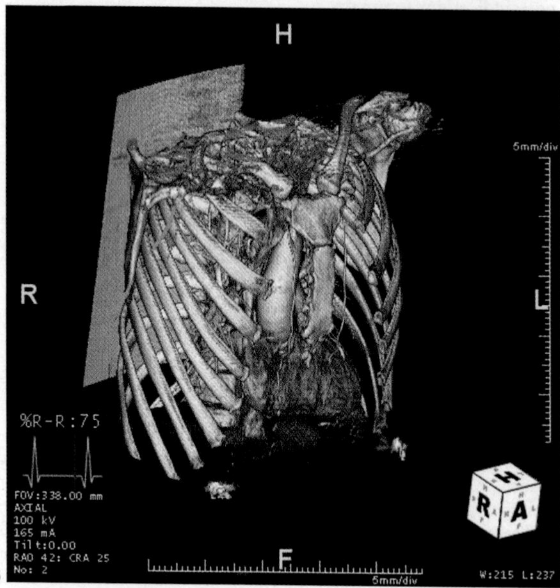

FIGURE 15.5 Three-dimensional (3D) computed tomographyic reconstruction for surgical planning. **A:** Location of the aorta in relation to the sternum predicts ease of access to the aortic valve via thoracotomy approach. **B:** Real-time 3D reconstruction with overlay of the planned skin incision in relation to the ascending aorta.

C. Subendocardial ischemia. Long-standing AS with severe LVH presents a management challenge. Intraoperative myocardial protection may be inadequate even with aggressive modern cardioplegia techniques, resulting in subendocardial ischemia manifested by diffuse ST segment elevation or depression, and in some instances by new-onset mitral regurgitation. The patients may also manifest ventricular arrhythmias that complicate hemodynamics. Consideration should be given to intra-aortic balloon counterpulsation or in extreme cases short-term extracorporeal membrane oxygenation.

VI. AORTIC VALVE INTERVENTIONS

A. Balloon valvuloplasty

Percutaneous balloon aortic valvuloplasty has a very limited role in the palliation of severe AS in patients otherwise too ill to undergo AVR. Patients treated with balloon aortic valvuloplasty alone have a markedly shorter survival than patients treated with valvuloplasty followed by surgery. Most benefits of the procedure are lost by 6 months after intervention. The primary limitations of balloon aortic valvuloplasty are the creation of AI, which may be very poorly tolerated by a hypertrophic ventricle, and restenosis. In large part, this approach has been supplanted by TAVR; however, there exist rare circumstances where BAV may make sense for palliation or as a diagnostic maneuver in very ill patients where the relative role of AS in the disease process is unclear.

B. Aortic valve surgery

Surgically important anatomic relations of the aortic valve include the base of the anterior mitral valve leaflet, the membranous septum, and the atrioventricular conduction system of the heart (Fig. 15.1). Knowledge of these relations is essential to safe aortic valve surgery, because injury may occur during valve debridement, suture placement, or secondary to distortion of the structures by an aortic prosthesis. Preoperative 3D imaging of the aortic valve and root by CT or MRI can provide important insight into the potential pitfalls at operation.

1. **Operative approach.** All primary AVR patients should be considered candidates for a minimally invasive approach until proven otherwise. A thorough preoperative work-up is essential. For pulmonic valve surgery, sternotomy is preferable as the position of the pulmonic valve is variable, and concomitant annular procedures may require more exposure than can be obtained via a mini approach.
   - **a.** Sternotomy. Sternotomy is generally required for concomitant coronary bypass, mitral valve or tricuspid valve surgery, extensive aortic arch surgery, MAZE procedure, or myectomy. Sternotomy should be strongly considered for aortic root surgery, especially aortic root reimplantation, unless the surgeon is experienced with coronary reimplantation via small incision (Fig. 15.6).
   - **b.** Upper hemisternotomy. This can be performed with a J incision to the right into the 4th intercostal space, or with an inverted T incision that can be made via the 3rd or 4th interspace for patients requiring aortic valve plus ascending aortic surgery, root enlargement, and extensive aortic valve repair. Concomitant hemiarch repair can be performed through this approach with a minimum of modification (Fig. 15.7).
   - **c.** Right minithoracotomy. This can be done for isolated AVR or aortic valve repair. Ascending aortoplasty is feasible in some patients. The ascending aorta should be free of calcification and significant root or ascending dilatation. Central aortic cannulation with peripheral venous cannulation is preferred. Femoral artery cannulation can be utilized if the descending aorta, iliacs, and femoral arteries are interrogated with CT prior to operation and are free of significant atherosclerosis (Fig. 15.8).
2. **Cardiopulmonary bypass.** With the exception of TAVR, all surgical approaches to the aortic valve and pulmonic valve require safe institution of cardiopulmonary bypass.

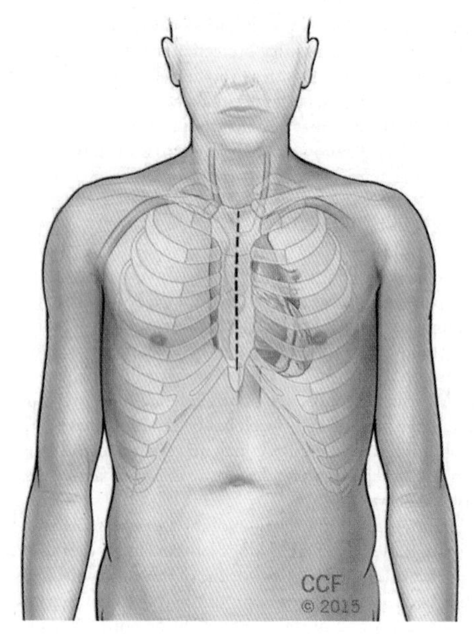

FIGURE 15.6 Sternotomy approach.

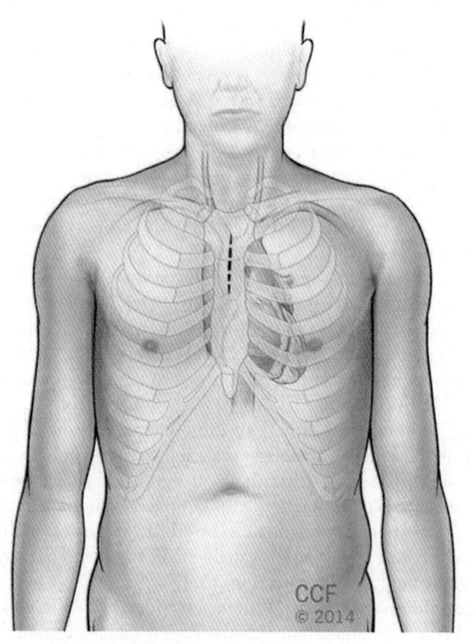

FIGURE 15.7 Upper hemisternotomy approach.

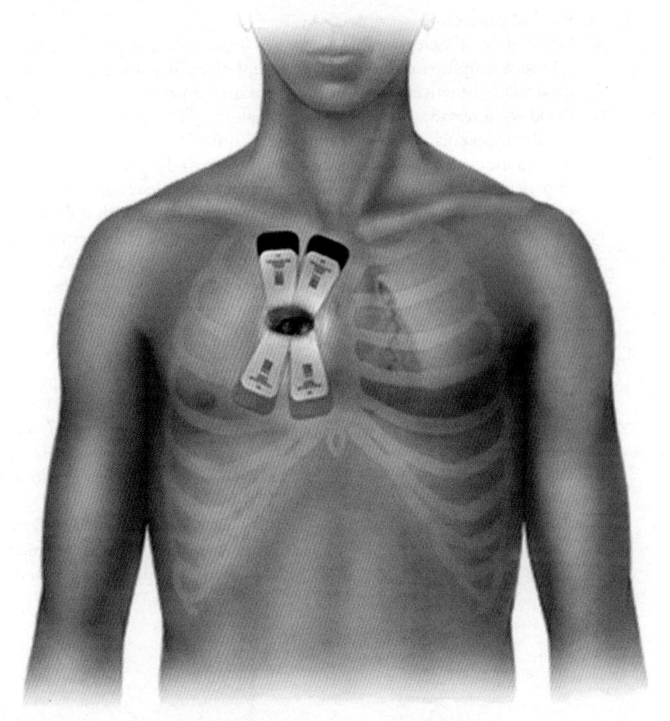

FIGURE 15.8 Right minithoracotomy approach.

a. Central aortic cannulation. This is preferred for most aortic and pulmonic valve surgery because it is safe and reproducible and avoids retrograde flow to the descending aorta.
b. Axillary artery cannulation. An 8-mm Dacron side graft is utilized in patients in whom concomitant distal ascending aortic surgery is anticipated secondary to arch aneurysm, dissection, or extensive aortic calcification where the possibility of circulatory arrest and aortic replacement is encountered.
c. Femoral artery. Retrograde perfusion of the iliac artery and descending aorta carries the possibility of debris entering the carotid circulation. Given the association of AS and aortic atherosclerosis, femoral cannulation should be avoided in most aortic and pulmonic valve operations. Exceptions may be made in young patients with normal vasculature undergoing minimally invasive operation by thoracotomy, and in the case of difficult reoperative surgery, especially with previous use of the axillary artery.
d. Venous cannulation is generally with a single cannula draining the right atrium directly, or inserted via the superior vena cava or over a wire via the femoral vein. Bicaval cannulation should be considered with difficult root anatomy as it allows for direct retrograde cardioplegia in the coronary sinus, simplifying protection of the heart while coronary buttons are prepared.

3. **Myocardial protection**
   a. Del Nido cardioplegia. This and other single-dose antegrade cardioplegia solutions simplify isolated aortic valve and ascending aortic surgery and are particularly beneficial via a minimally invasive approach.
   b. Buckberg antegrade and retrograde cardioplegia. This should be considered the standard approach for aortic and pulmonic valve surgery with or without AI. Retrograde cardioplegia can be used effectively to induce myocardial standstill in patients with severe AI, or in cases such as aortic dissection where delivery to the ascending aorta or coronary ostia may be fraught with difficulty.
   c. Beating heart surgery. In many cases, pulmonic valve replacement can be performed with the heart beating as long as bicaval cannulation is utilized and the right side of the heart is well suctioned to allow adequate visualization. More complex interventions on the pulmonic valve may benefit from an arrested heart.
4. **Aortic valve replacement**
   a. Approach to the valve. Once the heart is arrested, the valve may be approached via a transverse or oblique aortotomy. In general, the incision should be carried into the noncoronary sinus if root enlargement is contemplated. Transverse aortotomy is generally employed, and the sinotubular junction preserved, if aortic valve repair is planned. The aorta may be transected above the sinotubular junction if exposure is difficult (Fig. 15.9).
   b. Annular debridement. Complete debridement of annular calcium allows for optimal placement of the largest possible prosthesis. In particular in bicuspid valve patients, calcium may extend well below the annulus onto the anterior

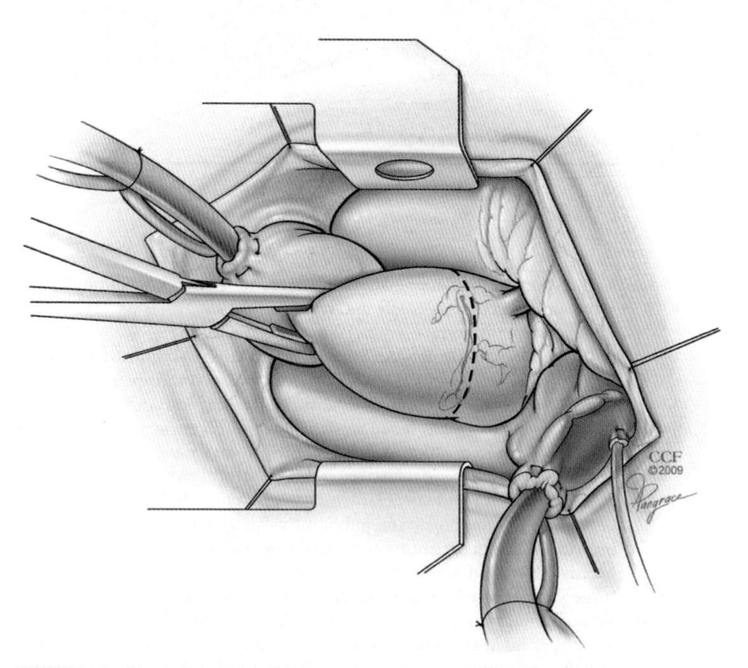

FIGURE 15.9 Approach to the aortic valve.

mitral valve leaflet. Such calcium is usually loosely attached to the underlying tissue and may be debrided completely with preservation of the soft tissue. In cases of invasive calcification, sufficient debridement should be completed to allow proper seating of the valve. Care must be taken to prevent embolization of calcific debris. Defects in the aorta or annulus are best repaired with tension-free technique using autologous pericardium before the valve is implanted.

c. Suture placement. Sutures can be interrupted, running, simple, mattress, or figure of 8. Care should be taken in the area of the membranous septum to avoid deep bites that can injure the conduction system.

d. Prosthesis choice. The multiple variables that can affect choice of prosthesis are beyond the scope of this chapter; however, several principles are worth considering. First, even in young patients, there is no difference in life expectancy for patients receiving tissue or mechanical valves. Tissue valves result in more reoperations for structural valve deterioration, and mechanical valves result in more complications related to bleeding or embolic events. Thus, the choice must be tailored carefully to the patient in consideration of age, activity level, anticipated valve size, and lifestyle expectations. Only in rare cases is a single prosthesis type suitable. For most patients with isolated aortic valve stenosis or regurgitation not amenable to repair, stented bovine pericardial valves, stented porcine valves, or mechanical bileaflet valves provide most proven durability and straightforward implantation.

e. Sutureless valves. These valves are essentially a hybrid between transcatheter aortic valves and traditional stented valves. They allow for rapid deployment of the prosthesis in a debrided annulus. As this technology evolves, it may facilitate the application of minimally invasive approaches to a wider variety of patients. At present, cost of these devices is significantly higher than standard valves, and early studies have shown a higher rate of pacemaker implantation.

f. Complete root replacement. This approach may be employed because of dilatation of the aortic root and annulus, or in some cases in a very small root to allow for a low gradient implant—a stentless porcine root or homograft valve. Coronary buttons are mobilized and the root prosthesis is sewn directly to the annulus. Coronary buttons are then attached to the side of the prosthetic root graft, porcine root, or homograft with fine suture. Care must be taken to avoid kinking of the coronary arteries that can result as root geometry is altered by the procedure. With the increasing use of bioprosthetic valves in young patients, it is important to consider factors relating to a likely second operation when considering root replacement. Explanting a full root whether a stentless porcine root or composite root graft and reimplanting a new prosthesis carries an increased risk of morbidity and mortality over redo AVR alone.

g. Root enlargement. As modern valve prostheses become more hemodynamically efficient, smaller valves can be implanted without adversely affecting the long-term success of the operation; however, root enlargement is still a viable option for patients with smaller aortic roots in whom a bioprosthetic valve is being implanted with the plan for future valve-in-valve TAVR if and when the valve degenerates. A simple root enlargement can be performed using autologous pericardium with a small incision in the aortic annulus in the area of the noncoronary sinus. This usually allows at least a 2 mm (one valve size) increase in the implanted valve.

h. Ross procedure. In this operation, the intact pulmonary valve is harvested and implanted in the aortic position, and the pulmonary valve is replaced with a cadaver allograft. In select experienced institutions, the Ross procedure is performed with excellent mortality and long-term durability. However, as bioprosthetic valve durability improves, the relative benefit of the Ross operation other than in very young patients with growth potential is debatable. The

Achilles heel of this operation remains the need to reconstruct the pulmonary outflow tract and valve with a homograft, and the inevitable need to reintervene on the degenerated pulmonary homograft. Percutaneous approaches have made this more palatable; however, the Ross procedure remains a relatively rare intervention in the spectrum of aortic valve disease.

i. Transcatheter aortic valve replacement. The principle of TAVR is fundamentally different from that of surgical AVR (SAVR) in that the existing aortic valve leaflets are preserved and serve to aid in fixation of the valve (Fig. 15.10). As a consequence of this design, the current crop of valves is well suited to the treatment of AS, where the presence of thickened, calcified leaflet tissue provides a firm substrate for anchoring the prosthesis. Transcatheter valves that rely on radial force for anchoring are less well suited to the treatment of AI, especially in the case of a dilated annulus.

Theoretically, placing an aortic valve prosthesis via a transcatheter route has the potential to eliminate some of the anatomic pitfalls inherent in open aortic valve surgery: sternal reentry in the setting of patent grafts, severely calcified ascending aorta, etc. There are unique considerations inherent in transcatheter valve implantation, as follows:

- Access to the valve can be obtained via transfemoral or transapical routes. Delivery of large devices via transfemoral approach can present a problem in patients with atherosclerotic iliac arteries. In early series of transfemoral valve implantation, access-related complications were a frequent cause of early mortality.
- Positioning and fixation. Currently available devices rely on a combination of fluoroscopy and transesophageal echocardiography for positioning. Small errors in positioning may result in inadequate fixation and subsequent device embolization into the ventricle or distal aorta. Newer devices allow for repositioning and even removal of a malpositioned valve and may abrogate this issue.
- Relation of the prosthesis to surrounding structures. Displacement of the calcified leaflets by stented prosthesis has the potential to obstruct blood flow to the coronary ostia. Radial force on the LV outflow tract has the potential to alter cardiac conduction and in some valve designs has led to higher pacemaker rates.

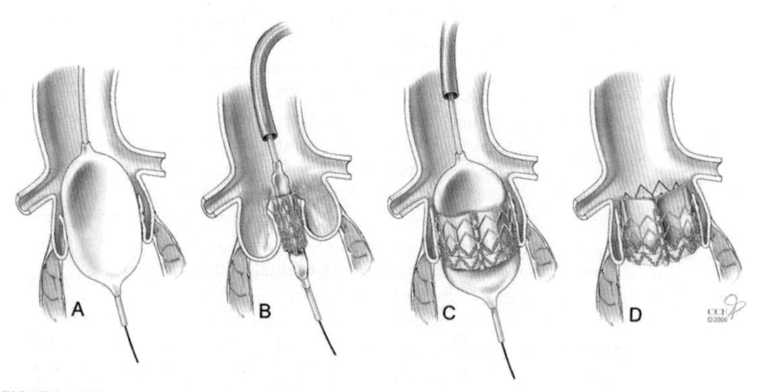

FIGURE 15.10 Implantation of a transcatheter aortic valve. **A-D** illustrate sequential events in placement of the valve.

Earlier device designs were subject to significant postprocedure AI, secondary to inadequate sealing of the valve to the leaflets. Newer valve designs incorporate sealing elements and have greatly reduced the incidence of significant AI, though it is higher than in SAVR.

5. **Aortic valve repair**

   a. Leaflet reduction and plication. The physiology of aortic regurgitation in bicuspid aortic valve disease is complex, involving differential length of the conjoined and reference aortic valve cusps, resulting in prolapse of the conjoined cusp, annular and sinotubular junction enlargement, and thickening and occasionally fenestration of the leaflets. Of regurgitant bicuspid valves without evidence of calcification, approximately two-thirds may be amenable to successful repair addressing both the leaflets and the annulus. The principle of repair is to make the length of the two leaflets equivalent, either by simple plication of the conjoined leaflet (Fig. 15.11), or by resecting and reconstructing the conjoined leaflet when the tissue is too bulky to plicate. The remaining commissures are then plicated with Cabrol mattress sutures in order to reduce annular dimension and increase the coaptation height at the leaflet edge. Care must be taken not to reduce the size of the valve orifice too much, resulting in stenosis.

      Standard repairs addressing the leaflets and commissures can have excellent durability in terms of freedom from recurrent insufficiency. Most late failures occur because of progressive stenosis; however, concern has been raised that this method of repair does not address the overall annular dilatation and may increase stress on the leaflets, leading many to advocate for aortic root reimplantation as the preferred repair technique in combination with leaflet repair.

   b. Aortic root remodeling and reimplantation (David procedure). For trileaflet aortic valves, regurgitation produced by dilatation of the annulus and sinotubular junction as is typical in Marfan syndrome can be very well corrected with aortic root reimplantation. Coronary arteries are mobilized as for a root replacement, and the leaflets and commissures preserved. The root is dissected

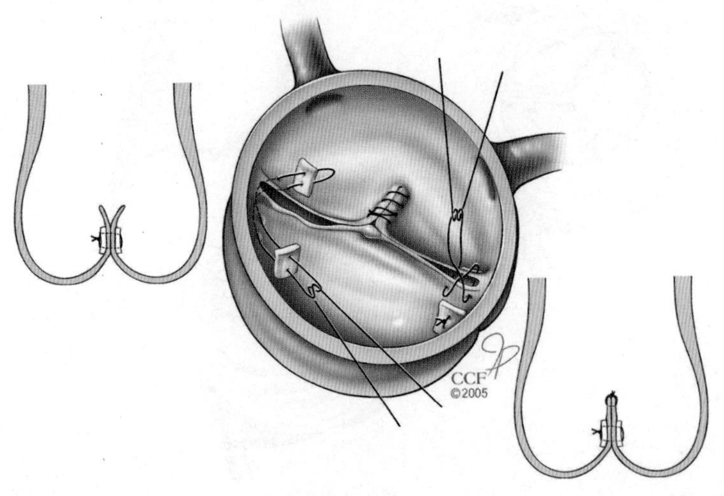

FIGURE 15.11 Bicuspid valve repair with leaflet plication.

free from surrounding tissue to the level of the annulus. The commissures and leaflets are then resuspended within a prosthetic graft, downsizing the annulus and intercommissural distance and providing adequate coaptation of the leaflets. Coronary arteries are then reattached to the graft. In the case of a bicuspid valve, leaflet reconstruction is performed in order to achieve equal length leaflets, and the commissures are aligned at 180 degrees in order to achieve a true bicuspid valve orientation.

Long-term durability of aortic root reimplantation has been excellent in experienced hands for tricuspid valves. Whether this approach will improve the durability of bicuspid aortic valve repairs is less clear.

c. Valve repair in endocarditis. Isolated leaflet perforation, as in the case of healed endocarditis, is amenable to autologous pericardial patch repair. Often, these lesions have thickened edges, facilitating suture placement in the normally thin and fragile aortic cusp tissue.

d. Commissural resuspension. Acute aortic dissection often displaces the commissures of the aortic valve centrally and toward the ventricle, which may result in severe AI. If the cusp morphology is normal, such valves may be successfully "resuspended" by restoring the integrity of the aortic wall at the level of the sinotubular junction. This can be accomplished using three layers of felt to reinforce the circumference of the aorta, without necessitating individual sutures in the commissures (Fig. 15.12).

6. Pulmonic valve replacement

a. Bioprosthetic valve implantation. In part because of decreased hemodynamic wear, bioprosthetic valve implantation in the pulmonic position is favored over mechanical valves. Valve-in-valve TAVR can be performed simply in the event of late valve failure. Large-sized valves are preferred. Especially in cases of previous tetralogy of Fallot repair with transannular patch, the annulus may be divided and a patch of autologous pericardium or bovine pericardium used to augment the size of the valve implanted.

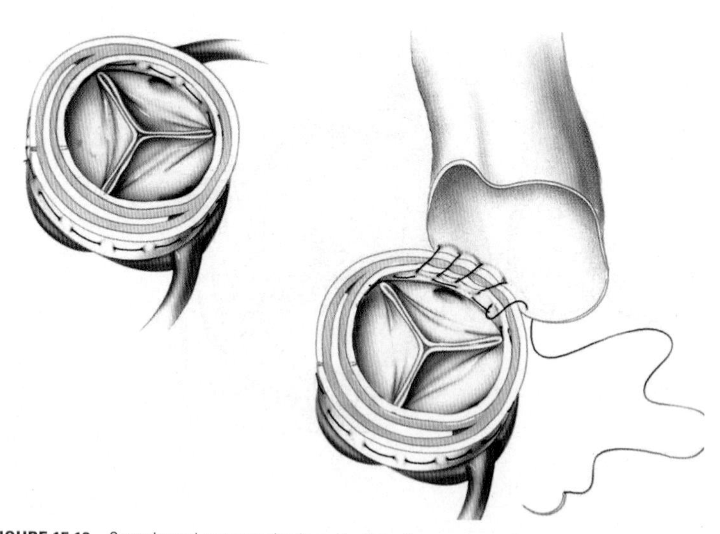

FIGURE 15.12 Commissural resuspension in aortic dissection.

b. Transcatheter implantation. Given the large number of homograft valves implanted in the pulmonic position for the treatment of congenital heart disease and Ross procedures, a large experience exists treating homograft failure with valve-in-valve transcatheter implantation. Standard aortic TAVR or dedicated valves such as bovine jugular venous valves have been used, often with multiple implants over several years, to avoid or postpone open surgery in the setting of multiple reoperations.

c. Reoperation for failed pulmonary homograft. In the modern era, open surgery for a failed pulmonary homograft is likely to be performed in a patient who has had multiple previous endovascular interventions, and so the calcified homograft must be removed carefully in order to avoid damage to the surrounding tissues, which may be adherent to the endovascular prosthesis. Reconstruction is usually accomplished with a new homograft, although valved conduits may be employed.

VII. OUTCOMES

A. Operative mortality

Early mortality after SAVR has been reported at 2% to 5% in large national databases. More recently, a number of series report mortality under 1% routinely in experienced centers. Risk factors for early mortality include redo operation, concomitant coronary bypass grafting, concomitant mitral valve replacement, and older age. Additional patient-related risk factors include decreased LV function, poor preoperative functional status, renal insufficiency, and atrial fibrillation. Causes of early mortality are myocardial infarction or cardiac failure in 58%, hemorrhage in 11%, infection in 7%, arrhythmia in 5%, and stroke in 4%.

B. Early complications

Serious early complications after SAVR include stroke in 1% to 2% of patients, mediastinal hemorrhage resulting in reoperation in 5% to 11%, wound infection in 1% to 2%, heart block requiring permanent pacemaker implantation in <1%, dialysis-dependent renal failure in 0.7%, prolonged ventilation in 3%, and perioperative myocardial infarction in 2%. Risks are similar for AVR or repair, although the risk of stroke may be increased in patients with a large calcium burden undergoing replacement. Prevention of stroke relies on meticulous removal of valve debris from the field and careful deairing following the procedure. Flooding the operative field with CO_2 may help displace air from the open cardiac chambers and is favored. Careful evaluation of the ascending aorta prior to cannulation and clamping are essential. Consideration for alternative cannulation or for TAVR in patients with ascending aortic atheroma or calcification may reduce stroke incidence.

C. Late complications

1. **Thromboembolism.** Incidence of thromboembolism has been reported to be 0.2% to 1.3% per patient-year for bioprosthetic valves in the aortic position without anticoagulation, versus 1.5% to 2.0% per patient-year for mechanical valves in patients on coumadin. The rate of significant hemorrhage is 0.3% per year for bioprostheses and 2% to 3% per patient-year for mechanical valves requiring warfarin. Elderly patients may be more prone to anticoagulant-related hemorrhage.
2. **Endocarditis.** Risk of late endocarditis (occurring after the first 6 months) is 0.5% to 1.0% per patient-year. Type of prosthesis is not likely related to endocarditis risk; however, aortic root abscess is more common with mechanical valves (65% of the total), versus 36% for porcine valves and 20% for homografts.
3. **Prosthetic valve dysfunction.** The rate of prosthetic valve dysfunction is related to age at implantation, valve gradient, and valve type. Newer valve models with more advanced anticalcification treatments may be less prone to structural valve deterioration. Very long-term durability of bovine pericardial valves has been documented even in young patients with stable valve gradients. Prosthetic valve

dysfunction in mechanical valves may occur secondary to pannus ingrowth under the valve that impinges on leaflet motion.

4. **Paravalvular leak.** Small leaks present at operation may close spontaneously after protamine administration. Sterile paravalvular leaks may occur at any time thereafter, even years later. Risk factors for paravalvular leak include endocarditis, prior operation, and large valve size. The overall incidence is 0.2% to 0.5%, many of which are associated with infection.
5. Less common complications include hemolysis, which is generally related to paravalvular leak but may occur with leaflet perforation or mechanical valves.
6. **Patient prosthesis mismatch (PPM).** This often misunderstood entity results from the fact that most implantable valves confer some degree of reduction in valve orifice area compared to a normal human semilunar valve. The effect of PPM on outcome is related to age, cardiac function, and degree of ventricular hypertrophy at the time of implant. Severe PPM in younger patients or those with severe LVH portends a significantly worse long-term survival and freedom from heart failure, whereas in elderly, less active patients the effect is minimal.

D. Long-term survival

Patients with AS can have a survival that is comparable to an age- and sex-matched patient population. Survival is negatively affected by decreased LV function, concomitant coronary disease, and renal disease. That younger patients fare worse than age-matched controls and that older patients have similar survival may suggest that younger patients undergo operation later in the course of disease, resulting in irreversible ventricular changes prior to AVR. Causes of death include heart failure, or sudden cardiac death in 42% to 83%, and valve-related complications such as hemorrhage, infection, or thromboembolism in 15%.

E. Symptomatic relief

Many patients have immediate symptomatic relief following the normal recovery from surgery. Patients with near-normal ventricular function may have significant improvement in exercise capacity immediately following operation. Those with low-flow, low-gradient AS or AI with dilated ventricles and poor EF may have a prolonged course of recovery of ventricular function. Failure to achieve symptom improvement in 6 months following aortic valve surgery with adequate technical result portends a worse prognosis.

F. Perspective

Refinements in surgical technique, device development particularly in TAVR, and patient care have resulted in dramatic reductions in operative risk for aortic valve surgery. Mounting evidence suggests that many so-called asymptomatic patients have markers for advanced disease and worse outcome after intervention. Many of these patients are not offered stress testing, and treatment is therefore delayed until the onset of symptoms, increasing risk and often resulting in undesirable lifestyle limitations from the patient's perspective. The excellent long-term durability of the current generation of bioprosthetic valves argues for a more aggressive strategy of early surgery, utilizing small incisions when possible and tailored to the needs of the patient.

KEY PEARLS

- The natural history of symptomatic severe AS is well characterized and all patients with symptoms should be considered for expedited percutaneous or surgical intervention.
- The appropriate treatment of asymptomatic severe AS patients is controversial. There is a risk of sudden cardiac death of approximately 1% per year, and of left ventricular remodeling. Approximately one-third of asymptomatic patients with severe AS will become symptomatic within 2 years and two-thirds of patients will become symptomatic within 5 years.

- Stress echocardiography is useful in asymptomatic severe AS patients to determine need for an operation by identifying patients with poor prognostic variables and for unmasking symptoms.
- Low-dose dobutamine echocardiography can identify contractile reserve as a ≥20% increase in stroke volume. The presence of contractile reserve is a powerful prognostic factor for TAVR or SAVR.
- The operative approach to AS and AR usually includes full sternotomy, upper ministernotomy, or right minithoracotomy. All primary aortic valve replacement patients should be considered candidates for a minimally invasive approach until proven otherwise.
- The choice of aortic prosthesis should be tailored carefully based on age, activity level, anticipated valve size, and lifestyle expectations. There is no difference in life expectancy for patients receiving tissue or mechanical valves. Tissue valves result in more reoperations for structural valve deterioration, and mechanical valves in more complications related to bleeding or embolic events.
- Aortic valve repair is feasible in approximately two-thirds of patients with bicuspid aortic valves and pure AR with good durability and freedom from AR. Restricted leaflets, cusp tissue deficiency, and calcification suggest a lower probability of successful repair.
- Pulmonary valve replacement is usually performed with a homograft or bioprosthetic valve via open surgery of percutaneous valve implantation, especially in congenital heart disease.
- Late complications of aortic valve surgery include thromboembolism, endocarditis, prosthetic valve dysfunction, paravalvular regurgitation, and patient prosthesis mismatch.

SUGGESTED READINGS

Borer JS, Herrold EM, Hochreiter C, et al. Natural history of left ventricular performance at rest and during exercise after aortic valve replacement for aortic regurgitation. *Circulation*. 1991;84:III133–III139.

Chan V, Lam BK, Rubens FD, et al. Long-term evaluation of biological versus mechanical prosthesis use at reoperative aortic valve replacement. *J Thorac Cardiovasc Surg*. 2012;144(1):146–151.

Clavel MA, Fuchs C, Burwash, IG, et al. Predictors of outcomes in low-flow, low-gradient aortic stenosis: results of the multicenter TOPAS study. *Circulation*. 2008;111:S234–S242.

Dal-Bianco JP, Khanderia BK, Mookadam F, et al. Management of asymptomatic severe aortic stenosis. *J Am Coll Cardiol*. 2008;52:1279–1292.

Das P, Rimington H, Chambers J. Exercise testing to stratify risk in aortic stenosis. *Eur Heart J*. 2005;26:1309–1313.

Fedak PW, Verma S, David TE, et al. Clinical update: clinical and pathophysiological implications of a bicuspid aortic valve. *Circulation*. 2002;106:900–904.

Galli D, Manuguerra R, Monaco R, et al. Understanding the structural features of symptomatic calcific aortic valve stenosis: a broad-spectrum clinico-pathologic study in 236 consecutive surgical cases. *Int J Cardiol*. 2017;228:364–374.

Iung B, Cahier A, Baron G, et al, Decision making in elderly patients with severe aortic stenosis: why are so many denied surgery? *Eur Heart J*. 2005;26:2714–2720.

Johnston DR, Atik FA, Rajeswaran J. Outcomes of less invasive J-incision approach to aortic valve surgery. *J Thorac Cardiovasc Surg*. 2012;144(4):852–858.

Johnston DR, Roselli EE. Minimally invasive aortic valve surgery: Cleveland Clinic experience. *Ann Cardiothorac Surg*. 2015;4(2):140–147.

Johnston DR, Soltesz EG, Vakil N, et al. Long-term durability of bioprosthetic aortic valves: implications from 12,569 implants. *Ann Thorac Surg*. 2015;99(4):1239–1247.

Lancellotti P, Lebois F, Simon M. Prognostic importance of quantitative exercise Doppler echocardiography in asymptomatic valvular aortic stenosis. *Circulation*. 2005;112:1377–1382.

Lembcke A, Kivelitz DE, Borges AC, et al. Quantification of aortic valve stenosis: head-to-head comparison of 64 slice spiral computed tomography with transesophageal and transthoracic echocardiography and cardiac catheterization. *Invest Radiol*. 2009;44(1):7–14.

Mentias A, Feng K, Alashi A, et al. Long-term outcomes in patients with aortic regurgitation and preserved left ventricular ejection fraction. *J Am Coll Cardiol*. 2016;68(20):2144–2153.

Mihaljevic T, Nowicki ER, Rajeswaran J, et al. Survival after valve replacement for aortic stenosis: implications for decision making. *J Thorac Cardiovasc Surg*. 2008;135:1270–1278.

Nishimura RA, Otto CM, Bonow RO, et al. 2014 AHA/ACC guideline for the management of patients with valvular heart disease: a report of the American College of Cardiology/American Heart Association Task Force on Practice Guidelines. *J Thorac Cardiovasc Surg*. 2014;148(1):e1–e132.

Pellika PA, Sarano ME, Nishimura RA, et al. Outcome of 622 adults with asymptomatic, hemodynamically significant aortic stenosis during prolonged follow-up. *Circulation*. 2005;111:3290–3295.

Pettersson GB, Crucean, AC, Savage R, et al. Toward predictable repair of regurgitant aortic valves: a systematic morphology-directed approach to bicommissural repair. *J Am Coll Cardiol*. 2008;51:40–49.

Ross DN. Replacement of the aortic valve with a pulmonary autograft: the "switch" operation. *Ann Thorac Surg*. 1991;52:1346–1350.

Ross J Jr, Braunwald E. Aortic stenosis. *Circulation*. 1968;38:61–67.

CHAPTER 16

Gösta B. Pettersson
Syed T. Hussain

Valve Surgery: Endocarditis

I. INTRODUCTION.

Infective endocarditis (IE) is the most severe and potentially devastating complication of heart valve disease, be it native valve (NVE), prosthetic valve (PVE), or infection on another cardiac device. Without treatment, IE is uniformly fatal, and the old concepts of acute, subacute, and chronic endocarditis only referred to the time it was anticipated to take before the patient died. Even in the current therapeutic era, with appropriate antibiotic therapy and surgical intervention, multicenter studies report in-hospital mortality of 15% to 20% and 1-year mortality approaching 40%. Patients with valve disease, prosthetic valves, cardiac devices, a history of IE, immuno suppression, dialysis, drug abuse, and other medical situations are at increased risk of IE. As a paradoxical effect of advances in medical and surgical therapy, the incidence of IE has increased during the past 30 years. This is due to an increase in the number of patients with risk factors for IE, including an increasing elderly population with degenerative valve disease and a rise in staphylococcal infections. It is extremely uncommon for normal valves to become infected, but it does happen.

The clinical scenarios presented by patients with IE are often very complex. At the same time, IE requires prompt diagnosis for early institution of antibiotic treatment and decision-making related to complications, including risk of embolism and need for and timing of high-risk surgery. IE patients require a multispecialty team approach: an infectious disease specialist, cardiologist, and cardiac surgeon constitute the core of this team, but input from other specialties, most often neurology, is often required. Execution of the operation with radical debridement and reconstruction of the heart and heart valves requires experience and special expertise. Despite advances in surgical techniques, operations for IE remain associated with the highest mortality of any valve disease, even at the most experienced centers.

II. PATHOGENESIS AND PATHOLOGY, MICROBIOLOGY, AND LEFT- VERSUS RIGHT-SIDED IE

A. Causative organism, position (aortic, mitral, or right-sided), and type of infected valve (NVE or PVE) are of great importance to pathology and prognosis. The factors responsible for the ability of the organisms to infect, survive, and destroy are called virulence factors, and include those that allow the organism to attach to the infection site, avoid the host's immune response, and produce destructive enzymes, toxins, protective substances, and other factors.

B. A valve becomes infected when circulating organisms adhere to damaged endothelium of a native or prosthetic valve. The organisms multiply, develop vegetations, and produce toxins and enzymes that disintegrate valve tissue and allow extravascular invasion.

C. A great variety of organisms can cause IE, and they differ with regard to virulence factors, which determine their aggressiveness. The microbiology of IE depends on whether the valve is native or prosthetic and whether the infection is community or hospital acquired. Staphylococci, streptococci, and enterococci are the most important causative organisms, responsible for approximately 85% of all IEs. Staphylococci and streptococci are the most common aggressive and destructive bacteria causing IE.

Although *Staphylococcus aureus* is more common with NVE, *Staphylococcus epidermidis* is a more common cause of PVE. Fungi form large vegetations but are usually less invasive, although *Aspergillus* IE is associated with development of mycotic aneurysms. We have recently described the progression and pathologic stages of NVE and in a PVE atlas (see Pettersson, Hussain, Shrestha, 2014).

D. Despite introduction of antibiotics, IE has remained notoriously difficult to treat, and even extended courses of high-dose antibiotics often fail to cure the infection. Recent research has provided a plausible explanation for this by introducing the biofilm hypothesis. Biofilm development and quorum sensing are social bacterial behaviors. Bacterial populations produce and live embedded in a self-produced, extracellular, polysaccharide slim matrix, and quorum sensing is a chemical cell-to-cell communication mechanism that synchronizes gene expression and activates the maturation and assembly of the biofilm in a coordinated manner. The biofilm provides protection against the host's immune system and is a difficult barrier for antimicrobials to penetrate. Ability to form biofilm is a characteristic of the bacteria commonly causing IE, including staphylococci, streptococci, and enterococci. Surgery effectively disrupts the biofilm and exposes residual bacteria to circulating antimicrobials, antibodies, and active immune cells.

E. Tissue disintegration and invasion caused by toxins and enzymes result in serious complications, including heart failure from valve regurgitation or fistulae. Extravascular invasion causes abscesses around the aortic root or in the atrioventricular (AV) groove, potentially leading to heart block. Embolism of pieces of vegetations can cause stroke, mycotic aneurysms, and other embolic phenomena. Destroyed tissue does not regrow; valves made leaky by bacterial destruction will not heal and become competent even if the infection is cured by antibiotics.

F. Outcomes after treatment of IE are often related to whether it is a native or a prosthetic valve infection. Prosthetic valve infections are generally more invasive and more difficult to treat and cure with antibiotics only. Formation of biofilm protecting the organisms offers an explanation to why surgery is more often needed for PVE.

G. When comparing aortic and mitral valve IE, we have observed that aortic valve IE is more invasive (true for both NVE and PVE) and that it is responsible for a higher proportion of prosthetic valve infections. Despite this, outcomes are worse after surgical treatment of mitral IE than after aortic IE. We identified three reasons why mitral IE is more difficult to deal with: Mitral valve patients are sicker, surgical anatomy is less favorable, and we do not have an allograft valve replacement alternative for the mitral valve. In another recent, as yet unpublished study, we looked at the difference in invasiveness between left-sided and right-sided IE and confirmed that right-sided IE is never invasive, although it is caused by the same aggressive organisms as *S. aureus*. Our hypothesis is that invasion is driven by high pressure, although oxygenated blood on the left side could also be a factor, because most bacteria that cause IE are aerobic.

H. Systemic emboli, with emboli to the brain being the most frequent and important, are very common in patients with left-sided IE. Although rare, systemic septic emboli can cause mycotic aneurysms in any artery, in any location, including the aorta. Right-sided IE frequently sends septic emboli to the lungs, with development of pulmonary abscesses.

III. THE VALUE OF SURGERY IN THE TREATMENT OF IE

A. Studies that question the value of surgery use methodology that takes into account "survival bias" and "referral bias"—the self-selection of patients surviving long enough to be considered for surgery—by looking at entire populations with IE to study whether or not addition of surgery improves outcomes. Surgeons at large referral centers are limited to studying patients who are still alive and referred with "surgical" complications; thus, referral and survival bias will always be an issue in outcome studies from such centers. However, with the current improved outcomes, there is general agreement, supported by guidelines, that surgery should play a major role in managing IE. Kang and coworkers recently published a randomized study specifically studying timing of surgery for IE and were able to provide evidence supporting early surgery (within 48 hours) rather than waiting for heart failure to develop. We have been proponents of early surgery for a long time, taking the patient to the operating room as soon as a surgical indication has been identified.

B. All patients diagnosed with IE are primarily treated with antibiotics, initially broad spectrum and then adjusted to sensitivity pattern once this is known. Antibiotics to which the organisms are sensitive suppress the infection, may prevent or halt further destruction, and, if treatment is initiated early enough, may cure the patient. Antibiotics will not, however, restore the integrity of damaged tissue and valves.

The hypothesis that IE is a biofilm-associated infection explains why it is difficult to treat this infection and its recurrence after seemingly successful treatment, and why surgery is often required for cure in addition to antibiotics. Surgery mechanically disrupts the biofilm and removes the vegetations, infected necrotic tissue, and foreign material and drains the infected areas, thereby improving the access of antimicrobials. In addition, valve repair or replacement restores valve function and cardiac integrity. Still, final cure is the result of antibiotics. Most experienced groups, including ours, are convinced that surgery is beneficial and are becoming increasingly aggressive about advocating earlier surgery rather than waiting for complications. This evolution is based on improved outcomes after surgery and the growing conviction that there is a small price to be paid for operating on patients with active infection, and duration of preoperative antibiotic treatment has no or minimal impact on outcomes.

IV. DIAGNOSIS OF IE

A. IE is suspected from the patient's history and symptoms. Clinical presentation varies according to the causative organism, preexisting cardiac disease, comorbidities, and complications. IE may present as an acute, rapidly progressive infection or as a subacute or chronic disease with recurrent episodes of fever and malaise. Fever, often associated with systemic symptoms of chills, night sweats, poor appetite, and weight loss, is a typical symptom. Clinical findings include a new murmur or a change in an existing murmur, and embolic phenomena like petechiae, Roth spots, Osler nodes, and Janeway lesions. Neurologic events with stroke are the most serious, occurring in 20% to 40% of all patients, whereas mycotic aneurysms are much less common. A high index of suspicion and low threshold to exclude IE are essential to diagnosis and early treatment. Echocardiography and blood cultures are the cornerstones of diagnosing IE.

B. Echocardiography remains the most important imaging modality in securing the diagnosis. Transesophageal echocardiography (TEE) is more sensitive than transthoracic echocardiography (TTE) and is the present gold standard diagnostic modality for documenting IE. Echocardiographic findings of IE include vegetations, periprosthetic leakage in patients with PVE, intracardiac fistulae, and abscess cavities. The echocardiographic examination is excellent at evaluating valve function, but less reliable for assessing severity and invasiveness of the infection. A negative echocardiogram does not exclude the diagnosis of IE. Echocardiography has a better yield in patients with NVE than PVE, and shadowing is a particular problem in patients with mechanical valve prosthesis. TTE must be performed first, but both TTE and TEE should be performed in the majority of cases of suspected or definite IE. The added value of cardiac computed tomography (CT) and magnetic resonance imaging (MRI) remains controversial. In most patients with IE, MRI will demonstrate abnormal consistency of tissue in the annulus.

C. Whenever possible, a bacteriologic diagnosis should be secured before starting antibiotics. When IE is suspected, ideally three or more blood cultures should be collected before antibiotics are initiated, and at least two should be obtained immediately from different peripheral sites. Additional blood cultures should be obtained a few hours later. Unless the patient is septic, it is appropriate to hold off on starting antibiotics until an adequate number of blood cultures have been collected. Blood cultures from separate sites are usually positive in patients with bacterial endocarditis; two positive cultures out of three is considered diagnostic. Although diagnostic methods have improved, cultures in patients with fastidious organisms or fungi may take more than 3 weeks to become positive. Cases of IE in which blood cultures are negative (10%) may reflect either that the patient had been treated with antibiotics before the blood culture was drawn or that the infection is caused by fastidious organisms. For cases caused by fastidious organisms, either serologic testing or valve polymerase chain reaction assay can identify the pathogen 60% of the time. Typical microorganisms causing IE include *Streptococcus viridans, Staphylococcus aureus, S. epidermidis, Streptococcus bovis,* a HACEK group organism (*Haemophilus* spp., *Actinobacillus actinomycetemcomitans, Cardiobacterium hominis, Eikenella* spp., and *Kingella kingae*), or community-acquired enterococci.

D. The modified Duke criteria (Table 16.1), based on clinical, echocardiographic, and microbiologic findings categorized as major and minor criteria, provide high sensitivity and specificity (~80% overall) for the diagnosis of IE. However, clinical judgment remains essential, especially in clinical scenarios with negative blood cultures, PVE, and so forth, where sensitivity of the Duke criteria is reduced.

V. INDICATIONS AND TIMING OF SURGERY

A. Patient management is discussed by a multispecialty team dedicated to managing patients with IE. This team should include a cardiologist, an infectious disease specialist, and a cardiac surgeon. A neurologist and sometimes a neurosurgeon become involved when neurologic complications are present, and a nephrologist may be needed to manage renal failure. A psychiatrist and a social worker help manage drug addicts. Other specialists are consulted as required for a particular patient. As per the 2014 American Heart Association/American College of Cardiology (AHA/ACC) guidelines for IE, decisions about timing of surgical interventions should be made by a multispecialty Heart Valve Team of cardiology, cardiothoracic surgery, and infectious disease specialists and is a class I recommendation.

B. Recommendations for diagnosis and treatment of IE based on 2014 AHA/ACC guidelines are presented in Figure 16.1. Standard indications for surgery in patients with IE are presented in Table 16.2. In patients with NVE, congestive heart failure is the most frequent and severe complication of IE and is a class I indication for surgery. Presence of invasive disease with extravascular extension and IE caused by "difficult to treat" organisms associated with continued fever and sepsis after institution of appropriate antibiotic therapy are reasons for early surgical intervention. Surgical treatment should be considered in patients with signs of congestive heart failure, acute valve dysfunction, invasion with paravalvular abscess or cardiac fistulae, recurrent systemic embolization, or persistent sepsis despite adequate antibiotic therapy for more than 4 to 5 days.

C. Surgery to prevent embolism in patients with large mobile vegetations is a more controversial indication. Location, size, and mobility of the vegetation; previous embolism; type of organism; and duration of antibiotic therapy influence the indication for surgery. Mobile large vegetations >10 mm on the anterior mitral valve leaflet have been proven to be associated with higher embolic risk. We have tended to be more aggressive in these cases as we have become more confident that the penalty for operating on patients with active IE is indeed low and the valve is usually possible to preserve.

D. For patients with uncomplicated, nonstaphylococcal, and late PVE, treatment with antibiotics alone may be worth trying, but often the infection will recur within a few months. In patients with less aggressive bacteria, for example, enterococci, vegetations may be miniscule and the infection noninvasive, thus making the diagnosis very difficult. Patients with invasive staphylococcal PVE and early PVE require early surgery.

E. Approximately half of patients with IE develop severe complications that sooner or later require an operation. Early surgery as advocated by Kang and coworkers and by our group means operating for any of these conditions before heart failure has

TABLE 16.1 Modified Duke Criteria for the Diagnosis of Infective Endocarditis (IE)

Major criteria

Blood culture positive for IE

- *Typical microorganisms consistent with IE from two separate blood cultures:*

  Viridans streptococci, S. bovis, HACEK group, *S. aureus;* or

  community-acquired enterococci, in the absence of a primary focus
- *Microorganisms consistent with IE from persistently positive blood cultures, defined as follows:*

  At least two positive cultures of blood samples drawn >12 hr apart; or

  All of three or a majority of ≥4 separate cultures of blood (with first and last sample drawn at least 1 hr apart)
- *Single positive blood culture for* Coxiella burnetii *or antiphase I immunoglobulin antibody titer >1: 800*

Evidence of endocardial involvement

- *Echocardiogram positive for IE (transesophageal echocardiography recommended in patients with prosthetic valves, rated at least "possible IE" by clinical criteria, or complicated IE [paravalvular abscess]; transthoracic echocardiography as first test in other patients), defined as follows:*

  Oscillating intracardiac mass on valve or supporting structures, in the path of regurgitant jets, or on implanted material in the absence of an alternative anatomic explanation; or

  Abscess; or

  New partial dehiscence of prosthetic valve

  New valvular regurgitation (worsening or changing of preexisting murmur not sufficient)

Minor criteria

- Predisposition: predisposing heart condition or injection drug use
- Fever: temperature >38°C
- Vascular phenomena: major arterial emboli, septic pulmonary infarcts, mycotic aneurysm, intracranial hemorrhage, conjunctival hemorrhages, and Janeway lesions
- Immunologic phenomena: glomerulonephritis, Osler nodes, Roth spots, and rheumatoid factor
- Microbiologic evidence: positive blood culture but does not meet a major criterion as noted above or serologic evidence of active infection with organism consistent with IE

Diagnosis of IE is definite in the presence of	**Diagnosis of IE is possible in the presence of**
Two major criteria, or	One major and one minor criteria, or
One major and three minor criteria, or	Three minor criteria
Five minor criteria	

Adapted from Li JS, Sexton DJ, Mick N, et al. Proposed modifications to the Duke criteria for the diagnosis of infective endocarditis. *Clin Infect Dis.* 2000;30:633–638, with permission of Oxford University Press; HACEK group (*Haemophilus spp. Actinobacillus actinomycetemcomitans, Cardiobacterium hominis, Eikenella spp., and Kingella kingae*).

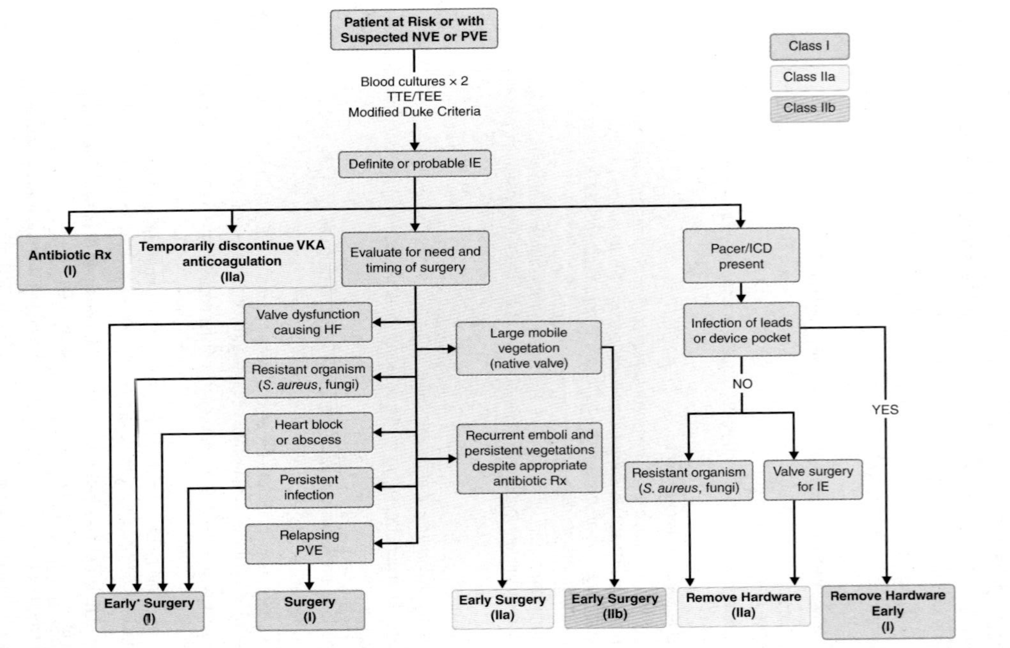

FIGURE 16.1 Diagnosis and treatment of IE. *Early surgery defined as during initial hospitalization before completion of a full therapeutic course of antibiotics. HF, heart failure; ICD, implantable cardioverter-defibrillator; IE, infective endocarditis; NVE, native valve endocarditis; PVE, prosthetic valve endocarditis; Rx, therapy; *S. aureus*, *Staphylococcus aureus*; TEE, transesophageal echocardiography; TTE, transthoracic echocardiography; VKA, vitamin K antagonist. (Reproduced with permission from Nishimura RA, Otto CM, Bonow RO, et al. 2014 AHA/ACC guideline for the management of patients with valvular heart disease: executive summary: a report of the American College of Cardiology/American Heart Association Task Force on Practice Guidelines. *Circulation*. 2014;129:2440–2492.)

TABLE 16.2 Indications for Surgery for IE

Class I Indications	Level of Evidence
Early surgery (during initial hospitalization before completion of a full therapeutic course of antibiotics) is indicated in patients with IE who present with valve dysfunction resulting in symptoms of heart failure.	B
Early surgery (during initial hospitalization before completion of a full therapeutic course of antibiotics) is indicated in patients with left-sided IE caused by *S. aureus*, fungal, or other highly resistant organisms.	B
Early surgery (during initial hospitalization before completion of a full therapeutic course of antibiotics) is indicated in patients with IE complicated by heart block, annular or aortic abscess, or destructive penetrating lesions.	B
Early surgery (during initial hospitalization before completion of a full therapeutic course of antibiotics) for IE is indicated in patients with evidence of persistent infection as manifested by persistent bacteremia or fevers lasting longer than 5–7 d after onset of appropriate antimicrobial therapy.	B
Surgery is recommended for patients with PVE and relapsing infection (defined as recurrence of bacteremia after a complete course of appropriate antibiotics and subsequently negative blood cultures) without other identifiable source for portal of infection.	B
Complete removal of pacemaker or defibrillator systems, including all leads and the generator, is indicated as part of the early management plan in patients with IE with documented infection of the device or leads.	B
Class IIa Indications	
Complete removal of pacemaker or defibrillator systems, including all leads and the generator, is reasonable in patients with valvular IE caused by *S. aureus* or fungi, even without evidence of device or lead infection.	B
Complete removal of pacemaker or defibrillator systems, including all leads and the generator, is reasonable in patients undergoing valve surgery for valvular IE.	B
Early surgery (during initial hospitalization before completion of a full therapeutic course of antibiotics) is reasonable in patients with IE who present with recurrent emboli and persistent vegetations despite appropriate antibiotic therapy.	B
Class IIB indications	
Early surgery (during initial hospitalization before completion of a full therapeutic course of antibiotics) may be considered in patients with NVE who exhibit mobile vegetations greater than 10 mm in length (with or without clinical evidence of embolic phenomenon).	B

IE, infective endocarditis; NVE, native valve endocarditis; PVE, prosthetic valve endocarditis. Adapted from 2014 AHA/ACC guidelines for the management of patients with valvular heart disease.

developed. In the study of Kang et al., the most frequent preventable complication in the conventional treatment group was embolic stroke. For this reason, once there is a surgical indication, surgery should not be delayed.

VI. PREOPERATIVE PATIENT MANAGEMENT AND PLANNING

A. When adequate blood cultures have been secured, an antibiotic regimen covering all suspected organisms should be initiated. Once the sensitivity of the organism has been confirmed, there is no additional benefit to delaying surgery to allow a longer period of preoperative antibiotic treatment. Outcomes are not related to the duration of antibiotic therapy before surgery. If the organism, however, happens to be insensitive to the antibiotics being administered at the time of surgery, the risk of recurrent infection is increased. Our infectious disease colleagues, however, have reassured us that the chance of that happening is very low provided that the diagnosis of IE was suspected preoperatively.

B. IE patients with neurologic symptoms who are scheduled for surgery should have neurologic evaluation and brain imaging, by either CT or MRI, within days of the planned operation to visualize any strokes and to determine if an infarct is ischemic or hemorrhagic. Imaging should be repeated in case of new or worsening symptoms. Because embolic events and strokes are so common in patients with IE, routine preoperative screening of asymptomatic patients, particularly those with high-risk vegetations, may be justified. The standard recommendation is that surgery should be delayed for 1 to 2 weeks in patients with nonhemorrhagic strokes and for 3 to 4 weeks in patients with hemorrhagic strokes to reduce the risk of further intracranial bleeding during heart surgery. We do not operate on patients with serious neurologic damage, unconscious patients, or those unable to follow simple commands until neurologic improvement has been demonstrated. Hemorrhagic lesions are associated with a higher probability of mycotic aneurysms, which often require treatment before valve surgery. Patients with intracranial bleeding must undergo cerebral angiography to exclude a mycotic aneurysm, although the yield will be low even in those with bleeding. For those with nonhemorrhagic embolic strokes, the main concerns are worsening the neurologic damage and hemorrhagic conversion of the infarct during the operation. The risk of worsening neurologic symptoms as a consequence of operation is time related, decreasing with increasing interval from the initial neurologic event. The risk of worsening the stroke symptoms must be weighed against the indications for surgery and the risk of additional emboli during the waiting period. If the patient is stable and risk of additional embolism deemed low, we try to delay surgery for 1 week, after which time we repeat brain imaging before operating.

Mycotic aneurysms in other places are uncommon but do occur, as do satellite infections (brain, spine, or splenic abscesses in left-sided IE, pulmonary abscesses in right-sided IE). Imaging with CT or MRI of the chest and abdomen may be justified in select cases, for example, in patients with *Aspergillus* IE.

Preoperative work-up should include cardiac catheterization in patients aged 40 years or older to exclude coronary disease on the basis of normal criteria for risk of coronary disease. Clinical judgment should be exercised in patients with large vegetations on the aortic valve where there is some concern about provoking embolic events and in patients with renal impairment when cardiac catheterization is not absolutely necessary for planning of the operation.

Safe sternal reentry in case of reoperation requires knowledge about structures at risk of injury, and all these patients should undergo chest CT without contrast; MRI does not provide the same information. When arterial structures such as the ascending aorta, a pseudoaneurysm, or an important graft are in direct contact with the sternum, consideration should be given to peripheral cannulation (preferably via the axillary artery) and institution of cardiopulmonary bypass before sternotomy.

VII. THE SURGERY

A. General principles

1. Objectives of surgery for IE are to prevent additional embolic events, to debride and remove all infected tissue and foreign material (disrupt the biofilm), and to restore functional valves and cardiac integrity. If infection is limited to valve cusps or leaflets (referred to as "simple" IE) of a native valve, replacement with either biologic or mechanical valve prosthesis according to the same principles as for noninfected valves is acceptable. There is no evidence that a bioprosthesis is better or worse than a mechanical valve with regard to risk of recurrent IE, but in patients with neurologic complications and for very sick patients, biologic valves may be preferable to avoid adding complexity to postoperative management by committing the patients to anticoagulation required for mechanical valves.
2. Patients with extravascular invasion beyond the cusps or leaflets require radical debridement and reconstruction, and this is easier to accomplish for the aortic valve and root than for the mitral valve. Aortic root infections are much simpler to expose and debride. The anatomy, access, and use of an allograft for reconstruction make both radical debridement and subsequent reconstruction easier with advanced aortic IE than with advanced mitral valve IE. Radical debridement with removal of all infected and necrotic tissue and foreign material is difficult to accomplish in mitral cases with AV groove invasion, necrosis, and abscess formation, and we do not have a reconstruction valve for the mitral position that is comparable to an aortic allograft.
3. Intraoperative TEE is mandatory in all cases of IE.

B. Aortic valve endocarditis

1. In every IE case, we look carefully for invasion because a small entry may hide an extensive extra-aortic spread of the infection (see Figure 16.2). Radical resection of all infected tissues and foreign material (prosthesis, pledgets, and sutures) is necessary, followed by reconstruction. If the patient has heart block of any degree, the infection is close to the AV node and bundle of His; a good understanding of the anatomy and mastery of different options for root reconstruction is required if these operations are to be safe and successful.
2. An aortic allograft is our preferred choice for reconstructing the aortic root, but use of an allograft is no substitute for radical removal of all infected tissues: Allografts are more resistant than prosthetic valves, but not immune to reinfection. We prefer untreated autologous pericardium when extra material is required.

C. Mitral valve endocarditis

1. Radical resection of all necrotic tissue is performed with caution, although all grossly infected tissue must be removed. When the infection involves mitral annular calcification, all infected calcium has to be debrided. Unaffected leaflets, chordae, and papillary muscles are preserved to allow repair, or to at least offer some support for the posterior annulus.
2. For NVE, repair is preferred and can be performed safely as long as sufficient tissue remains to guide the reconstruction. Standard repair techniques are applied. Successful repair can be achieved by an experienced surgeon in up to 80% of patients. Although it is desirable to avoid extra foreign material during surgery for IE, use of a prosthetic annuloplasty ring in NVE may be necessary to provide a durable repair and has a low risk of infection. The benefits of a good and durable repair outweigh the very low added risk of recurrent infection. If repair is not technically feasible and the valve must be replaced, the choice of valve follows the normal principles of valve surgery.
3. Fortunately, only a third of mitral IE cases are invasive, and the invasion is often shallow, even for PVE, and generally does not require extensive debridement and reconstruction. Deep invasion and destruction of the posterior annulus

require removal of all necrotic and devitalized tissue as well as old suture material. When invasion is deep into the AV groove, debridement must be performed with utmost care, mindful of the complex anatomic relationship in the area and need for reconstruction. Annulus reconstruction is performed with untreated autologous pericardium. Patching the entry to the cavity means the cavity is not drained and therefore has to be sterilized. From an infection standpoint, drainage to the atrium or the pericardium is preferable when possible. In most invasive cases, valve replacement is required. Occasionally, the posterior leaflet contour and chordae are preserved to allow repair of the annulus and leaflet, even in cases with posterior invasion.

VIII. DOUBLE-VALVE ENDOCARDITIS

Most double-valve IE cases are primarily aortic valve IE with jet or kissing lesions in the anterior mitral valve leaflet. These are localized secondary lesions, which can be easily dealt with by excision and an autologous pericardial patch. Destruction of the intervalvular fibrosa (IVF) usually occurs in the setting of PVE affecting both the aortic and mitral valves, although it can also occur with native valve infections. Radical debridement of infected tissue and foreign material may have to include all or parts of the IVF and require its reconstruction with autologous (or bovine) pericardium as well as replacement of both the aortic and mitral valves.

IX. RIGHT-SIDED IE

A. IE involving the right-sided valves, primarily the tricuspid valve and rarely the pulmonary valve, is an increasing problem that accounts for 5% to 10% of patients with IE.

B. Intravenous drug use remains a leading cause of right-sided IE in the Western world, despite both patient profile and the spectrum of causative organisms changing as a result of an increasingly aging population with degenerative valve disease, patients with prosthetic valves, those exposed to nosocomial infections, increasing cardiac interventions like pacers/defibrillators, and increasing staphylococcal infections. Decisions regarding surgery are affected by concerns about continued intravenous drug use and recurrent IE.

C. *S. aureus* is the dominant organism (60% to 90%); *Pseudomonas aeruginosa,* other gram-negative organisms, fungi, enterococci, streptococci, and polymicrobial infections are responsible for the rest. Infections on the right side of the heart are never invasive beyond the valve, so isolated right-sided IE responds better to antibiotic treatment and has low in-hospital mortality (<10%). Surgical treatment is required for large vegetations when the bacteremia cannot be cleared with antibiotics or when there is evidence of recurrent septic pulmonic emboli. Infected pacemaker leads need to be removed along with the pacemaker generator (Table 16.2). Pulling the leads from the generator pocket is associated with risk of serious damage to the tricuspid valve and veins, particularly if leads have been in place for a long time.

D. Strategies for surgery of tricuspid valve IE involve debridement of the infected area and the best possible valve repair (avoiding artificial material whenever possible) tailored to the individual patient. Valvectomy without prosthetic replacement is advocated only in extreme cases but is a possibility if pulmonary vascular resistance (PVR) is low. In patients with repeat pulmonic emboli, PVR and pulmonary artery pressure are likely to be elevated. Free tricuspid valve regurgitation is likely to result in right heart failure. Prosthetic valve replacement is the last resort if the valve cannot be repaired, but continued intravenous drug use is very likely to cause early PVE with need for repeat surgery. Placement of permanent epicardial leads should be considered if the tricuspid valve is replaced and continued need for pacing is anticipated.

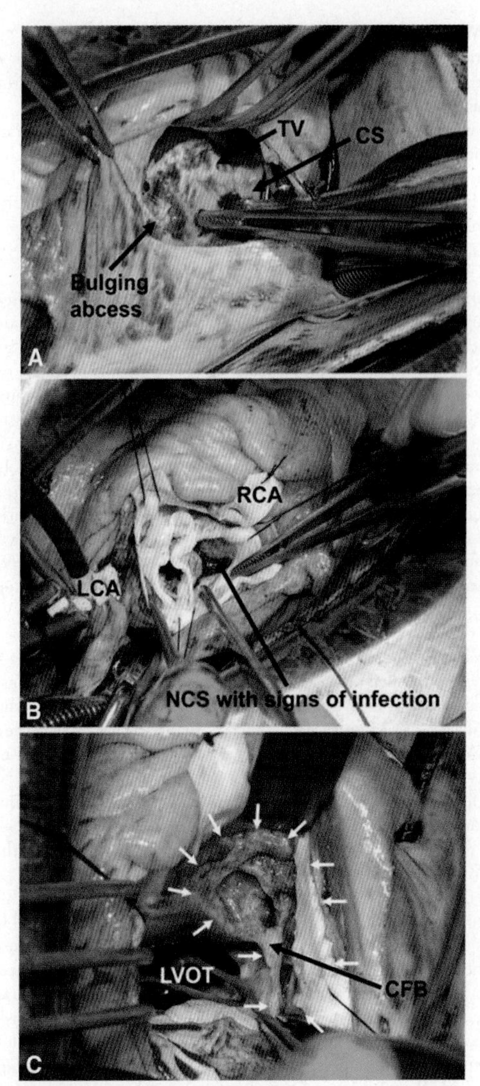

FIGURE 16.2 **A** and **B:** Aortic root abscess involving the noncoronary sinus (NCS) and presenting as a bulging abscess in the right atrium (RA) close to the atrioventricular (AV) node. **B:** The appearance of the aortic valve after transecting the aorta. Signs of infection and abscess are seen in the area of NCS. **C:** Left ventricular outflow tract (LVOT) view after the abscess is debrided *(white arrow)*; the bottom of the abscess is "behind" the central fibrous body. CFB, central fibrous body; CS, coronary sinus; LCA, left coronary artery; RCA, right coronary artery; TV, tricuspid valve.

X. POSTOPERATIVE COMPLICATIONS AND MANAGEMENT

A. Postoperative complications after surgery for active IE are common and include coagulopathy and bleeding requiring reoperations, vasoplegia, sepsis, stroke, multisystem organ failure, and heart block requiring a permanent pacemaker.

B. Patients with active IE routinely receive at least 6 weeks of postoperative intravenous antibiotics. For patients with fungal IE, lifelong oral antifungal therapy might be required. Possible primary and secondary foci of infection should be eradicated. IE patients have a greater risk of recurrent IE, and so patient education about prophylaxis is very important.

XI. OUTCOMES

Despite significant improvement in surgical results, in-hospital mortality among IE patients remains higher than after any other valve surgery. Surgical results depend on many variables, including patient characteristics, valve involved, timing of surgery, whether an emergency procedure is required, virulence of the organism, native or prosthetic IE, and whether the infection has extended into and beyond the valve anulus. The results of surgery for IE have improved over time. Variations in outcomes probably reflect variations in institution and surgeon experience in treating IE.

Traditionally, the factors associated with worse risk and prognoses have been PVE, presence of advanced disease like abscess, or aggressive organisms like *S. aureus.* We recently published our current results with surgery for IE. In 775 consecutive patients with active left-sided IE—413 with NVE and 362 with PVE—overall mortality was 8%, which is higher than for any other valve disease, but still better than previously reported. One- and 7-year survival was 81% and 60%, respectively. The results were worse for mitral IE than for aortic IE, but PVE was not associated with worse outcomes than NVE, even though PVE patients tend to be older and have more comorbidities.

A. Aortic Valve Endocarditis

In 2014, we published our current results of surgery for IE in 395 consecutive patients with isolated aortic valve active IE (Fig. 16.3). One hundred sixty-three patients had native valve IE and 232 prosthetic valve IE. Eighty-five percent of the prosthetic valve and 44% of the native valve IE patients had invasive disease, and overall operative mortality was 7%. Survival was similar after surgery for PVE and NVE. There was also no difference in survival between those with invasive versus noninvasive IE, which reflects our improved ability to master the surgery for invasive aortic valve IE, as we are able to debride the aortic root extensively and reconstruct it with an allograft.

B. Mitral Valve Endocarditis

Overall, the outcomes for patients requiring surgery for mitral valve IE were worse than for patients with aortic valve IE (Fig. 16.3). This is explained by mitral IE patients being sicker as well as the fact that invasive mitral disease is surgically more difficult to deal with. The results for valve repair are superior to those for valve replacement for mitral IE, with lower hospital mortality, improved long-term survival, better infection-free survival, and a reinfection rate of less than 1% per year. Patients who receive valve repair have less advanced disease, are less sick, and may experience long-term benefit from better preservation of left ventricular function associated with mitral valve repair. Patients with IE requiring valve replacement are the sickest patients with the most advanced and destructive disease.

With improved understanding of the disease and better management, both medical and surgical, the outcomes of patients with mitral PVE are improving and approaching those for mitral NVE. Outcomes are still worse for invasive mitral infection, and this is true for PVE and NVE. This is due to our limited ability to perform radical debridement, sterilization, and drainage of the infected area in patients with invasive disease into the AV groove. In addition, we lack an alternative mitral valve prosthesis that is equally optimal for IE, simple to implant, and as good as the allograft for the aortic valve.

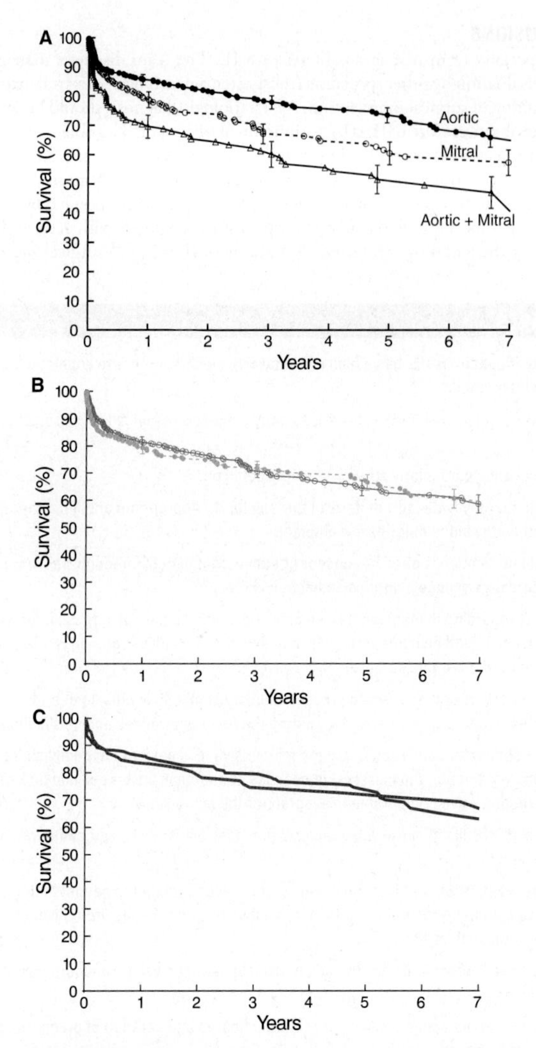

FIGURE 16.3 Survival after surgery for endocarditis. **A:** Survival after surgery for left-sided infective endocarditis (IE), stratified by the involved valve. Each *symbol* represents a death, and *vertical bars* represent the 68% confidence limits, equivalent to ±1 standard error in each figure. *Filled circles* indicate aortic valve IE alone; *open circles*, mitral valve IE alone; and *triangles*, aortic and mitral valve IE. Survival was significantly lower in the mitral and combined groups than in the isolated aortic patients ($p < 0.0001$). **B:** Survival after surgery for native *(solid green lines)* or prosthetic *(dashed orange lines)* aortic valve IE. **C:** Survival after surgery for invasive *(dashed red lines)* versus noninvasive *(solid blue lines)* aortic valve IE. (Adapted from Hussain ST, Shrestha NK, Gordon SM, et al. Residual patient, anatomic, and surgical obstacles in treating active left-sided infective endocarditis. *J Thorac Cardiovasc Surg*. 2014;148:981–988, with permission from Elsevier.)

XII. CONCLUSIONS

A multispecialty team manages patients with IE. The team discusses management and need for evaluation by other specialists (most often a neurologist or psychiatrist) and need for and timing of surgical intervention. A bacteriologic diagnosis should be secured before starting antibiotics. Cure of IE is by antimicrobial treatment. The objectives of surgery are to remove infected tissue and foreign material, prevent embolic events, and restore cardiac integrity and functional valves. To avoid further embolic complications and destruction and invasion, surgery is recommended as soon as a surgical indication has been established. There seems to be a minimal penalty for operating on patients with active infection. Understanding the pathology and surgical anatomy of IE is key to surgical success.

KEY PEARLS

- Infective endocarditis (IE) has a high mortality, even with appropriate antibiotic therapy and surgical intervention.
- High index of suspicion for IE is the key to early diagnosis, especially in cases of prosthetic valve IE.
- Embolic events, particularly strokes, are very common.
- Antibiotic therapy is the cornerstone of therapy for IE. Appropriate antibiotic therapy should be initiated *after* blood cultures are obtained.
- Surgical intervention is often needed for effective treatment of infection. There is no reason to wait for surgery once a surgical indication is present.
- Decisions regarding management strategies and optimal timing of surgical intervention are complex and should be made by a multispecialty team including cardiology, infectious disease, and cardiothoracic surgery.
- Objectives of surgery for IE are to prevent additional embolic events, to debride and remove all infected and foreign tissue, and to restore the functional valves and cardiac integrity.
- Radical debridement and reconstruction for invasive IE is easier to accomplish for the aortic valve and root than for the mitral valve because of anatomic limitations and lack of suitable reconstruction valve comparable to allograft for the mitral valve.
- For mitral IE, results of mitral valve repair, when possible, are superior compared with valve replacement.
- Outcomes remain worse for mitral versus aortic valve IE related to patient factors, inherent mitral valve anatomy in patients with invasive disease, and lack of alternative mitral valve prosthesis optimal for IE.
- With improved surgical results, the added risk of prosthetic valve endocarditis is neutralized for left-sided IE.
- Surgery during the active phase is not contraindicated and duration of preoperative antibiotic treatment is not critical.
- Cure of the infection requires adequate postoperative antibiotic treatment.

SUGGESTED READINGS

Baddour LM, Wilson WR, Bayer AS, et al. Infective endocarditis: diagnosis, antimicrobial therapy, and management of complications: a statement for healthcare professionals form the Committee on Rheumatic Fever, Endocarditis, and Kawasaki Disease, Council on Cardiovascular Disease in the Young, and the Councils on Clinical Cardiology, Stroke, and Cardiovascular Surgery and Anesthesia, American Herat Association: endorsed by Infectious Disease Society of America. *Circulation*. 2005;111:e394–e434.

Byrne JG, Rezai K, Sanchez JA, et al. Surgical management of endocarditis: the Society of Thoracic Surgeons clinical practice guidelines. *Ann Thorac Surg*. 2011;91:2012–2019.

David TE, Gavra G, Feindel CM, et al. Surgical treatment of active infective endocarditis: a continued challenge. *J Thorac Cardiovasc Surg*. 2007;133:144–149.

Gordon SM, Pettersson GB. Native-valve infective endocarditis—when does it require surgery? (editorial comments). *N Engl J Med*. 2012;366:2519–2521.

Habib G, Hoen B, Tornos P, et al. Guidelines on the prevention, diagnosis, and treatment of infective endocarditis (new version 2009): the Task Force on the Prevention, Diagnosis, and Treatment of Infective Endocarditis of the European Society of Cardiology (ESC). *Eur Heart J*. 2009;30:2369–2413.

Hoen B, Duval X. Clinical practice. Infective endocarditis. *N Engl J Med*. 2013;368:1425–1433.

Hussain ST, Shrestha NK, Gordon SM, et al. Residual patient, anatomic, and surgical obstacles in treating active left-sided infective endocarditis. *J Thorac Cardiovasc Surg*. 2014;148:981–988.

Kang D-H, Kim Y-J, Kim S-H, et al. Early surgery versus conventional treatment for infective endocarditis. *N Engl J Med*. 2012;366:2466–2473.

Li JS, Sexton DJ, Mick N, et al. Proposed modifications to the Duke criteria for the diagnosis of infective endocarditis. *Clin Infect Dis*. 2000;30:633–638.

Lytle BW, Sabik JF, Blackstone EH, et al. Reoperative cryopreserved root and ascending aorta replacement for acute aortic prosthetic valve endocarditis. *Ann Thorac Surg*. 2002;74:S1754–S1757.

Manne MB, Shrestha NK, Lytle BW, et al. Outcomes after surgical treatment of native and prosthetic valve infective endocarditis. *Ann Thorac Surg*. 2012;93:489–493.

Murdroch DR, Corey GR, Hoen B, et al. Clinical presentation, etiology, and outcome of infective endocarditis in the 21st century: the International Collaboration on Endocarditis-Prospective Cohort study. *Arch Intern Med*. 2009;169:463–473.

Musci M, Siniawski H, Pasic M, et al. Surgical treatment of right-sided active infective endocarditis with or without involvement of the left heart: 20 year single-center experience. *Eur J Cardiothorac Surg*. 2007;32:118–125.

Nishimura RA, Otto CM, Bonow RO, et al. 2014 AHA/ACC guideline for the management of patients with valvular heart disease: executive summary: a report of the American College of Cardiology/American Heart Association Task Force on Practice Guidelines. *Circulation*. 2014;129:2440–2492.

Pettersson GB, Hussain ST, Ramankutty RM, et al. Reconstruction of fibrous skeleton: technique, pitfalls and results. *Multimed Man Cardiothorac Surg*. 2014;2014. pii:mmu004. doi:10.1093/mmcts/mmu004.

Pettersson GB, Hussain ST, Shrestha NK, et al. Infective endocarditis: an atlas of disease progression for describing, staging, coding, and understanding the pathology. *J Thorac Cardiovasc Surg*. 2014;147:1142–1149.

Sheikh AM, Elhenawy AM, Maganti M, et al. Outcomes of surgical intervention for isolated active mitral valve endocarditis. *J Thorac Cardiovasc Surg*. 2009;137:110–116.

Thuny F, Beurtheret S, Mancini J, et al. The timing of surgery influences mortality and morbidity in adults with severe complicated infective endocarditis: a propensity analysis. *Eur Heart J*. 2011;32:2027–2033.

Thuny F, Grisoli D, Collart F, et al. Management of infective endocarditis: challenges and perspectives. *Lancet*. 2012;379:965–975.

SECTION IV

Multimodality Imaging and Cardiac Catheterization Laboratory Assessment

CHAPTER 17

Srikanth Koneru
Milind Y. Desai

Computed Tomography/Magnetic Resonance Imaging

I. INTRODUCTION

Multimodality imaging has been increasingly used to advance our knowledge of causes and consequences of valvular heart disease. Echocardiography is now the standard modality for evaluation of patients with valvular heart disease because it is widely accessible, cost-effective, and portable. However, there are significant limitations in precisely assessing the morphology and severity of valvular dysfunction especially in patients with poor acoustic windows. In addition, the assessment of valvular disease with echocardiography is operator dependent. Over the past two decades, cardiac computed tomography (CT) and magnetic resonance imaging (MRI) are emerging as alternative imaging modalities by allowing excellent visualization of the morphologic features and function of a wide range of valvular diseases.

In this chapter, we emphasize the role of cardiac CT and MRI in assessing cardiac valves, along with their role in preprocedural assessment.

II. AORTIC STENOSIS

A. Morphology

1. The morphology of the aortic valve is clearly assessed by echocardiography; however, it may be challenging to discern if the image quality is suboptimal or there is technical difficulty secondary to patient body habitus. In these patients, cardiac CT and MRI are immensely helpful to precisely assess the aortic valve structure.
2. In using cardiac CT to assess the aortic valve, both systolic and diastolic phases have to be evaluated carefully as there could be a bicuspid aortic valve with a raphe, which could mimic normal tricuspid leaflets in the diastolic phase. The raphe of a bicuspid aortic valve is usually indicative of a fusion line between the two leaflets of the bicuspid aortic valve (e.g., fusion of the left to right coronary cusps). A typical fish-mouth appearance is clearly viewed during the systolic phase of data acquisition. Most commonly, the two cusps of a bicuspid aortic valve are unequal in size because of congenital fusion of the leaflets. Rarely, no raphe is identified, and this type of bicuspid aortic valve is termed true or pure bicuspid aortic valve. It is important clinically to diagnose bicuspid or unicuspid and, on rare occasions, quadricuspid (4 leaflets) aortic valve, because this would signal a further evaluation of the patient's thoracic aorta to rule out associated thoracic aortic aneurysm, which could readily be evaluated within the same CT study.
3. Cardiac MRI has an advantage in evaluating young patients with suspected abnormal aortic valve morphology without the risk of radiation and also gives an excellent signal-to-noise ratio and better spatial resolution compared with transesophageal echocardiogram and transthoracic echocardiogram (TTE) for anatomic aortic valve assessment. Steady-state free precession (SSFP) acquisition with electrocardiography (ECG) gating is used to assess the aortic valve morphology. Once

again, cardiac MRI also has the advantage of enabling evaluation of the thoracic aorta for a possible aortopathy.

B. Aortic valve calcification

1. Slow progression of calcification along with sclerotic thickening of the aortic valve reduces aortic valve excursion and impedes left ventricular (LV) outflow. CT provides high spatial resolution in assessment of aortic annular and leaflet calcification. Aortic valve calcium is defined as calcification within the valve leaflet or aortic annulus. In CT images, calcific deposits are displayed as bright regions within the image and are quantified by using Agatston units (AUs). The threshold for a calcific lesion was set at a CT density of 130 Hounsfield units having an area $\geq$1 mm^2 with a density of 3 to 4 pixels. Area and volume of calcifications should be calculated per slice and summated. A recent study has shown that a calcium score $<$700 AU excludes severe aortic stenosis (AS) with a high negative predictive value and a score $>$2,000 AU suggests severe AS. However, according to the current guidelines, CT is not recommended for diagnosing AS, although calcification is the primary underlying pathology.
2. Measuring the aortic valve area planimetry by CT is also feasible and should be performed during midsystolic frames, ideally at 5% to 25% of the R-R interval to infer stenosis severity. Although CT is rarely used in clinical practice for this purpose, it has been shown to have a promising correlation with stenosis severity as assessed by TTE and is a useful guide in assessing the aortic valve when aortic valve calcification is seen on routine CT scans.
3. Cardiac MRI can be utilized in uncertain cases with inconclusive echocardiography results. The aortic valve planimetry can be performed from a series of sequential high-resolution SSFP or gradient echo cines acquired every 4 mm from a transverse plane. The smallest systolic opening during peak systole is planimetered. Low-dose dobutamine can be administered at the dose similar to echocardiography (up to 20 µg/kg/min) to differentiate pseudo-AS from true AS and also to assess contractile reserve. Cardiac MRI cannot quantify aortic valve calcification as there will be a signal void in the standard SSFP cine images.

C. Quantification of severity

1. Severity of AS can be assessed by echocardiography through measurement of transaortic valve flow velocity and insertion of the value into the continuity equation to obtain aortic valve area. The echocardiogram-based measure of aortic valve area is considered both reliable and accurate. However, it is increasingly common to underestimate transaortic flow velocity if the alignment of the transducer curser is not parallel to the flow, making it technically difficult to obtain the highest Doppler velocity.
2. Cardiac MRI has an advantage in this regard by allowing slice selection at any angle to measure an accurate flow velocity across the valve. Phase-contrast velocity mapping makes it possible to measure the flow of interest in an *en face* image of the aortic valve to determine the severity of the aortic valve stenosis by peak velocity. The phase-contrast imaging assesses the flow by calculating a shift of the precession between the stationary protons and protons moving in a magnetic field. The magnitude of this phase shift is proportional to the velocity of interest. The velocity must be sampled at 25 to 50 cm/s increments by setting the velocity encoding to reach the determined peak aortic valve velocity where there is no aliasing. A misalignment of more than 20 degrees between the phase direction and flow direction makes the velocities inaccurate. The functional and hemodynamic assessment of flow is not feasible and is still a research tool in the field of cardiac CT.

D. Assessing ventricular function

1. AS increases the afterload on the left ventricle, an effect that leads to compensatory LV hypertrophy. The chronicity of AS leads to ventricular dysfunction followed by irreversible LV injury, which is characterized histologically by fibrosis. Severity

and chronicity of AS can be assessed by measuring LV mass, volume, and ejection fraction. A reduced LV ejection fraction and increased LV mass have been associated with poor outcome in asymptomatic patients. The fast technical development of cardiac CT scanner hardware along with multisegmental image reconstruction has led to rapid improvement of spatial and temporal resolution and significantly faster cardiac scans. ECG-gated four-dimensional (4D) cine image reconstruction in systolic and diastolic phases can help assess LV functional parameters. The end-diastolic and end-systolic frames are used to calculate the LV volumes and ejection fraction, whereas an end-diastolic frame should be used to calculate LV mass. However, considering the accompanying contrast administration, radiation, and limited temporal resolution, referring a patient to cardiac CT only for evaluation of LV function is not warranted but adds important clinical information if the CT data are acquired for a different diagnostic utility (e.g., coronary artery disease, assessing aorta).

2. Cardiac MRI is very attractive in assessing LV function because there is no radiation exposure, though the risk of gadolinium is only evident in patients with renal dysfunction. A complete set of short-axis sequential cine images is acquired from base to apex (every 8 mm) using SSFP pulse sequence. The advantage of cardiac MRI is (1) it can assess LV and right ventricular (RV) function by planimetry of LV and RV volumes in end-diastole and end-systole slices, in a three-dimensional fashion without the need for geometric assumptions, and (2) the volumes are calculated by summing all the slices, thus determining ventricular stroke volume, cardiac output, and ejection fraction with standard equations. Furthermore, planimetry of epicardial contours can be performed on all the slices to obtain a highly accurate ventricular mass measurement. Late gadolinium-delayed enhancement imaging in patients with AS has shown patchy mid-wall enhancement in patients with severe stenosis. This likely reflects focal areas of fibrosis, which have also been correlated in autopsy studies, and has been associated with worse prognosis. Also, diffuse myocardial fibrosis can be quantified using T1 mapping and other newer MRI techniques currently being investigated.

E. Procedural assessment

1. Calcific and degenerative AS is a dynamic and progressive disease, with risk factors similar to atherosclerosis. Currently, there are no options to slow the progression of this disease, and the only solution is aortic valve replacement for advanced disease stages. Surgical aortic valve replacement is the treatment of choice for the majority of patients with severe symptomatic AS suitable for surgery. However, there are a significant number of patients with high operative mortality secondary to advanced age and comorbidities, as estimated from a number of different scoring systems such as the Society of Thoracic Surgeons (STS) risk estimate or EuroSCORE. The poor outcomes with medical management in patients with high surgical risk have led to the development of less invasive transcatheter interventional procedures, including percutaneous balloon aortic valvuloplasty and transcatheter valve replacement.
2. For the transcatheter approach to AS, the cardiac CT evaluation and imaging acquisition protocols are unique and are integrated into the work-up of transcatheter aortic valve replacement (TAVR) patients. They typically include imaging the entire aorta, including the aortic root, thoracoabdominal aorta, and iliofemoral arteries, along with a high-resolution (4D) root acquisitions for better detail of the valve/root imaging. ECG gating is critical to avoid image degeneration secondary to motion artifact as this could affect the precise measurement of the aortic root and annulus. The ECG gating could be achieved by either prospective gating or retrospective gating. Prospective gating has an advantage of reduced radiation exposure; however, it limits image acquisition to specific phases of the cardiac cycle. Though retrospective gating has the disadvantage of higher radiation exposure, it

has the advantage of acquiring the entire cardiac cycle to subsequently reconstruct images to a specific phase of the cycle. In addition, retrospective gating allows 4D image reconstruction of multiple image planes to evaluate the aortic root and annulus at different cardiac phases (i.e., aortic annulus during systolic phase) and helps to evaluate LV and left valvular function.

3. Radiation exposure is an important aspect to consider, though less concerning in the elderly patient population being evaluated for TAVR. Advanced scanner technology and imaging protocols allow a better image resolution with lower doses of radiation. Another critical aspect to consider is administration of contrast. Although contrast is necessary for precise measurement of luminal and annular diameters, the risk and benefit should be weighed before administering this in an elderly population with underlying renal dysfunction. A standard contrast dose of 80 to 120 mL is administered for a typical TAVR protocol. However, lower contrast-volume protocols are being evaluated; these use only 30 mL of contrast to visualize the aortic root with retrospective ECG gating, followed by a subsequent high-pitch data acquisition of the same contrast bolus. Alternatively, using an intra-arterial injection of contrast for iliofemoral CT angiography through a catheter left in place during coronary angiography may reduce the contrast required to <15 mL.
4. Annular measurements have been historically performed by using two-dimensional (2D) transthoracic or transesophageal echocardiography and aortic angiography, assuming the annulus is a circular orifice. From the procedural point of view, the annulus is defined as the plane at the lowest insertion point of the aortic valve leaflets, just above the LV outflow tract (LVOT). The acquired three-dimensional (3D) data from the CT scan are reconstructed along precisely defined 2D imaging planes perpendicular to the center axis, immediately below the hinge point of the aortic valve cusps. These double-oblique reconstructed planes reveal an ovoid to elliptical shape of the LVOT, from which the long- and short-axis diameters are measured, allowing for the calculation of the mean diameter. In addition, perimeter and area of the annulus can be obtained by planimetry, thus guiding the selection of correct prosthesis size and type (Fig. 17.1). Though currently there are no definite exclusion criteria based on the risk of coronary obstruction during TAVR, measuring the distance from the coronary ostia to the annulus helps in identifying patients at risk for coronary occlusion. The CoreValve (Medtronic, Minneapolis, MN) extends beyond the sinotubular junction into the aorta (in contrast to Edwards Lifesciences [Irvine, CA] valve), and hence measuring the ascending aorta should be part of the evaluation, as currently the maximal diameter of the proximal ascending aorta should not exceed 40, 42, and 43 mm for the three sizes of valves available.

   Finally, assessing the iliofemoral arteries for access is a major component of TAVR evaluation as this is the major route of delivery for the most commonly used devices. Vascular complications have emerged as the major cause of mortality and morbidity associated with percutaneous femoral interventions using older large sheaths (#22 French to #24 French) compared with the currently available vascular sheaths (#18 French). Assessing calcification is particularly important. If arranged in a circumferential or horseshoe-like pattern, such calcification limits arterial expandability to accommodate large-profile delivery sheaths, likely increasing the risk of dissection or perforation. CT provides multiple measurements throughout the course of the iliofemoral system bilaterally, with the minimum luminal diameter measured on each side and specific areas with reduced luminal size or plaque burden also assessed (Fig. 17.2).
5. Newer delivery systems, along with integrating CT into the TAVR work-up, further reduce the vascular complications, and in the setting of unfavorable iliofemoral anatomy, a subclavian or transapical approach may be selected.
6. Though the standard of care involves cardiac CT for TAVR evaluation, rarely cardiac MRI can be used for this purpose because it carries no risk of radiation, provides

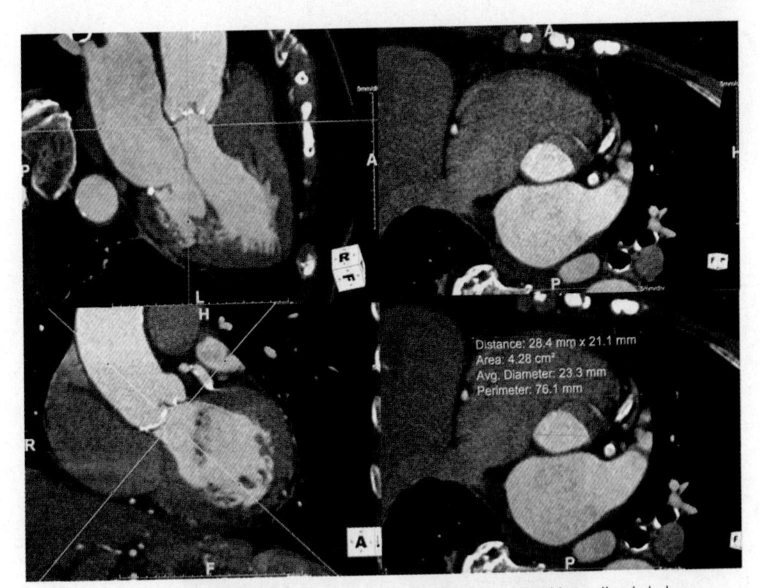

FIGURE 17.1 Measurement of annulus: The annulus is defined at the level immediately below the hinge points of the aortic valve leaflets. The double-oblique reconstruction planes reveal the ovoid-shaped annulus. The long and short diameters, along with the perimeter and area of the annulus are obtained.

superior hemodynamic information, and may be performed without contrast in patients with renal insufficiency. SSFP MRI sequences including the short axis at the level of the aortic valve, along with a 3D whole-heart image covering up to the ascending aorta, allow for reconstruction of the aortic annulus in orthogonal views, to precisely measure the aortic annular dimensions.

III. AORTIC REGURGITATION

A. Morphology

Bicuspid aortic valve and ectasia of the aortic root are the most common causes of aortic regurgitation (AR) in the developed countries, whereas rheumatic heart disease is more common in the developing countries. As mentioned earlier, the aorta and aortic valve structure are well visualized by both CT and MRI and can elucidate the mechanism of AR by demonstrating the valve cusp characteristics, and the status of aortic root and ascending aorta. Both imaging modalities demonstrate the regurgitant orifice in the case of moderate to severe AR. The area of the regurgitant orifice can be quantified with planimetry in the diastolic phase of the cardiac cycle and correlates with the severity of regurgitation estimated by echocardiography. An area of 0.28 cm^2 has a sensitivity and specificity of 90% and 91%, respectively, in detecting severe AR (Fig. 17.3). In MRI, the presence of a regurgitant jet can also be visualized in the long-axis LVOT cine images either through SSFP or by gradient echo (Fig. 17.4). This flow turbulence produces a signal void on the MRI cine images because of dephasing of protons. Early studies have shown some correlation between the signal void and the echocardiographic method of grading AR. A narrow jet width at the origin suggests lower degrees of regurgitation, whereas a wide jet with a core of high signal void

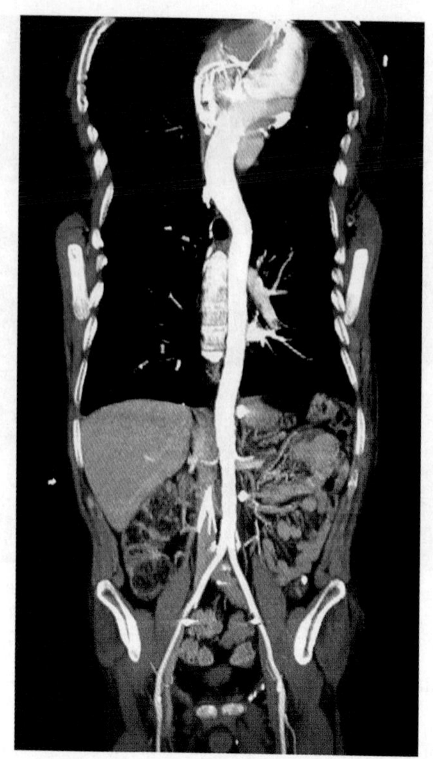

FIGURE 17.2 Assessing the iliofemoral arteries and aorta for evaluation of access. Centerline image processing of the iliac arteries allows assessment of the dimensions, calculation, and angulations.

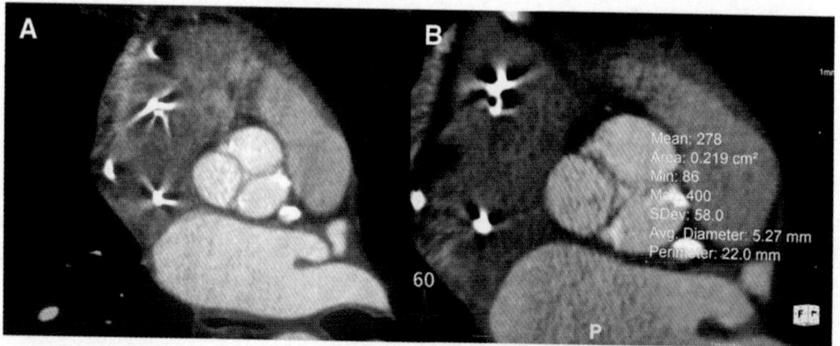

FIGURE 17.3 **A:** Using three-dimensional reconstruction along the cardiac cycle allows identification of the diastolic phase with aortic valve closure. A perpendicular plane at the aortic valve leaflet tips allows measurement of aortic regurgitant orifice area by planimetry. **B:** The measurement of aortic orifice area of 0.219 cm^2 corresponds to moderate aortic regurgitation, which was confirmed by echocardiography.

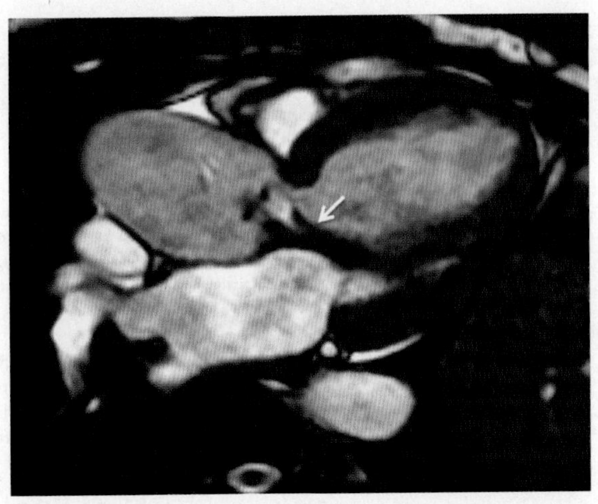

FIGURE 17.4 The steady-state free precession sequence showing signal void *(arrow)* in the left ventricular outflow tract view with eccentric jet of aortic regurgitation in diastole.

suggests more severe regurgitation. However, the signal void is highly dependent on the type of MRI pulse sequence parameters and can be misleading if it is the only method used to quantitate AR.

B. Quantification of severity

1. Cardiac MRI is an attractive tool for assessing AR because of its ability to quantify flow directly using through-plane phase-contrast velocity mapping, which does not rely on calculations from complex equations. The temporal resolution of the cardiac flow measurement is lower than the continuous-wave Doppler used in echocardiography, but is comparable for most flow and velocity quantification. Phase-offset errors due to eddy currents in the magnetic field can occur, affecting the background flow measurements. It is critical to ensure the image slice is at the magnet isocenter to minimize error.
2. The flow mapping image slice is placed just above the aortic valve to quantify both the forward and regurgitant flow in a single cardiac cycle. Placing the image slice much higher than the aortic valve level can underestimate the regurgitant volume, though this avoids the turbulent flow at the valve level. Phase-contrast method produces two sets of images, magnitude images and phase velocity maps. Magnitude images are used for anatomic orientation of the image slice and to identify the boundaries of the vessel images, and the phase maps encode the velocities within each pixel. Flow is derived through integration of the area over time and the velocity of each pixel per cardiac cycle. The instantaneous flow volume of each frame is plotted against the time of the cardiac cycle to integrate area under the curve for systole and diastole, by which regurgitant volume and regurgitant fraction (regurgitant volume/forward volume × 100%) can be obtained. The AR quantification using cardiac MRI is well correlated with echocardiographic and catheter-based quantification. Cardiac MRI quantification is the only technique that does not rely on any calculations and is the only true in vivo method of quantification of AR. Therefore, there is no better gold standard to compare its accuracy. The AR is quantified as severe when the regurgitant volume is ≥60 mL

or regurgitant fraction is ≥50%. Cardiac MRI quantification has recently been shown to predict need for valve replacement and symptom development with a regurgitant fraction of >33%, which provides the threshold for patients likely requiring surgery within the next few years.

3. Another less attractive indirect method of quantification of AR is through calculating both LV and RV volumes through acquiring multislice 2D SSFP short- and long-axis cine images and comparing the volumes of both the chambers. This method relies on the assumption of lack of any other significant valvular regurgitation or shunts, along with the assumption of precise contouring of both the chambers on multiple slices. This method is useful as an internal validation of the flow quantification or when the flow quantification cannot be performed.

C. **Assessing ventricular function**

1. AR causes volume overload of the left ventricle, followed by pressure overload from the increased wall stress. These changes are often chronic and slowly progressive, leading to LV dilatation and hypertrophy to preserve LV function during the long asymptomatic period. However, once the left ventricle continues to enlarge, decompensation occurs, followed by reversible and then irreversible ventricular dysfunction. Both excessive dilatation and reduced ventricular function are strong indicators of a poor prognosis. The ventricular volumes are optimally evaluated by obtaining multiple 2D SSFP cine images covering the ventricle; then a parallel stack of serial images (4 chambers) is acquired from base to apex with an 8-mm slice thickness and a slice gap of 2 mm. The volume from each image obtained from the stack is calculated as the area of endocardial tracing multiplied by the addition of image slice and interslice gap. All the slice volumes obtained from end-diastolic and end-systolic frames are summed, which will allow for calculating the stroke volume, cardiac output, and ejection fraction through standard equations. The end-diastolic volume index is used to analyze LV dilatation. Cardiac MRI is the most accurate and reproducible technique for assessing both LV and RV volumes and mass. Cardiac MRI–derived LV volumes also predict the onset of symptoms and other indications for surgery, though less strongly than quantification of the regurgitant severity.
2. Cardiac MRI is useful in quantification of AR, LV volumetric analysis, and determination of aortic root anatomy, along with having the advantage of getting all the information required without any contrast or radiation exposure, making it an attractive tool for assessing AR.
3. Although CT is not recommended for analysis of AR, the LV volume and mass may be analyzed by CT in patients assessed for aortic root dimensions or coronary artery disease, which could help in planning for more accurate diagnostic tests.

IV. MITRAL STENOSIS

Mitral valves are better visualized and assessed by echocardiography, particularly TEE, which remains the first-line technique given its higher spatial and temporal resolution compared with cardiac MRI or CT. However, cardiac MRI can be helpful in some patients with difficult echocardiographic windows. Cardiac MRI provides good visualization of the restricted mitral leaflets on the LVOT view, along with other cine images. Multiple thin slices can be obtained by positioning the image plane at the mitral valve tips to accurately perform planimetry of the orifice area during diastole. Similar to AS, diastolic flow and velocity can be obtained from the mitral valve through phase-contrast imaging, though when atrial fibrillation is present, the accuracy of the flow measurement is limited. Cardiac CT has the advantage of assessing calcification and thickening of the mitral leaflet and submitral apparatus for planning balloon mitral valvuloplasty. Mitral valve area can be calculated by dose modulation and acquiring the cardiac phase during diastole, which can be postprocessed and reconstructed in orthogonal planes to obtain a precise level of the leaflet tips at mid-diastole to measure the orifice area. However, its clinical use for this is limited.

V. MITRAL REGURGITATION

Echocardiography is the investigation of choice for assessing mitral regurgitation (MR). With their high spatial and temporal resolutions, TTE and TEE can easily evaluate the mechanism of regurgitation. Assessment of mitral leaflet morphology and valve function has improved further with newer-generation 3D TEE, giving the flexibility of postprocessing the data, analyzing 3D proximal isovelocity surface area, and reconstructing the acquired data in orthogonal planes to determine the precise severity of MR. Furthermore, 3D TEE can accurately localize the flail and prolapsing scallop of the mitral leaflets if mitral valve prolapse is the mechanism of MR. In some patients, symptoms and severity of MR assessed by echocardiography may not match, or the orientation of the regurgitant jet, such as with an eccentric jet, can make assessment by echocardiography difficult and unreliable. Cardiac MRI, and to some extent cardiac CT, may be able to provide useful information, and cardiac MRI can further validate the severity of MR quantified through other modalities.

A. Morphology

Mitral valve leaflets are interrogated with long-axis cine slices through each segment, specifically across the commissure, perpendicular to the edge of the leaflets at each scallop, to better visualize all segments of the leaflets. This provides long-axis views of all the leaflet scallops to provide an insight into the mechanisms (prolapse, thickening, restriction, flail) of MR. Cardiac MRI has the ability to characterize all the parts of the mitral apparatus including the papillary muscles, chordae, and individual scallops throughout the cardiac cycle. Acquiring thin slices (4 mm) parallel to the mitral annulus, placed at the mitral tips in systole, can provide direct visualization and measurement of the regurgitant orifice area. However, the complex shape of the mitral valve and annular motion during systole lead to difficulty in acquisition of images, which is not achievable in all patients.

Cardiac CT can also assess mitral valve morphology by acquisition of a data set during the entire cardiac cycle. Images are reconstructed in 4-chamber, 2-chamber, and 3-chamber views along with short-axis views to visualize the entire mitral apparatus. Cardiac CT has a sensitivity of 96% and specificity of 93% in accurately identifying mitral valve prolapse. Leaflets should be regarded as thickened if $>$2 mm in diameter, indicating myxomatous, degenerative, or inflammatory disease. Mitral annular calcification can also be visualized with a precise determination of its extension into the valve leaflets. Rarely, cardiac CT is extremely helpful to differentiate tumors from "caseous" mitral annular calcification.

B. Quantification of severity

1. Severity of MR is usually calculated indirectly by subtracting the aortic systolic flow from the LV stroke volume. In patients with MR, the total LV stroke volume is increased to compensate for the volume regurgitating into the left atrium; this volume can be calculated by acquiring serial SSFP cine images of short-axis stacks of the left ventricle from base to the apex followed by counting and measuring the LV volumes, as described earlier for LV volume assessment for AR. This provides the total LV volume, which comprises both stroke volume and mitral regurgitant volume. Calculating the stroke volume from the phase-contrast imaging of the aortic valve is done by placing the flow mapping slice at the level of the valve and acquiring both magnitude images and phase velocity maps as described earlier, in the aortic regurgitation section, to determine the stroke volume. Finally, subtracting the aortic forward flow (stroke volume) from the total LV volume equals the mitral regurgitant volume. Regurgitant fraction can be calculated by computing regurgitant volume/LV volume $\times$ 100%. This method of calculation relies on a combination of two different MRI techniques (phase contrast and counting LV

volumes through cine images), so care is required to minimize the errors while acquiring the flow sequences and LV contours. Also, this method can only be used to determine whether the MR is a single-valve lesion.

2. The quantification of MR correlates well with echocardiography and catheter-based assessment with good reproducibility. In addition, cardiac MRI quantification of MR provides a threshold for predicting the patients suitable for early mitral valve replacement or repair when the regurgitant fraction is 40% or greater. Large-scale clinical trials are required to validate and identify these patient populations.
3. Patients with acute myocardial infarction and associated MR as well as patients with chronic MR secondary to potential hibernating myocardium can be identified by cardiac MRI with the help of delayed enhancement imaging. This helps with decisions regarding the benefit and role of revascularization of the involved arterial territory and also whether valve repair or replacement versus revascularization alone will be required. Delayed enhancement imaging represents a noninvasive method to assess myocardial fibrosis. It has been shown that the presence of delayed enhancement on CMR is associated with less favorable outcomes in multiple cardiovascular diseases. Recent findings have suggested that lateral wall and papillary muscle infarct leads to a higher incidence of associated MR in patients with acute myocardial infarction. The lack of viability in the lateral wall of the left ventricle evaluated by delayed enhancement may suggest poor outcome with revascularization alone compared with accompanying mitral valve repair or replacement. Delayed enhancement imaging was also shown in patients with primary MR to be a marker of LV remodeling.
4. There are newer methods under clinical investigation to further strengthen cardiac MRI quantification of MR. One of these is 4D flow cardiac MRI for quantification of MR, which is independent of hemodynamic and geometric assumptions. It has the capability to retrospectively position the image plane in the direction of regurgitation and analyze multiple jets with separate image planes. However, no gold standard is currently available to validate 4D flow cardiac MRI. Clinicians are waiting for long-term clinical trials before including 4D flow quantification into everyday clinical cardiac MRI protocols.

C. **Procedural assessment**

1. Minimally invasive mitral valve repair (i.e., right thoracotomy and robotic approaches) has been proposed as an alternative technique for invasive open-heart surgery. However, because of the requirement for peripheral cardiopulmonary bypass, cardiac CT is utilized for preoperative assessment of systemic arterial and vascular anatomy to determine the risk of embolic complications and to assess coronary arteries. In patients anticipating minimally invasive surgeries, the presence of significant aortoiliac atherosclerosis may dictate a change to a more standard surgical approach with central cannulation.
2. Cardiac CT also provides an opportunity for precise measurement of the mitral valve orifice size used for upcoming transcatheter mitral valve implantation. Furthermore, cardiac CT can precisely assess mitral valve calcification before mitral valve balloon valvuloplasty for rheumatic mitral valve stenosis.

VI. PULMONARY STENOSIS

The pulmonary valve is a delicate semilunar valve with three cusps (anterior, right, and left) and lacks coronary ostia. Pulmonary stenosis is a congenital disorder in almost 95% of cases. Acquired pulmonary stenosis is extremely rare, with few cases noted secondary to rheumatic fever or carcinoid heart disease. Pulmonary stenosis may affect RV function by elevating RV pressure, resulting in RV hypertrophy, dilatation, and dysfunction. The pulmonary valve can be difficult to assess by echocardiography because of its location behind the sternum. RV function is also difficult to assess, particularly by volumetric analysis, secondary to its complex shape.

Cardiac CT is useful in detecting the poststenotic dilatation of the main and left pulmonary artery. Usually, the right pulmonary artery is normal in size, as the turbulent flow from pulmonary stenosis is directed posteriorly toward the left pulmonary artery. The 4D cine images may show restricted and thickened pulmonary valves. Similar to aortic valve area, pulmonary valve area measurement by planimetry is also feasible and should be performed during midsystolic frames to infer stenosis severity. RV function can also be analyzed using 4D cine retrospective imaging as described earlier, to precisely calculate RV volume and function. Cardiac CT can help in assessing the pulmonary valve and RV function. Its use for serial assessment is less valuable given concerns about radiation exposure.

Cardiac MRI is the gold standard for assessment of the pulmonary valve and RV outflow tract (RVOT). It facilitates easy identification of location (valvular, supravalvular, or subvalvular) and severity of pulmonary stenosis. Acquiring a precise cine RVOT image can help to qualitatively assess the severity of pulmonary stenosis by visualizing the stenotic jet and valve motion. Quantitative assessment and direct planimetry can be performed similar to AS. Peak velocities can also be obtained similar to AS through in-plane velocity mapping. RV function can be precisely measured by volumetric analysis as described earlier, for optimal surgical planning.

VII. PULMONARY REGURGITATION

Significant pulmonary regurgitation is most common in patients with congenital heart disease, largely in patients with surgically repaired tetralogy of Fallot. Trace to mild pulmonary regurgitation is a common finding in normal individuals. Cardiac MRI has transformed the accuracy of quantitative assessment of severity of pulmonary regurgitation and determination of RV volume and function. RVOT cine imaging can qualitatively predict the severity of regurgitation, though through-plane phase-contrast velocity mapping with the image slice just above the pulmonary valve, without any aliasing, can accurately quantify pulmonary regurgitation. A regurgitant fraction >40% is considered severe pulmonary regurgitation (Fig. 17.5).

Accurate measurement of RV volumes and function is important for timing of surgery. Abnormal septal motion gives an indirect measure of RV pressure and volume overload, particularly in short-axis cine images. Severe pulmonary regurgitation with an RV end-diastolic volume index <160 mL/m^2 predicts a greater chance of normalization of RV dimensions after pulmonary valve replacement.

Cardiac CT and cardiac MRI are increasingly being used in preinterventional planning for percutaneous pulmonary valve replacement using a stented prosthetic valve, as the accurate size and anatomy of the RVOT are important for determining procedural suitability. After a successful procedure, cardiac MRI can be used for serial assessment of valvular function. The flow quantification can be performed above the stent level.

VIII. TRICUSPID STENOSIS

The tricuspid valve apparatus consists of papillary muscles, chordae tendinae, annulus, and three leaflets (septal, anterior, and posterior). The tricuspid leaflets are usually thinner than the mitral valve leaflets.

The most common cause of tricuspid valve stenosis is rheumatic fever, followed by less common causes like congenital tricuspid atresia, infectious endocarditis, and carcinoid syndrome. Most common pathologic changes would include thickening, fibrosis, and commissural fusion, leading to progressive narrowing of the orifice area and to severe features of right heart failure. Although extremely rare and not a routine clinical practice, assessment of the tricuspid valve with cardiac CT or cardiac MRI

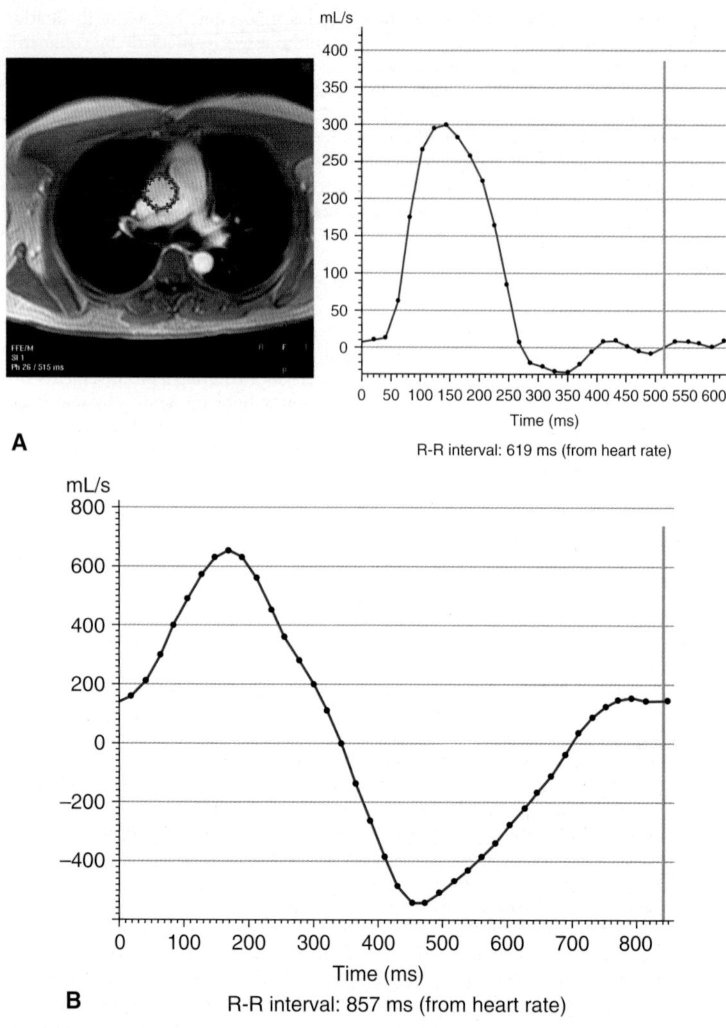

FIGURE 17.5 **A:** Phase-contrast imaging of the aorta to determine aortic stroke volume and flow. The area under the curve represents the volume of flow and can be calculated by the software. **B:** An extreme case of tetralogy of Fallot with surgical valvotomy showing severe free-flow pulmonary regurgitation in flow–time graph after integration of velocity in each voxel over one cardiac cycle, demonstrating forward flow above the zero line and regurgitant flow below the line.

can be employed when required. Cardiac CT can depict narrowed orifice area with thickened leaflets and associated right atrial enlargement, enlarged venae cavae, and hepatic venous congestion. Valve area can be measured by placement of an image slice through the valve tips in diastole, and the diastolic flow and velocity can be obtained from the tricuspid valve through phase-contrast imaging, though accuracy of the flow measurement is limited.

IX. TRICUSPID REGURGITATION

Tricuspid valve regurgitation is commonly secondary to RV and annular dilatation in response to pulmonary arterial hypertension. Cardiac CT can depict the morphologic changes in the leaflets and right side of the heart. The complete RV volume assessment can be performed, acquiring complete 4D cine imaging to precisely quantify RV volumes and ejection fraction. This method may be extremely useful in patients having contraindications to cardiac MRI (e.g., pacemaker/implantable cardioverter defibrillator).

Cardiac MRI is extremely valuable in assessing tricuspid regurgitation and underlying RV dysfunction. SSFP cine sequences are used for morphologic characterization of the leaflets, along with multiple cine slices at the level of the tricuspid valve, allowing for the assessment of leaflet morphology and abnormal attachment of the leaflets as seen in Ebstein anomaly. Qualitative assessment of the tricuspid valve can be achieved by acquiring in-plane velocity mapping in the RV long-axis cine images. However, the precise quantification of tricuspid regurgitation is achieved using RV stroke volume (calculated by measuring RV volumes) combined with flow measurement of the pulmonary valve (through-plane phase contrast) to acquire tricuspid regurgitant volume (RV stroke volume – pulmonary forward flow) and regurgitant fraction (regurgitant volume/RV stroke volume × 100%).

It is a challenge with echocardiography to precisely measure the anatomic and functional components of the right ventricle in patients with Ebstein anomaly. However, cardiac MRI can be used to precisely measure apical displacement of septal leaflet attachment and the redundancy of the anterior tricuspid leaflet, which helps to determine the approach of tricuspid repair versus replacement and exclude other associated congenital anomalies (commonly associated with atrial septal defect). Cardiac MRI is also a useful tool for serial follow-up, which aids in appropriate surgical planning. Cardiac CT with 4D cine retrospective imaging can give functional and morphologic information at the cost of higher radiation dose.

Percutaneous interventions for treating native tricuspid valve disease are currently lacking because of a lack of rigid landing zone for valve deployment and unusually variable annular dimensions. However, there are few case reports of degenerative bioprosthetic tricuspid valve conditions being successfully treated by transcatheter valve-in-valve implantation. Currently, there are no dedicated imaging protocols for preprocedural assessment of the tricuspid apparatus for percutaneous interventions.

X. PROSTHETIC VALVES

Cardiac CT is a valuable modality for assessing mechanical prosthetic valve dysfunction. This is achieved by obtaining a complete 3D and 4D cine imaging set to assess valve function in both diastolic and systolic phases of the cardiac cycle (Fig. 17.6). Cardiac CT has also been shown to be helpful in detection of prosthetic valve dysfunction, and these findings were directly correlated with surgical or autopsy findings. Surgical valve procedures may sometimes be confirmed by MRI (Fig. 17.7).

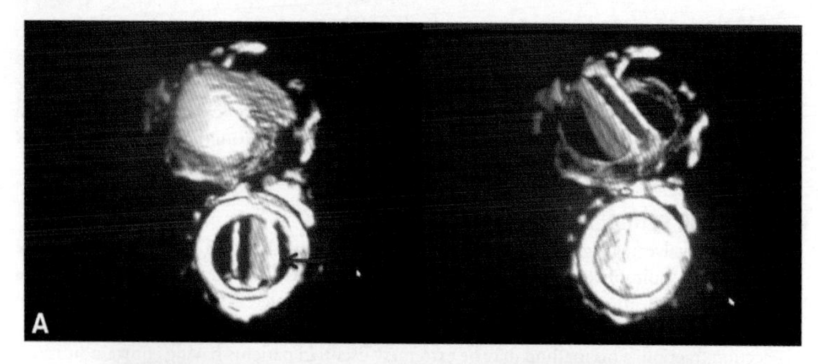

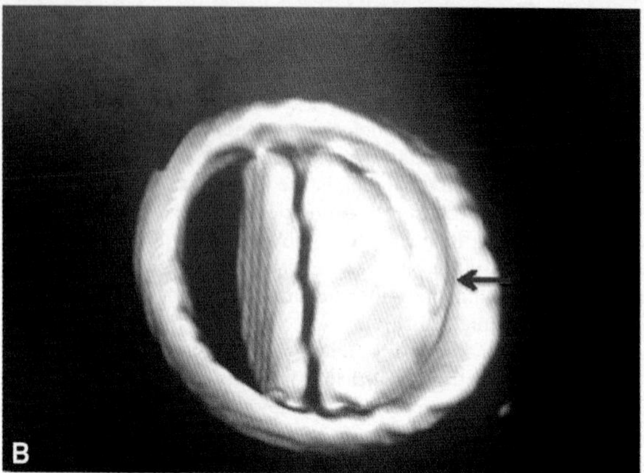

FIGURE 17.6 **A:** Three-dimensional (3D) volume-rendering technique (VRT) reconstruction of mechanical prosthetic valves permitting their evaluation in the mitral and aortic valve positions. Systolic phase showing partially restricted opening of the aortic leaflet *(arrow)* with normal mechanical mitral valve function in diastole and systole. **B:** 3D VRT showing completely restricted movement of one of the aortic valve discs during systole *(arrow)*.

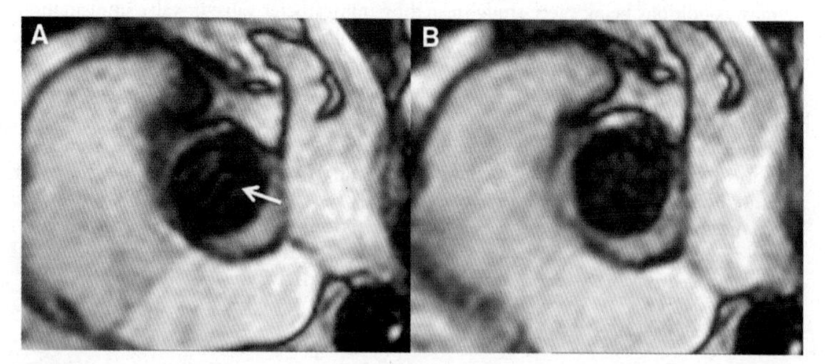

FIGURE 17.7 Steady-state free precession cine imaging depicting mechanical prosthetic valve in the aortic position in systole and diastole **(A, B)**. The *arrow* points to the prosthesis. In **A**, the opening of leaflets can be assessed.

KEY PEARLS

- In using cardiac CT to assess the aortic valve, both systolic and diastolic phases have to be evaluated carefully as there may be a bicuspid aortic valve with a raphe that could mimic normal tricuspid leaflets in diastolic phase.
- Bicuspid aortic valve (AV) should signal a further evaluation of a patient's thoracic aorta to rule out associated thoracic aortic aneurysm, which could readily be imaged within the same CT study.
- A calcium score <700 AU excludes severe AS with a high negative predictive value, and a score >2,000 AU suggests severe AS.
- ECG-gated 4D cine image reconstruction in systolic and diastolic phases can help assess left ventricular functional parameters.
- The advantage of cardiac MRI is that it can precisely assess LV and RV function by planimetry of LV and RV volumes in end-diastolic and end-systolic slices so that volumes can be calculated by summing all the slices, thus determining ventricular stroke volume, cardiac output, and ejection fraction with standard equations.
- Double-oblique reconstructed planes reveal an ovoid to elliptical shape of the LVOT, from which the long- and short-axis diameters can be measured, allowing for the calculation of the mean diameter, perimeter, and area of the annulus. This aids in the selection of correct prosthesis size and type.
- Assessing peripheral arterial calcification is particularly important for TAVR, as circumferential or horseshoe-like patterns limit arterial expandability to accommodate large-profile delivery sheaths, likely increasing the risk of dissection or perforation.
- SSFP MRI sequences including the short axis at the level of the aortic valve, along with a 3D whole-heart sequence covering up to the ascending aorta, allows reconstruction of the aortic annulus in orthogonal views to precisely measure the aortic annular dimensions for TAVR.
- Cardiac MRI is an attractive tool for assessing AR because of its ability to quantify flow directly using through-plane phase-contrast velocity mapping, which does not rely on calculations from complex equations.
- Both CT and MRI demonstrate the regurgitant orifice in moderate to severe AR. An area of 0.28 cm^2 has a sensitivity and specificity of 90% and 91%, respectively, in detecting severe AR.
- AR is quantified as severe when the regurgitant volume is ≥60 mL or regurgitant fraction is ≥50%.
- Cardiac MRI is useful in quantification of AR, LV volumetric analysis, and determination of aortic root anatomy, along with having the advantage of getting all the information required without any contrast or radiation exposure, which makes it an attractive tool for assessing AR.
- Cardiac CT has the advantage of being able to assess calcification and thickening of the mitral leaflet and submitral apparatus for planning balloon mitral valvuloplasty.
- Cardiac MRI quantification of MR provides the threshold for predicting patients suitable for early mitral valve replacement or repair when the regurgitant fraction is 40% or more.
- Lack of viability of the lateral wall of the left ventricle evaluated by delayed enhancement on MRI may suggest poor outcome with revascularization alone compared with accompanying mitral valve repair/replacement for patients with significant MR.
- Cardiac MRI is extremely valuable in assessing tricuspid regurgitation and underlying RV dysfunction.
- Cardiac CT is a valuable modality for assessing mechanical prosthetic valve dysfunction. This is achieved by obtaining complete 3D and 4D cine imaging to assess the valve function in both diastolic and systolic phases of the cardiac cycle.

SUGGESTED READINGS

Akat K, Borggrefe M, Kaden JJ. Aortic valve calcification: basic science to clinical practice. *Heart.* 2009;95:616–623.

Chatzimavroudis GP, Oshinski JN, Franch RH, et al. Quantification of the aortic regurgitant volume with magnetic resonance phase velocity mapping: a clinical investigation of the importance of imaging slice location. *J Heart Valve Dis.* 1998;7:94–101.

Chenot F, Montant P, Goffinet C, et al. Evaluation of anatomic valve opening and leaflet morphology in aortic valve bioprosthesis by using multidetector CT: comparison with transthoracic echocardiography. *Radiology.* 2010;255:377–385.

Cueff C, Serfaty JM, Cimadevilla C, et al. Measurement of aortic valve calcification using multislice computed tomography: correlation with hemodynamic severity of aortic stenosis and clinical implication for patients with low ejection fraction. *Heart.* 2011;97:721–726.

Debl K, Djavidani B, Buchner S, et al. Delayed hyper enhancement in magnetic resonance imaging of left ventricular hypertrophy caused by aortic stenosis and hypertrophic cardiomyopathy: visualization of focal fibrosis. *Heart.* 2006;92:1447–1451.

Gelfand EV, Hughes S, Hauser TH, et al. Severity of mitral and aortic regurgitation as assessed by cardiovascular magnetic resonance: optimizing correlation with Doppler echocardiography. *J Cardiovasc Magn Reson.* 2006;8:503–507.

Holmes DR Jr, Mack MJ, Kaul S, et al. 2012 ACCF/AATS/SCAI/STS expert consensus document on transcatheter aortic valve replacement. *J Am Coll Cardiol.* 2012;59(13):1200–1254.

Kapadia SR, Goel SS, Svensson L, et al. Characterization and outcome of patients with severe symptomatic aortic stenosis referred for percutaneous aortic valve replacement. *J Thorac Cardiovasc Surg.* 2009;137:1430–1435.

Koos R, Mahnken AH, Sinha AM, et al. Aortic valve calcification as a marker for aortic stenosis severity: assessment on 16-MDCT. *AJR Am J Roentgenol.* 2004;183:1813.

Laissy JP, Messika-Zeitoun D, Serfaty JM, et al. Comprehensive evaluation of preoperative patients with aortic valve stenosis: usefulness of cardiac multidetector computed tomography. *Heart.* 2007;93:1121–1125.

Maganti K, Rigolin VH, Sarano ME, et al. Valvular heart disease: diagnosis and management. *Mayo Clin Proc.* 2010;85(5):483–500.

Myerson SG, D'Arcy J, Mohiaddin R, et al. Aortic regurgitation quantification with cardiovascular magnetic resonance predicts clinical outcome. *Heart.* 2011;97:A93–A94.

Nietlispach F, Leipsic J, Al-Bugami S, et al. CT of the ilio-femoral arteries using direct aortic contrast injection: proof of feasibility in patients screened towards percutaneous aortic valve replacement. *Swiss Med Wkly.* 2009;139(31,32):458–462.

Nishimura RA, Otto CM, Bonow RO, et al. 2014 AHA/ACC guideline for the management of patients with valvular heart disease: executive summary: a report of the American College of Cardiology/American Heart Association Task Force on Practice Guidelines. *Circulation.* 2014:129.

Paelinck BP, Van Herck PL, Rodrigus I, et al. Comparison of magnetic resonance imaging of aortic valve stenosis and aortic root to multimodality imaging for selection of transcatheter aortic valve implantation candidazes. *Am J Cardiol.* 2011;108:92–98.

Sabet HY, Edwards WD, Tazelaar HD, et al. Congenitally bicuspid aortic valves: a surgical pathology study of 542 cases (1991 through 1996) and a literature review of 2,715 additional cases. *Mayo Clin Proc.* 1999;74:14–26.

Schoenhagen P, Hausleiter J, Achenbach S, et al. Computed tomography in the evaluation for transcatheter aortic valve implantation (TAVI). *Cardiovasc Diagn Ther.* 2011;1(1):44–56.

Sondergaard L, Stahlberg F, Thomsen C. Magnetic resonance imaging of valvular heart disease. *J Magn Reson Imaging.* 1999;10:627–638.

Tsai IC, Lin YK, Chang Y, et al. Correctness of multi-detector-row computed tomography for diagnosing mechanical prosthetic heart valve disorders using operative findings as a gold standard. *Eur Radiol.* 2009;19(4):857–867.

Van De Heyning CM, Magne J, Piérard LA, et al. Late gadolinium enhancement CMR in primary mitral regurgitation. *Eur J Clin Invest.* 2014;44(9):840–847.

CHAPTER 18

William J. Stewart

Intraprocedural Echocardiography in Valve Disease

I. INTRODUCTION. Echocardiography is an important component of the design and success of cardiovascular procedures in patients with structural heart disease. In this context, intraprocedural echocardiography (IPE) refers to imaging in the setting of procedures, including cardiac operations or transcatheter interventions. It is useful for defining the abnormal anatomy and physiology, guiding alignment and position of implanted devices, assessing valve regurgitation and stenosis after device deployment or surgery is done, and identifying postprocedural complications.

Intraoperative echocardiography (IOE) began in the early 1980s with left ventricular (LV) monitoring during noncardiac surgery. In the next decade, it expanded exponentially, spearheaded by its utility in valve repair for mitral regurgitation (MR). At this time, IOE is utilized in most cases of valve and congenital heart surgery. In adults, the method is mostly transesophageal echocardiography (TEE), and the majority of the persons doing the imaging are anesthesiologists. IOE is mandatory when unusual anatomic challenges or complex anatomic decisions are needed.

Similarly, the more recent advent of transcatheter structural interventions has introduced a new need for guidance by IPE. In most cases, TEE is used in a complementary tandem with fluoroscopy and angiography to achieve the desired goals. Echocardiographic images, fluoroscopic images, and pressure waveform data should all be easily viewable by all members of the multidisciplinary team.

TEE is useful in many transcatheter applications, including implantation of a prosthesis or device, and anatomic interventions such as balloon dilation, ablation, or puncture. Valve interventions and valve surgery benefit from imaging that can characterize soft tissue, which cannot be done with fluoroscopy alone. Table 18.1 lists a variety of procedures in the catheterization lab or operating room for which IPE has value, the most common of which will be described in this chapter. In transcatheter procedures done under light sedation (rather than general anesthesia), transthoracic echocardiography (TTE) may be of some limited value. However, TTE has reduced image quality and more potential to interfere with the sterile field. Because frequently the patient cannot be rolled onto their left side during these procedures, TTE is usually of insufficient quality to provide the precise assessments needed for IPE.

II. BASIC CONCEPTS OF INTRAPROCEDURAL ECHOCARDIOGRAPHY FOR GUIDANCE OF CARDIOVASCULAR PROCEDURES

For patients undergoing surgery involving cardiopulmonary bypass with cardioplegia, IPE is usually done before (prepump) and after (postpump) the heart is stopped. For most transcatheter procedures and off-pump surgeries performed with the heart beating, IPE is feasible throughout the procedure, including before (pre-IPE), during (intra-IPE), and after (post-IPE) the actual implantation or anatomic change. Its important ability is to guide the intervention and define its success or failure.

TABLE 18.1 Procedures or Problems for Which Intraprocedural Echocardiography Is Useful

- Surgical or transcatheter valve repair
- Surgical or transcatheter valve replacement
- Closure of defect or fistula, including paraprosthetic leak
- Hypotension or hemodynamic derangement of uncertain etiology
- Congenital heart surgery
- Complex procedures, which are new to the current interventional/operative team

A. **Before the procedure,** whether the surgical or transcatheter change in the patient's anatomy is made by implantation of a device or some other method, IPE has a role in defining the therapeutic plans. This includes determining the feasibility of the intervention, measuring the space where that intervention may occur, documenting the pretreatment magnitude of dysfunction, and defining other cardiovascular abnormalities that coexist with the primary problem(s). In most patients, IPE confirms the diagnoses made before the procedure. The imager should look carefully for changes in the anatomy that may have occurred since the preoperative imaging. This includes dysfunction of other valves, unexpected myocardial dysfunction, superimposed problems, or spontaneous improvement in the lesion(s) of importance. Incorporating these new findings into the procedural plans helps to avoid foibles and unintended outcomes.

   Even when the patient is already in the procedure room or operating room, the pre-IPE may change the ratio of risk versus benefit of performing the procedure at all. Even if the patient is already anesthetized or the incision is made, it is better to do the right thing, even if it is a new plan not anticipated preoperatively. The likely success and clinical outcome of doing the planned procedure may be altered if new abnormalities are found by the echocardiogram.

   Innovations in treatment of valvular heart disease are very much the purview of IPE. When the experience of the surgeon or interventionalist is less for a given procedure, especially when the procedure is new or the disease state is uncommon or complicated, IPE helps define the territory, clarify the feasibility, and avoid complications of the procedure. The accuracy of diagnosis at any phase depends on the ability to image the relevant anatomy and physiology and understand them.

B. **IPE at the moment of the intervention (intra-IPE):** Most transcatheter procedures, similar to on-pump cardiac surgery, are done with the heart beating, and so the imaging guidance provided by IPE includes the moment of implantation. The specific role of IPE is to guide the therapeutic activity to the correct location, at exactly the right angle and orientation. Many of these imaging objectives are specific for each procedure and will be discussed later in this chapter.

C. **Immediately after the procedure.** IPE is helpful in documenting the anatomic and physiologic success of the procedure(s), or determining the need for more work. Before leaving the operating room or procedure laboratory, it is useful to know about the new state of myocardial function, blood flow, and valve function. The frequency of treatment failure on the initial procedure varies with the mechanism and complexity of the original problem. If further interventional or surgical treatment is needed, the IPE is instrumental in defining and directing the available remedies. For surgery done on cardiopulmonary bypass, this entails a "second pump run." Another venue of IPE is identification of unanticipated emergencies. When patients have sudden hypotension, shock, or alteration of electrical or mechanical activity, online assessment can immediately define the nature of the aberration.

D. Completeness of study including 3DE: In most patients who are undergoing intraprocedural imaging, we recommend performing a complete TEE study, including a long- and short-axis view of every valve and each chamber, using structural imaging (black and white), color Doppler, and relevant spectral Doppler recordings for each valve or lesion. This enthusiasm for completeness must be tempered by the realities of clinical urgency and numerous patient-specific issues. Three-dimensional echocardiography (3DE) is now part of the technologic armamentarium of IPE. However, 3DE is sometimes cumbersome and time-consuming and is not always as versatile for making quick online decisions as 2D imaging. Still, 3DE has great utility in communicating anatomic details to a surgeon or interventionalist with less experience in tomographic imaging. It facilitates understanding the location and dynamic anatomy of the abnormal valve, sharpens expectations, and enhances success. 3DE often requires offline analysis of stored three-dimensional data sets.

E. Choice of echocardiographic imaging modalities: TEE is the most commonly used modality for IPE of valve procedures in the catheterization lab or operating room, but intraprocedural TTE, epicardial echocardiography, or intracardiac echocardiography (ICE) may be used in some cases. Rarely, these other modalities may be preferred, especially when there are contraindications or difficulties in placement of the TEE probe (such as esophageal disease), or when working on an anterior structure like the pulmonary valve. The inherent risks and potential adverse effects vary with each procedure, including potential esophageal trauma resulting from TEE, vascular trauma from ICE, or incomplete data from any of them. Epicardial echocardiography, placing a transducer on the surface of the heart, is an adequate substitute in open chest surgeries and may be superior to TEE in certain indications, such as assessment of hypertrophic cardiomyopathy or atheroma of the ascending aorta. Computerized tomography and magnetic resonance imaging would also be useful during valve procedures and operations; however, cost, space, speed, and radiation exposure presently make them impractical. A novel method has been developed that integrates echocardiography and fluoroscopy (EchoNavigator, Philips Healthcare, Best, the Netherlands) by marrying the two coordinate systems to visualize both modalities on one screen simultaneously. By tracking markers on specific points of interest on these combined images, guidance of transcatheter procedures is facilitated. What imaging modalities are chosen depends on the abilities and experience of the imaging team, and especially the ability of the surgeon or interventionalist to incorporate this information into decisions that will improve outcome.

F. Subjective and quantitative diagnosis

1. The images generated and diagnoses made with IPE are mostly interpreted subjectively. Some quantitative measurements can be made quickly at the time of image acquisition, at the cost of minor delay. At the ends of the spectrum of abnormalities (very good or very poor), such quantitation is often not necessary. However, in the moderate range of many abnormalities, specific measurements add substantially to the impact of imaging on procedural decisions. Measurements of diameter, area, or volume by tracing on selected IPE images may derive important information about the valve disease in question. Even when measurements are not accomplished during the procedure, it is often useful to store video clips, still frames, or 3D volume sets that would enable quantitation later. The learning curve of how to obtain the most relevant and reliable information efficiently often results from experience performing and interpreting echocardiography outside the catheterization lab or operating theater.
2. Before any IPE, the imager should be well versed with the patient's clinical picture, the current decisions at hand, the plans made by other clinicians, and the procedure that is anticipated. This usually entails direct review of the preprocedural imaging studies and goes way beyond just knowing the central diagnosis or the planned procedure. This working knowledge of the prior

findings helps the imager to identify new information during the pre-IPE, which would affect the plans.

3. When TEE is planned, it is important to be certain that there are no contraindications to esophageal endoscopy such as esophageal stenosis, esophageal cancer, or significant dysphagia. When these issues are raised, preoperative studies such as upper gastrointestinal endoscopy should be performed to decide if the TEE probe can be introduced safely.
4. The patient should be fasting before a TEE study and the risks, benefits, and alternatives to TEE reviewed with either the patient or family, and with the primary doctors involved. Compared with the minor additional risk of TEE probe insertion, much can be gained by online imaging.
5. In procedures where the patient will not have endotracheal intubation or general anesthesia, the decision to do a TEE is much less obvious. For example, procedures done under light sedation may be done with TEE, or with TTE, but the latter provides less value to the success of the procedure. Another issue affecting the decision to do without TEE is the intended position of the patient during the procedure. If the patient will be supine without an endotracheal tube, TEE requires frequent suctioning of the hypopharynx to prevent aspiration of saliva. The team must make a value judgment between the advantages of a less involved form of anesthesia with disadvantages of losing additional guidance that could be provided by TEE. Likewise, valve repair surgery may be done without intraoperative TEE, but the potential for finding problems with TEE still makes it a good choice.

III. INTRAPROCEDURAL ECHOCARDIOGRAPHY IN SPECIFIC OPERATIONS OR TRANSCATHETER PROCEDURES

A. IPE in mitral valve surgery

1. This is the bedrock of the invasive echocardiography movement of the last three decades (Table 18.2). The prepump TEE helps to define the mechanism and severity of MR before the surgery (Fig. 18.1). The surgeon must understand the dysfunction in order to enable successful repair. Pre-IPE contributes to a change in plans (sometimes minor) in about 15% of patients in our experience.
2. IPE can detect problems after the mitral repair, most commonly persistent MR. In most cases, we accept mild or no MR on the post-IPE and do further surgery if the MR is 3+ (moderately severe) or more. If it is 2+, we do further surgery if there is no contraindication, or we observe without decannulating, while giving an afterload challenge of boluses of phenylephrine to raise blood pressure. Also

TABLE 18.2 Utility of Echocardiography in Surgical Repair for Mitral Regurgitation

Prepump Transesophageal Echocardiography (TEE)—The "Road Map"

- Severity of regurgitation
- Mechanism of regurgitation, repairability
- Ventricular function, wall motion
- Abnormalities of other valves

Postpump TEE—The "Safety Net"

- Severity of mitral regurgitation
- Mitral systolic anterior motion
- New left ventricular dysfunction

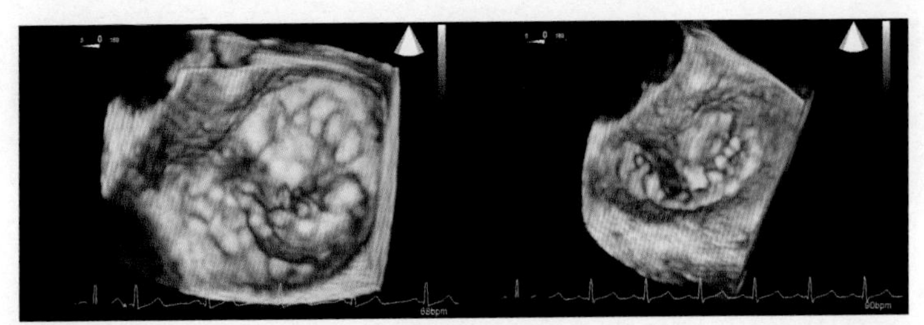

FIGURE 18.1 3D echo images from the left atrial viewpoint before (*left*) showing a flail portion of the middle scallop of the posterior leaflet, and (*right*) after surgical repair with quadrilateral resection of the flail portion, and placement of an annuloplasty device.

occurring with substantial frequency are new systolic anterior motion of the mitral valve and new wall motion abnormalities, particularly in the right coronary artery territory, due to its anterior ostium. A second run of cardiopulmonary bypass, to fix the problem(s) during the same thoracotomy, occurs in 3% to 6% of cases. Mitral valve replacement can be complicated by paravalvular leaks (PVLs) that are discernible by the postpump intraoperative TEE and are fixable on a second pump run.

3. Robotic mitral valve repair is done through a set of small right axillary incisions. This surgery entails no direct views of the beating heart other than a small portion of the right atrium, and so it is more dependent on TEE than an open chest procedure. The surgeon depends on TEE for observations of the adequacy of ventricular filling, presence of intracardiac air, and biventricular dysfunction.

B. IPE in transcatheter mitral procedures

1. In addition to balloon mitral valvotomy for mitral stenosis (Fig. 18.2), the most commonly used transcatheter procedure is valve repair using the MitraClip (Table 18.3). MR is reduced by using an implantable clip to approximate the two leaflet edges. This procedure is very technically demanding and cannot (or should

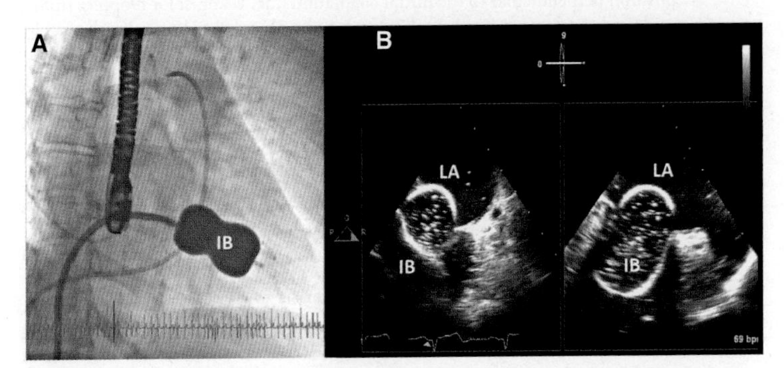

FIGURE 18.2 **A:** Fluoroscopic image during mitral balloon valvotomy in right anterior oblique projection, showing the Inoue balloon (IB) at the moment of maximum inflation displaying the neck of the balloon expanding the valve orifice. **B:** 2D X-plane images show the balloon projecting part way into the left atrium (LA). (Used by permission from Cavalcante JL, Rodriguez LL, Kapadia S, et al. Role of echocardiography in percutaneous mitral valve interventions. *JACC Cardiovasc Imaging*. 2012;5[7]:733–746.)

TABLE 18.3 Utility of Echocardiography in Transcatheter Repair of Mitral Regurgitation with the MitraClip

- Assess severity, mechanism, and location of mitral regurgitant jets
- Baseline assessment of other valves and biventricular function
- Guide trans-septal catheterization by watching indentation by the catheter
- Visualize direction and location of delivery catheter and arms of clip
- Demonstrate capture of leaflets by the clip
- Reassess amount of regurgitation after clip closure

not) be performed without continuous echocardiographic guidance. Because it does not visualize the mitral valve leaflets or the MR jets, fluoroscopy alone is not enough to guide the procedure. Initially, echocardiography is used to confirm that the anatomy is amenable to this procedure, including the severity of MR, its mechanism, LV size and function, the location and degree of flail or apical tethering, and absence of fibrotic commissural fusion. Intraprocedural TEE guides the location and increases the safety of the trans-septal catheterization. The site of interatrial septal puncture should be in its posterior and superior portion and is guided by watching with echocardiography the location where the tip of the trans-septal catheter indents the septum. The TEE short-axis view at the aortic valve level helps to visualize the anterior–posterior orientation, and a bicaval view the superior–inferior orientation. Using the mid esophageal four-chamber view, the indentation of the septum should be used to place the puncture site about 3.5 to 4.0 cm above the level of mitral coaptation in systole.

2. After the delivery catheter and valve (in closed position) are inserted into the left atrium, 3D echocardiography or biplane TEE is used to orient the catheter above the valve and parallel to mitral antegrade flow. After the clip is opened, 3D imaging from the left atrial view helps to orient the rotation of its arms to a position perpendicular to the mitral coaptation line. Using color Doppler from a midesophageal intercommissural 2D view or by 3D echocardiography, the precise medial–lateral location of the MR flow convergence is visualized, where the leaflets should be grasped with the clip. After the clip is inserted in the LV, a midesophageal long-axis view is used to verify mitral leaflet capture, which often requires multiple grasp attempts. TEE color Doppler is then used to determine if the MR has been reduced (Fig. 18.3) and identify the location of any persistent regurgitation. Multiple clips are often required to accomplish a good result, showing that the majority of the MR has been eliminated. Mitral valve antegrade velocity should then be evaluated by continuous wave (CW) Doppler and by catheter methods before release of the clip from the delivery system. A mean gradient of up to 5 mm Hg is acceptable, presuming reasonable heart rate control. 3D TEE can be used to planimeter and sum both orifices; an area of 1.5 cm^2 or above is desirable.
3. Additional transcatheter methods are under development to repair MR, including leaflet repair, ventricular remodeling, and both direct annuloplasty and indirect annuloplasty methods via the coronary sinus. These will also have substantial requirements for IPE guidance. Transcatheter mitral valve replacement methods are also being developed, all of which will likely require TEE and fluoroscopic guidance.

C. **IPE in transcatheter closure of paraprosthetic leaks:** Transcatheter closure of paraprosthetic mitral (Fig. 18.4) or aortic PVLs is also an important venue for intraprocedural TEE (Table 18.4). Whether the PVL was present after a transcatheter or surgical valve was implanted or not, transcatheter closure is sometimes an advisable

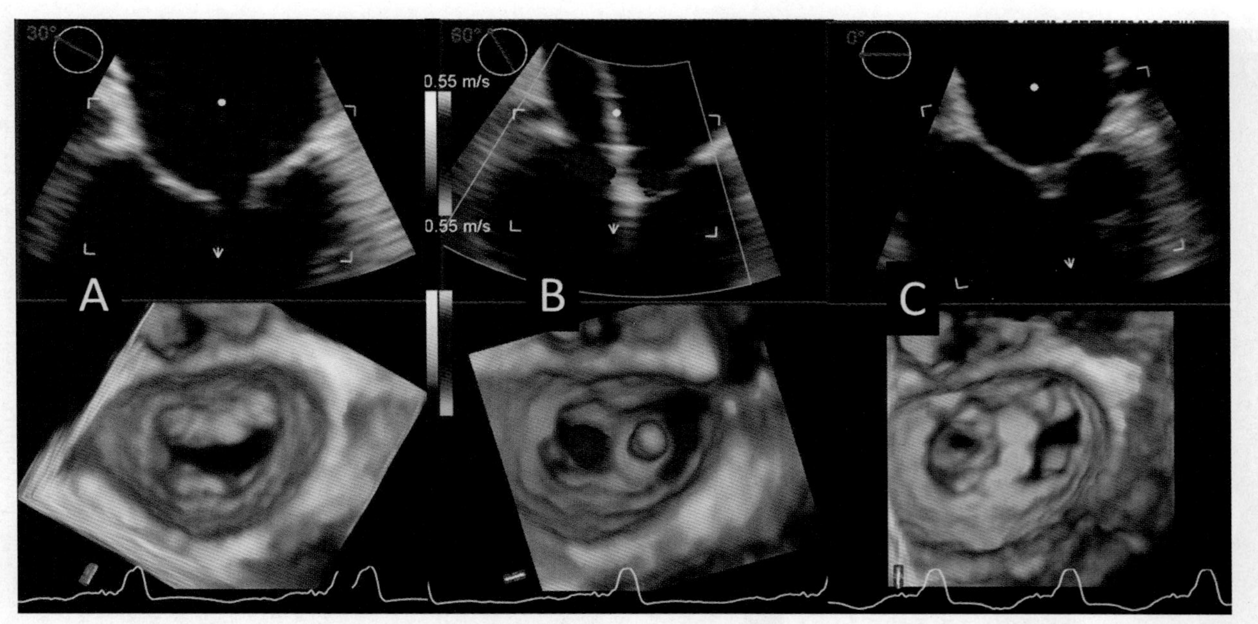

FIGURE 18.3 Transesophageal images in transcatheter repair in a patient with severe functional mitral regurgitation (MR). **A:** Before clip placement showing the apical tethering of normal leaflets. **B:** Color Doppler images during placement of the clip, showing reduction in the MR as the leaflets are grasped, while the delivery catheter is still attached. **C:** After removal of the delivery catheter, with the clip forming the double orifice valve during opening. In each pair, the midesophageal 2D image is above and the 3D image of the mitral valve viewed from the left atrial side is below.

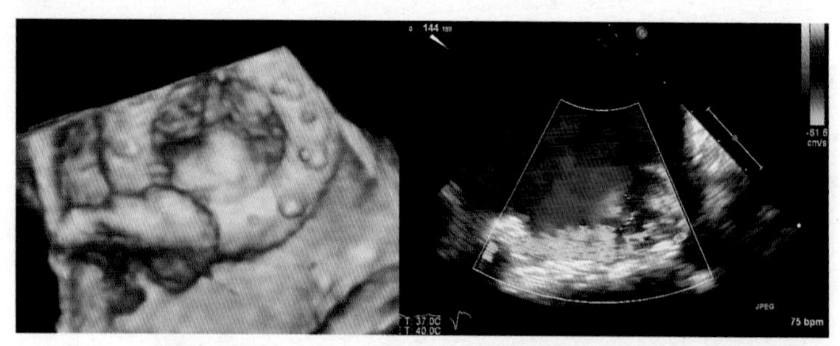

FIGURE 18.4 Transesophageal images in transcatheter repair of paravalvular regurgitation in a patient with a mitral bioprosthesis. 3D echo from the inverted left atrial perspective showing the occluder device still attached to the delivery catheter, adjacent to and outside the bioprosthetic stent (*left*). 2D color Doppler image showing the mitral regurgitation jet emerging outside the anterior portion of the bioprosthetic stent (*right*).

TABLE 18.4 Utility of Periprocedural Echocardiography in Device Closure of Paravalvular Regurgitation

- Define severity and location(s) of regurgitation
- Provide baseline on function of ventricles, pericardium, and other valves
- Exclude vegetations or thrombi
- Guide placement of wire and catheter(s)
- Define seating and stability of closure device
- Define function of prosthesis
- Locate and quantitate residual regurgitation
- Detect complications

option. In these patients, imaging is useful for determining the location and severity of the regurgitation and excluding concomitant thrombi or vegetations that could be dislodged. The location of the leak by color Doppler affects the choice of access, that is, from the trans-septal or trans-apical approach. The trajectory of the wire to enter the defect is guided primarily by TEE. Once a wire is placed across the site of regurgitation, it is useful to inflate a balloon within it, while assessing for reduction in the leak with color Doppler. As the closure device is inserted, IPE monitors the reduction in regurgitation and the motion of the prosthetic leaflets to avoid interference with their motion.

D. IPE in surgery for aortic valve disease

1. For surgical aortic valve replacement, the prepump intraoperative echocardiogram usually merely confirms what is already known. Although uncommon, the postpump intraoperative echocardiogram occasionally will find PVLs, new LV dysfunction, increases in MR, or dysfunction of other valves. In the newer sutureless valves, postpump IPE can define the location and "seating" of the valve as well as the potential for PVLs.

2. Surgical aortic valve repair is a reasonably common choice in patients with noncalcified regurgitant valves resulting from prolapse, often in patients with a bicuspid aortic valve. Repair is also a component of ascending aortic surgery where the aortic valve is resuspended, either combined with a supracoronary conduit or as a David procedure. Like those patients undergoing a Bentall procedure, reimplantation of the coronary arteries into the new conduit risks myocardial ischemia from coronary torsion, recognizable on IPE by new segmental LV dysfunction. Persistent regurgitation after aortic valve repair, leading to a second pump run, is more common than in mitral repair.

E. IPE in transcatheter procedures for aortic valve disease

1. The role of echocardiography (see Table 18.5) in patients with aortic stenosis starts well before the procedure itself, in determining candidacy for the procedure. Severity of the stenosis, outflow tract size, degree of regurgitation, ventricular function, and many other qualifying variables are first assessed. The LV outflow tract (LVOT) diameter by 2D echocardiography has been used for 40 years for continuity equation calculation of valve area. However, recent experience in transcatheter aortic valve replacement (TAVR) patients has shown that the cross-sectional shape of the subaortic area is elliptical in the majority of cases. As a result, 3D echocardiograpy and computed tomography are more accurate than 2D echocardiography in annulus sizing in order to plan the optimum size of the TAVR device.
   a. Intraprocedural echocardiography and fluoroscopy have complementary roles in TAVR. TEE begins with reassessing baseline structure and function, even if preprocedure information is complete. The imager(s) present should have a fresh knowledge of the baseline state for comparison so that it is apparent when a change occurs later in the procedure in amount of pericardial effusion, MR, right ventricular dysfunction, or segmental LV dysfunction. Intracardiac thrombi should be excluded. The ostium of the right coronary artery should be identified in the midesophageal long-axis view, whereas visualizing the left coronary ostia requires an X-plane derived from 3D TEE. If the distance from the hinge point of the aortic cusp to the coronary ostium is less than the length of the leaflet, there is a higher risk of coronary occlusion, and (at least) a wire should be placed into that coronary before balloon dilation. The LVOT should be remeasured and inspected for upper septal hypertrophy or severe nodular calcium within the aortic valve annulus that could cause postprocedural paravalvular regurgitation by preventing apposition of the valve skirt.
   b. Accurate sizing is important for optimum TAVR outcome. Undersizing the prosthesis can cause paravalvular aortic regurgitation (AR) or device migration. Oversizing can cause vascular complications, difficulty crossing the native valve, underexpansion, leaflet redundancy, central regurgitation, or reduction in valve durability.
   c. The second phase of TAVR implantation includes guidance of balloon dilation, and choosing the position and angulation of the device. Following the balloon procedure, native cusp mobility and AR severity should be reassessed. The starting position of the delivery catheter should be coaxial with the flow in the LVOT. The upper and lower ends of the device must be implanted at a specific depth in relationship to the aortic annulus, depending on the type of TAVR device. The most popular type of balloon expandable valve should be positioned with the ventricular edge of the prosthesis 2 to 4 mm below the annulus (Fig. 18.5), whereas the most popular type of self-expanding valve should start expansion with its lower edge 5 to 10 mm below the annular plane.
   d. During the implantation of a balloon expandable device, the patient is rapid paced to avoid extrusion of the device and the opened device should be solid and not mobile. The self-expanding devices give the interventionalist more opportunity to rethink the position and angulation while the valve is partially

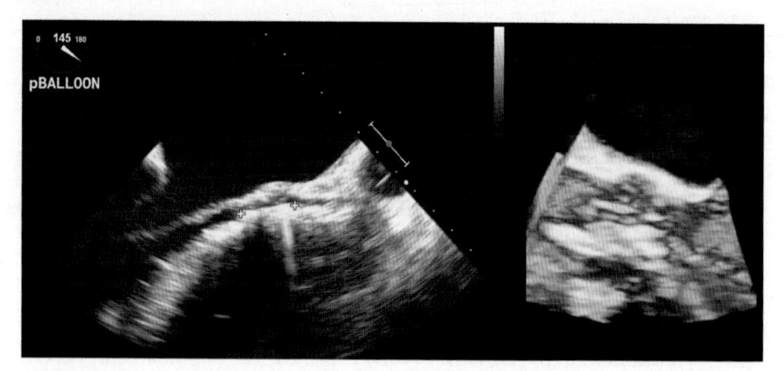

FIGURE 18.5 Intraprocedural transesophageal echo, by 2D (*left*) and 3D (*right*), after balloon dilation, showing positioning of the transcatheter aortic valve replacement, while it is still crimped on the catheter, prior to deployment. The calipers are shown on the upper and lower end of the crimped bioprosthetic valve.

deployed. Immediately after implantation, echocardiography is essential for determination of the severity and mechanism of AR, and measuring antegrade velocity and gradients. 3DE is useful for detection and quantification of central or paravalvular regurgitation, as mentioned earlier, which enables decisions about the need for postdilation or plug closure. Paravalvular regurgitation can sometimes be eliminated by postdilation. Central regurgitation is commonly seen while the delivery system is still across the valve and sometimes persists for a few minutes while the leaflets rebound from being crimped.

e. Qualitative assessment of AR severity after TAVR implantation incorporates assessment of proximal color Doppler jet dimensions, vena contracta, pressure half-time, CW Doppler density, descending aortic flow reversal, and Doppler comparison of antegrade stroke volumes. Three-dimensional echocardiography is useful to define the location, number, and circumferential extent of the paravalvular jets. The PVL is considered severe if 30% or more of the circumference of the device shows the presence of AR by color Doppler. Catheter-based hemodynamics and aortography are also a useful adjunct.

TABLE 18.5 Utility of Echocardiography in Transcatheter Aortic Valve Replacement

- Patient selection
- Prosthetic choice and sizing
- Aid balloon positioning for valvuloplasty
- Detect postvalvuloplasty aortic regurgitation
- Aid prosthesis positioning during implantation
- Confirm prosthesis function immediately after implantation
- Immediate detection of complications

2. TEE is also useful for detecting complications after TAVR implantation and directing their resolution. If the valve is deployed too low in the LVOT, it can become frankly loose within the left ventricle and require surgery, though sometimes it can be subsequently embolized distally into the aorta. In addition, deployment of the prosthesis too low can result in impingement on the anterior mitral leaflet, causing MR or leaflet erosion. If the TAVR device is deployed too high in the LVOT, it can cause paravalvular regurgitation or obstruction of the coronary artery ostia, or it can embolize distally. Coronary obstruction is identified by the appearance of new segmental or global LV dysfunction. Cardiac tamponade can occur from perforation of any wall of the left or right ventricle, aortic dissection, or rupture of the aortic annulus. New or increased MR can be characterized by echocardiography, which may be a clue to changes in LV geometry, dyssynchrony caused by right ventricular pacing, or direct structural distortion from the prosthesis impinging on the anterior mitral leaflet.
3. Annular rupture most commonly presents with new thickening of the intervalvular fibrosa. If severe right-to-left shunting across the atrial septal crossing is found, TEE can help in closing this with a clamshell device. Failure to cover the native aortic valve cusps with the TAVR device can allow them to project over the top of the prosthesis, which can cause persistent stenosis. Pericardial tamponade, visualized by TEE, is best managed by visualizing the effusion using TTE, to choose the site, depth, and needle angulation needed for pericardiocentesis. In cases of embolization of the prosthesis, fluoroscopy and echocardiography should be used to advance the prosthesis into the descending aorta, where it can be deployed, if side branch vessels are not compromised. If it cannot be oriented to allow opening during forward flow, the device can be compressed with a balloon, causing it to remain open throughout the cardiac cycle. Sometimes echocardiography is meritorious after TAVR implantation by defining that the hypotension is caused merely by hypovolemia.

F. **IPE in surgery for hypertrophic obstructive cardiomyopathy:** IPE is essential in surgery for LVOT obstruction, due to hypertrophic cardiomyopathy. The prepump TEE characterizes the systolic anterior motion, septal thickness, MR, and outflow tract velocity recorded by CW Doppler (Fig. 18.6). Gradients should be assessed

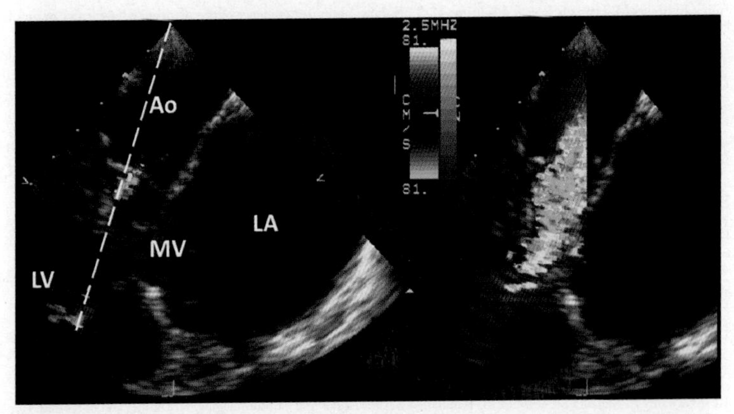

FIGURE 18.6 Epicardial color Doppler images in diastole (*left*) and systole (*right*) before myectomy in a patient with hypertrophic cardiomyopathy, showing the angle from which continuous wave Doppler recordings of LV outflow tract velocity are used to estimate gradients. Ao, ascending aorta; LA, left atrium; LV, left ventricle; MV, mitral valve.

by TEE or epicardial echocardiography, under basal euvolemic conditions, and during provocation, usually with infusion of isoproterenol. Persistence of significant obstruction is defined by a resting or inducible gradient above 40 to 50 mm Hg. Because dynamic obstruction is so load dependent, the post-IPE in this disorder leads to second pump runs in a higher percentage than any other kind of surgery.

IV. CONCLUSION

The expansion of surgical methods of valve repair and the increasing number of transcatheter approaches to patients with regurgitant as well as stenotic valvular disease have led to an increasing need for IPE to guide delivery of devices and monitor for anatomic and hemodynamic effects and complications. The most common current indications for IPE are TAVR, surgical and transcatheter nonprosthetic valve procedures, and closure of prosthetic paravalvular regurgitation. In the future, the armamentarium of catheter-based procedures and the need for intraprocedural echocardiographic guidance will likely expand.

KEY PEARLS

- The accuracy of diagnosis at any phase depends on the ability to image the relevant anatomy and understand the abnormal physiology.
- Imaging methods should be chosen on the basis of the abilities of the operative or interventional team to incorporate the information into decisions that will improve outcome.
- The frequency of treatment failure of the initial procedure (second pump runs or repeat interventions) varies with the mechanism and complexity of the original problem.
- Optimum imaging during catheter interventions or cardiac surgery requires judicious use of all modalities available with echocardiography, including 2D imaging, 2D color Doppler, 3D imaging, 3D color Doppler, and pulsed and continuous wave Doppler.

SUGGESTED READINGS

Altiok E, Becker M, Hamada S, et al. Real-time 3D TEE allows optimized guidance of percutaneous edge-to-edge repair of the mitral valve. *JACC Cardiovasc Imaging*. 2010;3:1196–1198.

Balzer J, van Hall S, Böring, YC, et al. New role of echocardiography in the Cath Lab: novel approaches of peri-interventional 3D echocardiography. *Curr Cardiovasc Imaging Rep*. 2013;6:445–453.

Cavalcante JL, Rodriguez LL, Kapadia S, et al. Role of echocardiography in percutaneous mitral valve interventions. *JACC Cardiovasc Imaging*. 2012;5(7):733–746.

Corti R, Biaggi P, Gaemperli O, et al. Integrated X-ray and echocardiography imaging for structural heart interventions. *EuroIntervention*. 2013;9:863–869.

Gao G, Penney G, Ma Y, et al. Registration of 3D trans-esophageal echocardiography to X-ray fluoroscopy using image-based probe tracking. *Med Image Anal*. 2012;16:38–49.

Goncalves A, Almeria C, Marcos-Alberca P, et al. Three-dimensional echocardiography in paravalvular aortic regurgitation assessment after transcatheter aortic valve implantation. *J Am Soc Echocardiogr*. 2012;25(1):47–55.

González-Gómez A, Zamorano JL. Imaging during transcatheter interventions for valvular heart disease. *EMJ Cardiol*. 2014;2:54–60.

Gripari P, Ewe SH, Fusini L, et al. Intraoperative 2D and 3D transoesophageal echocardiographic predictors of aortic regurgitation after transcatheter aortic valve implantation. *Heart*. 2012;98:1229–1236.

Hahn RT. Guidance of transcatheter aortic valve replacement by echocardiography. *Curr Cardiol Rep*. 2014;16(1):442.

Hahn RT, Little SH, Monaghan MJ, et al. Recommendations for comprehensive intraprocedural echocardiographic imaging during TAVR. *JACC Cardiovasc Imaging*. 2015;8(3):261–287.

Jayasuriya C, Moss RR, Munt B. Transcatheter aortic valve implantation in aortic stenosis: the role of echocardiography. *J Am Soc Echocardiogr*. 2011;24:15–27.

Krishnaswamy A, Kapadia SR, Tuzcu EM. Percutaneous paravalvular leak closure-imaging, techniques and outcomes. *Circ J*. 2013;77:19–27.

Leon MB, Smith CR, Mack M, et al. Transcatheter aortic-valve implantation for aortic stenosis in patients who cannot undergo surgery. *N Engl J Med*. 2010;363:1597–1607.

Ng AC, Delgado V, van der Kley F, et al. Comparison of aortic root dimensions and geometries before and after transcatheter aortic valve implantation by 2- and 3-dimensional transesophageal echocardiography and multislice computed tomography. *Circ Cardiovasc Imaging*. 2010;3(1):94–102.

Perk G, Kronzon I. Interventional echocardiography in structural heart disease. *Curr Cardiol Rep.* 2013;15:338.

Perk G, Lang RM, Garcia-Fernandez MA, et al. Use of real-time three-dimensional transesophageal echocardiography in intracardiac catheter-based interventions. *J Am Soc Echocardiogr.* 2009;22:865–882.

Pibarot P, Hahn RT, Weissman NJ, et al. Assessment of paravalvular regurgitation following TAVR: a proposal of unifying grading scheme. *JACC Cardiovasc Imaging.* 2015;8(3):340–360.

Siegel RJ, Luo H. Echocardiography in transcatheter aortic valve implantation and mitral valve clip. *Korean J Intern Med.* 2012;27(3):245–261.

Siegel RJ, Makkar R, Doumanian A, et al. Transcatheter aortic valve implantation three-dimensional echo monitoring and guidance. *Curr Cardiovasc Imaging Rep.* 2011;4:335–348.

Smith LA, Monaghan MJ. Monitoring of procedures: peri-interventional echo assessment for transcatheter aortic valve implantation. 2013;14(9):840–850.

Smith LA, Dworakowski R, Bhan A, et al. Real-time three-dimensional transesophageal echocardiography adds value to transcatheter aortic valve implantation. *J Am Soc Echocardiogr.* 2013;26:359–369.

Wunderlich NC, Beigel R, Siegel RJ. The role of echocardiography during mitral valve percutaneous interventions. *Cardiol Clin.* 2013;31:237–270.

Zamorano JL, Badano LP, Bruce C, et al. EAE/ASE recommendations for the use of echocardiography in new transcatheter interventions for valvular heart disease. *Eur Heart J.* 2011;32:2189–2214.

CHAPTER 19

Christine L. Jellis

3D Echocardiography

I. INTRODUCTION

One of the most significant developments in echocardiography over recent times has been the development and availability of three-dimensional (3D) echocardiography for practical clinical use. It has now become an integral aspect of both transthoracic and transesophageal cardiac assessment and provides complementary and incremental information over standard two-dimensional (2D) and M-mode echocardiographic techniques. Interchangeably referred to as 3D and four-dimensional (4D) imaging depending on vendor terminology, the additional dimension simply refers to 3D imaging in real time. High-quality 3D echocardiographic imaging is now routinely achieved in clinical practice, and 3D transesophageal assessment in particular has become an integral part of diagnosis and assessment of valvular heart disease.

II. INDICATIONS

3D echocardiography has revolutionized our morphologic and functional assessment of valvular heart disease. Progression in ultrasound and computer technologies has allowed us to achieve real-time direct visualization of valves and subvalvular apparatus from any orientation *en face* using a single-volume acquisition, thereby providing more realistic images with better reproducibility and improved scope for quantification.

A. Valvular assessment. Arguably, its most valuable contribution to valvular assessment has been our improved understanding of the complicated mitral valve, which can now be assessed from any spatial point of view. The 3D techniques pioneered for the mitral valve are now enabling better surgical planning for minimally invasive surgery and guiding of complex percutaneous procedures. Improved accuracy and reproducibility of distance and area measurements with 3D echocardiography means that it is now routinely employed for calculation of valve areas, annular dimensions, and preoperative planning.

B. Chamber size. Additionally, 3D full-volume technology has enabled us to more accurately assess cardiac chamber size. This has been particularly important in valvular conditions such as mitral and aortic regurgitation, where left ventricular enlargement may be an indication for surgery.

Common indications for valvular assessment with 3D echocardiography are listed in Table 19.1.

III. REIMBURSEMENT

The American Medical Association (AMA) has two Current Procedural Terminology (CPT) codes that can be used for 3D echocardiography. The ability to bill for 3D imaging and differentiation between the two billing codes is based upon performance of 3D reconstruction and whether the 3D reconstruction was performed online, on-cart, or offline on a remote workstation using postprocessing software. The two CPT codes are 76376 and 76377.

A. AMA descriptions for 3D CPT codes

1. **76376**: 3D rendering with interpretation and reporting of computed tomography (CT), magnetic resonance imaging (MRI), ultrasound, or other tomographic

TABLE 19.1 Common Indications for Valvular Assessment with Three-Dimensional Echocardiography

Indication	Aim of Three-Dimensional Echocardiographic Assessment
Assessment of valvular morphology	Determine congenital or acquired defects
Assessment of valvular stenosis or regurgitation	Determine mechanism and severity including prolapse/flail, perforation, prosthesis dehiscence, thrombus, pannus
Assessment of valvular masses	Determine etiology (e.g., infective endocarditis, tumors, postsurgical material)
Procedural planning	Accurate measurements and sizing before percutaneous or surgical valve procedures
Intraprocedural guidance	TAVR, valvuloplasty, edge-to-edge mitral valve clip, closure devices, valvular surgery
Postprocedural assessment	Evaluation for procedural success and complications
Assessment of associated factors	Ventricular volumes and function, left atrial and left atrial appendage thrombus

TAVR, transcatheter aortic valve replacement.

modality with image postprocessing under concurrent supervision, not requiring image postprocessing on an independent workstation.

In this scenario, the echocardiographic technician or echocardiologist performs 3D rendering using image postprocessing; however, the provider performs this directly on the echo machine and not on a separate workstation. This method is felt to be less labor and time intensive, and reimbursements for this on-cart method have been accordingly set lower.

a. 2015 Medicare Reimbursement Tech (facility reimbursement): $21.65
b. 2015 Medicare Reimbursement Pro (professional reimbursement): $21.65

2. **76377**: 3D rendering with interpretation and reporting of CT, MRI, ultrasound, or other tomographic modality with image postprocessing under concurrent supervision, requiring image postprocessing on an independent workstation.

   In this scenario, the echocardiographic technician or echocardiologist performs 3D rendering using image postprocessing; however, the provider performs the reformatting work on a remote, independent workstation with dedicated postprocessing software and capabilities. This method is felt to be more labor and time intensive and typically attracts higher hospital relative value units. Additional setup costs may also be incurred for the remote workstation and postprocessing software. Hence, reimbursements for this offline method have been set at a higher rate. Importantly, in order to bill using this code, the provider must clearly state that 3D rendering was performed on a separate workstation; otherwise, it may be downcoded to 76376.

   a. 2015 Medicare Reimbursement Tech (facility reimbursement): $61.53
   b. 2015 Medicare Reimbursement Pro (professional reimbursement): $61.53

IV. INSTRUMENTATION

A. History. Early iterations of 3D echocardiography relied on acquisition of 2D images with respiratory and electrocardiographic gating, in addition to information regarding transducer position and orientation. These data were then reconstructed offline to create a 3D image from a 2D data set. This method was time-consuming and reliant on specialized processing systems, thereby relegating the technique to largely research-based purposes.

B. Transducers. The ultimate success of 3D echocardiography technology centered on the progression from a sparse-array transducer to a full-matrix-array ultrasound transducer. This had previously been one of the most significant limiting factors in the roll out of this new echocardiographic application. Previously, the prohibitive size and limited number of crystal elements able to be incorporated into a reasonably sized 3D transducer limited spatial resolution and resulted in suboptimal image quality. These piezoelectric crystals both generate and receive ultrasound waves and are integral to ultrasound imaging. After substantial development and iterations of probes, new-generation transducers now incorporate upward of 3,000 tiny piezoelectric crystals, laser cut into equal squares and arranged in a matrix, thereby significantly enhancing image quality (Fig. 19.1).

C. Cost. Each 3D-capable echocardiographic machine has its own vendor and, sometimes, model-specific matrix-array transducer. Given the sophisticated microtechnology incorporated into these transducers, 3D probes are substantially more expensive than the corresponding standard 2D probes. Ongoing optimization of 3D matrix design has resulted in a progressive reduction in probe size with continued improvement in image quality.

D. Image processing. In addition to the transducer elements within the echocardiographic probe, newer probes also incorporate signal processing. This feature enables

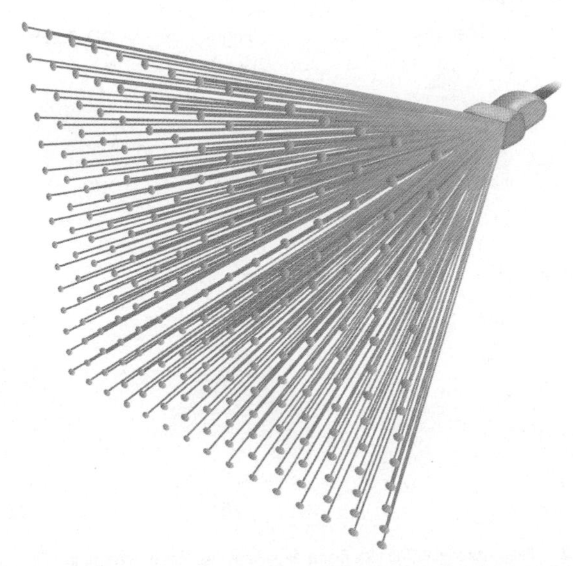

FIGURE 19.1 Full-matrix-array transducer, containing upward of 3,000 piezoelectric crystals cut into equal squares and arranged in a matrix, which both generate and receive ultrasound waves.

real-time online rendering of 3D images with a time resolution of approximately 50 ms (similar to a frame rate of 25 volumes per second). This allows performance of harmonic imaging, with better tissue penetration and contrast resolution. This online 3D rendering technique has superseded the offline 3D reconstruction technique for transthoracic imaging. However, 3D transesophageal echocardiography (TEE) remains in evolution and still relies on some 3D reconstruction techniques to compensate for the limitations of the miniaturized transesophageal probe. Online real-time 3D image availability using TEE remains a priority, particularly for valvular heart disease, where immediate image visualization can enable on-the-spot procedural guidance and intraoperative assessment.

V. TECHNIQUE

A. Current 3D echocardiographic rendering can be performed using three main methods (Fig. 19.2).

1. **Narrow-angle, real-time 3D imaging.** The first method involves online, real-time image acquisition of a specific volumetric sector, typically narrow angle ranging from 30 to 50 degrees in size. This method is particularly well suited to focused examination of smaller structures such as cardiac valves and can be zoomed or magnified, depending on the targeted spatial resolution. By limiting the size of the field of view, frame rate and imaging resolution can be optimized.
2. **Full-volume 3D imaging.** The second technique involves imaging of larger cardiac structures, whereby a full-volume data set needs to be acquired. Some newer platforms have introduced single-beat full-volume imaging, but traditionally this has been achieved by acquiring the data in four sectors during four consecutive heart beats, while maintaining the transducer in exactly the same position. The

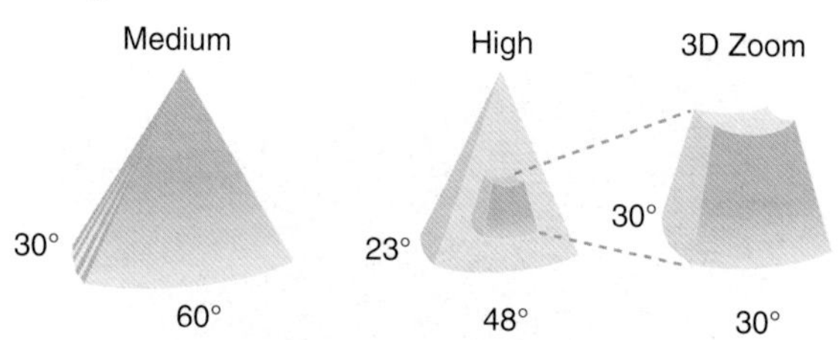

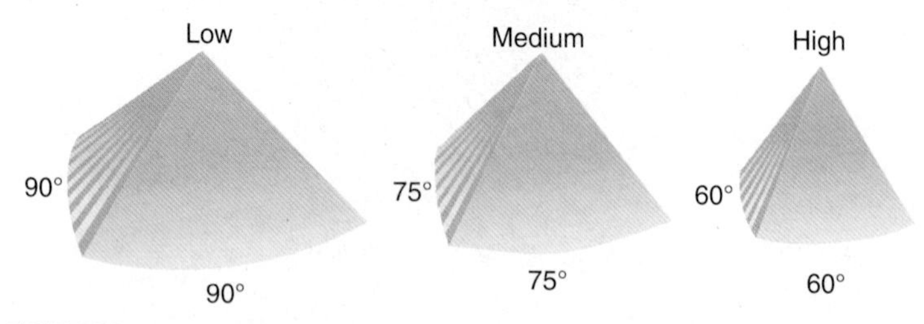

FIGURE 19.2 Ultrasound signals from the matrix-array transducer can be reconstructed to create a three-dimensional echocardiographic image. The narrower the image sector, the higher the frame rate and image resolution. (Redrawn with permission from Houck RC, Cooke JE, Gil EA. Live 3D echocardiography: a replacement for traditional 2D echocardiography? *AJR Am J Roentgenol.* 2006;187:1092–1106.)

four sectors of data are then combined to create a 3D data pyramid, although stitching artifact between these sectors can be problematic if there has been patient motion or variability in heart rate. Once the data pyramid is constructed, it can be cropped and manipulated on-cart or offline according to the structure of interest.

3. **Multiplanar reconstruction.** Last, multiplanar reconstruction (MPR) is an accurate and reproducible technique for quantification of detailed measurements including dimensions, circumference, and areas. This is particularly useful for assessment of preprocedural planning whereby patient's anatomical suitability can be established and prosthesis sizing can be determined. Different vendors have alternative iterations of this technique and reconstruction software, but primarily all involve volume segmentation of an image in three axes (*x*, *y*, and *z*). The positions of these axes are individually determined by the operator on the basis of the focus of interest, which is then demonstrated in a reconstructed 3D image. This can be performed on-cart or offline using postprocessing software on a remote workstation. Some aspects can be performed in real time, although more comprehensive quantitative analysis of measures such as length, area, and volume may require postprocessing. This technique is ideal for precise measurements of valve or annular areas, proximal isovelocity surface area (PISA), and vena contracta planimetry.

   It must always be emphasized that 3D imaging will be suboptimal in any situation where 2D image quality is limited. In most cases, appropriate acoustic windows for 3D imaging are even more challenging to achieve owing to the larger and typically more cumbersome 3D probe.

B. **Three-dimensional transesophageal echocardiography.** Real-time 3D TEE was made available for routine clinical use in 2007. The utility of 3D transthoracic echocardiography (TTE) for imaging of the mitral valve was first confirmed by publication in 2008. 3D TEE has much higher spatial resolution than 3D TTE and, as such, has become the mainstay of valvular imaging owing to its superior anatomic detail. When imaging the mitral valve by 3D TEE, the established convention is to display the valve from its left atrial aspect (surgeon's view), with the adjacent aortic valve orientated to the 12 o'clock position. This common logical approach has been advocated to create uniformity between studies and facilitate better communication between echocardiographers and surgeons. However, the ventricular aspect with a wide angle acquisition may be advantageous for assessment of chordae tendinae and papillary muscles, if these structures are not optimally visualized from a narrow-angled acquisition approach.

C. **3D color Doppler.** Optimal real-time 3D color Doppler imaging remains a technical challenge, particularly for TEE imaging owing to lower frame rates. Currently, acceptable temporal resolution with single heart beat acquisitions requires a frame rate of at least 16 volumes per second.

D. **Different vendors.** Each echocardiographic platform vendor has specific 3D technical features for image acquisition, optimization, and postprocessing. Generally, all include options for full-volume acquisition, real-time narrow-angle imaging with zoom feature, MPR techniques, 3D color Doppler, and cropping tools. The nomenclature for these features is vendor specific, which can lead to confusion for users. However, overall, the available technical options between platforms and software remain relatively similar in scope and quality. Currently, some variations exist between vendors with respect to 3D color Doppler frame rate and the ability to acquire full-volume data sets in a single beat. However, this variation appears unlikely to persist for long, with further updates in hardware and software always in development.

VI. LIMITATIONS

A. **Artifacts.** The quality of 3D echocardiography is dependent on the intrinsic quality of the ultrasound images and is subject to the same imaging artifacts faced in 2D imaging. These include technical factors, which can be more pronounced in 3D imaging and are related to machine gain settings, as well as patient issues involving electrocardiogram gating, respiration, and poor acoustic windows. Undergaining and overgaining can both impact the quality of 3D images, resulting in image dropout and blurriness, respectively. As outlined earlier, 3D multibeat acquisition techniques can be limited by stitch artifacts related to patient, respiratory, cardiac, or transducer motion. However, this is becoming less of an issue as more advanced and powerful 3D platforms are enabling single-beat acquisition of complete data sets for volume-rendered analysis, albeit at lower frame rates.

B. Frame rate. Currently, the relatively lower frame rates of 3D echocardiographic imaging detract from its spatial and temporal resolution. This means that some thinner and smaller structures may still be better delineated by 2D imaging at higher frame rates. Ongoing optimization of microprocessor technology is ameliorating this issue, by enabling further miniaturization of transducer size, along with faster data processing time.

C. Real-time imaging. Current 3D processors and matrix-array transducers are only able to perform real-time 3D imaging with relatively small (narrow-angle) fields of view. Ongoing development in this field will no doubt enable wider angle real-time imaging in the future. This will place less reliance on acquisition of full-volume data sets, which require time-consuming postprocessing, cropping, and analysis, without the clinical convenience and utility of real-time imaging, particularly for intraprocedural imaging.

D. Cost. The current cost of high-end echocardiographic machines with 3D capability, along with 3D probes, currently makes them more expensive relative to 2D-only platforms. Reimbursement for 3D acquisitions may negate some of this cost over time, but the setup costs or leasing plans may remain too prohibitive for some small centers or practices. Ideally, if a center could secure at least one machine with 3D echocardiography capability, this could be prioritized for valvular cases where arguably the most clinical benefit can be derived.

VII. STANDARD VIEWS

A. Imaging planes. Unlike conventional 2D echocardiographic imaging, 3D imaging is not governed by the same defined imaging planes. That being said, for real-time imaging using a narrow-angle field of view and 3D zoom mode, it is preferable to have the ultrasound beam perpendicular to the structure of interest. The resultant *en face* perspective (surgeon's view) allows assessment of the valve of interest in its entirety.

B. Transthoracic. Typically, images are initially optimized in two dimensions in the standard apical and parasternal acoustic windows. Activation of 3D mode imaging is then performed, with prespecification of the desired image field size (narrow or wide angle). A full-volume data set can be acquired for on-cart or offline manipulation, although typically this is used for larger structures including cardiac chambers for volume quantification. Valvular imaging is usually best performed with narrow-angle, real-time imaging to optimize frame rate. The images can then be manipulated or cropped to demonstrate the structure of interest in optimum orientation. Once adequately displayed, the 3D image can then be zoomed and acquired.

C. Transesophageal. 3D TEE imaging is also based on 2D images taken in the conventional planes. For valvular imaging, these are typically midesophageal views acquired at 0, 45, 60, 90, and 120 degrees. Once these images are optimized, the operator then switches to 3D imaging mode. Typically, 3D TEE, narrow-angle, real-time imaging is preferred as the valvular structures are relatively small, and this allows the frame rate to be enhanced. Once in 3D mode, the images can be cropped, rotated, and manipulated into nonconventional, off-axis orientations to adequately align the structure of interest *en face* and in its entirety.

VIII. CLINICAL APPLICATIONS—3D TRANSTHORACIC AND TRANSESOPHAGEAL ECHOCARDIOGRAPHY

In theory, 3D echocardiography can be employed for assessment of all valves and paravalvular structures; however, most incremental benefit has been achieved by imaging the mitral valve with 3D TEE.

A. Mitral valve

2D echocardiographic assessment of the mitral valve is complicated and multifaceted, perhaps reflecting that there is no good single method for quantification of either mitral stenosis or regurgitation severity. It requires identification of the pathology from multiple separate views, with subsequent extrapolation and mental reconstruction of the identified abnormality in three dimensions. Potentially, this type of imaging can also result in suboptimal visualization of the abnormality if it is not apparent on one of the standard 2D imaging planes.

Now for the first time with echocardiography, 3D imaging allows us to examine the mitral valve and subvalvular apparatus in its entirety and in any orientation relative to its surrounding structures, from both the atrial (so-called surgical view) and ventricular aspects. This obvious superiority in technique has been repeatedly recognized with both 3D TTE and TEE imaging. Thanks to 3D imaging, we now have a better appreciation of the saddle shape of the normal mitral valve annulus and asymmetric or symmetric alterations in this geometry, which can occur with different disease states such as ischemic or dilated cardiomyopathy, respectively. Greater anatomic detail also allows us to more precisely identify and localize valvular abnormalities, such as prolapse and flail of specific scallops, without rotational artifacts. Regions of prolapse are demonstrated as "bulging" segments into the left atrium (Fig. 19.3). Volumetric reconstruction can then color-code the region of prolapse to differentiate it from the normal surrounding leaflet. This technique is particularly useful for commissural pathology, which can be difficult to appreciate on 2D imaging. Ultimately, more accurate localization of pathology should result in better preoperative planning and potential interventional strategies. This can also influence the selection of surgeon and surgical technique, depending on the complexity of the lesion and the likelihood of successful valve repair.

By incorporating 3D color Doppler, we also have a better understanding of mitral valve dynamics. Not only will this likely influence procedural success, but, importantly, it may also impact upon the rates of successful valve repair able to be achieved.

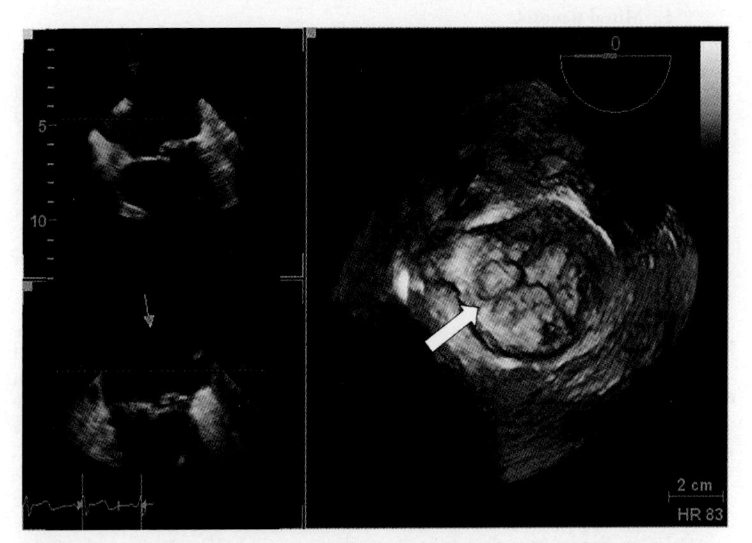

FIGURE 19.3 Three-dimensional transesophageal echocardiography *en face* reconstruction of the mitral valve demonstrating prolapse of the lateral and to a lesser degree the middle posterior leaflet scallops (P1 & P2) *(arrow)*.

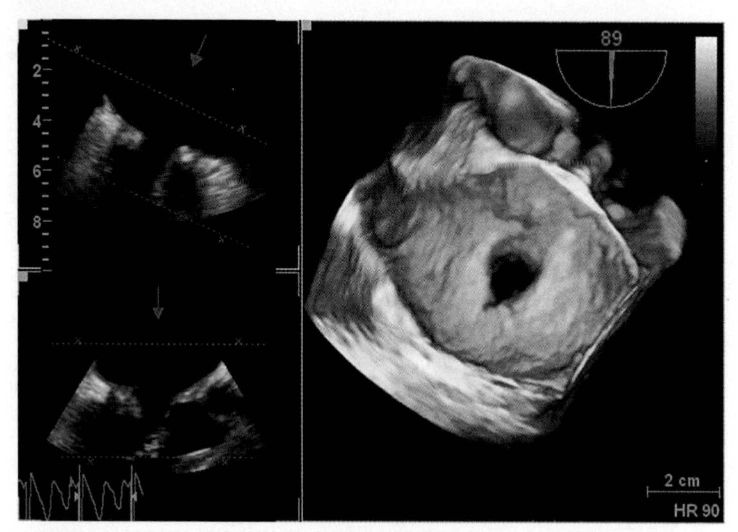

FIGURE 19.4 Three-dimensional transesophageal echocardiography zoom imaging of a previously repaired mitral valve with an annuloplasty ring in situ. An extensive inflammatory response to the ring resulted in severe mitral stenosis (peak and mean transvalvular gradients of 23 and 14 mm Hg, respectively), with severe global annular thickening extending onto the leaflet bases and restricting valve opening.

1. **Mitral stenosis**
   3D TTE *en face* rendering of the mitral valve enables direct visualization of the stenotic valve leaflets for qualitative valve assessment of etiology and severity. Regions of commissural fusion, leaflet tethering, thickening, and calcification can help determine the pathology involved, the suitability for valvuloplasty, and the likelihood of surgical repair (Fig. 19.4).

   Accurate planimetry for estimation of mitral valve area (MVA) is advisable using MPR techniques, whereby positioning of the narrowest cross-sectional area in the funnel-shaped orifice in three axes (*x*, *y*, and *z*) allows greater certainty that the smallest orifice area has been identified. This method has been found to correlate well with invasively determined MVA and gives more accurate estimates of MVA than traditional 2D TTE techniques.
2. **Mitral regurgitation**
   - **a.** The etiology of mitral valve pathology causing regurgitation can be more reliably established with 3D TEE, in comparison with corresponding 2D parameters. These 3D measures of regurgitant volume also correlate well with regurgitant fraction calculated from cardiac MRI quantitative flow data. These 3D results are also more closely matched with surgical findings especially for commissural and anterior leaflet disease.
   - **b.** In addition to the structural information provided by 3D imaging, the functional data available from 3D color Doppler imaging is incrementally important even at the lower frame rates often achieved. This is particularly important in the setting of mitral regurgitation. 3D color flow information can be used to precisely identify the location and quantitate the severity of mitral regurgitation via estimation of the jet orifice area and mitral regurgitant volume. Additionally, meaningful structural information about the underlying

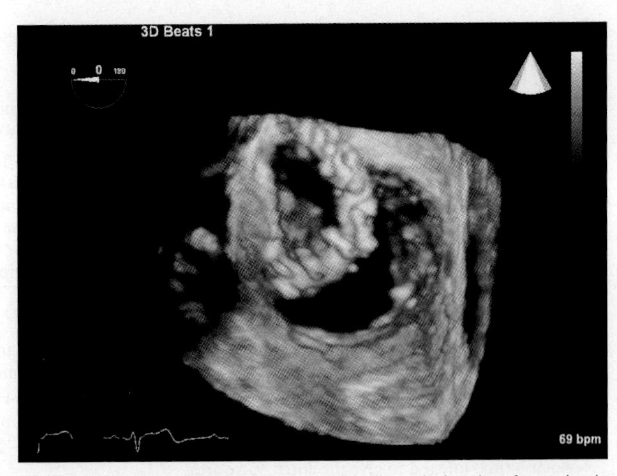

FIGURE 19.5 Three-dimensional transesophageal echocardiography imaging of a previously repaired mitral valve, demonstrating severe dehiscence of the annuloplasty ring, involving nearly 50% of its circumference.

etiology of regurgitation can be achieved simultaneously. 3D color Doppler imaging may help overcome the geometric assumptions made regarding flow convergence shape on 2D echocardiography, which can result in errors regarding estimation of mitral regurgitation severity. 3D color Doppler imaging has clearly demonstrated that in many situations the flow convergence zone (PISA) is not a simple hemisphere, but rather a more complex hemi-ellipsoid shape. 3D color Doppler can simultaneously demonstrate multiple jet orifices and eccentric jets, which may have been less apparent by 2D imaging, leading to an underappreciation of MR severity. 3D color Doppler imaging can also be used to determine the vena contracta area, from which the severity of mitral regurgitation can theoretically be extrapolated. However, this method may be limited by technical difficultly in determining the exact vena contracta position, especially in the setting of an eccentric jet.

c. In cases of prosthetic valve dehiscence, accurate identification of the origin of paravalvular leaks is imperative for determination of suitable management strategies (Fig. 19.5). Subsequently, real-time 3D echocardiographic guidance of percutaneous closure is an obvious advantage and should hopefully result in reduced procedural times and complication rates.

B. Aortic valve

The 3D structure of aortic valve, aortic annulus, and aortic root makes them ideal to assess with 3D echocardiography. Like the mitral valve, they are best demonstrated using 3D TEE with its increased spatial resolution; however, 3D TTE can provide clinically useful images. Due to its relatively small size, real-time, single-beat, narrow-angle image acquisition is feasible for detailed and accurate qualitative assessment of aortic valve morphology and function. Typically, the valve is orientated *en face* from the aortic aspect. This enables all cusps and potentially the coronary artery ostia to be identified. Detailed 3D assessment of aortic valve morphology enables better identification of cusp abnormalities including rarer entities such as quadricuspid and unicuspid valves, which are not always well seen using 2D echocardiography. This better spatial resolution also allows for better assessment and differentiation of small valve-related structures such as papillary fibroelastomas, Lambl's excrescences, and small vegetations.

1. **Aortic stenosis**

   2D echocardiographic measurements of aortic valve area are typically underestimated compared with 3D measurements, owing to the assumption that the left ventricular outflow tract (LVOT) is circular when using the continuity equation. Experience with 3D TEE has demonstrated that the LVOT is actually more elliptical and that it is more accurate to rely on planimetered LVOT area measured by 3D echocardiography and substitute this into the continuity equation:

$$\text{Aortic valve area (cm}^2\text{)} = \frac{\text{LVOT 3D area (cm}^2\text{)} \times \text{LVOT VTI (cm)}}{\text{Aortic valve VTI (cm)}}$$

   where LVOT = left ventricular outflow tract and VTI = velocity–time integral. Aortic valve area can also be estimated via 3D echocardiography using volumetric measurements or by direct valve planimetry. The volumetric technique involves using full-volume 3D data to determine left ventricular volumes and stroke volume. The 3D stroke volume is then divided by the aortic valve Doppler–derived velocity–time integral to give the aortic valve area.

$$\text{Aortic valve area (cm}^2\text{)} = \frac{\text{Left ventricular 3D stroke volume (cm}^3\text{)}}{\text{Aortic valve VTI (cm)}}$$

   Alternatively, direct valve planimetry can also be performed using MPR. This involves determining the narrowest cross-sectional area of the valve orifice in three axes (*x*, *y*, and *z*) with 2D image planes, then establishing the exact point at which the valve orifice area is smallest and reconstructing this in three dimensions. Accurate planimetry and distance measurements of this minimum area can then be directly performed on the 3D image on-cart or offline. All these methods have been found comparable to invasive measurements of valve area. Preferred techniques tend to be center specific, although 3D-valve planimetry using MPR is increasingly being employed, probably related to increasing experience with this technique in transcatheter aortic valve replacement (TAVR) trial and registry echocardiographic protocols.

   Cropping of 3D volume data sets in any orientation also allows identification of sub- and supravalvular stenosis. Qualitative assessment via 3D reconstruction of the LVOT and aortic root can identify the etiology of the stenosis, while MPR reconstruction can then provide additional quantitative assessment of the severity and exact location of stenosis. Assessment of valve-related stenosis should always be combined with complete transvalvular spectral Doppler assessment and estimate of left ventricular function to confirm agreement between transvalvular gradients and estimated aortic valve area. Disparity between parameters must be clarified as this may reflect low-flow low-gradient aortic stenosis or aortic pseudo-stenosis.

2. **Aortic regurgitation.** Severity of aortic regurgitation can often be technically challenging to determine. 3D echocardiography can provide useful adjunctive information to standard 2D parameters. Vena contracta cross-sectional area is a reliable indicator of the significance of aortic regurgitation. 3D color Doppler reconstruction of the vena contracta allows more accurate cross-sectional area estimation than that of 2D, which makes geometric assumptions that the regurgitant jet orifice is planar and round. This is particularly relevant in cases of valve asymmetry and jet eccentricity, such as seen with bicuspid aortic valves.

C. Tricuspid valve

3D echocardiography now enables the three leaflets of the tricuspid valve to be reliably visualized *en face* from either the right atrial or right ventricular aspects for the first time. Previously, 2D imaging was limited to demonstrating two out of three leaflets in any single plane. Anatomical reconstruction of the valve using the 3D technique has also enabled appreciation of the variability in leaflet size and the elliptical, saddle-shaped annulus, which were not previously well recognized. Simultaneous reconstruction of both atrioventricular valves in the same plane using cropping of full-volume 3D data has also reinforced the close relationship between the mitral and tricuspid valves and their geometric interdependence.

1. **Tricuspid stenosis.** The main advantage of 3D echocardiographic imaging in tricuspid stenosis is the ability to view the valve *en face* and see all valve leaflets simultaneously. Leaflet size, morphology, thickness, mobility, and calcification can be assessed and graded. The subvalvular leaflet apparatus can be similarly viewed from the right ventricular aspect. Similarly to the mitral valve, planimetry of the valve can then be performed using MPR techniques to ensure that the smallest estimated valve area is measured at exactly the narrowest valve orifice.
2. **Tricuspid regurgitation**
   a. Tricuspid valve abnormalities resulting in tricuspid regurgitation are substantially better appreciated by 3D echocardiography. This aids in more accurate identification of the pathologic etiology and also in determination of appropriate and feasible surgical treatment options. Leaflet prolapse and flail can be demonstrated in three dimensions in the same manner as for the mitral valve. This can be particularly useful in traumatic tricuspid regurgitation, where chest wall trauma can result in rupture of anterior leaflet chordae or the anterior papillary muscle, leading to severe acute tricuspid regurgitation. This requires immediate surgical repair, and so complete 3D preoperative assessment is essential to establish the extent of damage sustained and the best course of intervention. In addition to qualitative assessment of valve function and morphology, 3D color Doppler allows confirmation of regurgitation severity. Typically, this is performed by visually grading the color 3D jet; however, 3D vena contracta measurement is similarly possible. Unlike 2D, 3D echocardiography enables the jet to be accurately measured, at the correct level and without geometric assumptions, which is particularly important in situations where there are eccentric, elliptical, or multiple jets.
   b. Other congenital abnormalities such as Ebstein anomaly and atrioventricular canal defects can also be identified using narrow-volume zoomed imaging or by cropping full-volume data sets in any required orientation. Annular enlargement and increased geometrical sphericity can be appreciated in the setting of functional tricuspid regurgitation. Typically, this relates to increased annular anteroposterior dimension from right ventricular free-wall dilation. Accurate annular size is important preoperatively, when considering if the patient will benefit from an annuloplasty ring.
   c. Increased prevalence of pacemaker and implantable cardioversion device leads has also led to increased rates of associated tricuspid regurgitation. Primarily, this results from leaflet splinting from the pacing lead, although leaflet perforation and impingement of subvalvular apparatus have also been reported. 2D echocardiography is poor at tracking the course of the pacing lead and identifying which leaflet is involved. 3D echocardiography has much higher success rates (>90%) and has demonstrated that the posterior or septal leaflets are usually involved (Fig. 19.6).

D. **Pulmonic valve.** 2D echocardiographic assessment of the pulmonic valve is particularly challenging in most subjects due to the valve being positioned the furthest from the transducer on both TTE and TEE imaging. In addition, only two-valve leaflets can be demonstrated at any one time on standard 2D imaging planes. 3D echocardiography, therefore, provides a significant advantage by enabling the valve to be visualized *en face*, with all three valve leaflets displayed simultaneously. However, 3D assessment of the pulmonic valve still remains less successful than the other valves, as a result of

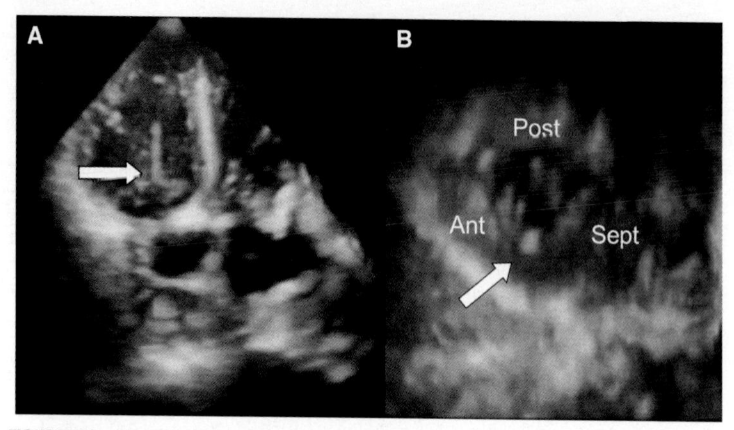

FIGURE 19.6 Three-dimensional full-volume reconstruction of the right heart, cropped to demonstrate the pacing lead *(white arrow)* traversing the tricuspid valve in a long-axis right ventricular optimized view **(A)** and a short-axis *en face* view **(B)** of the tricuspid valve from the right ventricular aspect. Tricuspid valve leaflets are labeled anterior *(Ant)*, septal *(Sept)*, and posterior *(Post)*.

the same echo-penetration issues plaguing 2D imaging, which result in suboptimal image quality from echo dropout. Overall, the pulmonic valve can be accurately demonstrated in three dimensions in approximately 60% of all echocardiograms.

1. **Pulmonary stenosis.** Congenital heart disease is the most common cause of pulmonary stenosis, although carcinoid disease can also result in significant restriction of leaflet opening and hemodynamically significant stenosis. Congenital stenosis can also involve supravalvular, subvalvular, or infundibular stenosis, such as that seen with a double-outlet right ventricle. Although adequate imaging of the right ventricular outflow tract and pulmonic valve is not possible in all subjects, when image quality is preserved, 3D images are accurate and provide useful information for diagnosis, functional assessment, and further interventional planning.
2. **Pulmonary regurgitation.** The etiology of clinically significant pulmonic regurgitation is also typically congenital heart disease or carcinoid valve disease. *En face* 3D imaging of all valve leaflets is relevant in both these situations to determine morphology and function. 3D echocardiography enables recognition of the thickened, restricted, and retracted leaflets typical for carcinoid valvulopathy. Valve mobility can be assessed, in addition to 3D color Doppler interrogation for determination of regurgitation severity. Like the other valves, regurgitation severity can be calculated using MPR techniques to accurately planimeter the vena contracta area. An additional advantage of 3D over 2D echocardiography is that the right ventricular outflow tract area can be accurately measured in any orientation, using 3D MPR techniques. This removes the assumption that the outflow tract is circular and allows the true area to be substituted into the continuity equation for more accurate calculation of the regurgitant volumes and fractions.

E. **Prosthetic valves**

1. 3D echocardiography and 3D TEE in particular have revolutionized the assessment of prosthetic valve function, along with diagnosis and assessment of associated complications. *En face* imaging provides detailed information about the entire valve structure simultaneously. This includes normal structures such as leaflets,

annular rings, and stent struts, as well as abnormal pathology such as vegetations, thrombi, or abnormal sutures. The addition of 3D color Doppler can also localize paravalvular leaks, valve dehiscence, and valvular regurgitation.

2. Prostheses in the mitral position are most reliably demonstrated by 3D TEE. Although conventional views may be hampered by valve shadowing, the ability of 3D cropping and acquisition in nonconventional imaging planes means that in most situations the mitral valve including all leaflets can be visualized regardless of original position or orientation. Aortic and tricuspid prosthetic rings are reliably demonstrated in three dimensions; however, the leaflets may be less well visualized. This may relate to the increased depth of the leaflets relative to the transducer or to technical factors associated with the angle of the ultrasound beam. Reliable 3D imaging of pulmonic valve prostheses is also currently limited. Ongoing optimization of 3D techniques and technology, with smaller transducers and higher frame rates, is required before all prosthetic valves can be adequately and reliably imaged at an adequate standard for diagnostic purposes.

F. **Endocarditis.** 3D TEE is a useful and complementary technique to 2D TEE for assessment of native and prosthetic valve endocarditis. However, the lower frame rates and reduced spatial resolution of 3D TEE relative to 2D TEE make it less sensitive for identification of smaller, highly mobile lesions. An advantage of 3D TEE is its ability to visualize the entire valve and therefore precisely identify the location of vegetation adherence and any associated leaflet, annular, or prosthetic complications. Off-axis imaging in any orientation using narrow-angle zoom images or cropping of 3D data sets also enables manipulation of image angles to best demonstrate the exact relationship of vegetations to valvular and nonvalvular structures. In some cases, this allows visualization of lesions not appreciable with 2D echocardiography. This may result in better mass characterization and differentiation of vegetations from other structures such as thrombi, prosthesis pannus, small tumors, or mobile suture material. 3D imaging is particularly useful and important for prosthetic valve dehiscence or paravalvular leaks, where images may require extensive rotation or manipulation to locate the precise defect and to plan and potentially guide percutaneous interventions. 3D color Doppler is also useful in this setting for quantification of regurgitant jets and identification of jet origins to localize valve pathology including perforations and prosthesis dehiscence.

G. **Congenital heart disease**

1. A further important clinical application of 3D echocardiography is congenital heart disease. The improved spatial orientation provided by 3D imaging not only identifies discrete structural abnormalities but also enables better conceptualization of these defects relative to the entire heart, while providing simultaneous functional information. In congenital valvular disease, this greater flexibility in off-axis imaging enables a better understanding of complex lesions and previous repairs. In some cases, this may negate the requirement for additional invasive catheterization or tomographic cardiac CT or MRI.

2. 3D echocardiography can be particularly helpful for direct visualization of structural abnormalities in conditions such as endocardial cushion defects with a cleft mitral valve, sub- and supravalvular stenosis, pulmonary valve pathology, and Ebstein anomaly. Preoperative assessment of these structures from nontraditional *en face* views may allow better determination of defect repairability and consideration of alternative operative strategies preoperatively.

IX. 3D ECHOCARDIOGRAPHY FOR PROCEDURAL PLANNING, GUIDANCE, AND OUTCOMES

A. **Transcatheter aortic valve replacement.** The utility of 3D echocardiography is perhaps best demonstrated in its central role for percutaneous aortic valve replacement. Arguably, this percutaneous technique would have been less available and less successful without the preoperative assessment and intraprocedural guidance provided by 3D TEE. The aortic valve lies in close proximity to several important structures and, hence, accuracy of distance and area measurements for any intervention in the region is crucial. Typically, this is best achieved using MPR techniques, whereby the smallest valve area, largest annular and root dimensions, and distance to the coronary ostia can all be accurately defined.

1. **Preprocedural assessment for TAVR**
   a. Preprocedural assessment involves complete qualitative assessment of aortic valve morphology and function by 2D and 3D TEE. MPR processing is then typically employed on-cart or offline to determine specific measurements, crucial to determine suitability for TAVR and for prosthesis sizing. The accuracy of these measurements is made feasible by the ability of 3D MPR to obtain perfect orthogonal alignment of the LVOT and the aortic annulus. Measurements include aortic annular dimensions (including distance, area, and circumference), distance from the aortic annulus to the coronary artery ostia, and smallest cross-sectional aortic valve area to confirm stenosis severity (Fig. 19.7). If the annulus is too small, too ovoid, or too large, significant procedural issues can result including annular rupture, paravalvular leak, or valve embolization. Oversized valves also potentially increase the risk of damage to the conduction system, which runs in close proximity to the aortic annulus. The currently available, purpose-designed, low-profile, percutaneous aortic valves typically range from 23 to 29 or 31 mm in size, depending on vendor. Suitable annular measurements for each sized valve vary slightly between manufacturers. However, for example, the Edwards SAPIEN three valves are suitable for a range of annular diameters between 18 and 27 mm and areas of 338 to 680 mm^2. Although the low-profile nature of the percutaneous valves means that they are relatively unlikely to obstruct coronary ostia, the annulus to coronary distance should be confirmed for suitability during the initial preprocedural assessment. Assessment of the length of the native valve leaflets is also important, relative to the annulus to coronary distance, as longer leaflets have potential for coronary ostia obstruction after TAVR deployment.
   b. The preprocedural MPR measurements performed for TAVR have been shown to be highly reproducible and correlate better with dimensions achieved via tomographic imaging with CT and MRI than 2D TEE measurements. Although 3D TEE annular measurements are consistently larger than by 2D echocardiography, they tend to run smaller than those achieved with CT and MRI. This needs to be remembered during selection of valve size. Most TAVR centers continue to perform preprocedural planning assessment with both 3D TEE and gated cardiac CT or noncontrast cardiac MRI (in the setting of renal dysfunction). Combining techniques provides confirmation of these important measurements and maintains the invaluable functional data provided by 3D TEE.
2. **Procedural TEE for TAVR.** Echocardiography remains integral for procedural guidance during TAVR. Typically, this involves TEE, but particularly in Europe, some centers are performing awake procedures with TTE assistance. Although valve positioning is predominantly determined by fluoroscopy, TEE remains useful for catheter guidance and confirming that the valve is appropriately sited and deployed. If a valve is deployed too far into the aortic root, the coronary ostia can become obstructed. Conversely, if the valve is positioned low in the LVOT, disruption to the geometry of the aortomitral curtain or impingement of the anterior mitral valve leaflet can result in mitral valve dysfunction and mitral regurgitation.
3. **Postprocedural TAVR.** The role of postprocedural echocardiography in TAVR is to monitor for specific complications including valvular or paravalvular aortic regurgitation, new wall motion abnormalities, and more serious sequelae such as annular rupture and pericardial effusion. Determination between valvular and paravalvular aortic regurgitant jets is not always clear on standard 2D color Doppler

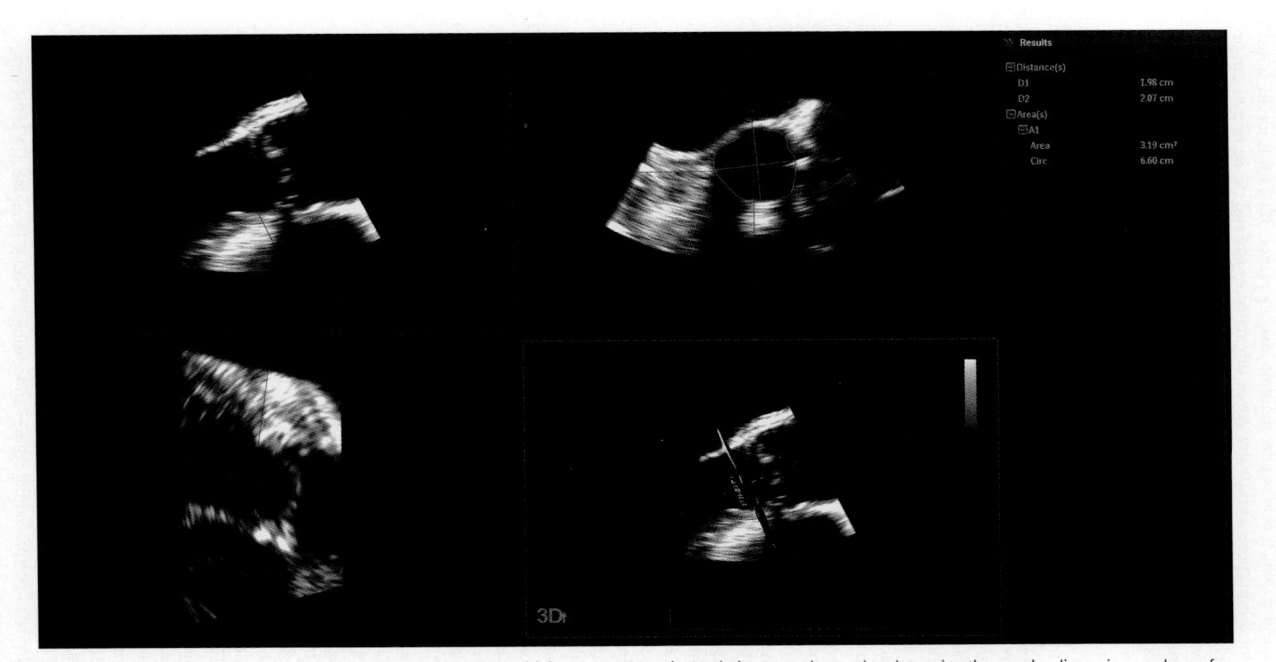

FIGURE 19.7 Three-dimensional transesophageal echocardiography multiplanar reconstruction techniques can be used to determine the annular dimensions and area for transcatheter aortic valve replacement sizing. This involves determining the cross-sectional area of the annulus in three axes (*x*, *y*, and *z*) with two-dimensional image planes and then creating a three-dimensional reconstruction from which accurate measurements can be directly performed on-cart or offline.

imaging, which may require multiple imaging planes. 3D TEE is ideally suited for this purpose, as the valve can be orientated *en face* and the jet origins can be identified with the addition of 3D color Doppler. Confidently demonstrating these jets and being able to demonstrate them online in real time during the procedure means that these results can be visually communicated to the interventionalist or surgeon in a clear and logical manner. In cases of significant aortic regurgitation or valve malposition, these results may then guide the operator with further intervention including valve-in-valve deployment or paravalvular closure devices. In the rare event of catastrophic complications such as annular rupture, prompt and accurate diagnosis by 3D echocardiography can save precious minutes and facilitate rapid resuscitation and surgical intervention.

B. Paravalvular closure devices

1. In this era of increasing percutaneous intervention, a multitude of percutaneous closure devices are now available. Increasingly, these devices are being successfully used for closure of paravalvular leaks. 3D echocardiography and 3D TEE in particular are crucial for these interventions. Preprocedure, 3D imaging enables accurate localization and sizing of single or multiple defects. 3D evaluation is particularly important for determining the defect shape as some large, elliptical, or asymmetrical defects are not suitable for device closure and need to be preemptively excluded from consideration and managed surgically. Imaging in two dimensions may infer a false degree of defect in geometrical symmetry and hence result in patients being inappropriately referred for device closure. The defect can be initially visualized in its entirety with 3D zoom or full-volume cropping techniques. MPR can then be used to make accurate defect measurements, and finally 3D color Doppler can quantify the leak size and confirm the leak position and direction. These accurate defect dimensions also assist with selection of device type and size.
2. Paravalvular leak closures for aortic and mitral valve prostheses are most common, related to the higher prevalence of left-sided valve replacements. Intraprocedure, like other percutaneous techniques, 3D TEE can be used for catheter guidance and device placement. Universally, in paravalvular leak closure the defect must be crossed by a guide wire to allow subsequent passage and deployment of the closure device in the appropriate position. The wire may be placed via an antegrade or retrograde approach, depending on the access site, defect location, and technical factors. Positioning of the guide wire using 2D techniques such as fluoroscopy or 2D TEE can at times be challenging, especially if the defect is small, has a large regurgitant jet, or is oblique in direction. Switching between different off-axis 2D imaging views can be cumbersome and add unnecessary complexity to these procedures, which could otherwise be guided by single *en face* 3D views. 3D imaging assists in these situations by demonstrating the defect and its surrounding structures, catheters, balloons, and devices in a simultaneous and more anatomically realistic fashion, thereby providing better geometrical orientation and guidance to the interventionalist.

C. Balloon valvuloplasty

1. Typically, balloon valvuloplasty is most commonly performed for rheumatic mitral stenosis, although in some situations aortic valve balloon valvuloplasty may be performed in a high-risk or unstable individual as a bridge to percutaneous or surgical aortic valve replacement. Fluoroscopic guidance has been traditionally employed for this technique; however, the increasing availability of intraprocedural 3D TEE has been a valuable addition. 3D imaging assists with guiding balloon placement and also for assessment of postprocedural results and complications. These include the degree of commissural splitting, presence of leaflet tears, and degree of postprocedural regurgitation using 3D color Doppler. 3D MPR imaging can also be employed to accurately determine the change between pre- and

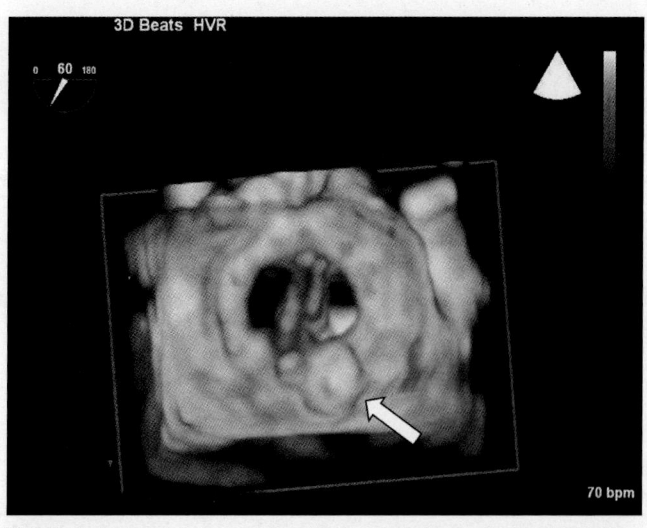

FIGURE 19.8 Three-dimensional transesophageal echocardiography zoom imaging demonstrates a bileaflet, mechanical mitral valve replacement with a vascular plug (Amplatzer Vascular Plug II device) deployed inferoposteriorly for percutaneous device closure of a paravalvular leak *(arrow)*. The patient had presented with a mild to moderate paravalvular leak, adjacent to the inferoposterior aspect of the mitral valve sewing ring, and associated hemolysis.

postprocedural valvular stenosis via planimetry. This method can be a useful alternative to 2D estimates of MVA immediately postvalvuloplasty, which tend to be less reliable and discrepant when compared with valve areas calculated using the Gorlin formula.

2. Appropriate patient selection and suitability for balloon valvuloplasty is paramount. Traditionally, this has been guided by the Wilkins score, which grades suitability for valvuloplasty on the basis of the amount of leaflet mobility and thickness, valvular calcification, and subvalvular thickening. Perceived weakness in the Wilkins score has resulted in the recent development of a 3D echocardiography-based score. This technique involves a more regional assessment of valvular abnormalities, by evaluating each leaflet segment and subvalvular apparatus individually. This includes separate assessment of the commissures, which are typically the most crucial determinants of procedural success. Each regional score is finally weighted according to its predetermined importance for procedural success, before the individual scores are summed to give a total score graded from 0 to 31. Mild mitral valve involvement was defined as a total score of $<$8 points, moderate mitral valve involvement as 8 to 13 points, and severe mitral valve involvement as $\geq$14 points. Hence, a score of $\leq$13 is considered optimal for successful valvuloplasty (Table 19.2).

D. Percutaneous edge-to-edge mitral valve clip repair

1. Percutaneous edge-to-edge clip repair of the mitral valve was approved in the United States in October 2013 for high-risk individuals with severe degenerative mitral regurgitation. This technique aims to use a single clip (or multiple clips) to join the leaflet tips of the anterior and posterior leaflets, thereby creating an Alfieri-type valve repair, with typically two-valve orifices. The repair results in a reduced total valve area, with improved leaflet competency and reduced regurgitation. 3D TEE is integral to all aspects of this intervention including preprocedural assessment

TABLE 19.2 Real-Time Three-Dimensional Echocardiography Regional Scoring of Mitral Valve Leaflets and Subvalvular Apparatus in Rheumatic Mitral Valve Stenosis

	Anterior Leaflet			Posterior Leaflet			
Leaflets	**A1**	**A2**	**A3**	**P1**	**P2**	**P3**	**Total Score**
Thickness (0 = normal, 1 = thickened)	0–1	0–1	0–1	0–1	0–1	0–1	0–6
Mobility (0 = normal, 1 = limited)	0–1	0–1	0–1	0–1	0–1	0–1	0–6
Calcification (0 = no, 1–2 = calcification)	0–2	0–1	0–2	0–2	0–1	0–2	0–10
Subvalvular Apparatus	**Proximal Third**		**Middle Third**		**Distal Third**		
Thickness (0 = normal, 1 = thickened)	0–1		0–1		0–1		0–3
Separation (0 = normal, 1 = partial, 2 = no)	0–2		0–2		0–2		0–6
							0–31

Taken from Anwar AM, Attia WM, Nosir YF, et al. Validation of a new score for the assessment of mitral stenosis using real-time three-dimensional echocardiography. *J Am Soc Echocardiogr.* 2010;23(1):13–22.

and planning, procedural guidance, and evaluation of procedural success and/or complications. Much of this process cannot be performed under standard fluoroscopic guidance, and 3D TTE is both inadequate and impractical in this setting.

2. 3D TEE allows *en face* imaging of the entire valve from the atrial or ventricular aspects, or even both views simultaneously. In combination with multiplanar imaging, this allows accurate multidimensional catheter guidance of clip placement to ensure appropriate grasping of both leaflets and suitable positioning of the clip with adequate coaptation zone. 3D imaging can also ensure that the clip is clear from surrounding structures and not tethered to subvalvular apparatus (Fig. 19.9).
3. The addition of 3D color Doppler imaging pre- and postprocedure is extremely useful. This technique can confirm the origin and severity of the original regurgitant jet and then ensure that the degree of regurgitation has sufficiently reduced postprocedure. Occasionally, persistent mitral regurgitation necessitates the deployment of a second (or even third) clip to ensure adequate leaflet coaptation. 3D guidance of clip deployment in this scenario becomes even more crucial, as there is an increased risk of subsequent clips and catheters becoming caught in subvalvular apparatus or dislodging the original clip. As always, 2D spectral Doppler remains an integral and complementary technique to 3D imaging for exclusion of procedural-related mitral stenosis.

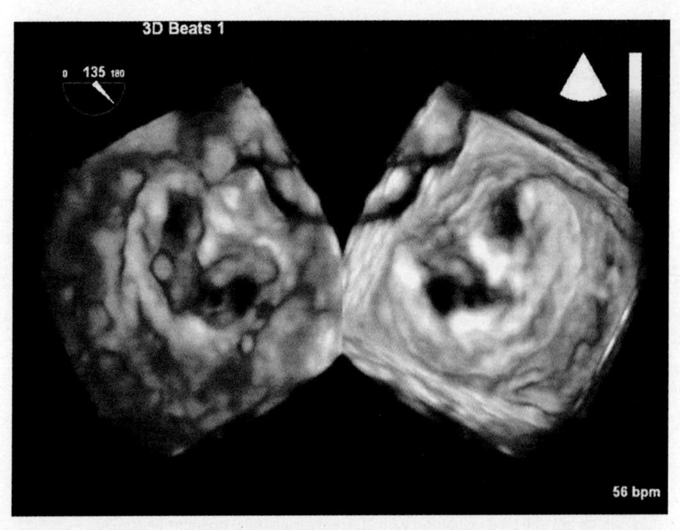

FIGURE 19.9 Percutaneous edge-to-edge clip repair of the mitral valve for severe degenerative mitral regurgitation with posterior leaflet prolapse, P2 flail and moderately severe pulmonary hypertension. Two adjacent clips were employed to adequately join the tips of the anterior and posterior leaflets. *En face* three-dimensional zoom imaging of the mitral valve demonstrates the Alfieri-type valve repair from the left ventricular *(left image)* and left atrial *(right image)* aspects, with subsequent creation of two-valve orifices.

E. **Perioperative valvular assessment.** These days, the majority of cardiac operating theaters have TEE available. Typically, the cardiac anesthesiologist or cardiologist will perform pre- and postoperative TEE assessment to confirm diagnosis and assess outcome of surgery once the patient has been weaned off cardiopulmonary bypass but before the chest is closed. 3D TEE is a useful adjunctive technique for these purposes and especially for assessment of paravalvular or valvular leaks and other valve-related problems such as mitral leaflet systolic anterior motion. Immediate and accurate recognition of these issues before the chest is closed means that the patient can be immediately put back on cardiopulmonary bypass and the problem rectified, leading to better postoperative outcomes. 3D echocardiographic demonstration of valves *en face* intraoperatively likely also facilitates better communication with surgeons who are used to this same perspective or "surgeon's view."

KEY PEARLS

- Three-dimensional (3D) echocardiography has revolutionized valvular assessment through its ability to view the valve *en face* from any orientation and in its entirety.
- Successful 3D echocardiography has been enabled by the progression from a sparse-array transducer to a full-matrix-array transducer, which now incorporates over 3,000 tiny piezoelectric crystals and provides significantly enhanced image quality.
- Microprocessor technology has allowed miniaturization of transducers, with faster data processing time, leading to incorporation of 3D technology into transesophageal echocardiography.

- Three main 3D echocardiographic methodologies include:
  - Real-time, narrow-angle 3D imaging with optional zoom and magnification features—typically useful for assessment of small structures such as valves and procedural guidance; higher frame rates result in better tissue penetration and contrast resolution.
  - Full-volume, large-angle 3D imaging—can be performed using single or multibeat image acquisition, usually employed for larger structures including volumetric assessment of cardiac chambers, and requires cropping and manipulation of the data pyramid.
  - Multiplanar reconstruction—segmentation of an image in three axes (*x*, *y*, and *z*) to create an orthogonally aligned image in three dimensions, which can facilitate precise measurements including length, area, and volume.
- 3D color Doppler imaging has been hampered by low frame rates; however, recent technical developments have improved time resolution and hence clinical utility.
- 3D imaging is subject to the same artifacts as two-dimensional (2D) imaging and will therefore be suboptimal in any situation where 2D image quality is limited.
- The frame rates of both 3D transthoracic echocardiography and transesophageal echocardiography are relatively lower than their 2D equivalents, resulting in comparatively lower spatial and temporal resolution. This means that 3D echocardiography is less sensitive for identification of small, highly mobile structures such as some vegetations and fibroelastomas, which are still best visualized with 2D transesophageal echocardiography.
- 3D echocardiography has proven invaluable for preprocedural assessment, intraprocedural guidance, and postprocedural evaluation of results and complications. In particular, transcatheter aortic valve replacement, percutaneous edge-to-edge mitral valve clip repair, and paravalvular device closure have all benefited from this technique.
- *En face* imaging of the valve structure with 3D echocardiography is particularly important for assessment of prosthetic valve dysfunction, dehiscence, and leaks. Images can be manipulated and rotated in any orientation to locate and size the defect and to plan and potentially guide percutaneous intervention.
- There have been increased implantations of pacemaker and implantable cardioversion devices over the past decade. 3D echocardiography is superior to 2D echocardiography for tracking the device leads within the right heart and identifying any valve-related lead complications such as leaflet splinting, perforation, or impingement of subvalvular apparatus, which may result in tricuspid regurgitation.

SUGGESTED READINGS

Anwar AM, Attia WM, Nosir YF, et al. Validation of a new score for the assessment of mitral stenosis using real-time three-dimensional echocardiography. *J Am Soc Echocardiogr.* 2010;23(1):13–22.

Breburda CS, Griffin BP, Pu M, et al. Three-dimensional echocardiographic planimetry of maximal regurgitant orifice area in myxomatous mitral regurgitation: intraoperative comparison with proximal flow convergence. *J Am Coll Cardiol.* 1998;32(2):432–437.

Iwakura K, Ito H, Kawano S, et al. Comparison of orifice area by transthoracic three-dimensional doppler echocardiography versus proximal isovelocity surface area (PISA) method for assessment of mitral regurgitation. *Am J Cardiol.* 2006;97(11):1630–1637.

Jilaihawi H, Doctor N, Kashif M, et al. Aortic annular sizing for transcatheter aortic valve replacement using cross-sectional 3-dimensional transesophageal echocardiography. *J Am Coll Cardiol.* 2013;61(9):908–916.

Kelly NF, Platts DG, Burstow DJ. Feasibility of pulmonary valve imaging using three-dimensional transthoracic echocardiography. *J Am Soc Echocardiogr.* 2010;23(10):1076–1080.

Langerveld J, Valocik G, Plokker HW, et al. Additional value of three-dimensional transesophageal echocardiography for patients with mitral valve stenosis undergoing balloon valvuloplasty. *J Am Soc Echocardiogr.* 2003;16(8):841–849.

Mediratta A, Addetia K, Yamat M, et al. 3D Echocardiographic location of implantable device leads and mechanism of associated tricuspid regurgitation. *JACC Cardiovasc Imaging.* 2014;7(4):337–347.

Messika-Zeitoun D, Serfaty JM, Brochet E, et al. Multimodal assessment of the aortic annulus diameter: implications for transcatheter aortic valve implantation. *J Am Coll Cardiol.* 2010;55(3):186–194.

Mori Y, Shiota T, Jones M, et al. Three-dimensional reconstruction of the color Doppler-imaged vena contracta for quantifying aortic regurgitation: studies in a chronic animal model. *Circulation.* 1999;99(12):1611–1617.

Nishimura RA, Otto CM, Bonow RO, et al; ACC/AHA Task Force Members. 2014 AHA/ACC guideline for the management of patients with valvular heart disease: executive summary: a report of the American College of Cardiology/American Heart Association Task Force on Practice Guidelines. *Circulation.* 2014;129(23):2440–2492.

Sugeng L, Shernan SK, Salgo IS, et al. Live 3-dimensional transesophageal echocardiography initial experience using the fully-sampled matrix array probe. *J Am Coll Cardiol.* 2008;52(6):446–449.

Sugeng L, Shernan SK, Weinert L, et al. Real-time three-dimensional transesophageal echocardiography in valve disease: comparison with surgical findings and evaluation of prosthetic valves. *J Am Soc Echocardiogr.* 2008;21(12):1347–1354.

Sugeng L, Weinert L, Lang RM. Real-time 3-dimensional color Doppler flow of mitral and tricuspid regurgitation: feasibility and initial quantitative comparison with 2-dimensional methods. *J Am Soc Echocardiogr.* 2007;20(9):1050–1057.

Zamorano J, Cordeiro P, Sugeng L, et al. Real-time three-dimensional echocardiography for rheumatic mitral valve stenosis evaluation: an accurate and novel approach. *J Am Coll Cardiol.* 2004;43(11):2091–2096.

CHAPTER 20

Grant W. Reed
Amar Krishnaswamy

Catheterization Hemodynamics and Formulae

I. INTRODUCTION.

Knowledge of the hemodynamic pressure waveforms and formulae used to diagnose valvular pathology can be a valuable tool in the management of valvular heart disease. As advances in cardiovascular imaging have decreased the need for routine invasive hemodynamic assessment, catheterization is typically reserved for patients with symptoms that are out of proportion to the severity of valvular pathology based on noninvasive testing. Additional patients that may benefit include those requiring precise assessment of valve gradients, valve areas, cardiac output (CO), or intracardiac pressures. Knowledge of normal hemodynamics is essential to interpret the hemodynamic tracings for common valvular pathologies, as discussed later.

II. NORMAL INVASIVE HEMODYNAMICS

A. Right heart catheterization. Right-sided hemodynamic pressure waveforms are obtained from right heart catheterization (RHC). During RHC, a balloon-tipped catheter (typically a 7 or 8 French Swan-Ganz) is inserted percutaneously through a venous sheath, most often placed in the internal jugular or common femoral veins; the subclavian vein is sometimes utilized, and in patients undergoing coronary angiography via the wrist a 5 French brachial vein Swan-Ganz may be floated. The catheter is passed sequentially through the central veins to the right atrium (RA), right ventricle (RV), and into one of the two main pulmonary arteries (PAs).

When the catheter tip is in a mid/distal PA branch, the inflated balloon serves to block anterograde flow and allows for an indirect measurement of pressure in the left atrium (LA), otherwise known as the pulmonary capillary wedge pressure (PCWP). In the absence of pulmonary vein stenosis, PCWP is a reasonable surrogate for LA pressure, which approximates left ventricular (LV) diastolic pressure in the absence of mitral stenosis (MS). Conversely, LA pressure can be directly measured via a transseptal puncture across the RA to the LA if the PCWP appears inaccurate in a given patient or more precise measurement of the LA pressure is necessary.

Aortic and LV hemodynamics are measured via left heart catheterization (LHC). This is usually accomplished with a pigtail catheter advanced to the aortic root and LV via a sheath in the radial artery or common femoral artery.

With these procedures, hemodynamic waveforms and oxygen saturations can be obtained in each of the cardiac chambers. This allows for the diagnosis of valvular disease, assessment of CO, intracardiac shunting, constrictive and restrictive cardiomyopathy, and many other conditions. Full descriptions of the RHC and LHC procedures are beyond the scope of this chapter, though details on calculation of CO are discussed further later.

1. Right atrial pressure.

a. An understanding of the normal pressure waveforms in each cardiac chamber is necessary for the proper interpretation of how these hemodynamic tracings change with valve disease. Normal pressure waveforms for each cardiac chamber,

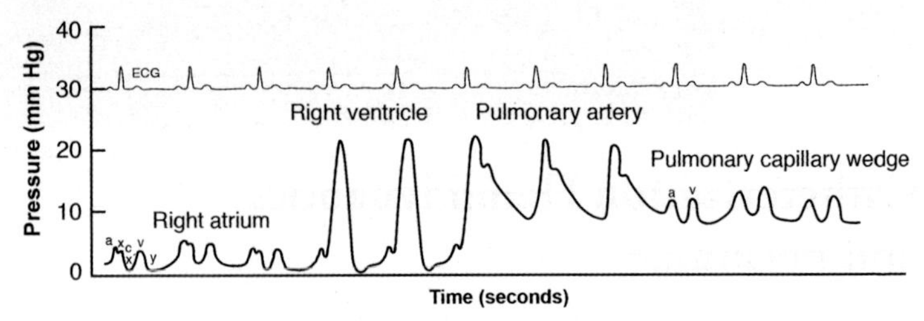

FIGURE 20.1 Normal hemodynamic tracings.

PCW, and pulmonary artery are displayed in Figure 20.1, and normal values are provided in Table 20.1.

b. Normal RA mean pressure is 2 to 6 mm Hg and is characterized by "a-," "c-," and "v-" waves, with "x-" and "y"-descents (Fig. 20.1). The a-wave represents pressure rise due to atrial contraction and follows the P-wave on electrocardiogram (ECG). The x-descent follows and represents atrial relaxation and sudden downward motion of the atrioventricular junction due to ventricular systole. The c-wave is next, which represents a subtle pressure rise due to closure of the tricuspid valve (TV) and motion toward the RA during ventricular systole. After the c-wave, the x-descent continues (and if the c-wave is present, it is termed the x′-descent). The final event is the v-wave, which represents passive venous filling during ventricular systole and corresponds to the T-wave on ECG.

c. During inspiration, intrathoracic pressure decreases, which increases venous return and right-sided filling; thus, the v-waves and y-descents become more

TABLE 20.1 Normal Hemodynamic Parameters

Parameter	Normal Pressure
RA	2–6 mm Hg
RV	20–30/2–8 mm Hg
PA	20–30/4–14 mm Hg
PCWP	4–14 mm Hg
LA	4–14 mm Hg
LV	90–140/10–16 mm Hg
Aorta	90–140/60–90 mm Hg
Cardiac output	5–6 L/min
Cardiac index	2.6–4.2 L/min/m^2

LA, left atrium; LV, left ventricle; PA, pulmonary artery; PCWP, pulmonary capillary wedge pressure; RA, right atrium; RV, right ventricle.

prominent. Additionally, while normally a-wave amplitude exceeds v-wave amplitude, certain pathologic conditions such as tricuspid regurgitation (TR) are associated with large v-waves. Finally, during atrial fibrillation, a-waves will not be seen.

2. **Right ventricular pressure.** The normal RV pressure is 20 to 30 systolic/2 to 8 diastolic mm Hg, with a rapid rise due to ventricular contraction during systole, and rapid decline with ventricular relaxation during diastole (Fig. 20.1). The diastolic pressure gradually rises due to RV filling during diastole. RA mean pressure should be within a few mm Hg of RV end-diastolic pressure (RVEDP), except in the presence of tricuspid stenosis (TS), in which case RA mean > RVEDP. Unlike the RA, there is not usually an a-wave seen on the RV tracing. If there is an a-wave, it will be seen just before RVEDP and is only seen in states of decreased RV compliance, such as volume overload, RV hypertrophy, or pulmonary hypertension.
3. **Pulmonary artery pressure**
   - **a.** Under normal circumstances, PA pressure is 20 to 30 systolic/4 to 14 diastolic mm Hg. Similar to other arterial waveforms, the PA tracing has a rapid rise, well-defined peak, a dicrotic notch (from pulmonic valve [PV] closure), and a well-defined nadir in diastole (Fig. 20.1). PA systolic pressure (PASP) should approximate RV systolic pressure (RVSP), unless there is pulmonic stenosis (PS), in which case RVSP > PASP. Furthermore, while PASP and RVSP are usually similar in magnitude, there is individual variability and these values may differ under normal conditions in certain patients.
   - **b.** Comparing the RV and PA tracings, important identifying features are the approximately 5 mm Hg increase in diastolic pressure from the RV to the PA, and the appearance of the dicrotic notch in the PA. Also, the events of the PA waveform are slightly delayed with regard to the ECG, with the PASP peaking within the T-wave on ECG.
4. **Pulmonary capillary wedge pressure**
   - **a.** The PCWP has a normal range of 4 to 14 mm Hg, and a-, c-, and v-waves similar to an atrial waveform (as it approximates LA hemodynamics) (Fig. 20.1). Unlike an atrial waveform, there is a delay in the pressure transmission from the LA across the pulmonary veins and pulmonary capillary bed. This delay usually places the a-wave after the QRS and v-wave after the T-wave on ECG. Additionally, unlike the RA tracing, the c-wave is not visible on the PCW tracing due to pressure dampening, and the v-wave typically exceeds the a-wave in amplitude.
   - **b.** The PCWP is typically reported as a mean with a normal value approximately 0 to 5 mm Hg lower than PA diastolic pressure, unless there is elevated pulmonary vascular resistance. Changes in thoracic pressure during the respiratory cycle alter the PCWP tracing baseline, and mean PCWP is typically measured at end expiration (corresponding to the "peaks" in normal patients, and "valleys" in patients intubated undergoing mechanical ventilation). It may be helpful in awake patients with substantial respiratory variation in pressure to simply hold their breath, but they should be advised not to take a deep breath (or exhale) before this hold.
   - **c.** While under ideal circumstances, PCWP approximates LA pressure (which approximates LVEDP), this rests on several assumptions, including no impedance of flow distally. PCWP will not correlate with LA pressure in the presence of pulmonary vein stenosis, and LA pressure will be a poor surrogate for LVEDP in patients with MS, severe mitral regurgitation (MR), severe AI, or poor LV compliance. Additionally, the presence of positive end-expiratory ventilation and improper RHC placement will decrease the reliability of the PCW tracing.
5. **Left ventricular pressure.** Normal LV pressure is 90 to 140 systolic/10 to 16 diastolic mm Hg, and similar to the RV waveform is characterized by a rapid

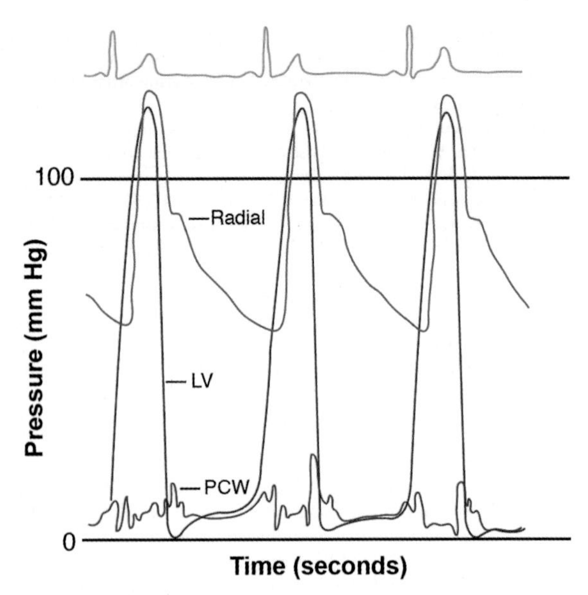

FIGURE 20.2 Simultaneous radial artery, left ventricular, and pulmonary capillary wedge pressure tracings.

upstroke and rapid decline. Diastolic pressure slowly rises during diastole to LVEDP, which is measured at end expiration just before the rapid upstroke during systole. Similar to the RV tracing, an a-wave is not usually seen except under circumstances of LV noncompliance. Simultaneous LV, arterial pressure, and PCWP are shown in Figure 20.2.

6. **Aortic pressure**
   a. Central aortic pressure is typically measured in the aortic root or ascending aorta, and normally measures 90 to 140 systolic/60 to 90 diastolic mm Hg. Similar to other arterial tracings, there is a rapid upstroke to a well-defined peak and gradual decline that is interrupted by a dicrotic notch, which is caused by closure of the aortic valve (AV).
   b. Aortic systolic pressure should equal LV systolic pressure in the absence of obstruction within the LV, at the level of the AV (i.e., aortic stenosis [AS]), or proximal aorta (i.e., supra-aortic membrane). While not normally seen, an "anacrotic" notch may be present during systolic pressure rise in patients with turbulent flow during ejection (i.e., severe AS).
   c. Simultaneous LV and aortic pressures are often measured when assessing for AS to determine transvalvular gradient (further discussed later). While femoral (or radial) arterial sheath pressures are sometimes substituted for central aortic pressures, differences between peripheral arterial sheath pressures and central aortic pressures are common. For instance, central aortic pressure may be higher than femoral (or radial) arterial sheath pressure in patients with peripheral arterial disease, sheath kinking, arterial tortuosity, or sheath thrombosis. Conversely, peripheral amplification of reflected arterial pressure waves may cause the peripheral arterial sheath pressure to be greater than central aortic pressure in certain individuals.

B. Measurement of cardiac output. Invasive assessment is the gold standard for determining CO. Normal CO increases in accordance to meet systemic oxygen demand. Thus, any factor that influences systemic oxygen demand influences CO. In the simplest terms, CO is the product of heart rate (HR) and stroke volume (SV):

$$CO = HR \times SV$$

As CO is greater with body size, CO is typically normalized to body surface area (BSA), resulting in the cardiac index (CI):

$$BSA\ (m^2) = \sqrt{((Ht\ [cm] \times Wt\ [kg])/3{,}600)}$$

$$CI = CO/BSA$$

Normal values for CO range between 5 and 6 L/min, whereas normal values for CI range between 2.6 and 4.2 L/min/m^2. The two major methods for determination of CO in the catheterization laboratory are the Fick technique and thermodilution technique.

1. **The Fick technique**
   a. The Fick equation is the most commonly used method for calculation of CO. The Fick equation is based on the principle that the total uptake (or release) of a substance by a tissue (i.e., lungs) is proportional to the blood flow to the tissue multiplied by arteriovenous (A-V) concentration difference of the substance. Assuming there is no intracardiac shunt, blood flow into the pulmonary circuit should equal blood flow into the LV and systemic circuit, thus:

$$CO\ (L/min) = \frac{O_2\ \text{consumption}\ (mL/min)}{(A\text{-}V)\ O_2\ \text{content difference}}$$

   b. O_2 consumption can be measured by subtracting the O_2 uptake from room air using a Douglas bag, metabolic hood, or a cardiopulmonary exercise testing machine. Given the limited availability, cost, and time involved in utilizing these methods, most laboratories use an assumed oxygen consumption of 125 mL/min/m^2, or 3 mL/min/kg.
   c. The A-V O_2 saturation difference across the lungs is then obtained by taking the difference between pulmonary venous blood O_2 saturation (or systemic arterial O_2 saturation, Sao_2) and the PA O_2 saturation (or "mixed venous" O_2 saturation, Svo_2). This difference is then multiplied by the O_2-carrying capacity of hemoglobin (Hb) to obtain the A-V O_2 content difference:

$$(A\text{-}V)\ O_2\ \text{content difference} = (Sao_2 - Svo_2) \times 1.36\ mL/O_2/g\ Hb \times g\ Hb/dL\ blood \times 10$$

   The final formula for calculation then becomes:

$$CO\ (L/min) = \frac{O_2\ \text{consumption}\ (mL/min)}{([SaO_2 - SVO_2] \times Hgb\ [g/dL] \times 1.36 \times 10)}$$

   d. Use of systemic arterial blood to estimate pulmonary venous blood O_2 content is typically acceptable in the absence of a shunt, as only a small amount of venous blood enters the arterial circuit within the heart via the thebesian veins. Use of central venous blood ($Scvo_2$ from the venae cavae [i.e., from a central line]) is less accurate. At rest, $Scvo_2$ is lower than Svo_2, as $Scvo_2$ contains only superior vena cava (SVC) blood (which has higher oxygen extraction from the brain), and Svo_2 contains both SVC and inferior vena cava blood.
2. **The thermodilution technique.** Alternatively, CO may be estimated via an indicator dilution method, most commonly via the thermodilution technique. During

thermodilution, a bolus of room-temperature saline is injected into the RA. The temperature of the blood in the PA is continuously measured by a thermistor on the end of the PA catheter (6 to 10 cm away) and graphed as a function of time. The resulting curve is analyzed by the computer, and CO is calculated via the basic premise that a slow temperature change corresponds to a low CO, and a quick temperature change corresponds to a high CO. Thus, the degree and speed of change in temperature are directly proportional to CO with the thermodilution technique. About three to four repeated measurements are taken to ensure accuracy.

3. **Comparison of the Fick and thermodilution techniques.** It is important to recognize the advantages and shortcomings of the Fick and thermodilution techniques when considering a method to calculate CO (or valve area). The Fick equation is most accurate when O_2 consumption can be directly measured, as actual O_2 consumption differs from the assumed 125 mL/min/m^2 by up to 25% in many patients, or even more in those with a systemic stressor (such as sepsis). Also, Fick is most accurate in patients with normal or low CO, as large A-V O_2 saturation differences (as in high CO states) are more likely to introduce error. In contrast, the thermodilution method is dependent on accurate measurement of blood and injectate temperature, and CO will be overestimated if the injectate temperature is inappropriately increased by allowing it to remain too long in the syringe or holding it by hand during injection. Similarly, the thermodilution technique is most accurate in normal or high-flow states due to warming of the blood by the cardiac chambers in low-flow states. Additionally, it is unreliable in the presence of severe TR.
4. **Other techniques.** Angiographic measurement of SV is possible via estimation of LV end-diastolic and end-systolic volumes via left ventriculography. When multiplied by HR at the time of ventriculography, this can estimate CO. However, this method is rarely used, as it is prone to error in patients with an irregular rhythm, and estimation of LV volume is challenging on angiography alone.

III. VALVULAR PATHOLOGY

A. Calculation of valve orifice area

1. **Gorlin formula.** Invasive calculation of valve orifice area (VOA) is most often performed via the Gorlin formula, which relies on the CO, mean pressure gradient across the valve (ΔP), and flow period (the portion of the cardiac cycle during which blood flows across the valve). Thus, the systolic ejection period (SEP) is used for the AV and PV, and the diastolic filling period (DFP) is used for the mitral valve (MV) and TV. Based on the Gorlin equation, calculation of VOA is:

$$\text{VOA} = \frac{\text{CO}/(\text{HR} \times \text{SEP or DFP})}{44.3 \times C \times \sqrt{\Delta P}}$$

where VOA is in cm^2, CO in mL/min, HR in beats/min, and SEP and DFP in sec/beat. C is an empiric constant of 1.0 for all valves except the MV, where it is 0.85.

2. **Hakki formula.** The Hakki formula is a simplified form of the Gorlin equation, based on the observation that at normal HR, the product of HR, SEP, or DFP is approximately 1 for most patients.

$$\text{VOA} = \frac{\text{CO (L/min)}}{\sqrt{\Delta P}}$$

A limitation of the Hakki formula is that SEP and DFP change markedly with tachycardia. To deal with this, Angel has suggested a correction for HR, such that the Hakki formula should be divided by 1.35 when the HR is >90 bpm for AS and <75 bpm for MS. For purposes of the cardiovascular boards, the Hakki equation should be all that is needed for calculation of VOA.

3. **Aortic valve resistance.** Another measure of severity of AS is aortic valve resistance (AVR), measured in a simplified form as:

$$\text{AVR} = (\text{dynes-s-cm}^{-5}) = \frac{(\text{LV-Ao}) \times 80}{(\text{CO} \times 2.5)}$$

where LV-Ao is the peak to peak AV gradient, 80 is a conversion factor, and 2.5 assumes an SEP of 40% of the R-R interval. Severe AS (VOA $<0.7\ \text{cm}^2$) corresponds to an AVR of ≥ 300 dynes-s-cm^{-5}.

B. Aortic stenosis

1. Echocardiography is usually adequate for the assessment of AS; however, invasive hemodynamic assessment may be necessary for patients in whom the echocardiographic degree of severity is not commensurate with symptoms or noninvasive tests are contradictory.

   The diagnosis of severe AS rests on measurement of the AV gradient, expressed as:

   a. Peak instantaneous gradient (obtained from Doppler flow velocity on echocardiography)
   b. Mean gradient (represented by the difference between the area under the curve during simultaneous Ao and LV pressure measurement) (Fig. 20.3)
   c. Peak-to-peak gradient (difference between maximum LV and Ao pressures), which approximates the echocardiographically obtained mean gradient

2. There are several possible techniques for measurement of peak or mean gradient (ΔP) during calculation of aortic VOA with the Gorlin or Hakki equations. For greatest accuracy, simultaneous measurement of LV and aortic root pressures should be obtained. Historically, this was performed through a two-catheter technique involving venous access and a subsequent transseptal puncture with direct measurement of LV pressures, and simultaneous measurement of arterial

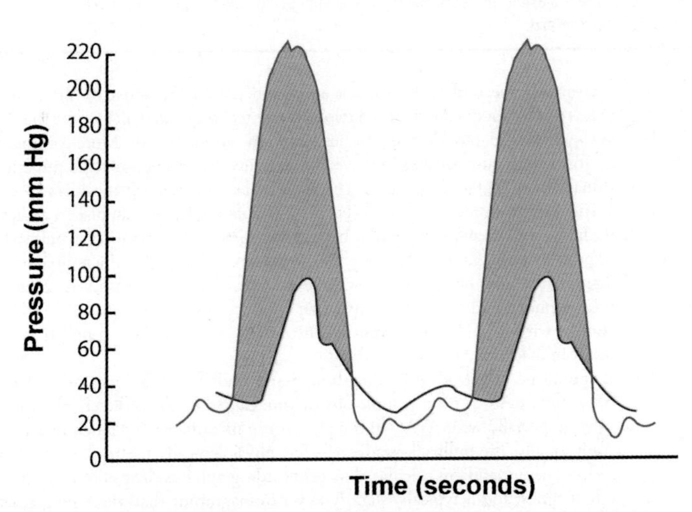

FIGURE 20.3 Simultaneous left ventricular (LV) and aortic tracings in severe aortic stenosis. Utilizing a dual-transducer pigtail catheter, pressure can be simultaneously obtained in the LV and aorta. The pressure difference between the two during systole is measured to calculate peak and mean gradients, which is subsequently used for valve orifice area calculations.

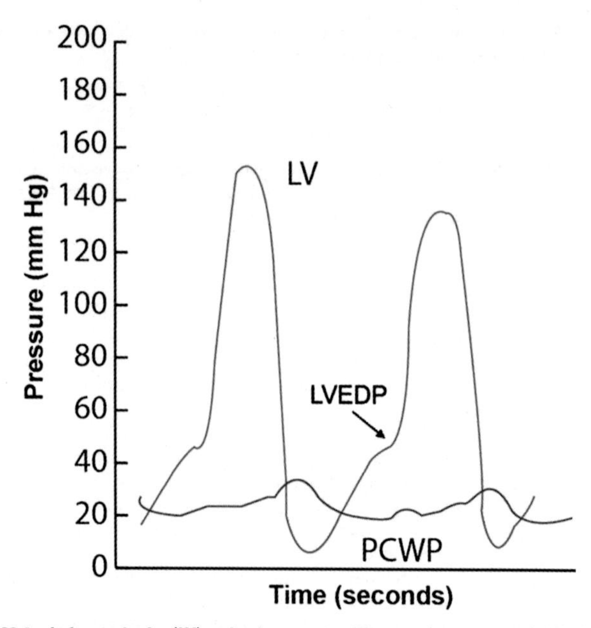

FIGURE 20.4 Left ventricular (LV) and pulmonary capillary wedge pressure (PCWP) in a patient with acute aortic insufficiency. Example of a patient with severe acute aortic insufficiency. Note that the LV end-diastolic pressure (LVEDP) is elevated to a greater degree than PCWP, indicating acute LV volume overload.

pressure via a second catheter in the aortic root. As an alternative to this, arterial access can be obtained twice for a two-catheter technique in which one catheter is advanced to the mid-LV and another placed in the aortic root. More commonly performed because it is less invasive and only involves a single arterial puncture, a dual-lumen pigtail (or Langston) catheter that simultaneously measures LV and aortic root pressures can be used (Fig. 20.3). Conversely, one can place a catheter in the LV and then quickly pull it back to the aortic root, obtaining a "pullback," or peak-to-peak gradient. However, it should be cautioned that the pullback may demonstrate an inherent inaccuracy due to a lack of simultaneous LV:Ao pressure measurement, and premature ventricular contractions (PVCs) caused by catheter contact with the LV and left ventricular outflow tract (LVOT) on pullback may result in inaccurate pressure readings.

3. It should be noted both the dual-lumen and pullback techniques may slightly overestimate AS, as there is some obstruction caused by the catheter crossing the valve (especially with AVA <0.6 cm^2 and use of catheters 7 French or larger). Additionally, the pullback gradient is less physiologically useful than the peak instantaneous gradient calculated by echocardiography, as the peaks occur at different times, and is typically slightly lower in magnitude than the echo gradient derived from peak instantaneous velocity.
4. Common sources of error in calculating the peak or mean pressure gradients are improper catheter placement (i.e., LVOT), low-flow states, and arrhythmia (atrial fibrillation or ventricular ectopy). Additionally, aortic VOA may be underestimated with concomitant severe aortic regurgitation (AR). Furthermore, the Gorlin

equation is quite flow dependent in low-flow states and becomes unreliable at CO <3 to 4 L/min. As such, patients with low-flow, low-gradient AS should be considered for measurement of pressure gradients after infusion of an inotropic agent (i.e., dobutamine) or sodium nitroprusside, which increase CO and allow for a more reliable VOA calculation. As with dobutamine stress echocardiography, in pseudo-AS the valve area will increase, whereas with truly severe AS the valve area will remain small.

5. In addition to the peak and mean gradients, there are several other characteristic hemodynamic abnormalities observed in severe AS. The aortic waveform often has a slow upstroke (*pulsus parvus et tardus*), but can be brisk in patients with calcified, noncompliant vessels. Turbulent flow across the valve may cause an anacrotic notch in the aortic upstroke, which is also often seen in severe AR. In cases in which LV pressure is measured via a retrograde approach placing a catheter across the AV, the profile of the catheter may make the obstruction worse. When the catheter is removed (i.e., during pullback), an increase in aortic pressure of at least 5 mm Hg may be seen (known as Carabello sign), though this is generally considered a historic vestige of using large (8 French or greater) catheters in patients with an AVA <0.6 cm^2.

C. Aortic valve regurgitation

1. Similar to patients with AS, invasive hemodynamic assessment of AR is indicated only when noninvasive tests are inconclusive or discrepant with clinical findings. Catheterization can be used to quantify the degree of AR using contrast injection, examination of the aortic pressure tracing, and simultaneous measurement of the LVEDP and aortic diastolic pressure.

2. In patients with significant AR, loss of the normal dicrotic notch or presence of an anacrotic notch may be seen. In acute AR, there is a marked, sudden rise in LVEDP and a fall in systolic blood pressure (SBP) due to a decline in SV. When regurgitant volume increases to the point that LVEDP = aortic diastolic blood pressure (DBP), this is called *diastasis*. By mid to late diastole, LVEDP may exceed LA (or PCW) pressure, resulting in premature closure of the MV (Fig. 20.4). In severe cases, LVEDP >> LA pressure, and there may be diastolic MR.

3. In contrast, chronic severe AR is associated with high aortic SBP (due to increased SV) and low aortic DBP (often <50 mm Hg), yielding a wide pulse pressure (often >100 mm Hg) (PP = SBP – DBP) (Fig. 20.5). The aortic DBP approaches LVEDP near the end of diastole. The systolic upstroke is usually rapid, due to increased LV contractility. In compensated chronic AR, LVEDP is usually normal or slightly elevated, as LV compliance has had time to adapt to chronically elevated LV volumes.

4. The severity of AR is graded on the basis of the amount of contrast regurgitation during aortography of the ascending aorta. To ensure accuracy, a pigtail catheter is placed in the aortic root 2 cm above the AV and a power injector should be used to inject approximately 20 to 30 mL of dye. While the left-anterior-oblique (LAO) projection is typically used to visualize the aorta and arch branch vessels, overlap of the cardiac silhouette with the descending aorta and/or fore-shortening of the LV in this projection may result in overestimation of the degree of AR. Therefore, a right-anterior-oblique (RAO) projection may be preferable (if biplane imaging is not available). The amount of contrast regurgitation is observed over 2 cardiac cycles, and the severity of AR graded as incomplete LV opacification (mild, 1+); moderate LV opacification < aortic root opacification (moderate, 2+); LV opacification = aortic root opacification within 2 cycles (moderate-severe, 3+); and immediate LV opacification > aortic root opacification (severe, 4+). Care should be taken to observe that the contrast opacifying the LV enters during diastole and not due to power-injection through the pigtail while the AV is open during systole.

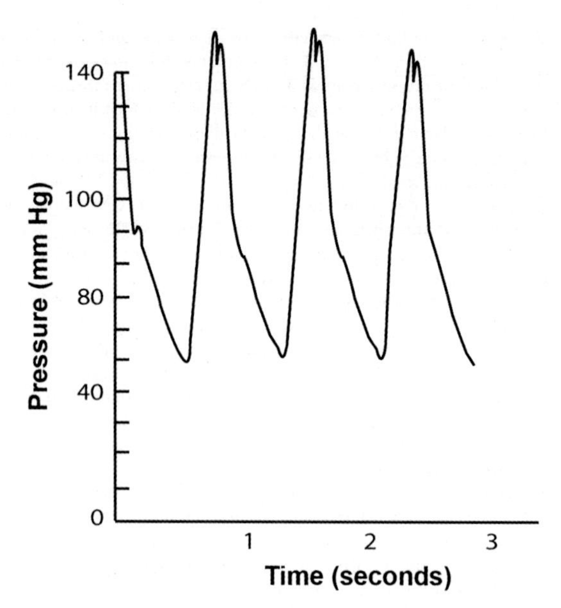

FIGURE 20.5 This is an example of aortic hemodynamics in a patient with chronic aortic insufficiency. Note the wide pulse pressure of approximately 110 mm Hg as well as the loss of a well-defined dicrotic notch in the diastolic portion of the tracing.

D. Mitral valve stenosis

1. The MV gradient is measured by taking simultaneous pressures in the LV and LA. This is most often accomplished by an arterial catheter placed in the LV and a venous catheter placed in the LA via transseptal puncture or with PCWP by RHC (Fig. 20.6). Though commonly done, use of PCWP to approximate LA pressure may be inaccurate in patients with pulmonary veno-occlusive disease (or pulmonary vein stenosis), may lead to overestimation of LA pressures with prosthetic MV stenosis, and can be difficult to interpret in patients with concomitant MR. Furthermore, the PCWP waveform is dampened in comparison with the LA pressure, and due to the delayed v-wave in the PCWP tracing (temporal delay), the DFP between the PCWP and the LV does not exactly match. Therefore, in patients for whom further management (e.g., surgery or balloon mitral valvuloplasty) is dependent on very accurate MV gradients, consideration should be given to direct LA pressure measurement. While managing fluid status in patients with MS and a PA catheter, it should be noted that the "true" PCWP/LA pressure is the measured PCWP minus the mean MV gradient.
2. The atrial waveform in MS depends on the severity of stenosis and pliability of the MV. The characteristic findings are presence of a pressure gradient in diastole between the LA (or PCWP) and LVEDP (Fig. 20.6). Under normal conditions, a small pressure gradient may be present in early diastole. As MS becomes more severe, a diastolic gradient develops that is typically greatest in early diastole. As mentioned earlier, the Gorlin equation for calculation of MV VOA is as follows:

$$\text{VOA} = \frac{\text{CO}/(\text{HR} \times \text{DFP})}{37.7 \times \sqrt{\Delta P}}$$

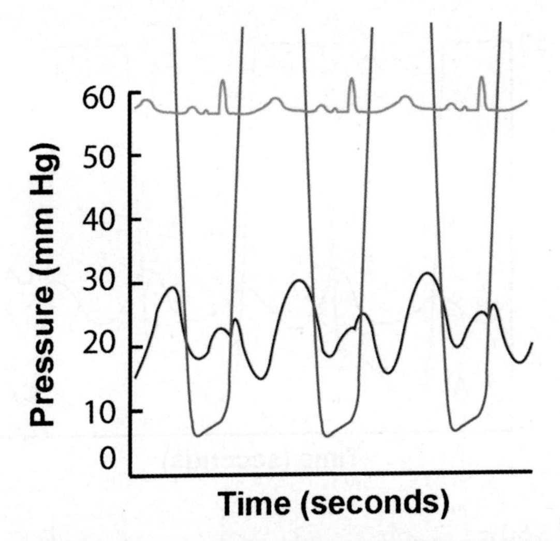

FIGURE 20.6 Simultaneous left ventricular (LV) and left atrial (LA) pressure measurement in mitral stenosis. Mitral stenosis may be assessed by transseptal puncture and measuring simultaneous pressures in the LA and LV. The severity of mitral stenosis is determined by calculation of the mean gradient across the valve, determined by the area between the LA and LV pressure tracings during diastole.

3. As with AS, the MV gradient (peak or mean) is dependent on HR, and higher gradients are observed with tachycardia. As such, when using the mean MV gradient in the Hakki equation, the VOA must be divided by 1.35 for HR <70 bpm (known as the Angel correction, as previously mentioned).
4. Characteristic features of hemodynamic LA or PCWP tracings in MS include a prominent "a" wave (due to atrial contraction against an obstructed valve) (Fig. 20.7 A) and/or a prominent "v" wave (due to LA filling occurring under a higher pressure, low-compliance state) (Fig. 20.7 B). Note that while "v" waves are more common in MR, they can be observed in severe MS as well.
5. There are several factors that may introduce error into MV VOA measurement. Ideally, CO should be measured simultaneously with the pressure gradients. Additionally, in the presence of concomitant MR, calculation of the MV VOA using only net forward flow will underestimate the actual VOA; this does not account for the diastolic flow across the valve due to MR.

E. Mitral valve regurgitation

1. Catheter-based hemodynamic assessment for MR is rarely needed and only indicated when noninvasive testing is inconclusive or symptoms out of proportion to echocardiographic findings. In acute MR, the classic finding is a large "v" wave on the LA or PCWP tracing (Fig. 20.8). This is similar in appearance to the "v" wave seen in MS; however, it is due to the large volume of regurgitation into the low-compliance LA. The amount of regurgitation will also elevate LV filling pressures, causing an increased LVEDP.
2. In chronic MR, LA compliance will increase over time, and thus the "v" wave will be smaller. Likewise, the LV increases its compliance over time to chronic volume overload similar to how it handles AR, and thus, filling pressures will not be as high as in acute MR.

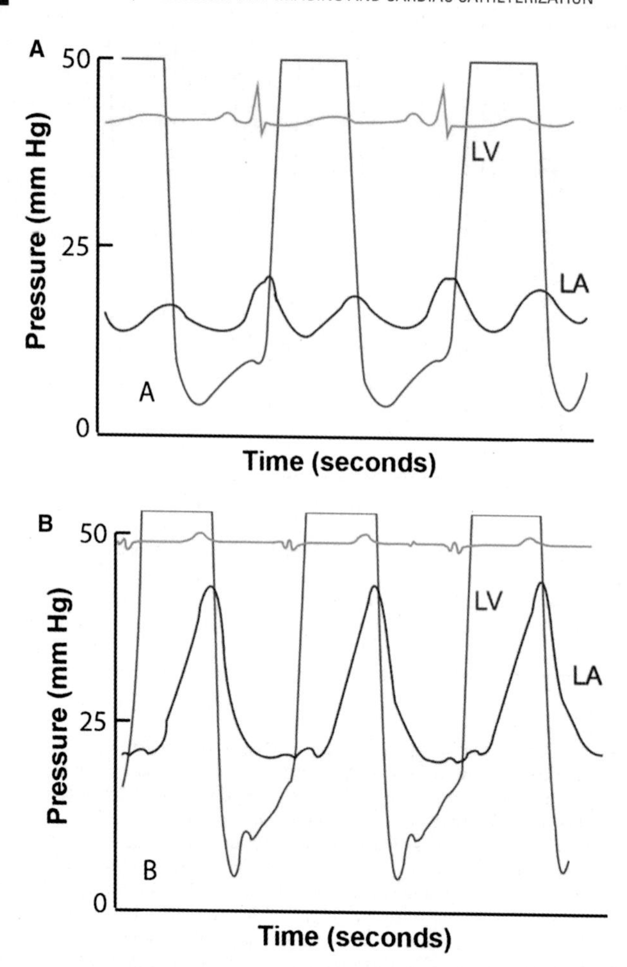

FIGURE 20.7 Hemodynamics of mitral stenosis and mitral regurgitation. A: In mitral stenosis, the "a"-wave may be accentuated in the left atrial (LA) or pulmonary capillary wedge pressure (PCWP) tracing. **B:** Similarly, in mitral stenosis there may be a large "v"-wave seen on LA or PCWP tracing. This may also be seen in mitral regurgitation. LV, left ventricle.

3. Similar to AR, ventriculography can be used to grade MR, and a similar scale is used: 1+ = transient, mild LA opacification, without LA enlargement; 2+ = moderate LA opacification < LV opacification, and without LA enlargement; 3+ = equal LA and LV opacification that takes at least 2 cycles to clear, with LA enlargement; 4+ = immediate LA > LV opacification with pulmonary vein filling, and LA enlargement. The camera should be placed in the RAO projection in order to visualize the LA, and care should be taken that the pigtail catheter is not entangled in the subvalvular apparatus (thereby causing iatrogenic MR). Additionally, PVCs induced by the catheter can result in LV contraction while the MV is open and may give a false impression of MR severity.

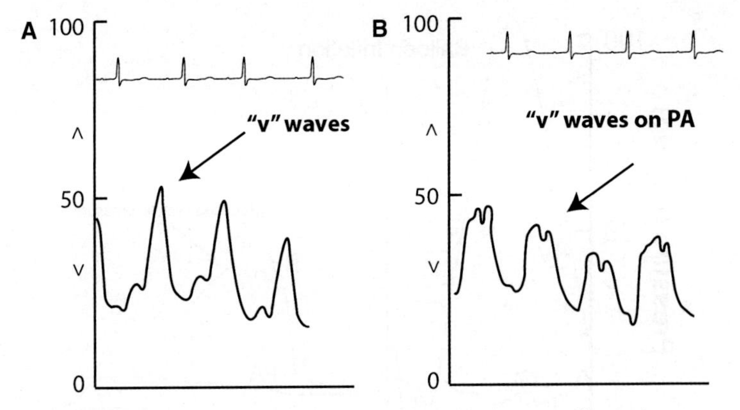

FIGURE 20.8 Example of "v"-waves of mitral regurgitation in the pulmonary capillary wedge pressure tracing **(A)** and transmitted to the pulmonary artery waveform **(B)**.

F. **Pulmonic valve stenosis**

1. PV stenosis is almost always due to congenital causes and rarely presents in adults. Most PS is due to fusion of the leaflets, and 85-90% of PS is treatable with balloon or surgical valvotomy.
2. Valvular PS causes a systolic pressure gradient across the PA and RV, whereas peripheral PS causes a gradient between the RV and a branch of the PA. For measurement of a pressure gradient in valvular PS, simultaneous PA pressure measurement and RV measurement is needed, either using two separate catheters or by exchanging a PA catheter over a wire for a dual-lumen pigtail catheter (with the distal ports in the PA and the proximal ports in the RV). The Gorlin and/or Hakki equations can be used for calculation of pulmonic VOA as with other valves. However, most clinicians classify the severity of PS and decision to pursue valvotomy on the basis of PV gradients alone. Current guidelines advise surgical or balloon valvuloplasty in asymptomatic patients once the mean systolic gradient is >40 mm Hg, and in symptomatic patients once the mean systolic gradient is >30 mm Hg. Outcomes with balloon valvuloplasty are generally good and PS does not often recur (Fig. 20.9).

G. **Pulmonic valve regurgitation.** Significant pulmonic valve regurgitation (PR) is uncommon and usually seen in congenital heart disease, as a consequence of surgical repair or valvuloplasty, or as a result of endocarditis. Patients with severe PR may have a widened PA pulse pressure, a fast dicrotic collapse, and rapid equilibration of the RVEDP and PA EDP. As the PA waveform appears similar to the RV, there is "ventricularization" of the PA tracing. Unlike in AR and MR, contrast injection is not useful in quantifying the severity of regurgitation in PR.

H. **Tricuspid valve stenosis.** Severe TS is uncommon and usually caused by rheumatic heart disease in association with MS. Rarely, it can be seen in other conditions, such as carcinoid syndrome. In TS, RA emptying is obstructed and RV filling impaired. As such, RA pressure is elevated, and patients may have a large "a" wave. Hemodynamic tracings demonstrate a diastolic gradient between the RA and RV. Similar with other valves, simultaneous measurement of RV and RA pressures allows for precise measurement of the TV gradient and calculation of tricuspid VOA via the Gorlin or Hakki equations. Like in AS or MS, concomitant TR will result in underestimation of the VOA because the actual transvalvular flow is confounded. It should be noted that the

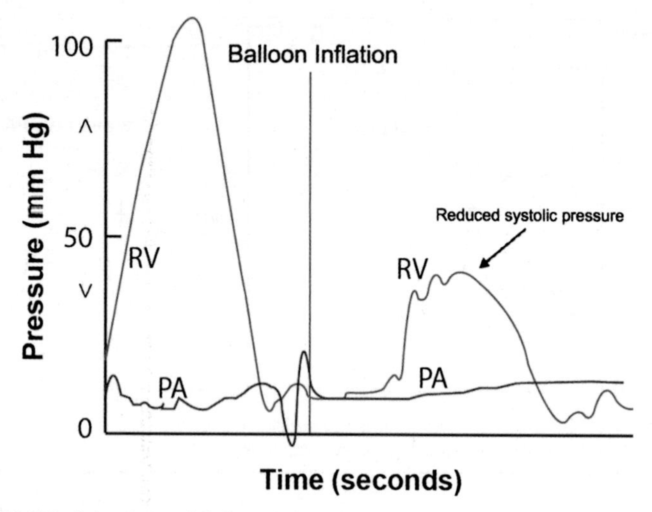

FIGURE 20.9 Pulmonic stenosis before and after balloon valvuloplasty. This is an example of reduction in right ventricular (RV) peak systolic pressure. PA, pulmonary artery.

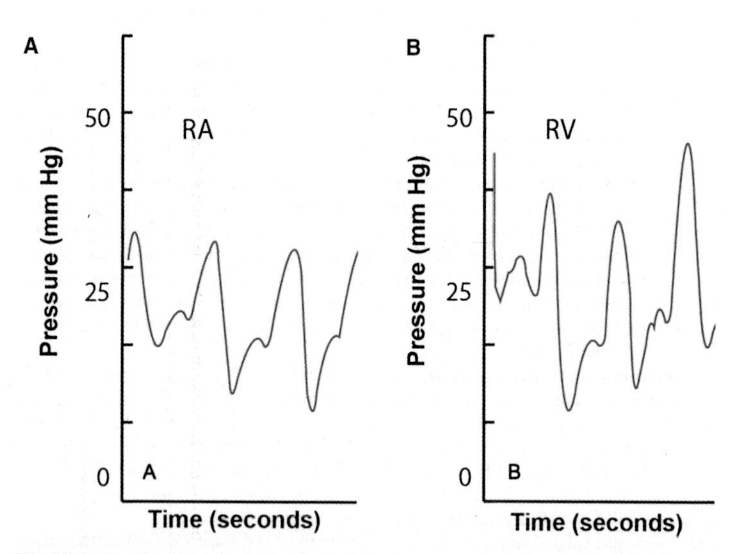

FIGURE 20.10 Tricuspid regurgitation. **A:** Similar to the left atrium with mitral regurgitation, there may be large "v"-waves visualized on the right atrial (RA) tracing in patients with significant tricuspid regurgitation, resulting in complete "ventricularization" of the RA tracing. **B:** The same patient's right ventricular (RV) pressure tracing.

Gorlin equation has not been validated in TS, although small series suggest that the calculated VOA correlates with the true valve area in patients who undergo surgery.

I. Tricuspid valve regurgitation

1. TR is the most common right-sided valvular problem, observed in many conditions including congenital abnormalities, rheumatic heart disease, pulmonary hypertension, and RV failure, among others. Mild TR is very commonly seen, yet of no clinical significance. Severe TR can cause RA and RV volume overload and eventual RV failure.
2. The hemodynamic findings of TR include RA pressure elevation, distortion of the RA pressure waveform, and corresponding elevation of jugular venous pressure. In TR, the x-descent is blunted, and eventually disappears as the severity of TR worsens. Eventually, the x-descent is replaced by a systolic wave corresponding to RV contraction, termed a *c-v* wave, with a "peak-dome" contour. The v-wave is followed by a brisk y-descent; thus, the RA waveform may appear similar to the RV waveform, and "ventricularization" may occur (Fig. 20.10). It should be noted that while supportive of severe TR, these findings are not always seen, especially in patients with atrial fibrillation and hypovolemia (as regurgitant volume is dependent on RV volume).

KEY PEARLS

- Invasive hemodynamic assessment of valve disease is indicated when results of noninvasive tests are inconclusive or discrepant with the clinical severity of valve disease.
- Knowledge of normal hemodynamic values and pressure waveforms is essential to interpret the pathologic hemodynamic findings in valvular heart disease.
- The most common technique used to calculate CO is the Fick equation:

$$\text{CO (L/min)} = \frac{O_2 \text{ consumption (mL/min)}}{([SaO_2 - SvO_2] \times \text{Hgb (g/dL)} \times 1.36 \times 10)}$$

  where most laboratories use an assumed value for O_2 consumption of 125 mL/min/m^2.
- An alternative for CO measurement is the thermodilution technique, which measures the change in temperature of PA blood over time after saline injection.
- Fick is less accurate in high-flow states, in situations of high O_2 demand (i.e., fever or sepsis), or intracardiac shunting. The thermodilution method is less accurate in low-flow states or in the presence of significant TR.
- The most widely used formula to calculate VOA of any valve is the Gorlin equation:

$$\text{VOA} = \frac{\text{CO/(HR} \times \text{SEP or DFP)}}{44.3 \times C \times \sqrt{(\Delta P)}}$$

  where *C* is an empiric constant of 1.0 for all valves except the MV, where it is 0.85.
- The Hakki formula is a simplified form of the Gorlin equation:

$$\text{VOA} = \frac{\text{CO (L/min)}}{\sqrt{\Delta P}}$$

To correct for HR, the Hakki formula should be divided by 1.35 when HR is >90 bpm for AS and <75 bpm for MS.

- Assessment of valve gradients across the AV is accomplished by simultaneous measurement of aortic root and LV pressures or a pullback gradient using a single catheter. Characteristic findings on hemodynamic tracings include pulsus parvus et tardus, an anacrotic notch, and Carabello sign (in critical AS or with large-sized catheters).
- In acute AR, there is a fall in SBP due to decreased SV, a sudden rise in LVEDP, and when LVEDP >> LA pressure, diastolic MR may occur. In contrast, in chronic AR there may be preserved SBP with a widened pulse pressure, and a normal to slightly elevated LVEDP due to gradual accommodation of LV compliance.
- Transvalvular gradients for MS are obtained with simultaneous LV pressure and LA (or PCWP) measurement. Classic findings are presence of a diastolic gradient greatest in early diastole, as well as prominent "a" and "v" waves on LA and/or PCWP tracings.
- In acute MR, there are typically large "v" waves on LA or PCWP tracings, which are smaller in chronic MR due to an increase in LA compliance over time.
- Severe AR and MR are graded on the basis of the amount of contrast regurgitation during sequential cardiac cycles.
- Both PS and PR are uncommonly encountered in adults. While valve area can be calculated via the Gorlin or Hakki equations, a mean systolic gradient >40 mm Hg in asymptomatic patients and >30 mm Hg in symptomatic patients is typically used as a threshold to pursue balloon valvuloplasty or surgery.
- In severe TS, there may be large "a" waves on RA tracing. In severe TR, there may be large c-v" waves with a "peak-dome" contour on RA and central venous pressure tracing.

SUGGESTED READINGS

Angel J, Soler-Soler J, Anivarro I, et al. Hemodynamic evaluation of stenotic cardiac valves, Part II: modification of the simplified valve formula for mitral and aortic valve area calculation. *Catet Cardiov Diagn*. 1985;11:127–138.

Biam DS, Grossman W, eds. *Cardiac Catheterization, Angiography and Intervention*. 5th ed. Philadelphia, PA: Lippincott Williams & Wilkins; 1996.

Hakki AH, Iskandrian AS, Bemis CE, et al. A simplified valve formula for the calculation of stenotic cardiac valve areas. *Circulation*. 1981;63:1050–1055.

Nishimura RA, Otto CM, Bonow RO, et al. 2014 AHA/ACC Guideline for the management of patients with valvular heart disease. *J Am Col Cardiol*. 2014;63(22):e57–e185.

Ragosta M. *Textbook of Clinical Hemodynamics*. 1st ed. Philadelphia, PA: Saunders; 2008.

SECTION V

Echocardiography and Cardiac Catheterization Cases and Calculations

CHAPTER 21

Terence Hill
Richard A. Grimm

Echocardiographic Calculations and Case Examples

I. INTRODUCTION

In this chapter, we will review the calculations used to quantitatively assess valvular stenosis and regurgitation by Doppler echocardiography. We will first review the necessary equations and data that must be acquired, along with how the results are calculated and used to assess valvular stenosis or regurgitation severity. We will also discuss potential pitfalls in performing these calculations. Finally, we will present several cases that demonstrate how to apply these calculations using real echocardiographic data.

II. CALCULATIONS: AORTIC VALVE

A. Aortic stenosis

1. Aortic stenosis (AS) severity is assessed by Doppler and two-dimensional (2D) echocardiographic imaging capabilities. Peak aortic flow velocity, peak aortic valve (AV) gradient, mean AV gradient, aortic valve area (AVA), and the dimensionless index (DI) all in combination with 2D appearance of the valve are required to derive a determination of stenosis severity. The aortic flow velocity is a measured variable that is acquired using continuous-wave (CW) Doppler echocardiography with the cursor aligned parallel to flow across the AV from either the apical 5-chamber (A5C) or apical 3-chamber (A3C) window. Additionally, data can be acquired from the right parasternal border, suprasternal notch, and subcostal windows. A dedicated Doppler Pedoff probe can be used to assure maximal velocities are obtained from each imaging plane. The highest values obtained, reported as Doppler velocities, are usually underestimated when images are off axis, as only the component of the velocity vector parallel to the Doppler signal is measured. The peak aortic gradient is calculated from the peak velocity, usually using the simplified Bernoulli equation (if subaortic velocity is <1.5 m/s):

$$\Delta P = 4V^2$$

where ΔP is the peak instantaneous gradient across the valve and V is the Doppler flow velocity. The mean aortic gradient is calculated as the mean velocity over time of left ventricular (LV) ejection.

2. The AVA is calculated by the continuity equation:

$$\text{AVA} = \text{CSA}_{(\text{LVOT})} \times \text{VTI}_{(\text{LVOT})}/\text{VTI}_{(\text{AV})}$$

3. The three main components of this equation include the LV outflow tract (LVOT) diameter, subaortic flow, and transvalvular flow (both approximated by the velocity–time integral or VTI). The LVOT diameter measurement is necessary to determine the cross-sectional area (CSA) of the LVOT. This is calculated from the LVOT diameter measured from the parasternal long-axis view just below the

AV. The LVOT is assumed to be circular, hence allowing for the calculation of the CSA as follows: $CSA_{LVOT} = (D_{(LVOT)}/2)^2 \times \pi$. VTI_{LVOT} is a representation of subvalvular systolic flow and is measured as the area under the Doppler velocity versus time curve during ventricular systole. The Doppler measurement for this parameter is obtained using pulsed wave (PW) Doppler across the AV (typically in the A5C or A3C window), with a sample volume located 0.5-1 cm on the ventricular side of the AV. VTI_{AV} is representative of flow across the AV and is obtained using CW Doppler across the AV, in multiple imaging windows, and measuring the area under the Doppler velocity versus time curve in systole. It is very important to note that the measured LVOT diameter has a major impact on the calculated valve area as the diameter is squared in the equation, and hence the potential error is magnified. In the event of uncertainty of measurement, one can simply report the ratio of subaortic to transvalvular maximum velocity, which is referred to as the velocity ratio or DI.

$$DI = V_{(LVOT)}/V_{(AV)}$$

4. Not infrequently, there will be a discrepancy between the calculated AVA, the DI, and the AV gradients, where an AVA calculated as <1.0 cm^2 and the gradients not being significantly elevated suggest severe disease. This can indicate a low-flow state, an error in measurement, or an error in Doppler velocity data sampling. Low-flow states can result from many causes, including an abnormally low LV systolic function, low output due to small ventricular cavities, atrial fibrillation, mitral regurgitation (MR), diastolic dysfunction, hypertensive heart disease, or increased valvuloarterial impedance. In order to appropriately identify these patients, it is important to calculate the stroke volume (SV) and index it to body size. The stroke volume index (SVI) is as follows (BSA = body surface area):

$$SVI = CSA_{(LVOT)} \times VTI_{(LVOT)}/BSA$$

5. Generally, a SVI of less than 35 mL/m^2 is consistent with a low-flow state. In patients with poor LV function, a dobutamine stress echocardiogram can be performed to determine if there is a fixed versus "pseudo"stenosis. This test either will confirm a truly severe AS (increase in gradient with persistently unchanged AVA) or can unmask pseudostenosis (no increase in gradient with an AVA that increases with dobutamine). Furthermore, the SVI can be calculated at rest and with stress. An increase in SV with dobutamine of greater than 20% is considered a favorable contractile reserve, whereas an increase in SV of less than 20% confers poor prognosis. Combining these variables, we can grade AS accordingly as shown in Table 21.1.
6. Common pitfalls in accurately determining AS severity are derived from improper or suboptimal Doppler sampling, and error in tracing or measurement of Doppler signals. Other pitfalls include confusing a mitral regurgitant jet signal by CW Doppler with a transvalvular aortic flow from an A5C view, which can happen if the CW tracing is misaligned to capture MR (which is in the same direction as the aortic flow). However, this can usually be recognized by the parabolic nature of the MR tracing, the longer duration of systole incorporating the isovolumic contraction and relaxation periods, as well as a peak velocity typically of at least 5 m/s. Additionally, the CW tracing can represent flow acceleration in a location along the beam other than the AV, usually from subaortic stenosis such as a subaortic membrane or LVOT obstruction (i.e., in hypertrophic cardiomyopathy). This error can be identified by examining the contour of the tracing, as in valvular stenosis the tracing will be triangular, while a dynamic LVOT obstruction is classically more "dagger" shaped. Careful assessment of the color flow Doppler map should be examined to ensure that the location of flow acceleration is at the valve

TABLE 21.1 Quantitative Assessment of Aortic Stenosis (AS)

	Aortic Sclerosis	Mild AS	Moderate AS	Severe AS
Peak velocity (m/s)	≤ 2.5	2.6–2.9	3.0–4.0	>4.0
Peak gradient (mm Hg)		27–34	35–64	>64
Mean gradient (mm Hg)		<20	20–40	>40
Aortic valve area (cm^2)		>1.5	1.0–1.5	<1.0
Dimensionless index		>0.5	0.25–0.5	<0.25

level consistent with valvular stenosis, as opposed to lower in the LVOT and more consistent with subvalvular stenosis. It may also be helpful to take several PW tracings from various points in the LV cavity to determine the location at which the velocity increases. Furthermore, attention should be paid to the morphology of the AV, as a very high gradient without significant calcification of the AV or restricted opening should prompt further scrutiny. Planimetry of the AV (usually in the parasternal short-axis [PSAX] window) can help, but is very operator dependent and prone to error in measurement. A typical LVOT diameter for patients with a trileaflet AV is approximately 2 cm, so for measurements significantly smaller or larger than 2 cm, the images should be reviewed with a particularly skeptical "eye." This should be a prime consideration when there is disagreement between the AVA and DI (which does not include the LVOT measurement).

B. Aortic insufficiency

1. While aortic insufficiency (AI) will frequently be assessed semiquantitatively, it can be quantitatively assessed by measuring the vena contracta (VC), calculating the regurgitant orifice area (ROA), as well as regurgitant volume (RV) and regurgitant fraction (RF) by volumetric methods. The VC is measured as the narrowest point in the regurgitant jet at the leaflet level in diastole, as observed on color flow Doppler, at a Nyquist limit of 50-60 cm/s. The ROA is a physiologic estimate of the regurgitant defect area that would be necessary to produce the amount of observed regurgitation. It is calculated by first measuring the proximal isovelocity surface area (PISA) radius obtained using color flow Doppler of the AI regurgitant jet. The PISA is observed as a hemispherical color flow disturbance within the regurgitant jet on the aortic side of the valve. After measuring the PISA (typically in the right parasternal or A3C window), the ROA is calculated as follows:

$$\text{ROA} = 2\pi(r_{\text{PISA}})^2 \times V_{\text{aliasing}}/V_{\text{AI Jet}}$$

where r_{PISA} is the measured radius of the PISA (as described earlier), V_{aliasing} is the Nyquist limit set when the PISA is measured, and $V_{\text{AI Jet}}$ is the peak velocity of the AI jet, measured using the CW Doppler sampling across the AV. The RV and RF are calculations of the approximate total volume (RV) or percentage (RF) of blood flow through the regurgitant orifice compared with the total SV ejected from the left ventricle. In a normal heart with no regurgitant valves, the blood entering the left ventricle through the mitral valve (MV) is equal to the blood exiting the left ventricle through the AV. The SV is the quantity of blood that exits and enters the heart on each and every beat. Therefore, in a normal heart:

$$SV_{LVOT} = SV_{MV\ Inflow}$$

because all blood enters through the MV and exits through the LVOT (AV). The SV moving through any portion of the heart is defined as

$$SV = CSA_{area\ of\ interest} \times VTI_{area\ of\ interest}$$

and

$$CSA = 2\pi r^2$$

Therefore, substituting these equations, for the normal heart:

$$\pi r_{LVOT}^2 \times VTI_{LVOT} = \pi r_{MV}^2 \times VTI_{MV\ inflow}$$

where r_{LVOT} is the LVOT radius, r_{MV} is the MV radius, and $VTI_{MV\ inflow}$ is the VTI of the MV inflow. The MV radius is calculated from the annular diameter, which is measured in the apical 4-chamber (A4C) window during mid-diastole (just after the leaflets begin to close). The VTI of the MV inflow is measured by positioning the sample volume of the PW Doppler cursor just inside of the MV. In the case of AI, blood enters the heart both from the regurgitant lesion (the volume of AI is defined as the RV) and through the MV, while both the RV and the mitral inflow exit through the LVOT. Therefore, for AI:

$$\pi r_{LVOT}^2 \times VTI_{LVOT} = \pi r_{MV}^2 \times VTI_{MV\ inflow} + RV$$

$$RV = \pi r_{LVOT}^2 \times VTI_{LVOT} - \pi r_{MV}^2 \times VTI_{MV\ inflow}$$

2. Once the RV is determined, RF is calculated as the ratio of the RV to the total SV (which for AI is the LVOT SV):

$$RF = RV/(\pi r_{LVOT}^2 \times VTI_{LVOT}) \times 100.$$

3. Alternatively, RV can be calculated using the ROA (calculated from the PISA) and the VTI of the AI jet, using the equation:

$$RV = ROA \times VTI_{AI\ Jet}$$

This equation can be somewhat less cumbersome, but relies on an accurately measured ROA and accurately sampled and measured AI Doppler signal. Severity of AI can be described quantitatively using Table 21.2.

TABLE 21.2 Quantitative Assessment of Aortic Insufficiency

Parameter	Mild	Moderate	Severe
VC (cm)	<0.3 (<25% LVOT diameter)	0.31–0.6	>0.6 (>65% LVOT diameter)
ROA (cm^2)	<0.10	0.1–0.29	≥ 0.30
RV (mL)	<30	30–59	≥ 60
RF (%)	<30	30–49	≥ 50

LVOT, left ventricular outflow tract; RF, regurgitant fraction; RV, regurgitant volume; ROA regurgitant orifice area; VC, vena contracta.

4. In aortic regurgitation, Doppler quantification has several potential sources of measurement error typically related to suboptimal image quality or acquisition technique. When there are multiple or eccentric AI jets, the VC can be under- or overestimated. The PISA can frequently be a challenge to measure as the hemisphere of the isovelocity flow is often difficult to identify. Additionally, measurement using PISA does not perform as well in patients with aneurysmal ascending aortas, or with cusp perforation or commissural leak. These limitations primarily apply to noncentral and eccentrically directed jets of regurgitation.
5. RV and RF measurements using PW Doppler volumetric techniques are accurate only in the absence of any significant MR or intracardiac shunt. For these calculations to be most accurate, the only inflow into the ventricle needs to come through the MV, and the only outflow through the AV. Furthermore, the equations rely on several different measurements including both the LVOT and MV annulus, which are assumed to be circular (a less valid assumption particularly for the MV). Any significant measurement error can cause wide variation in this calculation. Again, when assessing AV insufficiency it is important to remember that the length of the AI jet by color flow mapping does not correlate well with severity. Finally, flow reversal in the proximal descending aorta may result from other disease conditions such as patent ductus arteriosus or arteriovenous fistula. As a reminder, an integrative approach, incorporating several of these parameters, is the rule in echocardiography whenever generating an overall assessment of valvular dysfunction severity.

III. CALCULATIONS: MITRAL VALVE

A. Mitral regurgitation

1. MR is interpreted in a similar manner to AI, yet quantitative measurements are used more commonly with MR than they are with AI. This is largely related to the fact that MR is more amenable to PISA identification and measurement. The ROA for MR is calculated using similar parameters as the ROA for AI:

$$\text{ROA} = 2\pi(r_{\text{PISA}})^2 \times V_{\text{aliasing}}/V_{\text{MR jet}}$$

Notably, when the Nyquist limit is set to 40, and the velocity of the MR jet is 5 m/s (which represents a 100 mm Hg pressure difference between LV and left atrium, as is a usual measurement for this value), the equation simplifies to:

$$\text{ROA} = (r_{\text{PISA}})^2/2$$

The RV and RF are calculated similarly to the method described earlier for AI. Notably, however, because the MV is leaking, the SV of the MV inflow represents the total inflow, with the outflow being the SV_{LVOT} and SV_{MR} (which is the RV for the MV). Therefore,

$$\text{RV} = \text{SV}_{\text{MV Inflow}} - \text{SV}_{\text{LVOT}}$$

$$\text{RV} = \pi r_{\text{MV}}^2 \times \text{VTI}_{\text{MV inflow}} - \pi r_{\text{LVOT}}^2 \times \text{VTI}_{\text{LVOT}}$$

The total SV is now equal to the $SV_{\text{MV inflow}}$, and so the RF is calculated as:

$$\text{RF} = \text{RV}/(\pi r_{\text{MV}}^2 \times \text{VTI}_{\text{MV inflow}}) \times 100$$

As with AI, the RV can also be calculated using the ROA, where

$$\text{RV} = \text{ROA} \times \text{VTI}_{\text{MV jet}}$$

MR severity is described using the parameters mentioned in Table 21.3.

2. Pitfalls in measuring MR are similar to those in measuring AI. The PISA method may underestimate the ROA if suboptimally acquired or in multiple jets, or overestimate the MR severity in eccentric jets where constraint of the LV wall/myocardium deforms the isovelocity flow fields, as the equation assumes a perfectly

TABLE 21.3 Quantitative Assessment of Mitral Regurgitation

Parameter	Mild	Moderate	Severe
Vena contracta width (cm)	<0.3	0.3–0.69	≥ 0.7
Regurgitant volume (mL)	<30	30–59	≥ 60
Regurgitant fraction	<30	30–49	≥ 50
Effective regurgitant orifice area (cm^2)	<0.2	0.2–0.39	≥ 0.4

hemispheric PISA. Transesophageal echocardiography (TEE) may help to define anatomy more precisely. Also, the RF and RV measurements fail when there is significant aortic regurgitation, as they assume that the only flow into the LV on each heartbeat comes through the MV. Furthermore, when calculated using the inflow SV and outflow SV, the annular area equations assume a circular MV and AV annulus, which can be an additional source of error.

B. Mitral stenosis

1. Mitral stenosis severity is typically derived on the basis of quantification of the transmitral valve gradient and the MV area (MVA), similar to that of AS. The peak gradient (which is even less useful in describing mitral stenosis severity than it is in describing AS) is measured from the A4C window using a CW Doppler sampling across the MV. The mean gradient is measured as the integral of the CW tracing across the MV (both the E- and A-waves are included) during the diastolic filling period. MVA is best quantified directly as measured by planimetry (2D or 3D) or estimated using the empirically derived pressure half-time (PHT) formula:

$$MVA = 220/PHT$$

To measure the PHT, a line is drawn tracing the deceleration of the E-wave of the mitral inflow tracing from PW Doppler usually from the A4C window. The PHT is the calculated time it would take for the maximum value to become half. Because of the limitations of PHT, direct planimetry of the MV is measured from the PSAX. While planimetry can be very accurate, it requires technical acquisition and measurement expertise, as an accurate valve area must be traced precisely at the leaflet tips in a plane perpendicular to the mitral orifice. Off-axis or out-of-plane images will lead to inaccurate measurement (usually overestimation). Furthermore, windows can be limited because of calcification in degenerative MS. These limitations of planimetry can be overcome utilizing three-dimensional echocardiography, and in fact this is considered the optimal and preferred method for echocardiographic assessment of mitral stenosis severity, although it is not universally available. MV stenosis is classified using the parameters outlined in Table 21.4.

TABLE 21.4 Classification of Mitral Stenosis

Parameter	Progressive	Severe	Very Severe
Valve area (cm^2)	>1.5	≤ 1.5	<1.0
Mean gradient	<5	>5–10	>10

2. Errors in measuring mitral stenosis severity by transmitral Doppler gradients may arise owing to the fact that mitral stenosis is dependent to some extent on loading conditions and can increase with increasing LV afterload (i.e., hypertension). Likewise, gradients can be underestimated in sedated patients or hypotensive patients. Heart rate also effects loading conditions and should be noted when gradients are measured and taken into account when comparing serial echocardiograms. Planimetry, by either the 2D or 3D method, is limited by image quality and hence equipment quality and operator experience. Three-dimensional and biplane imaging can help ensure the valve area is measured at the proper location at the inflow level, and ultimately TEE may provide better image quality. Importantly, mitral stenosis commonly coexists with MR; yet, provided it is not severe, it does not typically significantly affect the mean valve gradient, valve area based on planimetry, or valve area based on PHT. It will, however, increase the peak gradient.

IV. TRICUSPID VALVE

A. While tricuspid valve regurgitation (TR) is most typically assessed semiqualitatively using an integrated methodology similar to MR assessment, it can be assessed quantitatively by using the VC and PISA methods, both of which are directly measured typically from an A4C window or reverse A4C window (i.e., LV on the left side of the screen). More complex calculations such as RF, RV, and ROA are not well validated and rarely used to determine the severity of TR (Table 21.5).

B. Tricuspid stenosis, although uncommon, can be assessed quantitatively using Doppler and 2D methodology similar to that applied to the MV. CW Doppler sampling is optimally aligned with flow across the tricuspid valve to enable measurement of the mean valvular gradient and PHT. These measurements are obtained in a similar fashion to mitral stenosis using acoustic windows optimized to align the CW Doppler cursor most parallel to flow. Tricuspid stenosis is not graded as mild, moderate, or severe like other valvular stenosis. Generally, it is graded as significant when the mean gradient is >5 mm Hg and a PHT >190 ms.

TABLE 21.5 Quantitative Assessment of Tricuspid Regurgitation

Parameter	Mild	Moderate	Severe
Vena contracta width (mm)[a]	Not defined	<7	≥7
Proximal isovelocity surface area radius (cm)[b]	≤0.5	0.6–0.9	>0.9

[a]With Nyquist limit at 50 to 60 cm/s.
[b]With baseline shift of Nyquist limit to 28 cm/s.

V. PULMONIC VALVE

A. Pulmonic stenosis severity is assessed using Doppler methodology and by sampling the peak and mean transpulmonic flow velocity, as well as incorporating the 2D appearance of the valve. The maximum velocity is typically optimally sampled from the PSAX window. The peak gradient is calculated from the peak velocity and converted to pressure using the Bernoulli equation in the same manner as for AS. Valve area and mean gradients are typically not calculated and are not included in the generally accepted definitions for pulmonary stenosis severity (Table 21.6).

B. Pulmonic insufficiency (PI) is typically assessed semiquantitatively primarily because of the availability of less critical data supporting quantitative analysis for PI, relative lower prevalence particularly in the adult population, and relatively lesser significance

TABLE 21.6 Assessment of Pulmonic Stenosis

Parameter	Mild	Moderate	Severe
Peak velocity (m/s)	<3	3–4	>4
Peak gradient (mm Hg)	<36	36–64	>64

hemodynamically. Owing somewhat to the relative difficulty and experience in imaging the pulmonic valve and the fact that significant PI is less common than the higher pressure left-sided valvular regurgitant lesions. Measurements are less well validated and therefore infrequently used in pulmonary regurgitation.

C. Because right-sided (tricuspid and pulmonic) valve regurgitation severity is usually measured more qualitatively and semiquantitatively than quantitatively, there are fewer pitfalls with regard to calculations, although several pitfalls exist relative to qualitative assessment. Measurement of the VC with TR has similar pitfalls as described previously with aortic and mitral regurgitation, and tricuspid regurgitant jets are frequently eccentric. The measurement of stenosis and regurgitation in these right-sided valves is also frequently limited by difficulty in obtaining optimal, on-axis imaging in part due to the relatively low prevalence of significant pulmonic and tricuspid pathology finding, hence a lesser experience in imaging particularly in adult echocardiography laboratories.

VI. CASE-BASED EXAMPLES

Case 1. A 65-year-old man undergoes a transthoracic echocardiogram for suspected AS. Figures 21.1 to 21.3 are representative images from the echocardiogram.

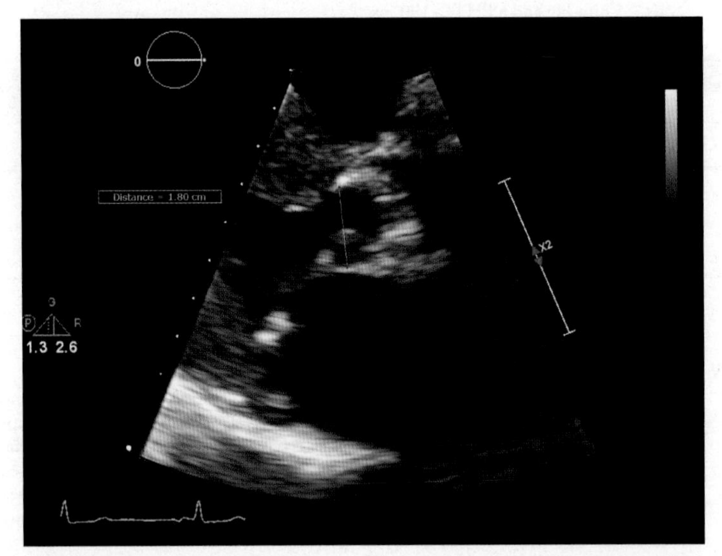

FIGURE 21.1 Parasternal long-axis view of left ventricular outflow tract (LVOT) during systole to measure the LVOT dimension at its maximum.

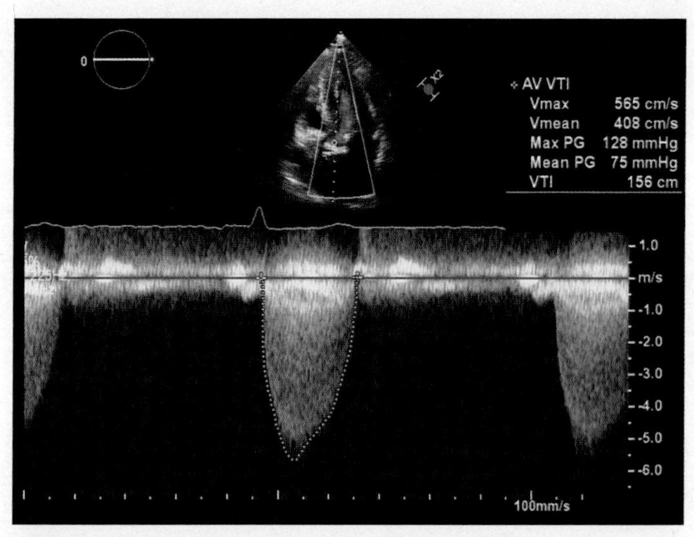

FIGURE 21.2 Apical 5-chamber continuous-wave Doppler through aortic valve.

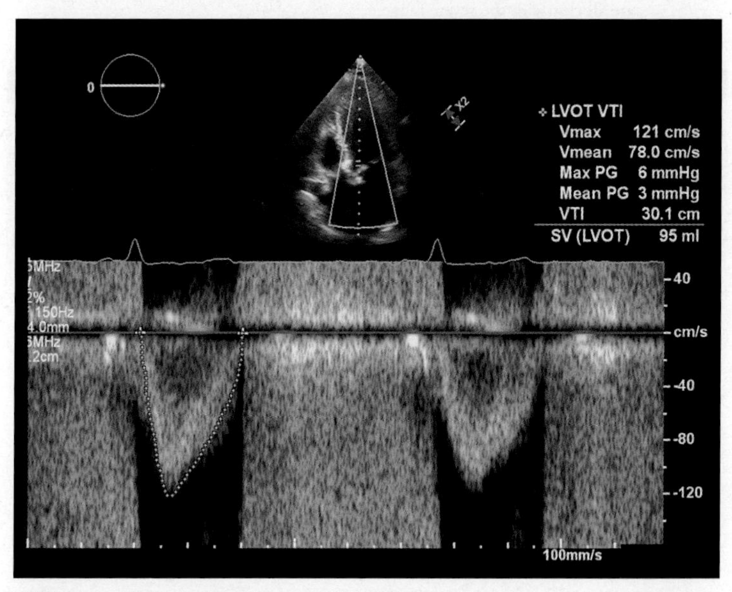

FIGURE 21.3 Apical 5-chamber PW Doppler of left ventricular outflow tract. Note the significant turbulent diastolic flow in this image, which here is related to aortic insufficiency. Note that the outer edge of the modal velocities (brightest) portion of the pulsed wave Doppler jet should be traced as seen in this image. In addition, a spectral Doppler profile without significant spectral distortion should be obtained.

1. To determine the severity of AS, we would calculate the peak and mean valve gradient, as well as the DI and AVA. We calculate the AVA by using the peak velocity measured in Figure 21.2.

$$\text{Peak gradient} = 4V^2$$

$$\text{Peak gradient} = 4 \times (5.65\ \text{m/s})^2 = 128\ \text{mm Hg}$$

2. Note that in this calculation, the velocity must be in m/s (i.e., we must convert from cm/s as reported). The mean gradient is calculated by the image acquisition software as the integral of the CW AV tracing (also Fig. 21.2), which is 75 mm Hg. The AVA is calculated using the LVOT measurement (Fig. 21.1), the AV VTI (Fig. 21.2), and the LVOT VTI (Fig. 21.3), using the continuity equation:

$$\text{AVA} = \text{CSA}_{(\text{LVOT})} \times \text{VTI}_{(\text{LVOT})}/\text{VTI}_{(\text{AV})}$$

$$\text{AVA} = \pi(\text{D}_{\text{LVOT}}/2)^2 \times \text{VTI}_{(\text{LVOT})}/\text{VTI}_{(\text{AV})}$$

$$\text{AVA} = \pi(1.8\ \text{cm}/2)^2 \times 30.1\ \text{cm}/156\ \text{cm} = 0.49\ \text{cm}^2$$

3. The DI is calculated as follows:

$$\text{DI} = V_{(\text{LVOT})}/V_{(\text{AV})}$$

$$\text{DI} = 121\ \text{cm/s}/565\ \text{cm/s}$$

$$\text{DI} = 0.21$$

4. In this case, the peak and mean gradients (128 and 75 mm Hg), AVA, and DI are all clearly in the severe range.

KEY PEARLS

- The LVOT dimension is squared in the continuity equation, and so accurate measurement is essential.
- Optimal site of measurement of the LVOT diameter is typically 1 cm below the AV in systole.
- The DI is an easy check against inaccuracy in this measurement and is typically 0.25 or less in severe AS.

Case 2. An 85-year-old man is referred for echocardiography for AS. His body surface area is 2.05 m^2. Figures 21.4 to 21.6 are representative images from this patient.

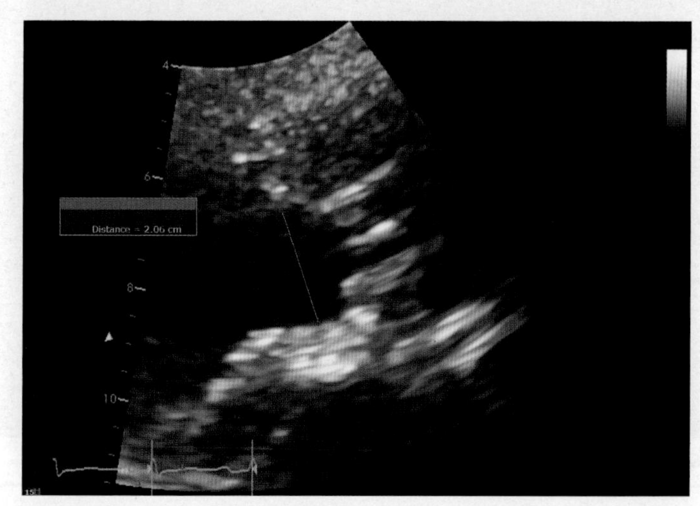

FIGURE 21.4 Parasternal long-axis view of the left ventricular outflow tract.

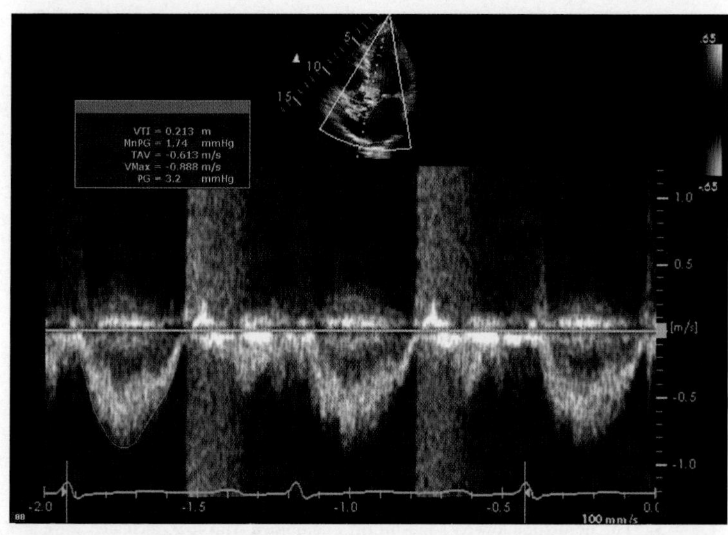

FIGURE 21.5 Left ventricular outflow tract velocity–time integral from the apical 5-chamber window.

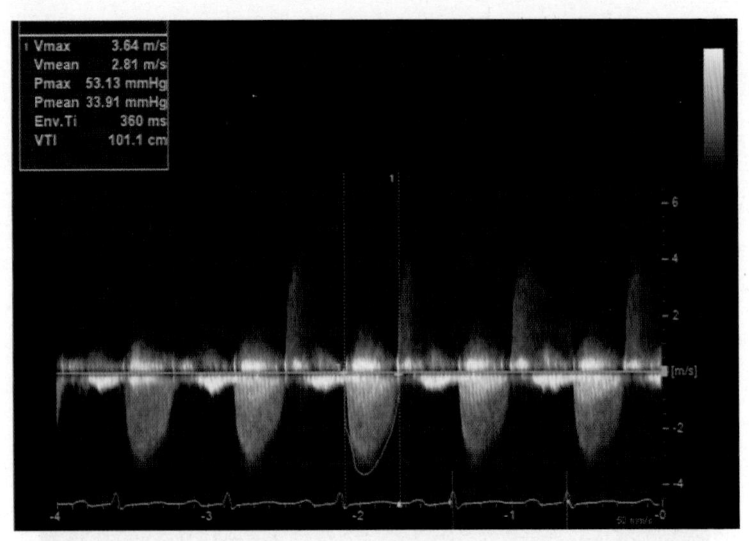

FIGURE 21.6 Continuous wave Doppler tracing from the right sternal border (using Pedoff probe).

1. As shown in Case 1, the peak gradient is calculated from the AV peak velocity, and mean AV velocity from integrating the CW tracing across the AV. Both calculations are done here automatically by the acquisition software and are displayed in Figure 21.6. The AVA is calculated using the continuity equation:

$$AVA = \pi(D_{LVOT}/2)^2 \times VTI_{(LVOT)}/VTI_{(AV)}$$

$$AVA = \pi(2.06/2)^2 \times (21.3/101.1) = 0.70\ cm^2.$$

2. Again, the LVOT diameter is measured from the PLAX view (Fig. 21.4), and the LVOT and AV VTI and maximum velocities from the PW tracing at the LVOT and CW tracing across the AV (Figs. 21.5 and 21.6, respectively). The DI is calculated as follows:

$$DI = V_{(LVOT)}/V_{(AV)}$$

$$DI = 21.3/101.1 = 0.21$$

In this situation, the gradients and AV velocity do not meet criteria for severe AS (mean gradient is <40 mm Hg and peak velocity <4 m/s), but the DI and calculated AVA suggest severe AS. The next step (as discussed earlier) is to calculate the SVI to evaluate for low-flow, low-gradient AS:

$$SVI = (CSA_{(LVOT)} \times VTI_{(LVOT)})/BSA$$

$$SVI = \pi(2.06/2)^2 \times (21.3)/2.05m^2 = 34\ mL/m^2$$

3. The borderline low SVI (34 mL/m^2) combined with low calculated valve area and DI confirms low-flow, low-gradient AS. This patient has a normal ejection fraction (images not shown) and therefore is diagnosed with paradoxical low-flow, low-gradient severe AS. The calcified appearance of the valve (notable on Fig. 21.4) also serves to confirm the diagnosis of severe AS.

KEY PEARLS

- If there is a discrepancy between the calculated valve area and AV gradients, the next step is to assess the SVI to look for low-flow, low-gradient AS. A SVI of <35 mL/m^2 suggests low flow through the AV.
- Low-flow, low-gradient AS can exist because of low left ventricular ejection fraction or because of low SV despite a normal ejection fraction.
- As always, 2D and color flow Doppler parameters help to confirm that true AS exists.

Case 3. An 82-year-old woman is being followed for AS. She has an initial echocardiogram, which reveals a peak gradient of 48 mm Hg, mean gradient 25 mm Hg, AVA of 0.62 cm^2, and DI of 0.24 Her SVI is 24 mL/m^2, her BSA is 1.99m^2, and her LVOT diameter is 1.8 cm (Figs. 21.7 to 21.9A and B). The LVEF in this patient was reduced.

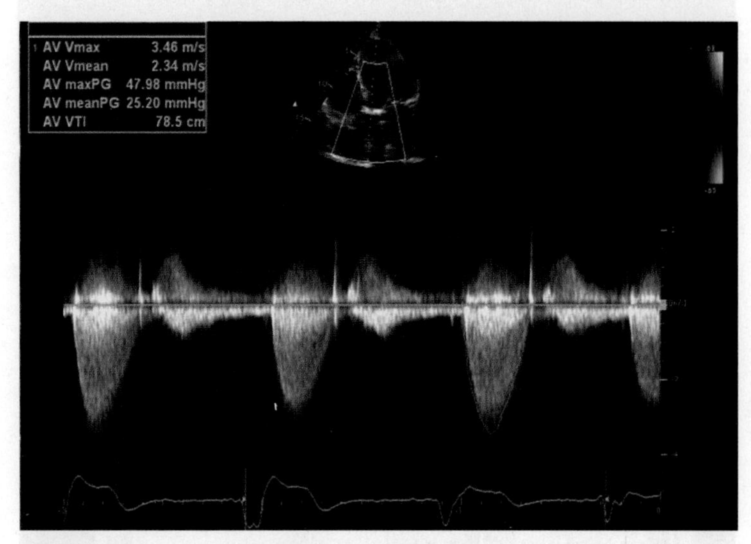

FIGURE 21.7 Continuous-wave aortic valve tracing from apical 5-chamber before dobutamine administration.

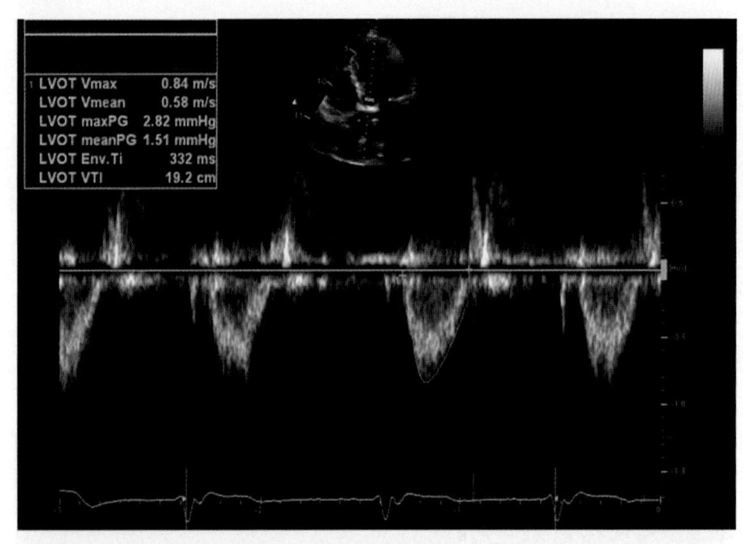

FIGURE 21.8 Pulsed wave tracing of left ventricular outflow tract from apical 5-chamber window before dobutamine administration.

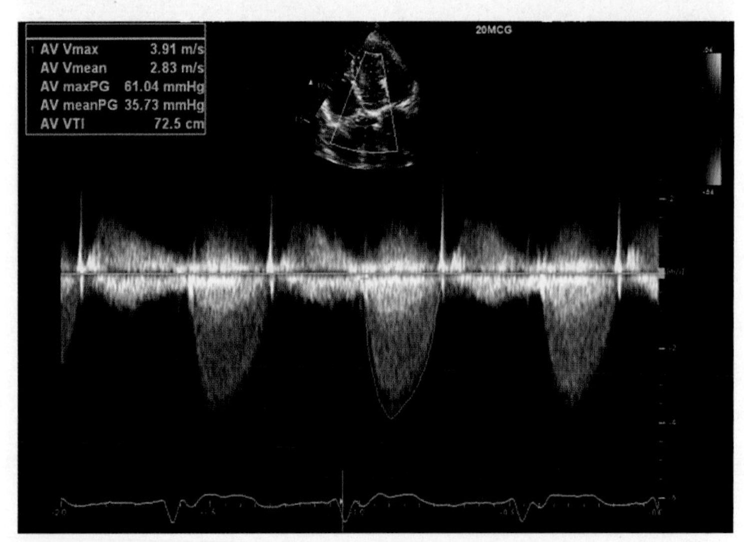

FIGURE 21.9 **A:** Continuous wave tracing across the aortic valve from the apical 5-chamber (A5C) window at maximum dobutamine dose of 20 μg/kg/min. **B:** Puled wave tracing of left ventricular outflow tract from the A5C window at maximum dobutamine dose of 20 μg/kg/min.

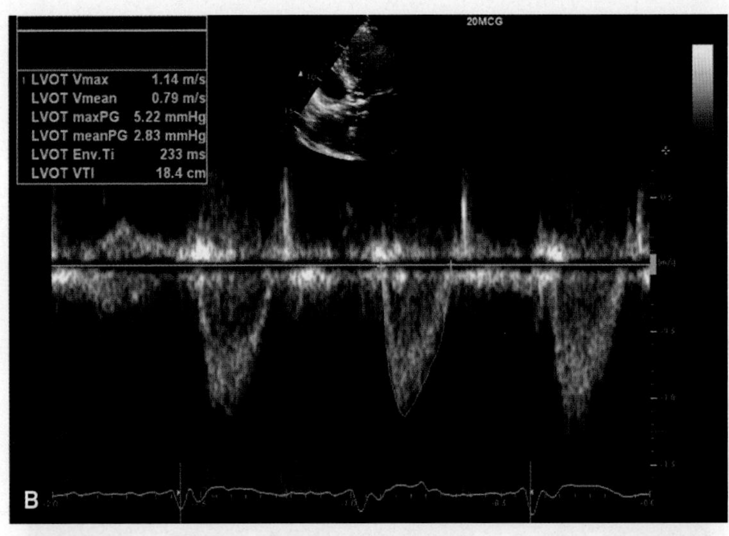

FIGURE 21.9 *(continued)*

1. In reviewing this study, we must calculate the peak and mean AV gradients before and after dobutamine, the SV before and after dobutamine, and the AVA before and after dobutamine. Before dobutamine, her AV gradients are peak 48 mm Hg and mean 25 mm Hg. These increase to 61 mm Hg peak and 36 mm Hg mean post dobutamine. Pre dobutamine, the AVA calculates to:

$$AVA = \pi(D_{LVOT}/2)^2 \times VTI_{(LVOT)}/VTI_{(AV)}$$

$$AVA = \pi(1.8\text{ cm}/2)^2 \times (19.2\text{ cm}/78.5\text{ cm}) = 0.62\text{ cm}^2$$

   a. Post dobutamine, the AVA calculates to:

$$AVA = \pi(1.8\text{ cm}/2)^2 \times (18.4\text{ cm}/72.5\text{ cm}) = 0.64\text{ cm}^2$$

   b. Before dobutamine, the SV calculates to:

$$SV = \pi r_{LVOT}^2 \times VTI_{LVOT}$$

$$SV = \pi(1.8\text{ cm}/2)^2 \times 19.2\text{ cm} = 49\text{ mL}$$

   c. After dobutamine, it calculates to:

$$SV = \pi(1.8\text{ cm}/2)^2 \times 18.4\text{ cm} = 47\text{ mL (no increase)}$$

2. In summary, with this patient, we have a low calculated AVA (in the severe range) with gradients that are in the moderate range and a low LV ejection fraction. With dobutamine, we first see an increase in gradients right at the severe range and maintenance of a valve area in the severe range. This confirms that we have true AS. However, we do not see significant contractile reserve, as the SV does not increase. This is a negative prognostic sign.

KEY PEARLS

- Dobutamine stress echo can be used to assess for suspected AS in patients with low ejection fraction, low SVI (<35 mL/m²), and low calculated valve area.
- In true AS, the gradient will increase and AVA will stay similar, while in pseudo-AS, the gradients will stay the same and calculated valve area will increase as flow increases.
- An increase in SV of >20% with dobutamine indicates contractile reserve, which is a positive prognostic marker.

Case 4. A 56-year-old woman undergoes echocardiography for MR. Following are representative images. Not shown is the LVOT VTI (measured in a similar manner to the prior cases), which is 21 cm, and LVOT diameter, which measures 2.4 cm (see Figs. 21.10 to 21.13).

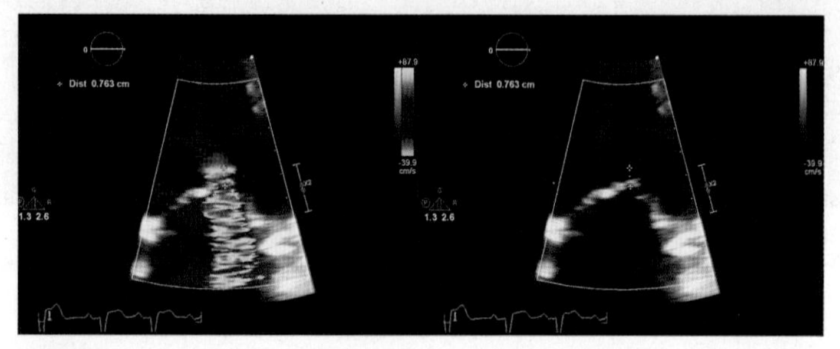

FIGURE 21.10 Apical 4-chamber (A4C) window demonstrating measurement of the mitral regurgitation proximal isovelocity surface area.

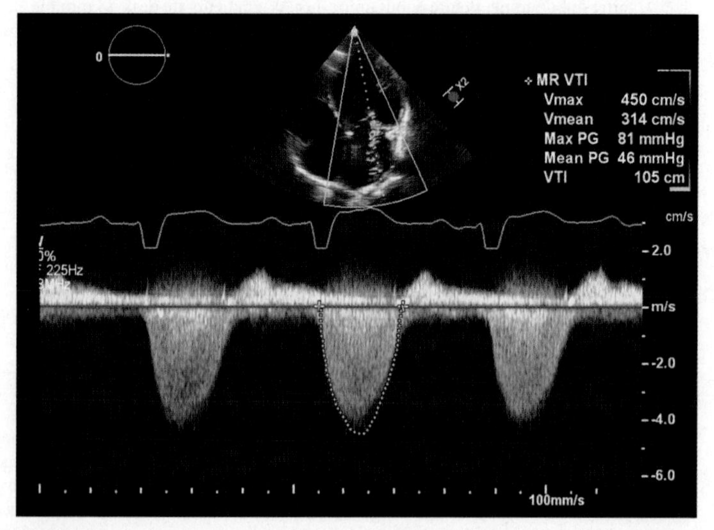

FIGURE 21.11 Continuous wave tracing from apical 4-chamber window showing mitral regurgitation velocity–time integral measurement.

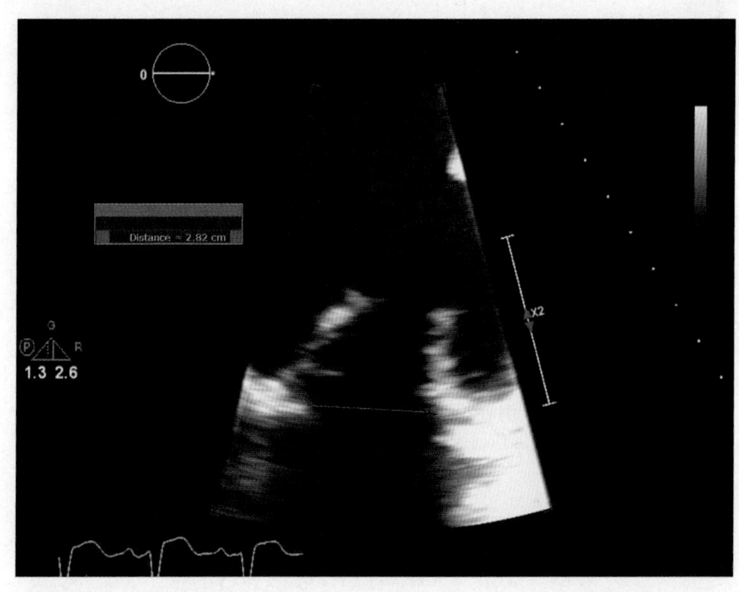

FIGURE 21.12 Apical 4-chamber with measurement of the mitral valve annulus diameter.

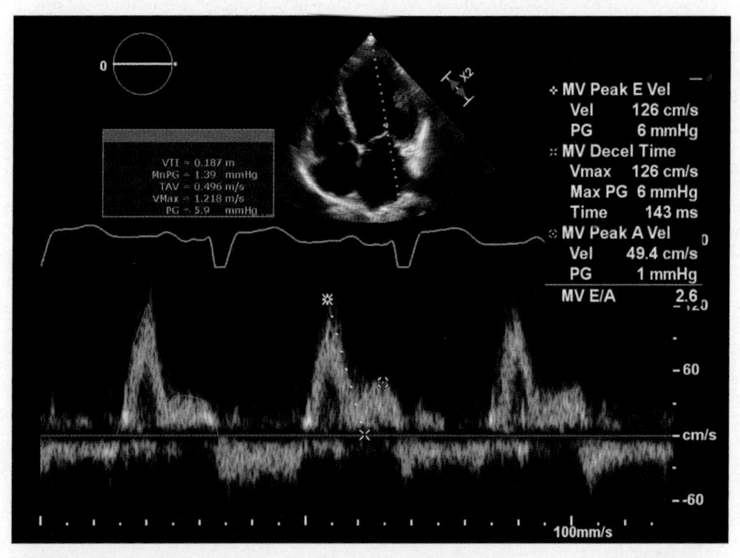

FIGURE 21.13 Pulsed wave Doppler measuring the mitral valve inflow.

1. As discussed earlier, we will characterize the MR severity on the basis of the ROA, RF, and RV. The ROA is calculated using the measured PISA (Fig. 21.10):

$$ROA = 2\pi(r_{PISA})^2 \times V_{aliasing}/V_{MR\ Jet}$$

2. While the Nyquist limit in this case is close to 40 cm/s (39.9), the maximum MR velocity is only 4.5 m/s, and so the simplified equation, $ROA = (r_{PISA})^2/2$, may underestimate the degree of MR. Therefore, we will use the full equation:

$$ROA = 2\pi(r_{PISA})^2 \times V_{aliasing}/V_{MV\ Jet}$$

$$ROA = 2\pi(0.76\ cm)^2 \times (39.9\ cm/s)/(450\ cm/s)$$

$$ROA = 0.32\ cm^2$$

   a. We can calculate the RF using the equation:

$$RV = ROA \times VTI_{MV\ Jet}$$

   b. The VTI of the MR jet is measured in Figure 21.11. Substituting in the measurements yields

$$RV = ROA \times VTI_{MV\ Jet}$$

$$RV = 0.32\ cm^2 \times 105\ cm = 34\ mL$$

3. Alternatively, we can calculate the RV using volumetric methods and comparing the LV inflow and outflow measurements according to the equation:

$$RV = \pi r_{MV}^{\ 2} \times VTI_{MV\ inflow} - \pi r_{LVOT}^{\ 2} \times VTI_{LVOT}$$

4. We measure the VTI of the MV inflow in Figure 21.13, the MV annulus in Figure 21.12, and the LVOT VTI and diameter are not shown, but measured to be 21 and 2.4 cm, respectively. Substituting these numbers,

$$RV = \pi r_{MV}^{\ 2} \times VTI_{MV\ inflow} - \pi r_{LVOT}^{\ 2} \times VTI_{LVOT}$$

$$RV = (\pi(2.82\ cm/2)^2 \times 18.7\ cm) - (\pi(2.4\ cm/2)^2 \times 21\ cm) = 22\ mL$$

5. This result in this case, is not too similar to the value obtained using the PISA and ROA method. The RF is calculated by comparing the RV to the total SV.

$$RF = RV/(\pi r_{MV\ annulus}^{\ 2} \times VTI_{MV\ inflow}) \times 100$$

$$RF = 22\ cm^3/(\pi(2.82\ cm/2)^2 \times 18.7\ cm) \times 100 = 18\%$$

6. Overall, when referenced to Table 21.3, these calculations suggest mild to moderate MR.

KEY PEARLS

- MR can be quantified using the PISA method to calculate ROA and RV, or volumetric methods to calculate RV and RF.
- Volumetric methods are fraught with error as they require multiple measurements, two of which (the LVOT diameter and MV annulus diameter) are squared. Additionally, they fail if concomitant AR or intracardiac shunting is present.
- The simplified ROA equation can ONLY be used if the MR maximum velocity is close to 5.0 m/s, and the Nyquist limit is set near 40 cm/s.
- Calculation of stroke volume through the mitral valve can be done assuming a circular or elliptical shape, with various methods, but is subject to error related to multiple measurements.

Case 5. A 51-year-old man undergoes echocardiography for AI. The following are representative images from this patient seen in Figures 21.14 to 21.16.

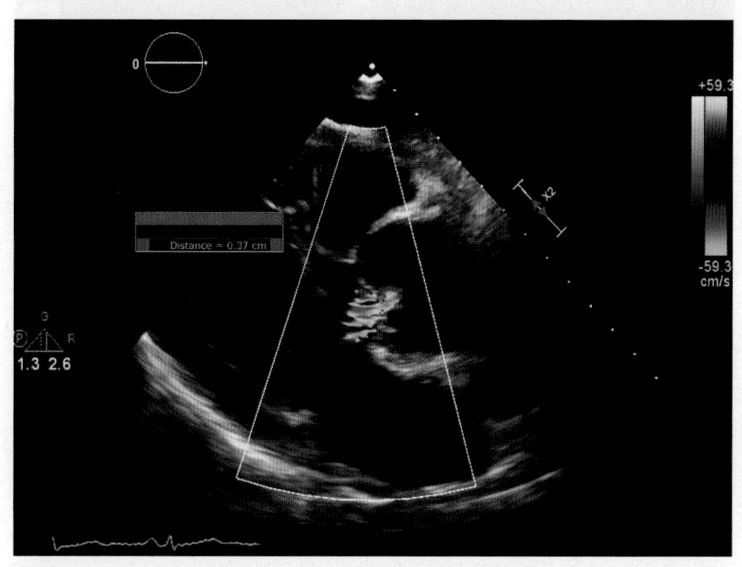

FIGURE 21.14 Parasternal long-axis view with measured vena contracta.

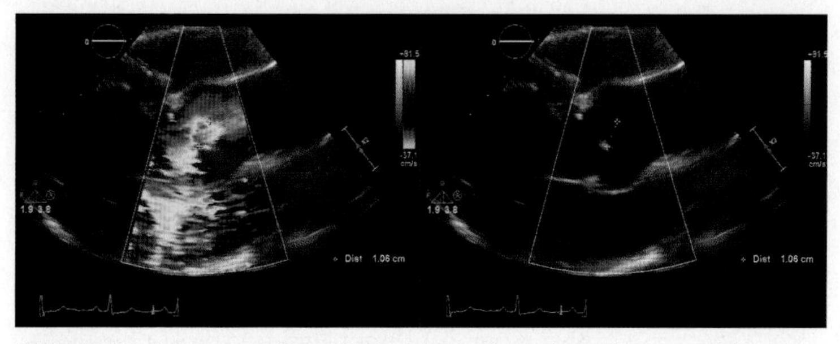

FIGURE 21.15 Right parasternal long-axis image showing the aortic regurgitation proximal isovelocity surface area.

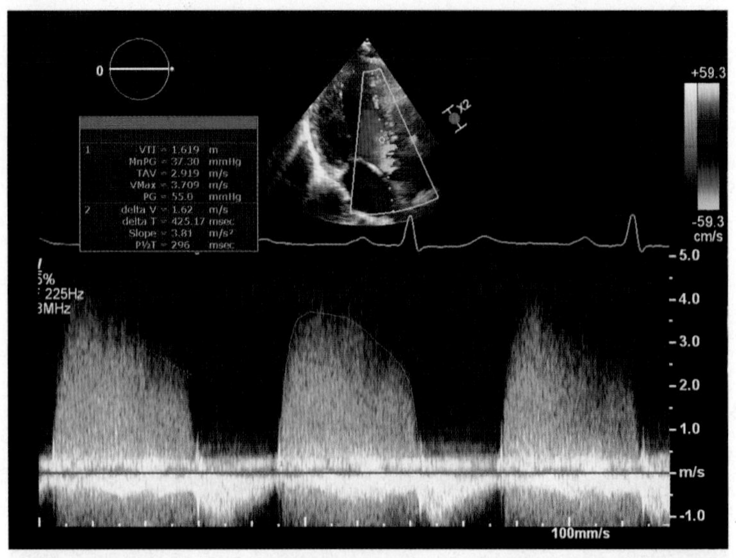

FIGURE 21.16 Figure 21.16 CW Doppler tracing from the A3C window showing the measurement of the AI jet VTI, AI jet peak velocity and AI jet deceleration time.

1. Here, we will use the measured VC and calculated ROA, RF, and RV to describe the severity of AI. The VC measures to 0.37 cm as shown in Figure 21.14. The ROA is calculated using the PISA measured in Figure 21.15 and AI jet peak velocity measured in Figure 21.16.

$$\text{ROA} = 2\pi(r_{\text{PISA}})^2 \times V_{\text{aliasing}}/V_{\text{AI Jet}}$$

$$\text{ROA} = 2\pi(1.06 \text{ cm})^2 \times (37.1 \text{ cm/s}/370 \text{ cm/s}) = 0.71 \text{ cm}^2$$

2. The RV is then calculated using the AI VTI measurement (also measured in Fig. 21.16)

$$\text{RV} = \text{ROA} \times \text{VTI}_{\text{AI Jet}}$$

$$\text{RV} = 0.71 \text{ cm}^2 \times 162 \text{ cm} = 115 \text{ mL}$$

3. As for MR, we can also calculate the RV by comparing the MV inflow SV and AV outflow SV according to the equation:

$$\text{RV} = \pi r_{\text{LVOT}}^{\ 2} \times \text{VTI}_{\text{LVOT}} - \pi r_{\text{MV}}^{\ 2} \times \text{VTI}_{\text{MV inflow}}$$

4. In this patient, the LVOT diameter and LVOT VTI (measured in the same way as in Case 1) are 2.3 cm and 34 cm, respectively. The MV diameter and MV inflow VTI (measured as in Case 4) are 2.4 cm and 20 cm, respectively. Therefore,

$$\text{RV} = \pi r_{\text{LVOT}}^{\ 2} \times \text{VTI}_{\text{LVOT}} - \pi r_{\text{MV}}^{\ 2} \times \text{VTI}_{\text{MV inflow}}$$

$$\text{RV} = \pi(2.3 \text{ cm}/2)^2 \times 34 \text{ cm} - \pi(2.4 \text{ cm}/2)^2 \times 20 \text{ cm} = 51 \text{ mL}$$

5. The RF is calculated from the RV and total SV. Note that in the case of AI, the total SV is the SV exiting the LV (whereas for MR, it is the SV entering the LV).

$$\text{RF} = \text{RV}/(\pi r_{\text{LVOT}}^{\ 2} \times \text{VTI}_{\text{LVOT}}) \times 100$$

$$\text{RF} = 51 \text{ mL}/(\pi(2.3/2)^2 \times 34) \times 100 = 36\%$$

6. There is a large discrepancy between the severity of the AI when calculated by the PISA method (suggesting severe AI) and volumetric method (suggesting moderate AI). This highlights the dependence of volumetric calculations on the measurement of many parameters that leads to many sources of error. We would need to combine these measurements with the appearance of the valve on color flow Doppler and other measurements such as the PHT, at 296 ms (Fig. 21.16) in the moderate range and the VC (Fig. 21.14), which in this case at 0.37 cm is in the moderate range as well. Overall, the degree of aortic regurgitation here is probably moderate to severe.

KEY PEARLS

- AI can be assessed with similar parameters as mitral insufficiency, though the PISA is more difficult to measure.
- Nonquantitative measurements (LV size, density of the AI jet on CW, etc.) are very important in the measurement of AI, given complexity and error induced with calculated variables.

Case 6. A 62-year-old woman is referred for echocardiography to evaluate mitral stenosis. The following images are taken from this patient and are shown in Figures 21.17 and 21.18.

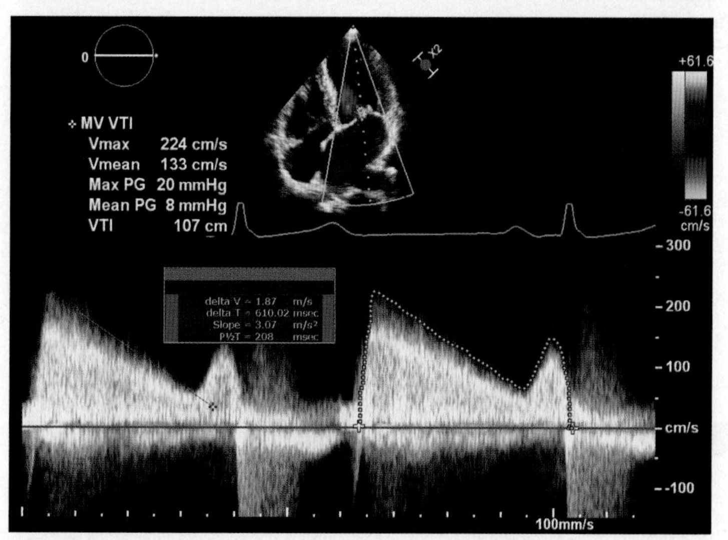

FIGURE 21.17 Continuous wave tracing through the mitral valve from the apical 4-chamber window showing the deceleration time, pressure half-time, and mitral valve gradient measurement.

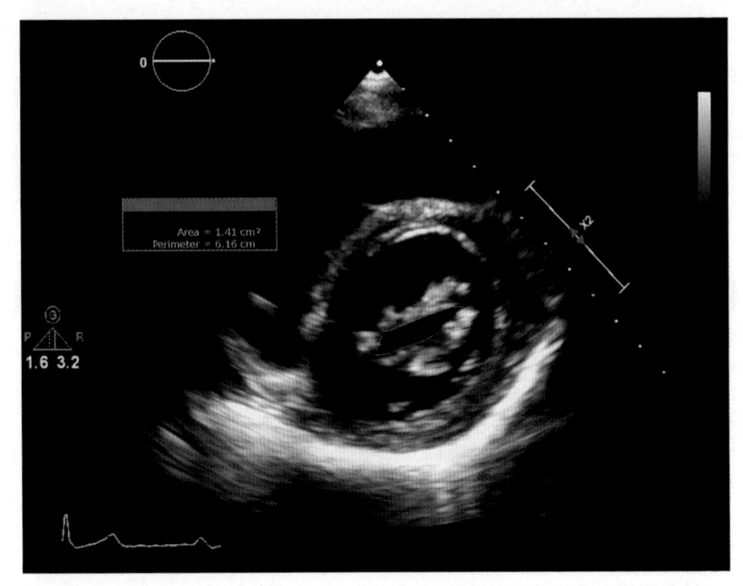

FIGURE 21.18 Planimetry of the mitral valve orifice from the PSAX.

1. As discussed previously, mitral stenosis is usually quantified on echocardiography on the basis of mean valve gradient and valve area, which is directly measured and calculated. The mean gradient is calculated by integrating the CW tracing across the valve (Fig. 21.16). The valve area measurement is shown in Figure 21.18, and calculated valve area by PHT is calculated using the empirically derived formula:

$$\text{MVA} = 220/\text{PHT}$$

$$\text{MVA} = 220/208 = 1.05\ \text{cm}^2$$

2. These measurements (mean gradient 8 mm Hg, MVA 1.41 cm^2 by planimetry and 1.05 cm^2 by PHT) are consistent with severe mitral stenosis. Based on the most recent valve guidelines, MVA $<$ 1.5 cm2 is now considered severe mitral stenosis.

KEY PEARLS

- MV gradient is technically the simplest and most reproducible measurement for assessing mitral stenosis.
- Planimetry of the MV orifice area is possible on transthoracic echocardiography, but requires precise axis imaging at the leaflet tips. Otherwise, the area will be overestimated.
- Three-dimensional echocardiography can be helpful for more precise planimetry of mitral valve area.

VII. CONCLUSION

We have demonstrated and given examples of how echocardiography, particularly Doppler echocardiography, can provide a powerful tool to measure valvular stenosis and regurgitation quantitatively. We have also identified the pitfalls and key points in measurements. As with all empiric calculations, the accuracy depends heavily on the parameters being measured appropriately, and even a small inaccuracy can be multiplied as the equations are computed. Overall, it is important to take into account the calculated echocardiographic parameters, the overall 2D and color Doppler images, and the clinical scenario to arrive at the proper diagnosis.

KEY REFERENCES

Baumgartner H, Hung J, Bermejo J, et al. Echocardiographic assessment of valve stenosis: EAE/ASE recommendations for clinical practice. *Eur J Echocardiogr*. 2009;10(1):1–25.

Monin JL, Quere JP, Monchi M, et al. Low-gradient aortic stenosis: operative risk stratification and predictors for long-term outcome: a multicenter study using dobutamine stress hemodynamics. *Circulation*. 2003;108(3):319–324.

Nishimura RA, Otto CM, Bonow RO, et al. 2014 AHA/ACC guideline for the management of patients with valvular heart disease: a report of the American College of Cardiology/American Heart Association Task Force on practice guidelines. *J Am Coll Cardiol*. 2014;63(22):e57–e185.

Thavendiranathan P, Phelan D, Collier P, et al. Quantitative assessment of mitral regurgitation: how best to do it. *JACC Cardiovasc Imaging*. 2012;5(11):1161–1175.

Zoghbi WA, Enriquez-Sarano M, Foster E, et al. Recommendations for evaluation of the severity of native valvular regurgitation with two-dimensional and Doppler echocardiography. *J Am Soc Echocardiogr*. 2003;16(7):777–802.

CHAPTER 22

Joseph Campbell
E. Murat Tuzcu

Cardiac Cases and Calculations

I. INTRODUCTION. Over the past several decades, the field of interventional cardiology has seen the emergence of several novel percutaneous therapies aimed at treating individuals with advanced valvular disease. Accounting for the complexity of the decision-making process in evaluating and treating these patients, the current iteration of the American College of Cardiology (ACC)/American Heart Association (AHA) guidelines advocates a multidisciplinary approach to management through the establishment of heart teams. Integral to this process is the ability of the team to obtain a thorough clinical and laboratory assessment. This requires physicians who care for these patients to be familiar with the scope of relevant invasive and noninvasive techniques used to determine the hemodynamic significance of the relevant valvular pathology. With this in mind, the focus of this chapter will be to review the fundamental methods for assessing valvular disease in the cardiac catheterization laboratory both through discussing commonly used techniques and providing case-based examples.

II. INDICATIONS

Advances in the field of Doppler echocardiography have resulted in the ability to obtain accurate and reproducible hemodynamic data noninvasively, thereby obviating the need for routine cardiac catheterization in the evaluation of all patients with valvular heart disease. Despite this, there are still several scenarios in which an invasive hemodynamic assessment can be beneficial.

A. Inconclusive noninvasive testing: either suboptimal image quality or discrepancy between bedside clinical assessment and echocardiographic findings.

B. Use of dobutamine in patients with presumed low-flow low-gradient aortic stenosis to distinguish between pseudo and true aortic stenosis, as well as to assess contractile reserve in cases where this is incompletely evaluated, or information that is unable to be assessed by noninvasive means.

C. Assess response to percutaneous structural interventions, including assessment of valve area, pressure gradients, and other relevant hemodynamic data immediately before and after the procedure.

D. Assessment of valvular prosthesis when noninvasive evaluation is inadequate due to poor image acquisition.

III. OVERVIEW OF COMMON CALCULATIONS

In the following section, we will briefly review the common methods used in the cardiac catheterization laboratory to assess patients with valvular heart disease. For additional information, as well as a review of normal hemodynamics, please refer to Chapter 20.

A. Valve area

Accurate assessment of mean pressure gradient and valve area is imperative in order to determine the hemodynamic significance of stenotic valvular lesions and thus guide the decision on appropriate timing for intervention. The Gorlin formula is used for valve area calculations. For a quick calculation, an abbreviated formula developed by Hakki is used.

1. **Gorlin equation**
   a. In 1951, Gorlin developed a hydraulic formula intended to provide a mechanism to invasively determine valve orifice area. This formula requires precise determination of several key variables:
      i. Flow across a valve (during systole for aortic valve and diastole for mitral valve), which is equal to cardiac output (CO) divided by the product of heart rate (HR) and either systolic ejection period (SEP) or diastolic filling period (DFP).
      ii. Mean pressure gradient (ΔP) averaged over 5 or 10 cardiac cycles depending on whether a patient is in sinus rhythm versus atrial fibrillation, respectively.
   b. These variables are then used to determine valve area according to the following equation:

$$\text{Valve area} = \frac{\text{CO}/(\text{HR} \times \text{SEP or DFP})}{44.3 \times C \times \sqrt{\Delta P}}$$

   where CO = cardiac output (mL/min), HR = heart rate, SEP and DFP = systolic ejection period and diastolic filling period, respectively, C = constant, and ΔP = mean pressure gradient (mm Hg)

   c. Gorlin validated this formula by comparing calculated values with measured mitral valve area (MVA) values in 11 patients (6 at autopsy and 5 during surgery). In this study, he noted a good correlation (within 0.2 cm2) between the calculated and measured valve areas.
   d. Using these data, an empiric constant of 0.7 was derived for calculation of mitral valve area. Once left ventricular end-diastolic pressure (LVEDP) could be routinely measured, this value was adjusted to 0.85. The empiric constant has not been determined for aortic stenosis and an assumed value of 1 has been assigned. For patients with pulmonic and tricuspid stenosis, valve area is not routinely used, and mean pressure gradients are the predominant mechanism used to determine severity.
   e. Using the Gorlin formula, MVA and aortic valve area (AVA) can be calculated as:

$$\text{MVA} = \frac{\text{CO}/(\text{HR} \times \text{DFP})}{37.7 \times \sqrt{\Delta P}}$$

$$\text{AVA} = \frac{\text{CO}/(\text{HR} \times \text{SEP})}{44.3 \times \sqrt{\Delta P}}$$

   f. Examples:
      i. Mitral stenosis: Assume a calculated Fick CO of 4.0 L/min, HR of 100 bpm, DFP 0.40 sec/beat, and ΔP of 25 mm Hg

$$\text{MVA} = \frac{4000/(100 \times 0.40)}{44.3 \times 0.85 \times \sqrt{25}} = 0.5\ \text{cm}^2$$

      ii. Aortic stenosis: Assume a calculated Fick CO of 5 L/min, HR of 100 bpm, SEP 0.20 sec/beat, and ΔP of 64 mm Hg

$$\text{AVA} = \frac{5000/(100 \times 0.20)}{44.3 \times 1.0 \times \sqrt{64}} = 0.7\ \text{cm}^2$$

2. Hakki equation

a. In an effort to simplify the process of invasive valve area calculation, Hakki et al. studied 100 consecutive patients (60 with aortic stenosis and 40 with mitral stenosis) who underwent combined left and right heart catheterization with calculation of valve area using the Gorlin equation. They observed that at normal HR, the product of HR, SEP or DFP, the constant, and 44.3 closely approximates 1,000 over a wide range of valve areas. With this in mind, they simplified the equation as follows:

$$\text{Valve area} = \frac{\text{CO}}{\sqrt{P}}$$

where CO = cardiac output (L/min) and P = pressure gradient (mm Hg)

Using this equation, they noted a positive correlation between valve area calculations derived using the Gorlin and Hakki equations for patients with both aortic stenosis ($r = 0.96$) and mitral stenosis ($r = 0.94$).

b. In patients with aortic stenosis, the correlation was positive whether mean gradient or peak-to-peak gradient was used.

c. Care must be used when using this formula in patients with tachycardia, as the relative time spent in systole and diastole may change sufficiently at high HRs to render the basic assumptions used to derive this formula invalid.

d. Examples:

i. Mitral stenosis: Using the above values of CO = 4.0 L/min and ΔP of 25 mm Hg

$$\text{MVA} = \frac{4.0}{\sqrt{25}} = 0.8 \text{ cm}^2$$

ii. Aortic stenosis: Using the above values of CO = 5.0 L/min and ΔP of 64 mm Hg

$$\text{AVA} = \frac{5.0}{\sqrt{64}} = 0.6 \text{ cm}^2$$

B. Pressure gradients

As the cardiac valve becomes progressively narrower and resistance to flow consequently rises, higher pressure gradients are required in order to maintain adequate tissue perfusion. Although echocardiography has become the standard for determining these values in clinical practice, there are still scenarios where these calculations must be done in the cardiac catheterization laboratory. In these select cases, pressure gradients are directly measured rather than being indirectly obtained noninvasively using the simplified Bernoulli or continuity equation. If done with close attention being paid to best practice standards, such as the use of dual-lumen pigtail catheters with simultaneous LV to aortic pressure measurements for aortic stenosis, these measurements should be more accurate than the gradients obtained noninvasively. Failure to strictly adhere to these standards may result in inaccurate data acquisition and thereby clinical assessment.

1. Aortic stenosis

a. The LV–aortic gradient may be reported as:

i. Peak-to-peak gradient: refers to the difference between the peak aortic measurement and the peak LV measurement. Given that they are not temporally related, this measurement does not carry any physiologic significance, though it is often used to approximate mean gradient.

ii. Peak instantaneous gradient: represents the peak gradient that exists between the LV and aorta at any given point in time during the period of systolic ejection.

iii. Mean gradient: determined by integrating the area under the curve of the simultaneous LV–aortic pressure waveform. This measurement is the most reliable way for expressing the pressure gradient and the form used in calculating valve area via the Gorlin equation.

b. Technique:

i. Simultaneous LV–peripheral artery tracing: limited by both temporal delay and peripheral amplification of pulse waveform.

(a) Folland et al. directly compared simultaneous LV–aortic with LV–femoral arterial tracings and observed that in tracings that did not adjust for temporal delay, gradient was overestimated by a mean of 9 mm Hg, whereas the adjusted tracings underestimated gradient by a mean of 10 mm Hg.

ii. Simultaneous LV–aortic tracing via transseptal catheterization: Method of choice with mechanical aortic valves, in some cases when precise measurements of LV outflow tract (LVOT) gradients are needed (i.e., in patients with HOCM), or when the left ventricle is unable to be accessed via a retrograde approach.

(a) Limited use given invasiveness and consequent potential for complications.

iii. Simultaneous LV–aortic tracing via retrograde LV catheterization: This is the most common and preferred method. It can be done using a dual-lumen pigtail catheter or a single-lumen pigtail catheter in the aorta in combination with either a high-fidelity pressure wire or additional single-lumen pigtail catheter in the left ventricle.

2. Mitral stenosis

a. The mean gradient across the mitral valve may be determined either through direct left atrial (LA) cannulation via a transseptal puncture or using pulmonary capillary wedge pressure (PCWP) as a correlate for LA pressure.

i. Schoenfeld et al. studied 12 patients with prosthetic mitral stenosis and determined that the use of PCWP in this population consistently led to the overestimation of the mean gradient (13.2 mm Hg vs. 6.7 mm Hg) and consequent underestimation of MVA (mean 1.29 cm^2 vs. 1.89 cm^2). They postulated that this may have been due to (1) phasic delay in the PCWP V wave resulting in a higher mean diastolic pressure relative to the pressure obtained via use of direct LA pressure and/or (2) the recording of a dampened pulmonary artery pressure rather than a true PCWP tracing in patients with pulmonary hypertension.

IV. ANGIOGRAPHIC ASSESSMENT OF AORTIC AND MITRAL REGURGITATION

Although most commonly done through the use of Doppler echocardiography, there are certain scenarios when the use of angiography is needed to assess the degree of aortic or mitral regurgitation. The angiographic assessment of valvular regurgitation using the Sellers criteria for both the aortic and mitral valve is as follows:

A. Sellers criteria

1. 1+: Faint opacification of proximal chamber which clears with each beat

2. 2+: Mild opacification of proximal chamber which clears within a few beats

3. 3+: Moderate opacification of entire proximal chamber of equal intensity to the distal chamber

4. 4+: Intense opacification of proximal chamber to a greater degree than the distal chamber

V. AORTIC REGURGITATION INDEX

Given the correlation of increasing degrees of aortic regurgitation (AR) with post–transcatheter aortic valve replacement (TAVR) mortality, precise assessment of AR is crucial as a routine part of intraoperative care in this patient population. This remains difficult despite the routine use of invasive hemodynamics, aortography, as well as transesophageal echocardiography (TEE). Although not yet widely used in clinical practice, the AR index and time-integrated (TIAR) index were developed to help improve the accuracy by which postimplantation AR is measured.

A. AR index: Requires simultaneous determination of systolic blood pressure (SBP), diastolic blood pressure (DBP), as well as LVEDP, which are related as follows:

$$\text{AR index} = \frac{\text{DBP} - \text{LVEDP}}{\text{SBP}} \times 100$$

1. The complementary value of the AR index was prospectively assessed in 146 high-risk patients (mean Society of Thoracic Surgeons score = 9.8 ± 7.3%) who underwent implantation of a Medtronic CoreValve prosthesis. In this study, the AR index incrementally decreased with worsening AR and independently predicted 1-year mortality in patients with an AR index <25.

B. TIAR index: Attempts to improve the accuracy of the above assessment by integrating the representative pressures throughout their corresponding time in the cardiac cycle. It requires precise calculation of the LV-aorta (Ao) diastolic pressure time integral (DPTI) and LV systolic pressure time integral (SPTI).

1. LV-Ao DPTI: Represented by the integrated area between the central aortic and LV pressure waveforms during diastole.
2. LV SPTI: Calculated by integrating the area under the LV pressure waveform during systole.
3. These measurements can then be related to determine the TIAR index as follows:

$$\text{TIAR index} = \frac{\text{LV-Ao DPTI}}{\text{LV SPTI}} \times 100$$

4. In a study of 64 patients with severe aortic stenosis who underwent implantation of a Sapien valve, a TIAR index <80 predicted the presence of more than mild aortic insufficiency (AI) with a sensitivity of 86% and specificity of 83%. Furthermore, using receiver operating characteristic curve assessment, the TIAR index was associated with improved diagnostic accuracy compared to the AR index.

VI. FLUOROSCOPIC ASSESSMENT OF MECHANICAL VALVES

Occasionally, when either the presence of significant artifact limits the visualization of mechanical valves or falsely elevated noninvasive gradients are suspected due to pressure recovery, the use of fluoroscopic methods can be employed. This involves meticulously imaging the valve in a projection perpendicular to the plane of opening and closing of the prosthesis. Using these images, opening and closing angles can then be calculated and compared with standard values to determine whether or not significant obstruction is present (Fig. 22.1).

VII. REGURGITANT VOLUME AND REGURGITANT FRACTION

This concept was borne out of the desire to have a mechanism for quantitatively assessing valvular regurgitation in the cardiac catheterization laboratory. First described in 1963 by Sandler et al., it relies on the determination of the total LV stroke volume (TSV) as well as the effective forward stroke volume (FSV). Although not widely used, it will be briefly discussed here.

A. TSV: Defined as the difference between end-diastolic and end-systolic volumes as determined by left ventriculography.

B. FSV: Calculated by dividing CO (as determined by either Fick or thermodilution techniques, which measures effective forward flow) by HR.

C. These variables are then related according to the following equation to calculate regurgitant volume (RV):

$$\text{RV} = \text{TSV} - \text{FSV}$$

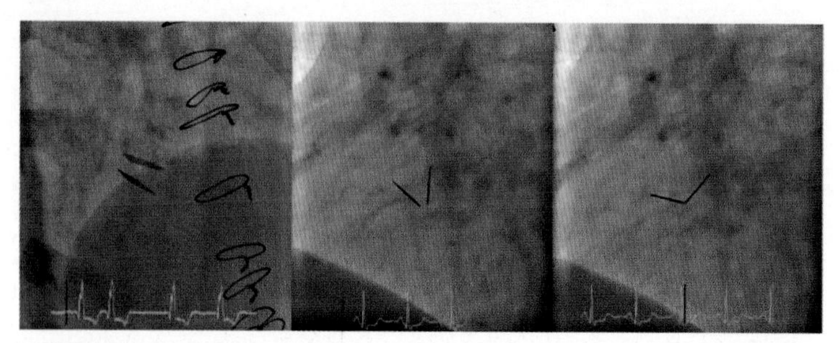

FIGURE 22.1 Fluoroscopic assessment of mechanical valves: In the left panel, it is evident that the image is obtained at an oblique angle, which would result in an inaccurate assessment of valve opening and closing. The center and right panels demonstrate proper orientation for measuring opening and closing angles in a separate patient with a mechanical aortic valve. The opening and closing angles represent the angle formed between the two leaflets in systole and diastole, respectively. These measurements can be compared to standard values in order to determine whether or not restriction is present.

D. Using this information, regurgitant fraction (RF) can then be determined:

$$RF = (TSV - FSV)/TSV$$

E. Using this equation, mild = <20%, moderate = 21% to 40%, moderately severe = 41% to 60%, and severe = >60%.

F. Limitations:

1. Can be time-consuming and requires the use of highly sophisticated computerized software for calculating ventricular volumes.
2. The operator must ensure that representative volumes are obtained, as they may differ during each beat in the cardiac cycle. Of note, accurate volumes cannot be obtained in scenarios with variable R-R intervals, such as atrial fibrillation or frequent ectopic beats.
3. Error can also be introduced through inherent limitations involved in standard methods used to calculate CO.
4. The degree of valvular regurgitation is dependent on loading conditions of the LV, and as such, the operator must ensure that these remain consistent throughout the course of the procedure when measurements are being obtained.

VIII. CASE-BASED EXAMPLES

The remainder of the chapter will focus on case-based scenarios aimed at illustrating the clinical utility of the above techniques using a variety of hemodynamic loading conditions and provocative measures relevant to clinical practice. In addition to the above discussion, reference to Chapters 20 and 23 is encouraged to complement the information presented in the cases.

A. Aortic valve

Case 1: Normal flow with high gradient. A 68-year-old woman presented for further evaluation of worsening dyspnea on exertion. Her medical history is notable for hypertension, hyperlipidemia, pulmonary hypertension, moderately severe tricuspid regurgitation, heart failure with preserved ejection fraction (EF), and moderate aortic stenosis. She underwent a transthoracic echocardiogram, which demonstrated EF 65% with right ventricular systolic pressure 100 mm Hg, 3+ tricuspid regurgitation, and moderately severe aortic stenosis with mean gradient 33 mm Hg and AVA 1.0 cm^2.

In order to further investigate the etiology of her symptoms, the patient was taken to the cardiac catheterization laboratory. Coronary angiography did not demonstrate any obstructive coronary artery disease (CAD). Right heart catheterization and simultaneous LV aortic pressure measurements were obtained using a dual-lumen pigtail catheter with the following results as shown in Figure 22.2.

Right artery (mm Hg)	9
Right ventricle (mm Hg)	92/10
Pulmonary artery (mm Hg)	92/32 (60)
PCWP (mm Hg)	25
Fick CO (L/min)	4.7
Mean LV-aortic gradient (mm Hg)	42
HR (beats/min)	75
SEP (msec)	25
Stroke volume (mL/beat)	63
Stroke volume index	37

Using the above data,

$$AVA = \frac{4700/(75 \times 0.25)}{44.3 \times 1.0 \times \sqrt{42}} = 0.9 \text{ cm}^2$$

FIGURE 22.2

KEY PEARLS

- ACC/AHA guidelines support the use of cardiac catheterization to determine severity of aortic stenosis when there is a discrepancy between the clinical assessment and results of noninvasive tests.
- Due to inaccuracies that can result from peripheral amplification of the arterial pressure waveform as well as a time delay between LV and peripheral arterial pressure, peripheral arterial pressure should not be substituted for central aortic pressure. Instead, simultaneous LV–aortic pressure should be obtained, with the most common method being through the use of a dual-lumen pigtail catheter.
- After high-quality measurements are obtained and verified, catheter pullback should be recorded for two reasons:
  1. Confirm lack of a pressure gradient in the aorta between the two-catheter lumens, which would indicate a technical issue with either the catheter or transducer system and thereby affect the accuracy of the pressure measurements.
  2. Exclude the presence of a concomitant LVOT gradient.

Case 2: Pressure recovery with mechanical valve. An 88-year-old man presented for further evaluation of progressive dyspnea. His medical history is notable for hypertension, hyperlipidemia, COPD, and severe aortic stenosis s/p AVR with a 24-mm St. Jude valve. Transthoracic echocardiogram was done and demonstrated EF of 55% with a mean gradient of 60 mm Hg and AVA 0.7 cm^2. TEE was severely limited due to shadowing from the mechanical prosthesis and as such fluoroscopic assessment was performed demonstrating appropriate excursion of the mechanical discs. Subsequently, simultaneous LV–aortic pressure gradients were obtained following a transseptal puncture. This yielded a mean gradient of 25 mm Hg across the mechanical valve, thereby confirming the presence of moderate aortic stenosis. Following intensification of his bronchodilator regimen, the patient's dyspnea improved.

KEY PEARLS

- In addition to shadowing, noninvasive assessment of mechanical prostheses can be limited due to the concept of pressure recovery.
- Flow through a normally functioning tilting disc bileaflet mechanical aortic valve occurs through a small central orifice as well as two lateral orifices. Therefore, a localized high-pressure gradient may be created as blood accelerates through this central orifice with rapid pressure recovery in the central aorta distal to this.
- Because the velocity recorded using continuous-wave Doppler represents the highest value present along the direction of the ultrasound beam, pressure recovery cannot be accounted for and thus the pressure gradient measured by echocardiography will reflect the velocity of blood flow between the LV and central orifice and not necessarily that between the LV and aorta. This may ultimately result in a falsely elevated transvalvular pressure gradient despite normal prosthetic valvular function.
- When pressure recovery is suspected, fluoroscopic assessment should be pursued. If valve opening is restricted significantly, then the diagnosis of severe prosthetic AS can be made. If this is not the case, then proceeding with an invasive assessment is indicated. Because invasive pressure gradients are directly obtained by catheters positioned proximal and distal to the valve, error introduced by pressure recovery can be avoided and a definitive diagnosis can be made.

Case 3: Low-flow low-gradient with contractile reserve. A 78-year-old female was referred for progressive fatigue. Her medical history is notable for hypertension, hyperlipidemia, CAD with prior drug-eluting stent (DES) to the proximal left anterior descending (LAD) artery, atrial fibrillation, and symptomatic bradycardia status postplacement of a dual-chamber pacemaker. She was recently hospitalized with pulmonary edema at which time she was noted to have a decline in her EF from 55% to 35%. This echocardiogram was also notable for a severely calcified aortic valve with a peak gradient of 36 mm Hg, a mean gradient of 16 mm Hg, AVA 0.86 cm^2, and trivial AI. Given the decline in EF, she underwent a coronary angiogram, which demonstrated a patent LAD stent. Subsequently, simultaneous LV–aortic pressure gradients were obtained using a dual-lumen pigtail catheter both at rest and following infusion of up to 20 mcg/kg/min of dobutamine, with the results as shown in Figure 22.3.

	Rest	Dobutamine 20 mcg/kg/min
Cardiac output (L/min)	3.9	5.8
Heart rate (bpm)	70	85
SEP (msec)	0.31	0.30
Mean gradient (mm Hg)	25	43
Stroke volume (mL/beat)	56	68

Using the above data,

$$AVA_{rest} = \frac{3900/(70 \times 0.31)}{44.3 \times 1.0 \times \sqrt{25}} = 0.8 \text{ cm}^2$$

$$AVA_{stress} = \frac{5800/(85 \times 0.30)}{44.3 \times 1.0 \times \sqrt{43}} = 0.8 \text{ cm}^2$$

FIGURE 22.3

KEY PEARLS

- Low-flow low-gradient severe AS with LV dysfunction represents a subset of patients with EF <50%, AVA <1.0 cm^2, and mean gradient <40 mm Hg.
- Invasive hemodynamic assessment with a dobutamine challenge in patients with concomitant LV dysfunction and AS can be helpful to distinguish between several different phenotypes:
  - Low-flow low-gradient severe AS with contractile reserve: Increase in gradient with stable AVA and augmentation of stroke volume by ≥20%.
  - Low-flow low-gradient severe AS without contractile reserve: No change or increase in gradient with stable AVA and failure of stroke volume to augment by ≥20%.
  - Pseudo-aortic stenosis: Increase in the AVA with a variable change in the mean gradient.
- Although this information can often be obtained on a dobutamine stress echocardiogram, the invasive route is typically pursued if these results are thought to be inadequate or in patients with critical CAD who require revascularization before dobutamine challenge.
- Invasive hemodynamic assessment with dobutamine is contraindicated in patients with severe left main stenosis, active coronary ischemia, ventricular arrhythmias, and acute decompensated heart failure. Before the study is performed, these situations should be addressed (i.e., with percutaneous coronary intervention [PCI] and diuresis, respectively).

Case 4: Low-flow low-gradient without contractile reserve. A 71-year-old man presented for further evaluation of worsening dyspnea on exertion and lower extremity edema. His medical history is notable for hypertension, hyperlipidemia, diabetes, and rheumatic heart disease with prior mitral valve replacement. He recently underwent a transthoracic echocardiogram, which demonstrated EF of 20% with a well-seated mechanical mitral prosthesis and moderately severe aortic stenosis (peak gradient 42 mm Hg, mean gradient 26 mm Hg, AVA of 1.0 cm^2) and 1+ AI. Subsequent TEE demonstrated AVA of 1.5 cm^2 by both two-dimensional and three-dimensional planimetry. Coronary angiography demonstrated no significant atherosclerotic CAD. Contrast-enhanced gated computed tomography (CT) demonstrated aortic valve calcium score of 1800 Agatston units. Given concern for low-flow low-gradient aortic stenosis, simultaneous LV–aortic pressure measurements using a dual-lumen pigtail catheter were obtained both at rest and with infusion of up to 20 mcg/kg/min of dobutamine, with the results as shown in Figure 22.4.

	Rest	Dobutamine 20 mcg/kg/min
Cardiac output (L/min)	4.0	4.7
Heart rate (bpm)	80	94
SEP (msec)	25	24
Mean gradient (mm Hg)	14	28
Stroke volume (mL/beat)	50	50

Using the above data,

$$AVA_{rest} = \frac{4000/(80 \times 0.25)}{44.3 \times 1.0 \times \sqrt{14}} = 1.2\ \text{cm}^2$$

$$AVA_{stress} = \frac{4700/(94 \times 0.24)}{44.3 \times 1.0 \times \sqrt{28}} = 0.9\ \text{cm}^2$$

FIGURE 22.4

KEY PEARLS

- This case represents low-flow low-gradient severe AS without contractile reserve. Notice that with the infusion of dobutamine, the valve area decreased to 0.9 cm^2, which is consistent with severe aortic stenosis. Despite this, the stroke volume failed to increase by 20%, which is indicative of a lack of contractile reserve.
- In a study of 136 patients with severe low-flow low-gradient AS, operative mortality was 5% in patients with and 33% in patients without contractile reserve. In the group with contractile reserve, survival was improved with AVR, and although a similar trend was seen in patients without contractile reserve, it did not meet statistical significance. Mean gradient <20 mm Hg at baseline and lack of contractile reserve independently predicted operative mortality. Given the high operative mortality in patients without contractile reserve, using response to dobutamine infusion is helpful, as part of the overall risk assessment when deciding whether or not to pursue AVR.
- Herrmann et al. studied 530 patients in the PARTNER cohort with low-flow AS and noted a higher mortality in this subgroup when compared with patients with normal flow (47% vs. 34%). In both high-risk and inoperable patients, intervention resulted in improved survival. Low-flow AS was an independent predictor of mortality, but the same was not true for either EF or gradients.
- In patients without contractile reserve, in whom the decision regarding intervention is more complex, assessment of aortic valve calcium by CT and/or fluoroscopy can be of benefit. Higher degrees of calcification have been shown to be associated with increased long-term mortality, and such patients may derive a greater benefit from intervention when compared with individuals with less calcification.

Case 5: Pseudo-aortic stenosis. A 76-year-old man was referred for further evaluation of progressive dyspnea on exertion and decline in his LV function. His medical history is notable for hypertension, hyperlipidemia, CAD status postcoronary artery bypass grafting (left internal mammary artery [LIMA] to LAD, saphenous vein graft [SVG] to OM1, and SVG to posterior descending artery [PDA]), and aortic stenosis. Over the past 6 months, he has noted progressive shortness of breath with his daily activities and as a result had been hospitalized several times for decompensated heart failure. During his most recent hospitalization, his EF was noted to be 25% from a baseline of 50%, with mildly calcified aortic valve with peak gradient 36 mm Hg, mean gradient 20 mm Hg, AVA of 0.9 cm^2, and no AI. Given concern for significant distal left main trunk stenosis, the patient was taken to the cardiac catheterization laboratory for further assessment of his CAD, as well as hemodynamic evaluation of his aortic stenosis. After demonstrating a fractional flow reserve of 0.93 across the distal left main stenosis, simultaneous LV–aortic pressures were obtained using a dual-lumen pigtail catheter both at rest and with up to 20 mcg/kg/min of dobutamine, with the results as shown in Figure 22.5.

	Rest	Dobutamine 20 mcg/kg/min
Cardiac output (L/min)	3.5	7.0
Heart rate (bpm)	80	91
SEP (msec)	26	22
Mean gradient (mm Hg)	17	30

Using the above data,

$$AVArest = \frac{3500/(80 \times 0.26)}{44.3 \times 1.0 \times \sqrt{17}} = 0.9\ cm^2$$

$$AVAstress = \frac{7000/(91 \times 0.22)}{44.3 \times 1.0 \times \sqrt{30}} = 1.4\ cm^2$$

FIGURE 22.5

KEY PEARLS

- This example highlights the propensity of the Gorlin equation to underestimate true AVA in low-flow states.
- Inspection of the degree of aortic valve calcification as well as the response of the mean pressure gradient and AVA following dobutamine challenge can help elucidate if true versus pseudo-aortic stenosis is present. In patients with pseudo-aortic stenosis, as contractility is augmented, the aortic valve opens more fully, and AVA increases.
- This is of great importance, as AVR or TAVR would not be of clinical utility given that the LV dysfunction is not related to AS.

Case 6: Severe aortic stenosis with mechanical mitral and aortic valves. A 57-year-old woman was referred for further management of progressive dyspnea on exertion and lower extremity edema. Her medical history is notable for rheumatic valvular disease with severe mitral and aortic stenosis status postmitral and aortic valve replacement with mechanical valves. Transthoracic echocardiogram and TEE were done and demonstrated EF of 35% with elevated gradients across the aortic valve suggestive of severe prosthetic aortic stenosis, albeit limited by poor visualization of the valve. In order to further investigate this, the patient was taken to the cardiac catheterization laboratory for fluoroscopic assessment of the aortic valve with the results demonstrated in Figure 22.6. The aortic valve is a bileaflet valve, and an opening angle of 35 degrees is very abnormal. Opening angles for bileaflet valves are usually in the range of 80 to 85 degrees.

Opening angle (degrees)	38
Closing angle (degrees)	138

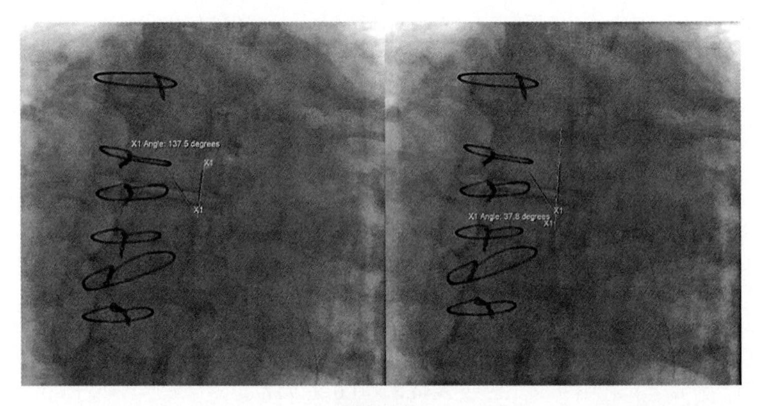

FIGURE 22.6

KEY PEARLS

- Direct LV cannulation by standard means is not feasible in the presence of concomitant mechanical aortic and mitral prostheses. In this scenario, directly measuring opening and closing valve angles using fluoroscopy and comparing the results to published values can confirm a diagnosis of severe prosthetic AS. In extraordinarily rare circumstances where the degree of AS is still in doubt after all other methods, LVEDP can be directly measured by apical puncture.
- When making these measurements, it is critical to image in a plane perpendicular to valve opening and closing.

Case 7: Patient–prosthesis mismatch. A 69-year-old woman was referred for further management of progressive chest pain and shortness of breath. Her medical history is notable for prior bioprosthetic AVR in 2002 due to severe AS with redo AVR in 2011 using a 19-mm bioprosthesis, CAD status postcoronary artery bypass grafting (LIMA to LAD and SVG to PDA) with subsequent DES placement to proximal right coronary artery (RCA), and interstitial lung disease due to asbestosis. Transthoracic echocardiogram demonstrated EF of 40% and prosthetic aortic valve with peak gradient 38 mm Hg, mean gradient 24 mm Hg, and 1+ AI. Due to her chest pain, a coronary angiogram was performed and demonstrated patent LIMA to LAD and no obstructive disease in the RCA or left circumflex artery. Simultaneous LV–aortic pressure gradients were obtained using a dual-lumen pigtail catheter both at rest and following infusion of up to 20 mcg/kg/min of dobutamine, with the results as shown in Figure 22.7. Of note, the BSA was 2.0 m^2.

	Rest	**Dobutamine 20 mcg/kg/min**
Cardiac output (L/min)	3.7	6.8
Heart rate (bpm)	80	94
SEP (msec)	21	23
Mean gradient (mm Hg)	25	65

Using the above data,

$$AVA_{rest} = \frac{3700/(80 \times 0.21)}{44.3 \times 1.0 \times \sqrt{25}} = 1.0 \text{ cm}^2$$

$$AVA_{stress} = \frac{6800/(94 \times 0.23)}{44.3 \times 1.0 \times \sqrt{65}} = 0.9 \text{ cm}^2$$

FIGURE 22.7

KEY PEARLS

- Although the above invasive data would support a diagnosis of severe low-flow low-gradient AS, it is important to consider alternate explanations for the presence of elevated transvalvular gradients.
- Patient–prosthesis mismatch (PPM) occurs when the effective orifice area (EOA) of the valve is too small relative to the patient's body size, which results in abnormally elevated pressure gradients across the prosthetic valve. An indexed EOA can be calculated by dividing EOA by the patient's body surface area. The thresholds for mild, moderate, and severe PPM are >0.85 cm^2/m^2, between 0.85 cm^2/m^2 and 0.65 cm^2/m^2, and <0.65 cm^2/m^2, respectively. Especially prone to this phenomenon are 19 mm valves. In patients with a small aortic root, clinically significant PPM can be avoided by either using a stentless valve or performing an aortic root enlargement.
- Given concern for PPM, the patient subsequently underwent a TEE, which was notable for mildly calcified aortic valve leaflets that appeared to be opening well. By planimetry, AVA was calculated at 1.2 cm^2 with an indexed value of 0.6 cm^2/m^2. Taken together, the elevated gradients were thought to be due to severe PPM.

Case 8: Severe aortic stenosis with severe AR. A 73-year-old woman presented for further evaluation of worsening shortness of breath and fatigue. Her medical history is notable for Hodgkin lymphoma with prior chest wall radiation, CAD status postcoronary artery bypass grafting (LIMA to LAD, SVG to OM1, and SVG to PDA), and severe COPD requiring continuous O_2 at 5 L/min. Transthoracic echocardiogram demonstrated EF of 60% and a heavily calcified aortic valve with peak gradient 64 mm Hg, mean gradient 43 mm Hg, AVA of 0.9 cm^2, and 4+ central AI. AVA by direct planimetry on TEE was 0.8 cm^2. Because the patient was not deemed to be a surgical candidate, she was brought to the cardiac catheterization laboratory for transcatheter AVR. Baseline hemodynamics before valve deployment are as shown in Figure 22.8.

Fick CO (L/min)	3.5
Mean LV–aortic gradient (mm Hg)	45
HR (beats/min)	75
SEP (msec)	0.25

Using the above data,

$$AVA = \frac{3500/(75 \times 0.25)}{44.3 \times 1.0 \times \sqrt{45}} = 0.6\ cm^2$$

FIGURE 22.8

KEY PEARLS

- Although the noninvasive data clearly demonstrate severe AS/AI and thereby establish an indication for intervention, the baseline data here are shown as they demonstrate the limitation of the Gorlin equation in assessing patients with concomitant stenosis and regurgitation.
- Assessment of cardiac output by either thermodilution or Fick, in patients with severe AS and concomitant AI or MR will not take into account the regurgitant flow. This will lead to an underestimation of true systolic flow, and therefore AVA.

Case 9: Balloon aortic valvuloplasty. An 88-year-old man was admitted to the hospital with acute on chronic LV diastolic heart failure complicated by acute hypoxemic respiratory failure and acute on chronic renal insufficiency. His medical history is notable for CAD with prior PCI to the LAD, chronic kidney disease, COPD with an FEV1 of 1.0 L, and severe aortic stenosis. Transthoracic echocardiogram demonstrated an EF of 55% and a heavily calcified aortic valve with peak gradient 110 mm Hg, mean gradient 64 mm Hg, AVA of 0.5 cm^2, and trace AI. After several days of aggressive intravenous diuresis and treatment with sodium nitroprusside, the patient's respiratory status improved and his renal function returned to baseline. He was subsequently taken to the cardiac catheterization lab for balloon aortic valvuloplasty with the preprocedure and postprocedure hemodynamics shown in Figure 22.9.

	Preprocedure	Postprocedure
Cardiac output (L/min)	4.0	5.5
Peak-to-peak gradient (mm Hg)	60	25
LVEDP (mm Hg)	25	21
Central aortic diastolic BP (mm Hg)	70	73

Using the above data,

$$AVA_{pre} = \frac{4.0}{\sqrt{60}} = 0.5\ \text{cm}^2$$

$$AVA_{post} = \frac{5.5}{\sqrt{25}} = 1.1\ \text{cm}^2$$

FIGURE 22.9

KEY PEARLS

- Given its accuracy and ease of use, the Hakki equation is often used as a method to quickly calculate valve area in the procedural setting.
- Although traditionally the use of mean gradient is advocated when performing calculations with the Gorlin equation, calculated AVA was demonstrated to be reasonably accurate whether peak-to-peak or mean gradients were used.
- Caution must be exercised in patients with tachycardia, as the assumptions built into the derivation of the Hakki equation may be compromised at faster heart rates.

Case 10: Severe paravalvular AI. An 87-year-old man was referred for further evaluation of worsening dyspnea on exertion and fatigue. His medical history is notable for hypertension, CAD with prior coronary artery bypass grafting (LIMA to LAD and SVG to RCA), and chronic kidney disease with a baseline creatinine of 2.0 mg/dL. Transthoracic echocardiogram demonstrated an EF of 55% and severe AS with mean gradient of 56 mm Hg and AVA of 0.7 cm^2. The patient was subsequently referred for TAVR. Following valve deployment, the patient was noted to have a wide pulse pressure and at least moderate AI on aortography. TEE demonstrated a very eccentric posterior jet of AI, which appeared to be 2 to 3+ in severity. Hemodynamics are shown in Figure 22.10.

BP (mm Hg)	110/40
LVEDP (mm Hg)	30

Using the above data,

$$\text{AR index} = \frac{40 - 30}{110} \times 100 = 9$$

FIGURE 22.10

Based on the aggregate data, the patient was determined to have severe paravalvular AI. This persisted despite serial balloon dilations, and he thus underwent prompt valve-in-valve TAVR with reduction of the AI to trivial in severity.

KEY PEARLS

- Determination of AI severity in the procedural setting can be complex and currently relies on integration of hemodynamic data, aortography, as well as assessment by TEE.
- When the degree of AR is unclear using the routine methods of assessment, the AR index can be useful to help clarify this question. As the severity of AI increases, the AR index decreases.
- The AR index also carries prognostic importance independent of AI severity, with an AR index <25 being associated with increased 1-year mortality among patients undergoing TAVR.

B. Mitral valve

Case 11: Balloon mitral valvuloplasty. A 65-year-old woman presented for further evaluation of progressive shortness of breath. Her medical history is notable for rheumatic mitral valve stenosis s/p closed mitral commissurotomy and severe restrictive lung disease. She was recently hospitalized for new-onset atrial fibrillation, which required urgent direct current cardioversion. Transthoracic echocardiogram confirms an EF of 60%, severe rheumatic mitral stenosis with peak gradient 26 mm Hg, mean gradient 11 mm Hg, 1+ MR, and Wilkins echo score of 6. She was subsequently taken to the cardiac catheterization laboratory for balloon mitral valvotomy (BMV). Hemodynamics before and after the procedure are noted in Figure 22.11.

	Preprocedure	Postprocedure
Cardiac output (L/min)	3.0	3.5
Heart rate (bpm)	65	65
DFP (msec)	35	34
Mean gradient (mm Hg)	14	3

Using the above data,

$$MVA_{pre} = \frac{3000/(65 \times 0.35)}{44.3 \times 0.85 \times \sqrt{14}} = 1.0 \text{ cm}^2$$

$$MVA_{post} = \frac{3500/(65 \times 0.34)}{44.3 \times 0.85 \times \sqrt{3}} = 2.4 \text{ cm}^2$$

FIGURE 22.11

KEY PEARLS

- Prior to a BMV, a TEE is essential to exclude the presence of a LA thrombus and >2+ MR, both of which would be contraindications to the procedure.
- Phasic delay in the PCWP "v" wave may lead to error when measuring mean mitral valve gradient. This is especially pertinent to patients with prosthetic mitral valves, in whom the use of PCWP may lead to significant underestimation of MVA.
- In addition to a hemodynamic assessment, observation for fluoroscopically visible calcification is important. In a study of 328 patients with severe mitral stenosis undergoing BMV at Massachusetts General Hospital, a successful procedural outcome (defined as MVA >1.5 cm^2 without significant MR or right-to-left shunting) was achieved in 62% of patients without, and 52% of patients with mitral valve calcification (33% and 35% with 3+ and 4+ calcification, respectively). Event-free survival at 2 years was also worse in patients with mitral valve calcification compared to without calcification (63% vs. 88%), and became more pronounced with greater degrees of calcification.

Case 12: Severe mitral regurgitation. An 82-year-old man was referred for further management of dyspnea. His medical history is notable for CAD with prior coronary artery bypass grafting (LIMA to diagonal and right internal mammary artery to left circumflex). He has noted progressive dyspnea over the past year. Transthoracic echocardiogram and TEE demonstrated EF of 50% with 3+ MR. Cardiac catheterization demonstrated patent grafts. Left ventriculography was performed and RF was calculated using the hemodynamics in Figure 22.12.

Fick CO (L/min)	3.5
TSV (mL/beat)	118
HR (beats/min)	85

Using the above data,

$$RF = \frac{118 - 41}{118} \times 100 = 65\%$$

FIGURE 22.12

Owing to the patient's advanced age and prior sternotomy, he was deemed to be high risk for surgery and was referred for percutaneous mitral valve repair. Following the placement of a mitral clip, the MR was shown to decrease to 2+.

KEY PEARLS

- In order to obtain accurate estimation of end-systolic and end-diastolic volumes, the patient must be in sinus rhythm without a significant amount of ectopy, as variations in R–R interval can compromise the integrity of this calculation.
- The presence of a RF >60% confirms the diagnosis of severe MR. Although this calculation carries historical importance, it is rarely used today in clinical practice.
- The presence of large "v" waves on either a LA or PCWP tracing is another ancillary hemodynamic finding in patients with severe MR. If present, one would expect it to improve after intervention. (See Chapter 23, Figures 23.14 and 23.15 in the *Atlas of Hemodynamic Tracings* for the representative hemodynamic waveforms.)

C. **Tricuspid valve**

Case 13: Severe prosthetic tricuspid stenosis. A 65-year-old man was admitted with acute on chronic right ventricular systolic heart failure. Due to morbid obesity and significant respiratory variation, accurate gradients could not be obtained on transthoracic echocardiogram, though there was suspicion for severe tricuspid stenosis. As such, he was brought to the cardiac catheterization laboratory, where simultaneous RA–RV (right atrium–right ventricle) pressures were obtained using a dual-lumen pigtail catheter. Hemodynamic results are shown in Figure 22.13.

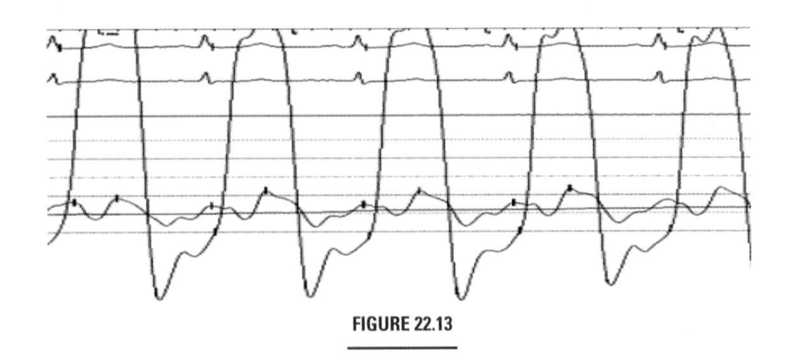

FIGURE 22.13

Mean RA–RV gradient was determined to be 9 mm Hg. The patient subsequently underwent transcatheter tricuspid valve replacement.

KEY PEARL

- Invasive assessment of tricuspid stenosis involves assessment of a simultaneous RA-to-RV mean pressure gradient. Assessment of tricuspid valve area via the Gorlin equation is not routinely done. A mean gradient >5 to 10 mm Hg usually signifies severe tricuspid stenosis.

D. **Pulmonic valve**

Case 14: Severe pulmonic stenosis with severe pulmonic insufficiency. A 43-year-old woman was referred for further management of dyspnea and palpitations. Her medical history is notable for complex congenital heart disease including congenital pulmonic stenosis, atrial septal defect (ASD), and PDA for which she underwent pulmonary valvotomy, ASD closure, and PDA ligation as a child, with subsequent pulmonary homograft placement due to valvular degeneration with severe pulmonic insufficiency. She also required mechanical AVR and aortic root replacement in the setting of severe AI and aortic aneurysm. Transthoracic echocardiogram demonstrated mildly decreased right ventricular systolic function, as well as severe pulmonic stenosis and 2+ pulmonic insufficiency. She was subsequently taken to the cardiac catheterization where peak and mean gradients across the pulmonic valve were 85 and 52 mm Hg, respectively. Pulmonary angiogram is shown in Figure 22.14.

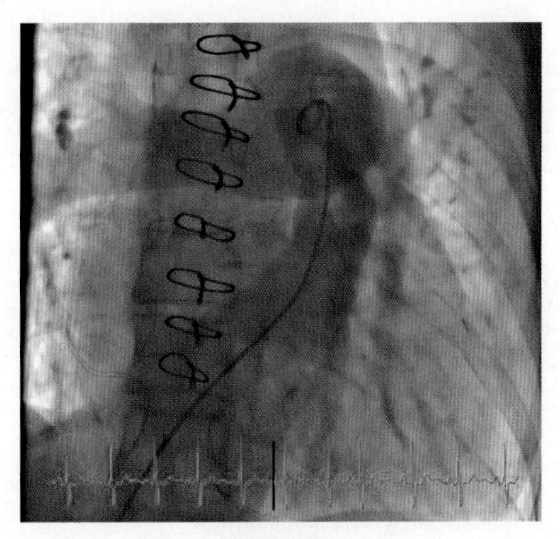

FIGURE 22.14

KEY PEARL

- The assessment of the degree of pulmonic stenosis and regurgitation can be made both with the use of pulmonary angiography and through the measurement of pressure gradients. A mean gradient >50 mm Hg, as seen in this patient, is considered to be severe. The degree of pulmonic regurgitation is graded according to visual assessment. Assessment of valve area and the use of RFs are not routinely done in clinical practice.

IX. CONCLUSION

Although the evaluation of patients with valvular heart disease is often done using noninvasive imaging modalities, there are several scenarios in which an invasive hemodynamic study can be of particular benefit. A thorough understanding of when to pursue cardiac catheterization in this patient population as well as the relative strengths and limitations is of critical importance to those who care for patients with advanced valvular disease.

SUGGESTED READINGS

Bache RJ, Wang Y, Jorgensen CR. Hemodynamic effects of exercise in isolated valvular aortic stenosis. *Circulation.* 1971;44:1003–1013.

Bugan B, Kapadia S, Svensson L, et al. Novel hemodynamic index for assessment of aortic regurgitation after transcatheter aortic valve replacement. *Catheter Cardiovasc Interv.* 2015;86:E174–E179.

Burwash IG, Thomas DD, Sadahiro M, et al. Dependence of Gorlin formula and continuity equation valve areas on transvalvular volume flow rate in valvular aortic stenosis. *Circulation.* 1994;89:827–835.

Carabello BA, Barry WH, Grossman W. Changes in arterial pressure during left heart pullback in patients with aortic stenosis: a sign of severe aortic stenosis. *Am J Cardiol.* 1979;44:424–427.

Folland ED, Parisi AF, Carbone C. Is peripheral arterial pressure a satisfactory substitute for ascending aortic pressure when measuring aortic valve gradients? *J Am Coll Cardiol.* 1984;4:1207–1212.

Galan A, Zoghbi WA, Quiñones MA. Determination of severity of valvular aortic stenosis by Doppler echocardiography and relation of findings to clinical outcome and agreement with hemodynamic measurements determined at cardiac catheterization. *Am J Cardiol.* 1991;67:1007–1012.

Gorlin R, Gorlin SG. Hydraulic formula for calculation of the area of the stenotic mitral valve, other cardiac valves, and central circulatory shunts. I. *Am Heart J.* 1951;41:1–29.
Hakki AH, Iskandrian AS, Bemis CE, et al. A simplified valve formula for the calculation of stenotic cardiac valve areas. *Circulation.* 1981;63:1050–1055.
Herrmann HC, Pibarot P, Hueter I, et al. Predictors of mortality and outcomes of therapy in low-flow severe aortic stenosis: a Placement of Aortic Transcatheter Valves (PARTNER) trial analysis. *Circulation.* 2013;127:2316–2326.
Monin JL, Quéré JP, Monchi M, et al. Low-gradient aortic stenosis: operative risk stratification and predictors for long-term outcome: a multicenter study using dobutamine stress hemodynamics. *Circulation.* 2003;108:319–324.
Nishimura RA, Grantham JA, Connolly HM, et al. Low-output, low-gradient aortic stenosis in patients with depressed left ventricular systolic function: the clinical utility of the dobutamine challenge in the catheterization laboratory. *Circulation.* 2002;106:809–813.
Nishimura RA, Otto CM, Bonow RO, et al. 2014 AHA/ACC guideline for the management of patients with valvular heart disease: a report of the American College of Cardiology/American Heart Association Task Force on Practice Guidelines. *J Am Coll Cardiol.* 2014;63:e57–e185.
Nishimura RA, Rihal CS, Tajik AJ, et al. Accurate measurement of the transmitral gradient in patients with mitral stenosis: a simultaneous catheterization and Doppler echocardiographic study. *J Am Coll Cardiol.* 1994;24:152–158.
Oh JK1, Taliercio CP, Holmes DR Jr, et al. Prediction of the severity of aortic stenosis by Doppler aortic valve area determination: prospective Doppler-catheterization correlation in 100 patients. *J Am Coll Cardiol.* 1988;11:1227–1234.
Schoenfeld MH, Palacios IF, Hutter AM Jr, et al. Underestimation of prosthetic mitral valve areas: role of transseptal catheterization in avoiding unnecessary repeat mitral valve surgery. *J Am Coll Cardiol.* 1985;5:1387–1392.
Sellers RD, Levy MJ, Amplatz K, et al. Left retrograde cardioangiography in acquired cardiac disease: technic, indications, and interpretations in 700 cases. *Am J Cardiol.* 1964;14:437–447.
Sinning J, Hammerstingl C, Vasa-Nicotera M, et al. Aortic regurgitation index defines severity of peri-prosthetic regurgitation and predicts outcome in patients after transcatheter aortic valve implantation. *J Am Coll Cardiol.* 2012;59:1134–1141.
Tuzcu EM, Block PC, Griffin B, et al. Percutaneous mitral balloon valvotomy in patients with calcific mitral stenosis: immediate and long-term outcome. *J Am Coll Cardiol.* 1994;23:1604–1609.

KEY REVIEWS

Carabello BA. Advances in the hemodynamic assessment of stenotic cardiac valves. *J Am Coll Cardiol.* 1987;10:912–919.
Nishimura RA, Carabello BA. Hemodynamics in the cardiac catheterization laboratory of the 21st century. *Circulation.* 2012;125:2138–2150.

RELEVANT BOOK CHAPTERS

Carabello BA, Grossman W. Calculation of stenotic valve orifice area. In: Moscucci M, ed. *Grossman & Baim's Cardiac Catheterization, Angiography, and Intervention.* 8th ed. Philadelphia, PA: Lippincott Williams & Wilkins; 2014:272–283.
Ragosta M. Aortic valve disease. In: Ragosta M, ed. *Textbook of Clinical Hemodynamics.* Philadelphia, PA: WB Saunders Elsevier; 2008:68–90.
Ragosta M. Mitral valve disorders. In: Ragosta M, ed. *Textbook of Clinical Hemodynamics.* Philadelphia, PA: WB Saunders Elsevier; 2008:50–67.

SECTION VI

Atlas of Cardiac Catheterization Laboratory Hemodynamics

CHAPTER 23

Andrew L. Goodman

Atlas of Hemodynamic Tracings

I. INTRODUCTION

The first human cardiac catheterization is credited to Werner Forssmann who performed a right heart self-catheterization in 1929. Over the next 50 years, invasive hemodynamic assessment in the cardiac catheterization laboratory provided critical clinical data for the management of patients with structural heart disease. During the 1980s, the improvement in two-dimensional echocardiography and Doppler echocardiography allowed for a noninvasive assessment of patients with structural heart disease and shifted the evaluation of these patients from the catheterization laboratory to the echocardiography laboratory. However, it is important to note that despite the advances in echocardiography, there are inherent limitations to noninvasive hemodynamic assessment. Current guideline recommendations suggest that hemodynamic assessment in the catheterization laboratory be performed when noninvasive assessment is inconclusive or when there is a discrepancy between the severity of a patient's symptoms and noninvasive testing. With the evolution of structural heart disease percutaneous intervention in the catheterization laboratory (transcatheter aortic valve replacement [TAVR], percutaneous mitral valve repair, balloon valvuloplasty), there has been a resurgence in the need for careful hemodynamic assessment both before and following these complex interventions. This chapter will provide a careful overview of the typical waveform tracings encountered on both right and left heart catheterization as well as typical findings encountered during percutaneous structural interventions.

II. NORMAL HEMODYNAMIC PRESSURE WAVEFORMS

See Figures 23.1 through 23.4; Table 23.1.

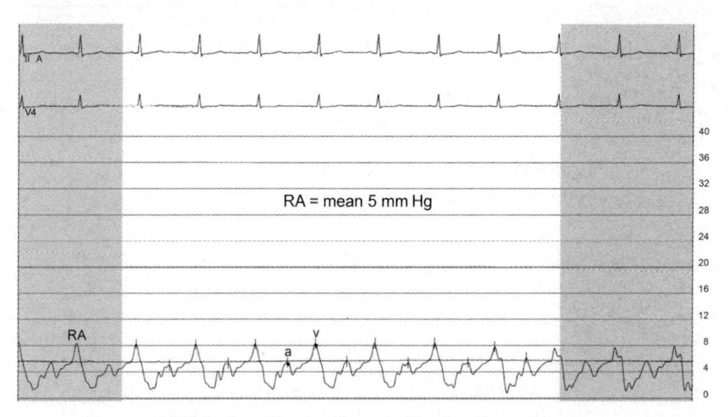

FIGURE 23.1 Normal right atrial (RA) waveform tracing.

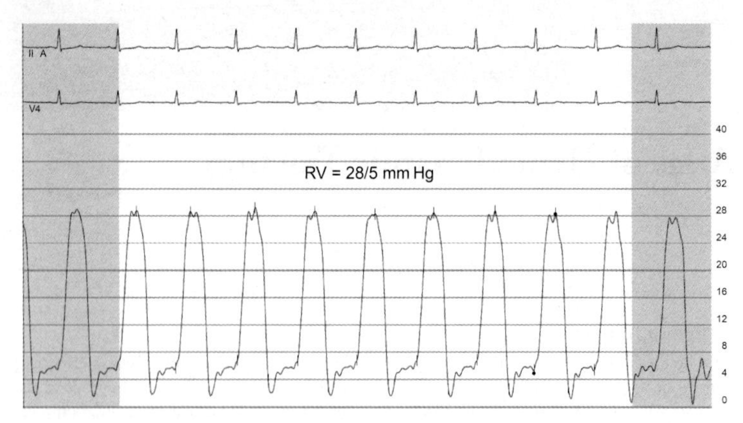

FIGURE 23.2 Normal right ventricular (RV) waveform tracing.

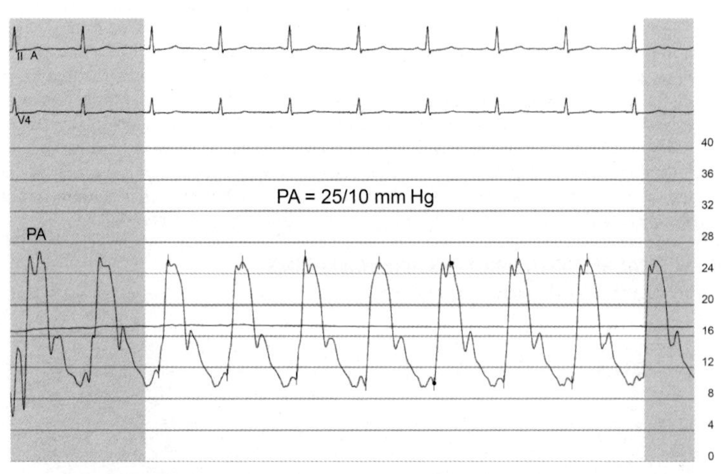

FIGURE 23.3 Normal pulmonary artery (PA) waveform tracing.

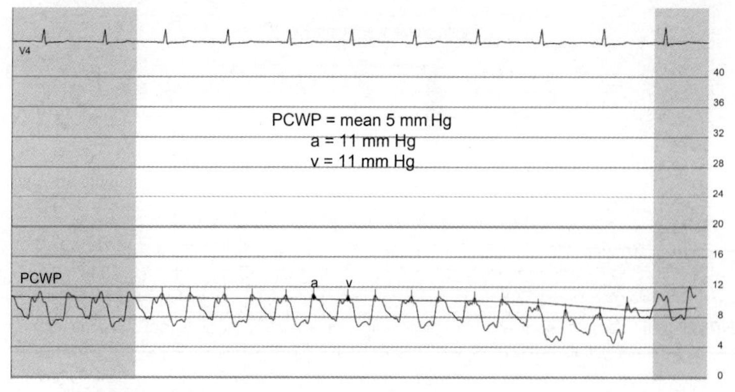

FIGURE 23.4 Normal pulmonary capillary wedge pressure (PCWP) waveform tracing.

TABLE 23.1 Normal Values

Structure/Measurement	Normal Values (mm Hg)
Right atrium	Mean: 0–9
Right ventricle	Systolic: 15–30
	Diastolic: 0–8
Pulmonary artery	Systolic: 15–30
	Diastolic: 2–12
Pulmonary capillary wedge pressure	Mean: 6–12
Left atrium	Mean: 6–12
Left ventricle	Systolic: 100–120
	Diastolic: 6–12
Aorta	Systolic: 100–120
	Diastolic: 60–80

III. VALVULAR STENOSIS

A. Aortic stenosis. Simultaneous left ventricular (LV) and ascending aorta (Ao) waveform analysis is the optimal technique to assess aortic stenosis (AS). Analysis of these waveforms allows for calculation of the peak-to-peak gradient as well as the mean transvalvular gradient. The mean gradient is the integrated gradient between the left ventricle and the Ao over the entire systolic period and is the recommended value to assess the severity of obstruction (Figs. 23.5 to 23.7).

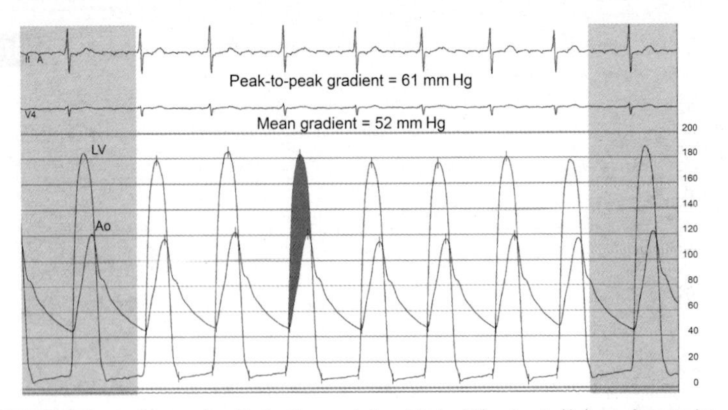

FIGURE 23.5 Aortic stenosis with simultaneous left ventricular (LV) and aorta (Ao) waveform tracing.

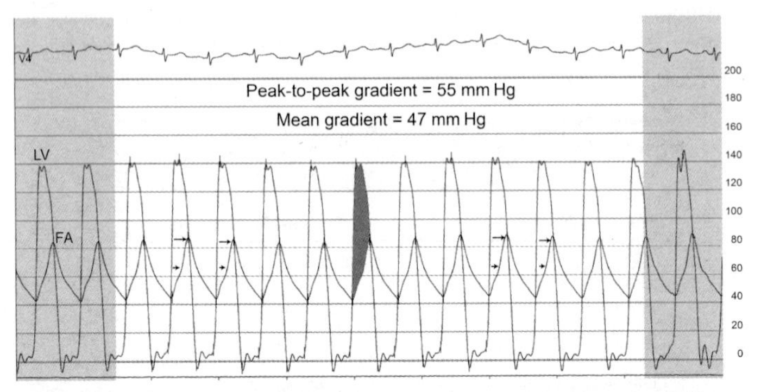

FIGURE 23.6 Aortic stenosis (AS) with simultaneous femoral artery (FA) and left ventricular (LV) waveform tracing. Note temporal delay in peak FA pressure, which may lead to false elevation in mean gradient and overestimation of AS severity.

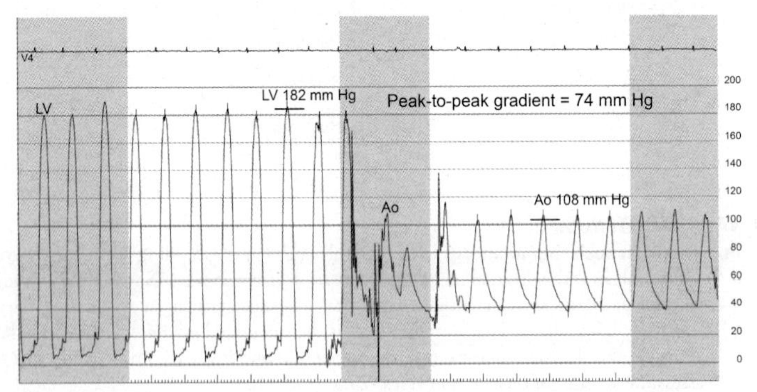

FIGURE 23.7 Aortic stenosis with pullback method from left ventricle (LV) to aorta (Ao) to calculate peak-to-peak gradient.

B. Mitral stenosis. Invasive assessment of mitral stenosis is typically performed with simultaneous LV and pulmonary capillary wedge pressure (PCWP) waveform analysis to calculate the mean transvalvular gradient. While the mean PCWP typically reflects the mean left atrial pressure, it is important to note the limitations of this approach (Figs. 23.8 and 23.9).

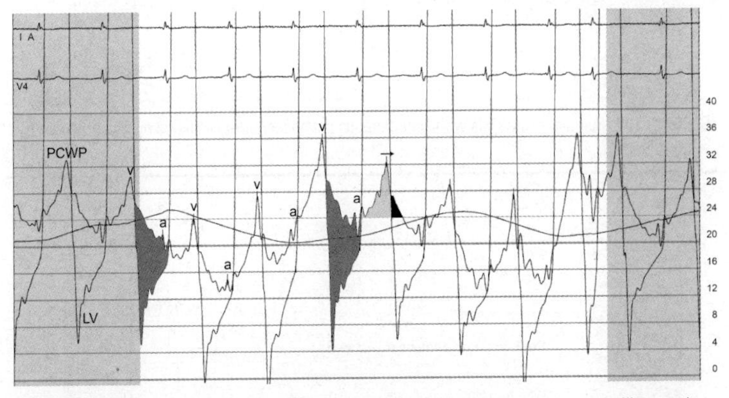

FIGURE 23.8 Mitral stenosis with simultaneous left ventricular (LV) and pulmonary capillary wedge pressure (PCWP) waveform tracing.

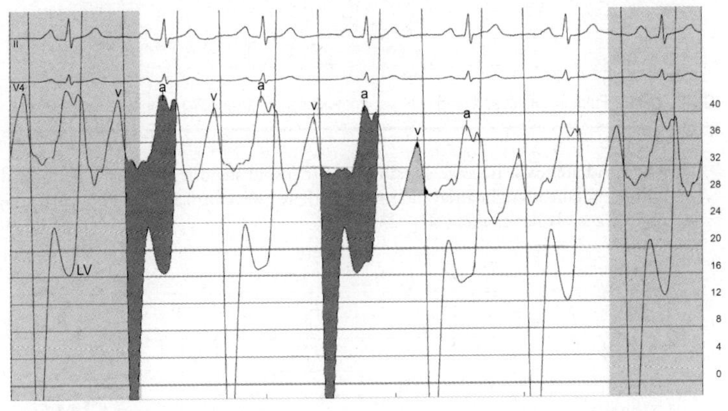

FIGURE 23.9 Mitral stenosis with simultaneous left ventricular (LV) and left atrial (LA) waveform tracing. Note the difference between using pulmonary capillary wedge pressure and LA pressure in gradient calculation given the delay in transmission of the LA pressure across the pulmonary vasculature *(shaded graphic in black seen in Figure 23.8)*. This can lead to a falsely elevated transvalvular gradient and overestimation of valve stenosis severity.

C. Pulmonic stenosis. Two-dimensional echocardiography with continuous wave Doppler examination characterizes the severity and anatomic abnormalities in cases of pulmonary stenosis. Catheter-derived transvalvular gradients are typically obtained during pulmonary valvuloplasty; the pre– and post–catheter-derived peak-to-peak gradients are measured (Figs. 23.10 and 23.11).

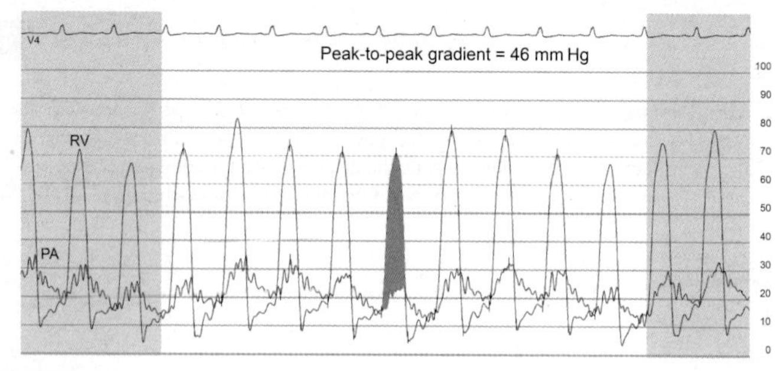

FIGURE 23.10 Pulmonary stenosis with simultaneous pulmonary artery (PA) and right ventricular (RV) waveform tracing.

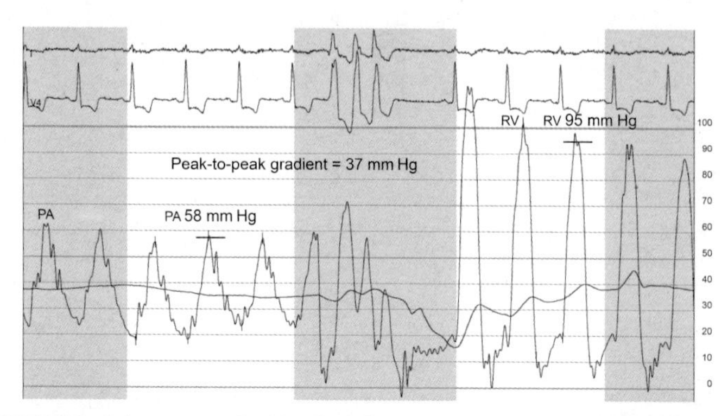

FIGURE 23.11 Pulmonary stenosis with pullback from pulmonary artery (PA) to right ventricle (RV).

D. Tricuspid stenosis. Invasive assessment of tricuspid stenosis is typically performed with simultaneous right atrial and right ventricular waveform analysis to calculate the mean transvalvular gradient (Fig. 23.12).

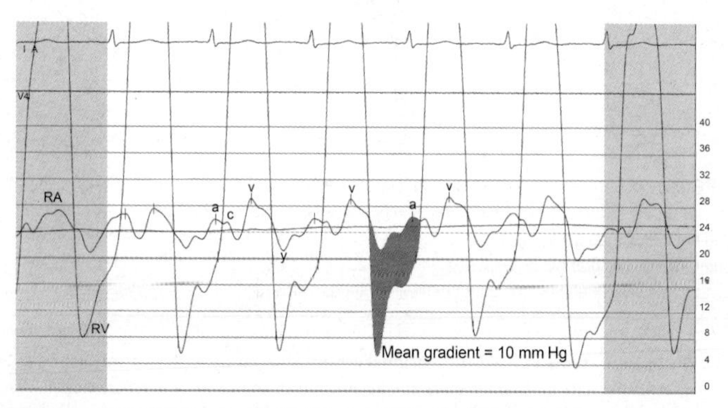

FIGURE 23.12 Tricuspid stenosis with simultaneous right atrial (RA) and right ventricular (RV) waveform tracing.

IV. VALVULAR REGURGITATION

Comprehensive evaluation of valvular regurgitation is often performed noninvasively with echocardiography before the patient's arrival to the catheterization lab. Angiography can be helpful in classifying the severity of valvular regurgitation when there is a discrepancy between the patient's symptoms and noninvasive testing. Hemodynamic evaluation is particularly useful in the periprocedural period of percutaneous structural interventions (balloon aortic valvuloplasty, TAVR, etc.).

A. Aortic regurgitation

See Figure 23.13.

B. Mitral regurgitation

See Figures 23.14 and 23.15.

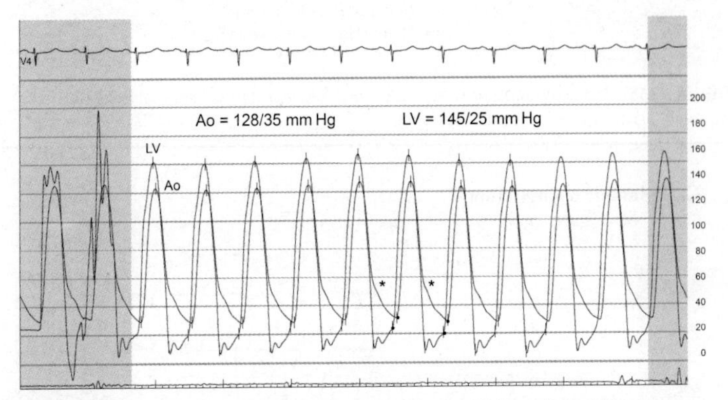

FIGURE 23.13 Severe acute aortic regurgitation with simultaneous left ventricular (LV) and aorta (Ao) waveform tracing. Note the loss of the dicrotic notch (*) on the Ao waveform, the low Ao diastolic pressure, and elevated LV end-diastolic pressure.

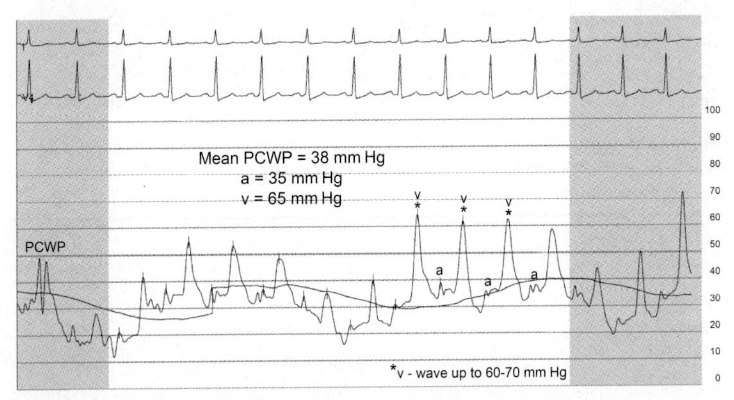

FIGURE 23.14 Mitral regurgitation with pulmonary capillary wedge pressure (PCWP) waveform tracing. Note the presence of large v-waves on the PCWP tracing.

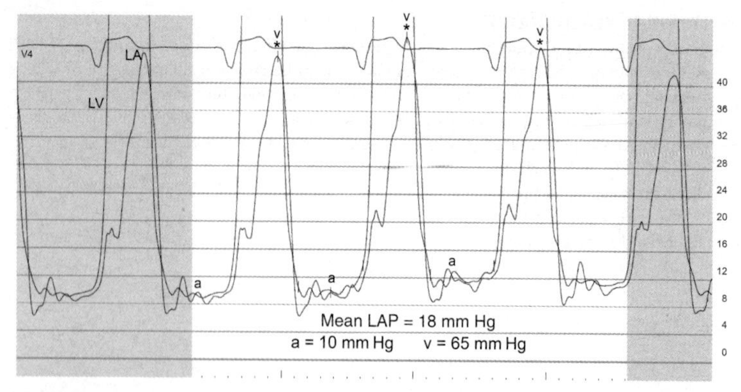

FIGURE 23.15 Mitral regurgitation with simultaneous left atrial (LA) and left ventricular (LV) waveform tracing. Large v-waves are again noted.

C. Pulmonic regurgitation

See Figure 23.16.

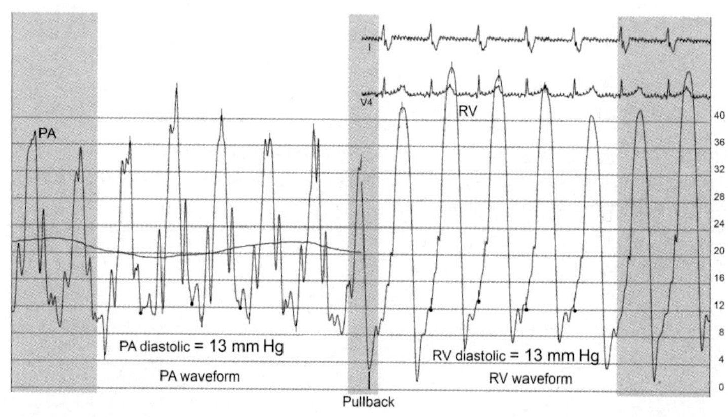

FIGURE 23.16 Pulmonic regurgitation with pullback from pulmonary artery (PA) to right ventricle (RV). Note the low PA diastolic pressure and elevation in RV end-diastolic pressure. PA and RV diastolic pressures are equalized.

D. Tricuspid regurgitation

See Figures 23.17A and B.

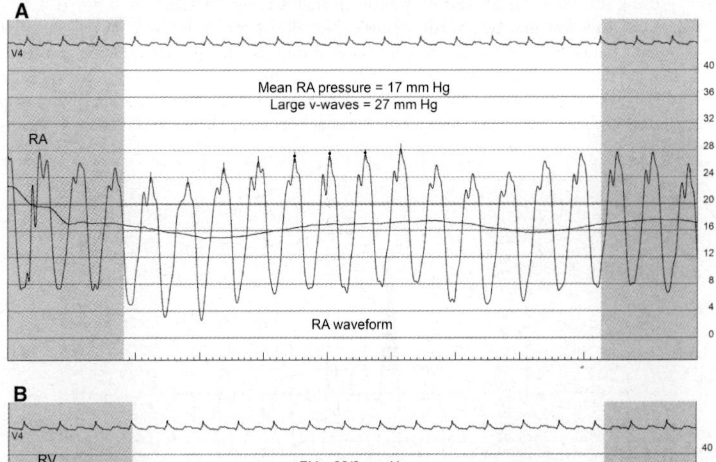

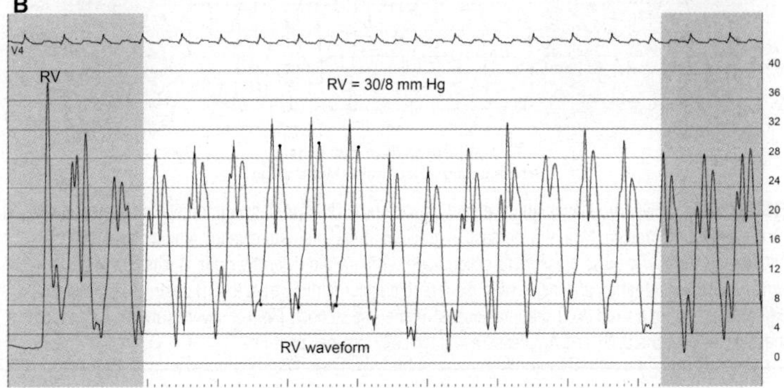

FIGURE 23.17 **A:** Tricuspid regurgitation (TR) with right atrial (RA) waveform tracing. Note the large v-waves on the RA tracing with "ventricularization" of the RA waveform. **B:** TR with right ventricular (RV) waveform tracing.

V. SPECIAL CIRCUMSTANCES

A. Hypertrophic obstructive cardiomyopathy (HOCM). HOCM is characterized by a dynamic left ventricular outflow tract (LVOT) obstruction, which can be evaluated using simultaneous LV and Ao waveform analysis (Fig. 23.18).

B. Low-flow, low-gradient aortic stenosis. Not all patients with severe AS will manifest high transvalvular gradients. In patients with impaired LV systolic function, gradients may be low (mean gradient <40 mm Hg) due to "true-AS" or "pseudo-AS," and it can be difficult to differentiate these two. Invasive assessment in the catheterization lab can help differentiate these two entities with the use of dobutamine. There is also a subset of patients

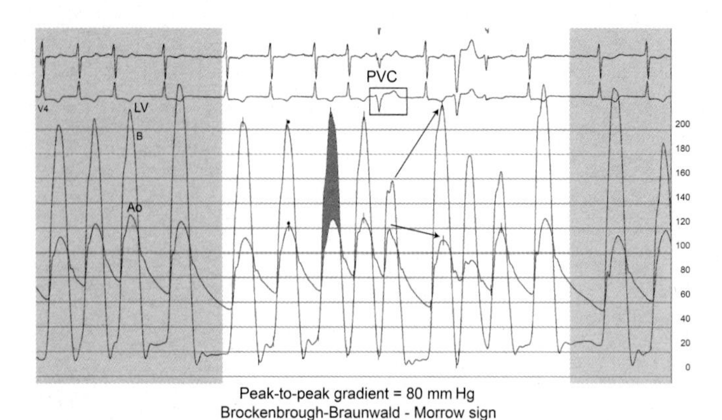

FIGURE 23.18 Hypertrophic obstructive cardiomyopathy (HOCM) with simultaneous left ventricular–aorta (LV-Ao) waveform tracing. Note the increase in gradient after a premature ventricular contraction (PVC) with a reduction in Ao pulse pressure (Brockenbrough–Braunwald–Morrow sign). This is due to post-PVC extrasystolic accentuation and increase in the left ventricular outflow tract (LVOT) obstruction. This can be differentiated from a fixed LVOT gradient (subvalvular aortic stenosis [AS]) or severe valvular AS because in these cases both the LVOT and Ao pressure will typically increase post-PVC.

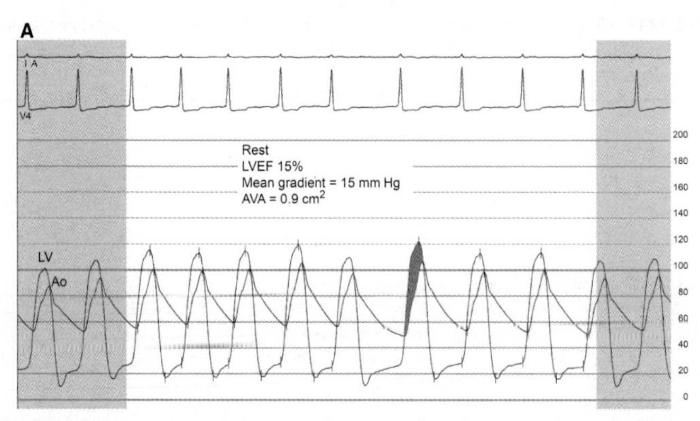

FIGURE 23.19 **A:** "Pseudo-aortic stenosis (AS)" with simultaneous left ventricular–aorta (LV-Ao) pressures before dobutamine infusion. **B:** "Pseudo-AS" with simultaneous LV-Ao pressures during dobutamine infusion. AVA, aortic valve area; LVEF, left ventricular ejection fraction.

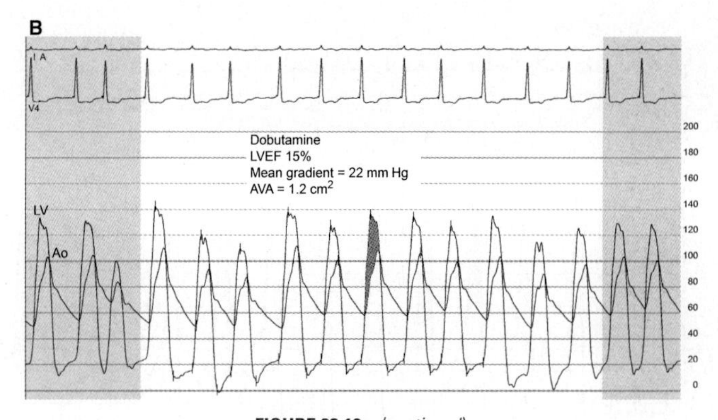

FIGURE 23.19 *(continued)*

with low-gradient AS with preserved LV systolic function due to a paradoxical low-flow state (low-flow, low-gradient [LFLG]). In some of these patients, the low-flow state may be precipitated by increased afterload, and invasive assessment with intravenous vasodilators may unmask the severity of AS (Figs. 23.19 to 23.21). Typically LFLG AS is defined as an effective orifice area $\leq$ 1.0 cm^2, mean transvalvular gradient $<$ 40 mm Hg, and a low LVEF $\leq$ 40%. Paradoxical LFLG AS refers to preserved LVEF with an SV index $<$ 35 ml/m^2.

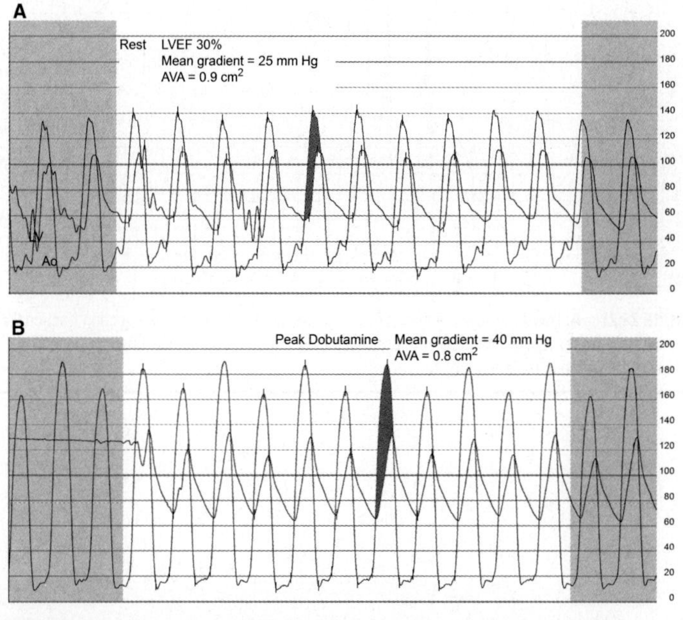

FIGURE 23.20 **A:** "True aortic stenosis (AS)" with simultaneous left ventricular–aorta (LV-Ao) pressure before dobutamine infusion. **B:** "True-AS" with simultaneous LV-Ao pressure during dobutamine infusion. AVA, aortic valve area; LVEF, left ventricular ejection fraction.

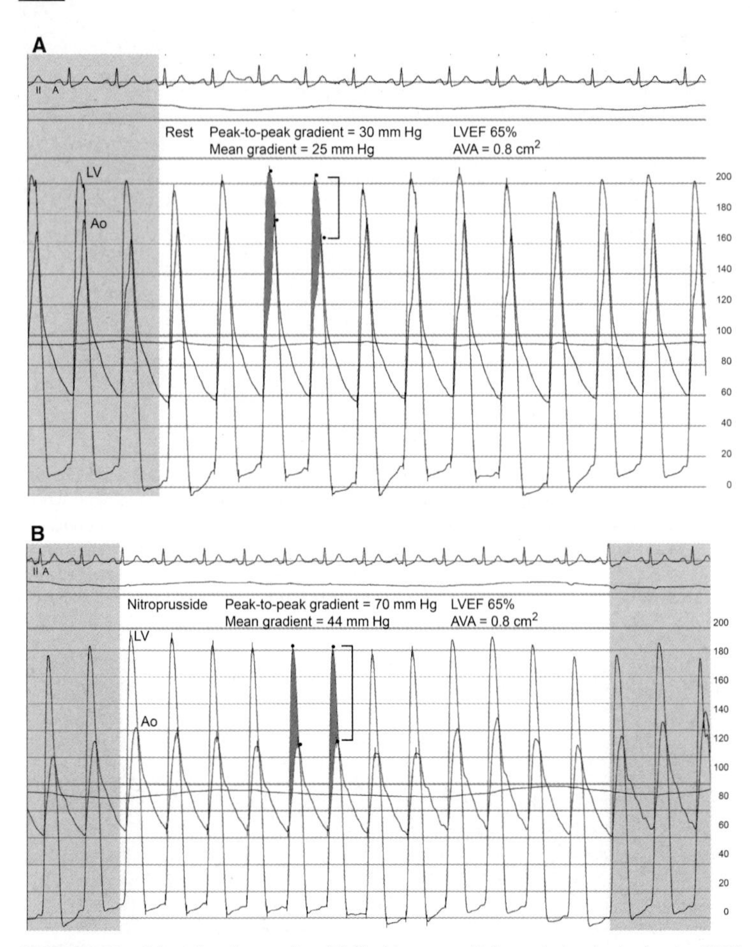

FIGURE 23.21 **A:** Low-flow, low-gradient (LFLG) with preserved left ventricular ejection fraction (LVEF) before nitroprusside infusion. **B:** LFLG with preserved LVEF during nitroprusside infusion. Ao, aorta; AVA, aortic valve area; LV, left ventricle.

VI. HEMODYNAMIC TRACINGS DURING PERCUTANEOUS STRUCTURAL INTERVENTION

A. Balloon aortic valvuloplasty

See Figures 23.22A and B.

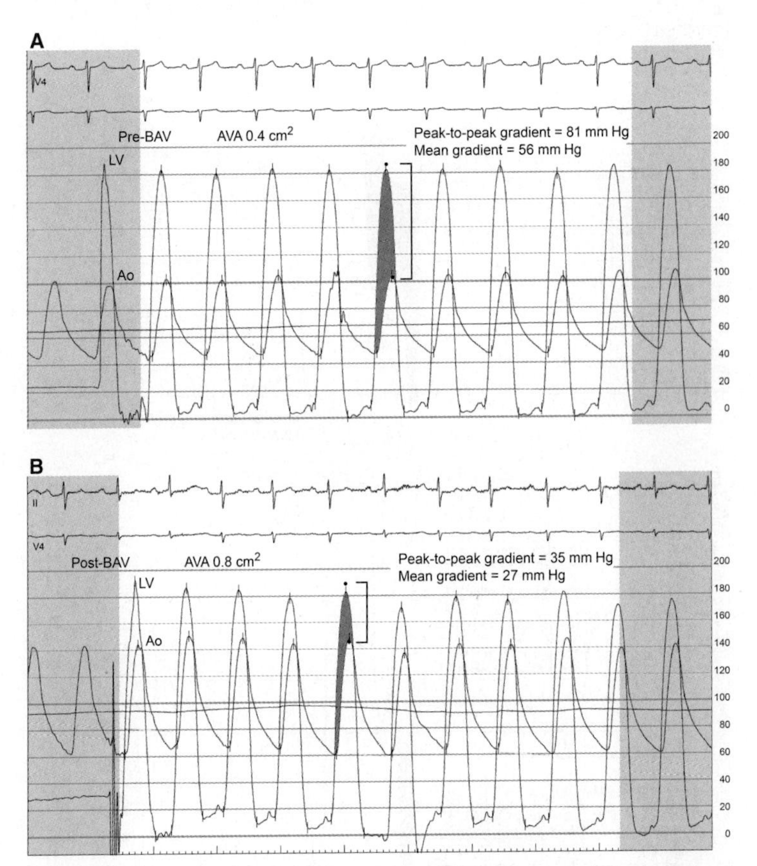

FIGURE 23.22 **A:** Simultaneous left ventricular (LV)–aorta (Ao) waveform tracing before balloon aortic valvuloplasty (BAV) showing a mean gradient of 56 mm Hg and an aortic valve area (AVA) of 0.4 cm^2. **B:** Simultaneous LV-Ao waveform tracing after BAV with a 22 mm balloon showing a decline in the mean gradient to 27 mm Hg and increase in AVA to 0.8 cm^2.

B. Balloon mitral valvuloplasty

See Figures 23.23A and B.

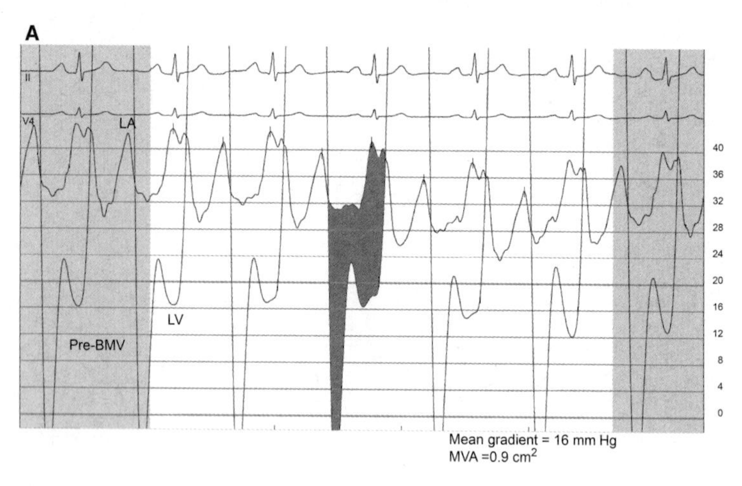

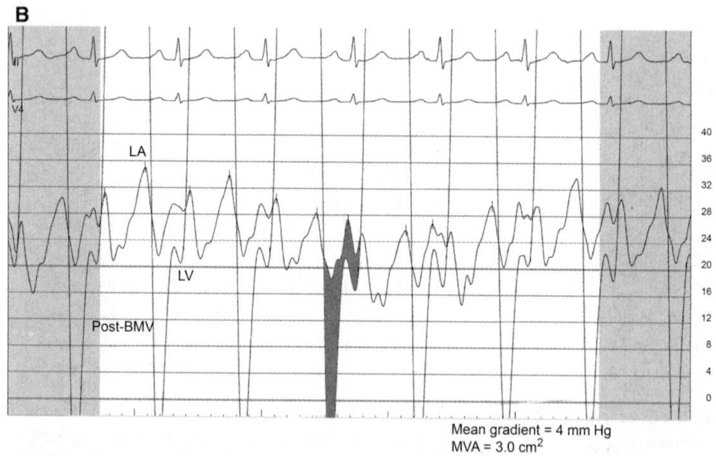

FIGURE 23.23 **A:** Simultaneous left atrial (LA)–left ventricular (LV) waveform tracing before balloon mitral valvuloplasty (BMV) showing a mean gradient of 16 mm Hg and a mitral valve area (MVA) of 0.9 cm^2. **B:** Simultaneous LA-LV waveform tracing after BMV with a 26-mm balloon showing a reduction in the mean gradient to 4 mm Hg and increase in MVA to 3.0 cm^2.

C. **Balloon pulmonary valvuloplasty**

See Figures 23.24A and B.

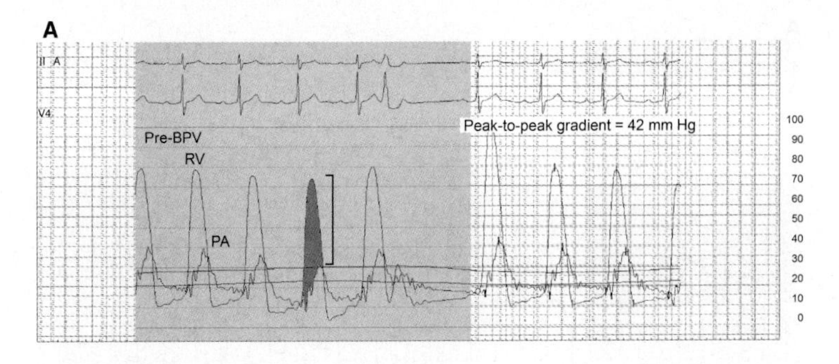

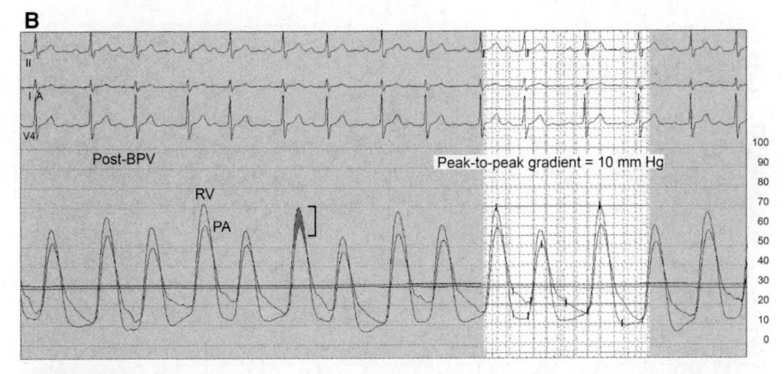

FIGURE 23.24 **A:** Simultaneous pulmonary artery (PA)–right ventricular (RV) waveform tracing before balloon pulmonary valvuloplasty (BPV) showing a peak-to-peak gradient of 42 mm Hg. **B:** Simultaneous PA-RV waveform tracing after successful BPV with a 26-mm balloon showing a reduction in the peak-to-peak gradient to 10 mm Hg.

D. Alcohol septal ablation

See Figures 23.25A and B.

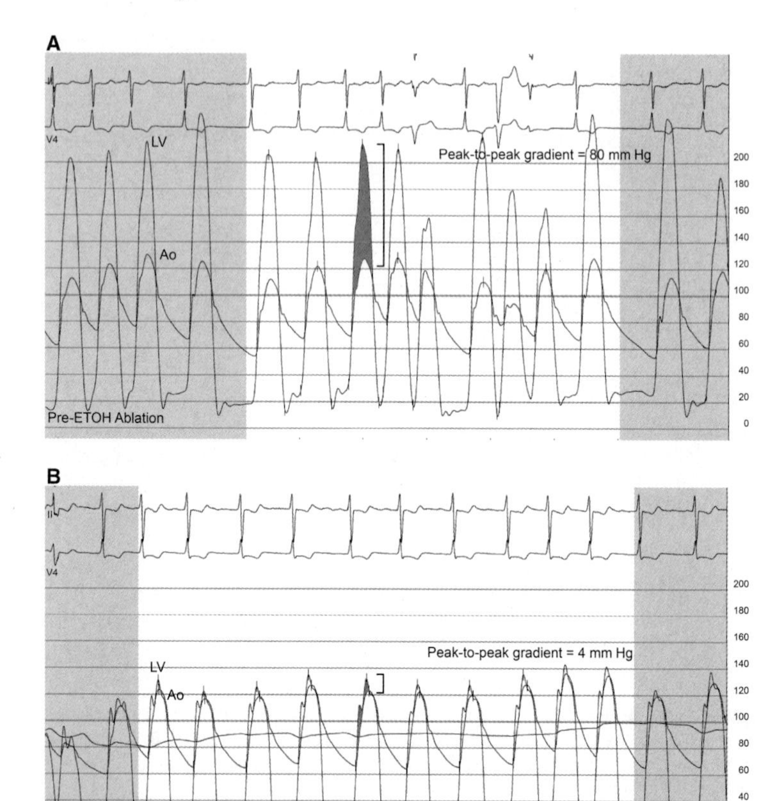

FIGURE 23.25 **A:** Simultaneous left ventricular (LV)–aorta (Ao) waveform tracing before ethyl alcohol (ETOH) septal ablation showing a dynamic peak-to-peak gradient of 80 mm Hg. **B:** Simultaneous LV-Ao waveform tracing after successful ETOH septal ablation showing a dramatic reduction in the LVOT gradient.

E. Percutaneous mitral valve repair

See Figures 23.26A and B.

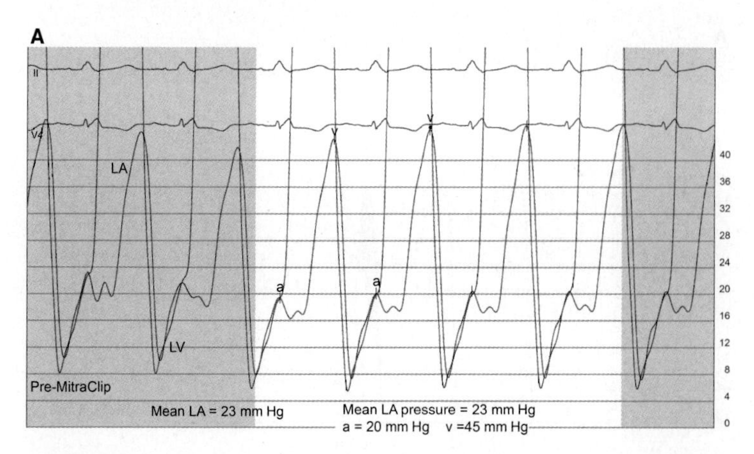

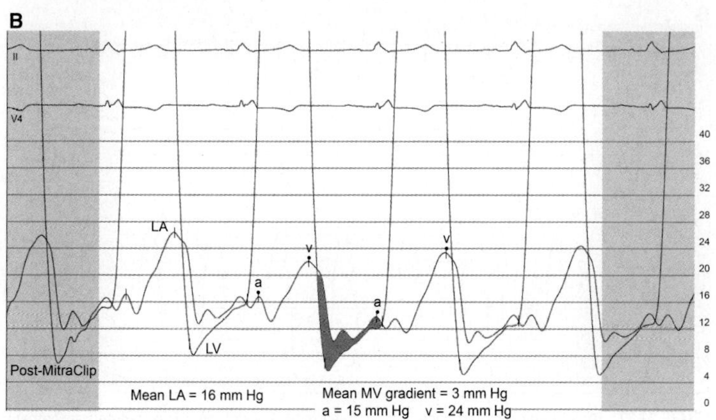

FIGURE 23.26 **A:** Simultaneous left atrial (LA)–left ventricular (LV) waveform tracing before percutaneous mitral valve repair. Note the predominant v-waves approaching 50 mm Hg. **B:** Simultaneous LA-LV waveform tracing following successful MitraClip placement. Note the dramatic reduction in the v-waves, overall reduction in LA mean pressure, and absence of a significant transmitral diastolic gradient.

F. Transcatheter aortic valve replacement

See Figures 23.27 and 23.28.

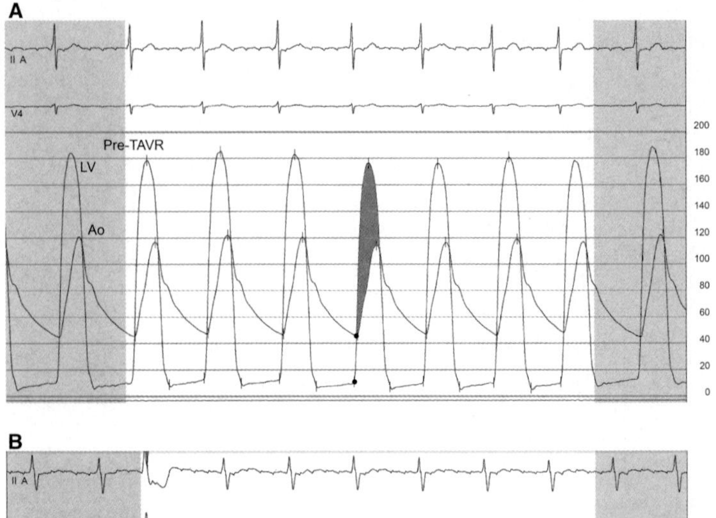

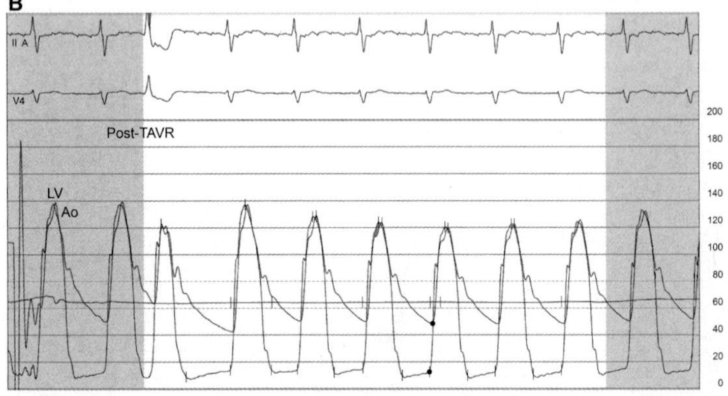

FIGURE 23.27 **A:** Simultaneous left ventricular (LV)–aorta (Ao) waveform tracing before transcatheter aortic valve replacement (TAVR) showing a mean transvalvular gradient of 52 mm Hg and aortic valve area (AVA) 0.7 cm^2. **B:** Simultaneous LV-Ao waveform tracing following successful placement of a transcatheter aortic valve. Note the absence of residual transvalvular gradient, preserved dicrotic notch on the Ao waveform, and low LV end-diastolic pressure; these are all key hemodynamic parameters to review following TAVR.

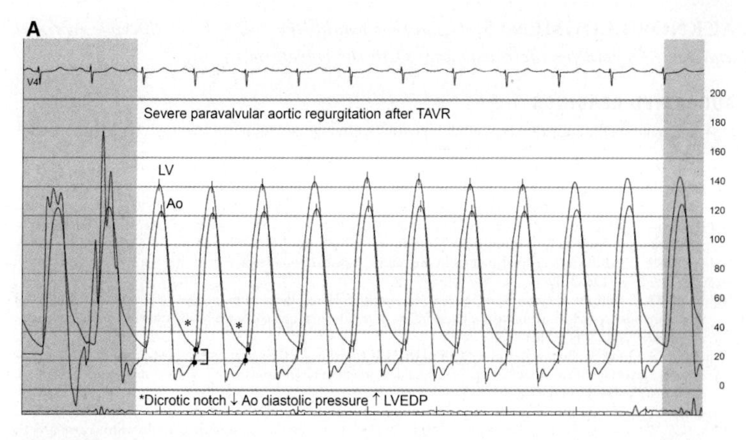

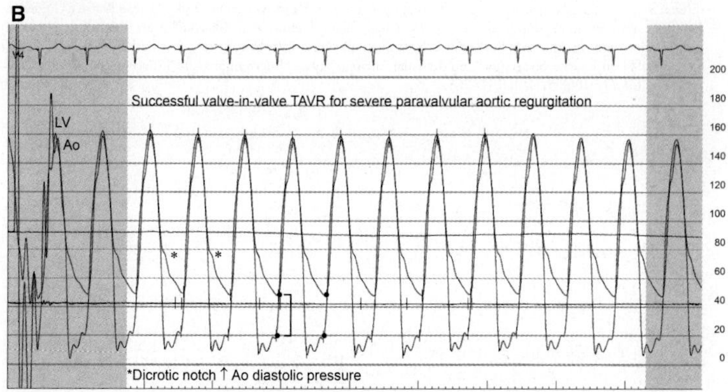

FIGURE 23.28 **A:** Simultaneous left ventricular (LV)–aorta (Ao) waveform tracing following placement of a transcatheter aortic valve, which was associated with severe paravalvular aortic insufficiency. Contrast this waveform tracing with that of Figure 23.27B. Note the loss of the Ao dicrotic notch, reduced Ao diastolic pressure, and increased LV end-diastolic pressure (LVEDP); these are all key findings with significant acute paravalvular leak. **B:** Simultaneous LV-Ao waveform tracing following successful placement of a second transcatheter aortic valve (valve-in-valve) in the same patient. Note the return of the dicrotic notch and increase in the Ao diastolic pressure.TAVR, transcatheter aortic valve replacement.

ACKNOWLEDGMENTS: *The author would like to thank Dr. Shikhar Agarwal and Terri Obrian for their assistance with the waveform tracings.*

SUGGESTED READINGS

Eleid MF, Nishimura RA, Sorajja P, et al. Systemic hypertension in low-gradient severe aortic stenosis with preserved ejection fraction. *Circulation*. 2013;128(12):1349–1353.

Forssmann W. *Experiments on Myself: Memoirs of a Surgeon in Germany*. New York, NY: St. Martin's Press; 1974.

Hachicha Z, Dumesil JG, Bogaty P, et al. Paradoxical low-flow, low-gradient severe aortic stenosis despite preserved ejection fraction is associated with higher afterload and reduced survival. *Circulation*. 2007;115(22):2856–2864.

Lou JL, Menon V. Right heart catheterization. In: Griffin BP, ed. *Manual of Cardiovascular Medicine*. 4th ed. Philadelphia, PA: Lippincott Williams & Wilkins; 2013:977–991.

Nishimura RA, Carabello BA. Hemodynamics in the cardiac catheterization laboratory of the 21st century. *Circulation*. 2012;125(17):2138–2150.

Nishimura RA, Grantham A, Connolly HM, et al. Low-output, low-gradient aortic stenosis in patients with depressed left ventricular systolic function: the clinical utility of the dobutamine challenge in the catheterization laboratory. *Circulation*. 2002;106(7):809–813.

Nishimura RA, Otto CM, Bonow RO, et al. 2014 AHA/ACC guideline for the management of patients with valvular heart disease: a report of the American College of Cardiology/American Heart Association Task Force on Practice Guidelines. *J Am Coll Cardiol*. 2014;63(22):e57–e185.

Ragosta M. *Textbook of Clinical Hemodynamics*. Philadelphia, PA: Saunders; 2008.

Warnes CA, Williams RG, Bashore TM, et al. ACC/AHA 2008 guidelines for the management of adults with congenital heart disease: a report of the American College of Cardiology/American Heart Association Task Force on Practice Guidelines (writing committee to develop guidelines on the management of adults with congenital heart disease): developed in collaboration with the American Society of Echocardiography, Heart Rhythm Society, International Society for Adult Congenital Heart Disease, Society for Cardiovascular Angiography and Interventions, and Society of Thoracic Surgeons. *J Am Coll Cardiol*. 2008;52(23):e143–263.

INDEX

Page numbers followed by t indicate table; those in *italics* indicate figure

B

C

N

P

Q

R